Pioneering Paths in the Study of Families: The Lives and Careers of Family Scholars

Pioneering Paths in the Study of Families: The Lives and Careers of Family Scholars has been previously published as *Marriage & Family Review*, Volume 30, Number 3 2000; Volume 30, Number 4 2001; Volume 31, Numbers 1/2/3/4 2001; and Volume 32, Numbers 1/2 2001.

Pioneering Paths in the Study of Families: The Lives and Careers of Family Scholars

Suzanne K. Steinmetz
Gary W. Peterson

Pioneering Paths in the Study of Families: The Lives and Careers of Family Scholars has been previously published as *Marriage & Family Review*, Volume 30, Number 3 2000; Volume 30, Number 4 2001; Volume 31, Numbers 1/2/3/4 2001; and Volume 32, Numbers 1/2 2001.

Routledge
Taylor & Francis Group
LONDON AND NEW YORK

First published 2002 by The Haworth Press, Inc.

Published 2019 by Routledge
2 Park Square, Milton Park, Abingdon, Oxon OX14 4RN
605 Third Avenue, New York, NY 10017

Routledge is an imprint of the Taylor & Francis Group, an informa business

Pioneering Paths in the Study of Families: The Lives and Careers of Family Scholars has been previously published as *Marriage & Family Review*, Volume 30, Number 3 2000; Volume 30, Number 4 2001; Volume 31, Numbers 1/2/3/4 2001; and Volume 32, Numbers 1/2 2001.

Cover design by Jennifer Gaska

Library of Congress Cataloging-in-Publication Data

Pioneering paths in the study of families : the lives and careers of family scholars / [edited by] Suzanne K. Steinmetz, Gary W. Peterson.
p. cm.
"Previously published as Marriage & family review, volume 30, number 3 2000; volume 30, number 4 2001; volume 31, numbers 1/2/3/4 2001; and volume 32, numbers 1/2 2001."
Includes bibliographical references and index.
ISBN 0-7890-2088-2 (alk. paper) – ISBN 0-7890-2089-0 (pbk : alk. paper)
1. Family–Research. 2. Family life education. 3. Sociologists–Biography. 4. Home economists–Biography. I. Steinmetz, Suzanne K. II. Peterson, Gary W. III. Marriage & family review.
HQ10 .P56 2003
306.85'07'2–dc21

2002152625

ISBN 978-0-7890-2088-8 (hbk)

Pioneering Paths in the Study of Families: The Lives and Careers of Family Scholars

CONTENTS

ABOUT THE EDITORS

Suzanne K. Steinmetz, PhD, MSW, DAPA, is Professor and former Chair of Sociology at Indiana University-Purdue University at Indianapolis (IUPUI). She is certified as a civil and family mediator and, with her husband, mediates neighborhood disputes for Indianapolis Superior Courts. Dr. Steinmetz does pro bono therapy with a focus on individuals with a diagnosis of Dissociative Identity Disorder. Credited as being one of the founders of the field of family violence, she was the first scholar to bring the problems of battered husbands and elder abuse into the public arena as a result of her Congressional testimony in 1978. She has served on the Board of Directors of the Society for the Study for Social Problems and was President of both the University of Delaware's and Indiana University's chapters of Sigma Xi, the National Science Society. Dr. Steinmetz has authored two research monographs, *Duty Bound: Elder Abuse and Family Care* and *Cycle of Violence: Assertive, Aggressive and Abusive Family Interaction*, and is also co-author of *Behind Closed Doors: Violence in American Families* and *Marriage and Family Reality: Historical and Contemporary Analysis* She is also co-editor of *Family Support Systems Across the Life Span, Violence in the Family, Concepts and Definitions of Family for the 21st Century*, and *Fatherhood: Research, Interventions and Policies*. In addition, she is a co-editor of *Handbook of Marriage and the Family* (1st and 2nd editions) and *Sourcebook of Family Theory and Methods: A Contextual Approach*, two major reference books in the discipline. Steinmetz has also authored over 75 additional publications and is currently working on annotating a text written by Tongo Takebe, an early 20th century Japanese theorist.

Gary W. Peterson, PhD, is Head and Profesor, Department of Child and Family Studies, College of Human Ecology, University of Tennessee, Knoxville. He is former Chair and Professor, Department of Human Development, Washington State University, Pullman, Washington, and is former Professor and Chair of the Department of Sociology at Arizona State University. He is also former Chair of the Department of Family Resources and Human Development at Arizona State University. Dr. Peterson's general area of research and scholarly expertise is adolescent development within the context of family and parent-child relationships. Currently, he is analyzing the impact of ethnic and cultural issues in samples of adolescents from the People's Republic of China, Russia, India, Mexico, Chile, and the U.S. Previous research using samples from the U.S. examined health issued in Mexican-American populations of adolescents and young adults as well as influences on the life plans of low-income, rural youth from Appalachian areas of the United States. Peterson's research papers have appeared in such publications as *Journal of Marriage and the Family, Family Relations, Journal of Adolescent Research, Youth and Society, Family Science Review, Family Process*, and *Family Issues*. He was co-editor of *Handbook of Marriage and the Family* (2nd ed.) and *Adolescents in Families*. Major review articles on parent-child and parent-adolescent relationships have appeared in several books including *Advances in Adolescent Development, Handbook for Family Diversity, Handbook of Marriage and the Family* (1st and 2nd editions), and *Families Across Time: A Life Course Perspective*. Dr. Peterson has been a guest editor for special issues of several research journals and has been a member of the Board of Directors for the National Council on Family Relations.

Preface

Academic fields of study are often thought of in the abstract as theoretical perspectives, bodies of knowledge, and methodological approaches that are used to reveal and accumulate new knowledge about particular phenomena of interest. Current texts in the social sciences often describe their respective disciplines or fields of study in terms of a history of ideas, somewhat free of personalized input, momentary creativity, serendipity, and accident. Following this trend, methods and survey courses in the social sciences often convey an image of careful precision, hypothesis testing, and the gradual accumulation of knowledge through the elegant procedures of science. Viewing the evolution of a field of study in this manner creates the image of large communities of scholars acting more or less collectively to structure both descriptive and explanatory bodies of knowledge. Within the diverse fields of study that focus on families, there is certainly considerable truth in this "macro-level image" of the purely intellectual and positivistic basis for the creation of knowledge.

Another way of viewing the growth of academic fields of study, however, occurs at the micro–rather than the macro–level of analysis. This way of viewing the knowledge creation process involves examining the lives of scholars who generated ideas about family processes, development, transitions, and linkages with society. From this perspective, the evolution of knowledge about families is a much more subjective process, shaped by such things as the family experiences, traumatic life events, personal determination, commitment to scholarship, individual creativity, connections with mentors, unanticipated choices, and chance events in the lives of productive scholars. As a consequence of this micro-level perspective, the knowledge creation process becomes an "insider's view" in which things do not appear quite so cumulative, neat, formula-based, and inevitable.

This is certainly the view provided throughout this collection of autobiographical essays of prominent family scholars in a variety of fields. Important issues include: What was their county of origin and who were their ancestors, that is, their own family heritage? With whom did they have experiences that caused these scholars to think in particular ways about families? What historic events, social changes, or cohort effects provided life experiences and values that impacted their work? Where did the "lens" come from through which they organized information and interpreted family phenomena? Who or what were the major scholars, the academic significant others, and the events in their professional lives that influenced them? Was most of their story one of success, the "straight-A student" progressing forward toward inevitable leadership in their chosen endeavors? Or was their experience one of being shaped by initial failures, troubling obstacles, a good measure of happenstance, or even sheer dumb luck?

Through these autobiographies we can gain insights into how an interdisciplinary (multidisciplinary) field is "socially constructed," shaped by individual creativity, distal and proximal life events, and the significant others with whom they interacted. Of particular importance is a person's academic lineage, or the scholarly heritage of those who contribute to a field of study. Specifically one's academic roots–that is, whom a person studied under and who influenced their thinking about families–is a powerful force in the micro-analysis of academic fields. Ever since Alex Haley's *Roots* (1974) burst onto the scene as historical fiction and a television miniseries in the 1970s, the public has become increasingly aware of the ancestral basis for a person's current actions. One's academic heritage is conveyed through several mechanisms, some of which involve intellectual ideas, but other components of which involve the compelling influence of certain forceful personalities, including such prominent mentors as Ernest Burgess, Wesley Burr, Harold Christensen, Gerald Handel, Reuben Hill, Ira Reiss, and Marvin Sussman.

One form of academic heritage is particularly captured by the idea "school of thought," identified with either a particular institution or a collection of interrelated constructs having pervasive influence within one or more fields of study. We can speak of "schools of thought" such as the "Chicago School," so famous for the type of theory and methodology that became know as Symbolic Interaction–the basic substance of which is described in the essays by Bernard Farber, Gerald Handel, and Sheldon Stryker.

Another kind of academic heritage may be conveyed, not simply by a single theoretical perspective like symbolic interaction or systems theory, but more through the impact of a specific academic program, such as that which developed at the University of Minnesota. A single sociology department, in this case, brought together the extraordinary talents of Reuben Hill, Murray Straus, Irv Tallman, and Ira Reiss for a period of national prominence. This collection of scholars produced, in turn, such prominent successors as Joan Aldous, Wesley Burr, Viktor Gecas, Brent Miller, Harold Grotevant, and Gary Lee. These individuals continue to shape our field today through contributions to the field and training the next generation of scholars. Tracing such academic lineages in this manner helps us to understand how academic perspectives can be transmitted across generations and continue to shape our contemporary thinking about families.

If one reads the essays of scholars like Sussman, Stryker, Feldman, Chilman, Duvall, Tallman, Lopata, Farber, Handel, Neubeck, Reiss and Christensen, a fairly representative picture of our field during its earliest days is portrayed. In fact, in some instances, these scholars were either the founders of our field or were only one academic generation removed from its origins! The autobiographies of authors such as Burr, Fox, Gecas, Elder, Scanzoni, and Aldous, to name just a few, in turn provide insights into a middle generation of scholars who had links to the past, but made major contributions during a time of tremendous growth in our knowledge about families. Finally, this collection also provides an array of somewhat younger, entrepreneurial scholars from multiple disciplines who are currently at peak levels of productivity during a time when the study of families has truly become a key part of the larger social science industry. Some of these, e.g., Allen and La Rossa, demonstrate the growth in stature of qualitative research, while others, such as Conger, Lamb, Schumm, Steinberg, and Grotevant, demonstrate how the study of families has entered a time of highly sophisticated research, driven by large collaborative projects with extensive external funding.

As I (Steinmetz) was writing my portion of this introduction, I could reflect back on my interaction with the authors that I personally knew and how they influenced me in many direct and indirect ways. I will list only a few. Evelyn Duvall sent me a request for a reprint of my first journal article–the request is framed and hangs on the wall in my office. Early in my career, Margaret Feldman invited me to speak at Ithaca and I stayed in her home with its wonderful collection of African art. I remember Helena Lopata and I skipping out of a particularly strange evening of entertainment at an NCFR conference (men with faces painted on their stomachs). When I contributed to *Contemporary Theories About the Family* (Burr, Hill, Nye and Reiss, 1978), the editors as well as many of the contributors were extremely helpful in providing advice and guidance. My last interaction with Bernie Farber was teaching him how to send his essay via an e-mail attachment. He was so pleased when it worked! Marvin Sussman has always been a major mentor and advisor; it would be hard to imagine how different my academic life might have been without him. And last, but not least, Gary (Pete) Peterson is a good friend and valuable collaborator.

The other "I" (Peterson) owes much to many others for opportunities sent my way that contributed to a personally satisfying career. First on my list would be John DeFrain, who encouraged me to pursue higher education, and Bert Adams, who gave me key advice at a time of transition during my graduate studies. I owe much to Wesley Burr for teaching me the importance of family theory and to Reuben Hill for being the personification of what family scholarship should mean to us all. Boyd Rollins provided me, in turn, with research skills, a model of the persistent, careful social scientist, and the importance of being a good colleague. Still others of major importance were Marvin Sussman and Suzanne Steinmetz, who provided me with valuable opportunities to write challenging book chapters and assume major editorial roles. Finally, former students like Stephan Wilson, Kevin Bush, and Andrew Supple have kept me energized about scholarship, despite the demands of challenging administrative roles.

The overall message in these pages, therefore, is that academic fields of study are human endeavors created not only by great intellectual traditions, but also by everyday interactions and some unpredictability. What we have today is a body of knowledge about families that resulted, in part, from the collective activities of scholars, but also from the acts of individuals who responded somewhat differently to the "family world," based, to a significant extent, on their own experiences.

Suzanne K. Steinmetz
Gary W. Peterson

PART I
CROSSING BOUNDARIES

Crossing Boundaries: An Introduction to the Lives of Family Scholars

Suzanne K. Steinmetz
Gary W. Peterson

This volume is devoted to autobiographical essays by scholars in family studies and child development from a variety of disciplines. Marvin Sussman, as the Founding Editor of *Marriage & Family Review,* initiated this project in the early 1990s. For a variety of reasons, however, the project never came to fruition according to the original schedule.

When we (Suzanne Steinmetz and Gary Peterson) took over as Co-Editors of *Marriage & Family Review,* we found the dozen or so existing essays with much additional work needed before completion. To make the project easier for participants, Dr. Sussman had provided blank audio tapes and invited several scholars to provide oral histories. Some scholars had provided typed essays, whereas others provided the audio tapes for Marvin to type. Some essays were only a dozen or so pages in length, whereas others were in excess of 100 pages.

The developmental stage of these essays varied from fleshed-out outlines, to more lengthy first drafts, to polished essays. No matter what the stage of development, however, all required updating. Marvin had originally organized the scholars' essays by the stage of the individual's career. Wes Burr, for example, who retired last year, was considered to be in "mid-career," whereas I (Sue Steinmetz) was considered to be in my "early career." Dr. Sussman and his cohort (all now in various stages of post-retirement or perhaps "post-career") were considered to be in "late career." Clearly, things had changed over the past decade and some serious rethinking was needed to "restart" the project.

However, even in their rough and dated condition, it was obvious to us that the family and early educational experiences of our academic forebears (i.e., foremothers and forefathers) had considerable influence on the academic research, teaching, and advocacy of their own and subsequent scholarly generations. Furthermore, many of the scholars representing a later career cohort had often studied with notable founders or predesescessors in the fields of Sociology, Home Economics (Human Ecology), Child Development, and Family Studies. Thus, these essays provided insights into academic life during earlier years for these fields of scholarship. Great insight also is provided in these essays about how our thinking about families and family members has evolved. Much like the primary focus of these scholars (i.e., families), each generation of scholars socializes (in their role as "academic parents") their successors and continues, therefore, to have influence on the scholarship produced by their "academic offspring."

We subsequently decided to resurrect the project and expand the number of scholars involved. The expansion would not only involve "younger scholars," but also scholars who were more clearly identified with a diversity of fields, including Child Development, Psychology, Sociology, and Family Studies. The downside of this tremendous expansion (from about 12 to over 40 essays), however, was that it would no longer be possible to publish them as a single issue of *Marriage & Family Review.* Instead, they would now be published in sequential issues of the journal and, subsequently, as an edited volume by The Haworth Press, Inc. This was truly becoming a much larger, but also very interesting project.

The next issue to be addressed was how to organize these essays. First, organizing them by cohort did not seem appropriate because many of the older scholars had been in various stages of retirement for 20-25 years. We then considered organizing the essays by discipline, but many scholars crossed several disciplines. We also considered organizing them by theoretical perspectives, but this proved problematic, not only because of the diverse disciplines, but also because some scholars could not easily be identified with a particular theoretical perspective. We then considered a schema in which scholars would be organized by the topic for which they are known–an approach that proved to be extremely difficult. Not only did the Co-Editors have different ideas regarding how a scholar was known (which reflected the aspect of a scholar's work with which we were most familiar), but also many scholars had written on diverse topics that made categorization almost impossible.

Finally, we settled on using themes that seemed to emerge in reading the authors' essays as a way to organize the essays. The first group, which we have called "Crossing Boundaries," was most typical of Gecas, Lamb, Neubeck, McCubbin, and Lopata, who crossed international borders and immigrated to the U.S. The inclusion of McCubbin, who was born and raised in Hawaii before it became a state, was based on his essay in which his early roots as a Hawaiian descendent makes his case more similar to that of an immigrant rather than someone raised in the continental U.S. We also included Marvin Sussman's essay in this group because of two factors, the first being that his essay fits the overall theme in a metaphorical sense–his career is characterized by crossing many boundaries to attain prominence in interdisciplinary scholarship on families. Second, with his role as Founding Editor of *Marriage & Family Review* and as the individual who originated this autobiographical project, it seemed appropriate to include his autobiography in the first group of essays.

Marvin Sussman, in his own autobiographical essay, has chosen to compare his life to a classical journey in Greek mythology–the theme of the heroic individual struggling valiantly against powerful, even overwhelming forces for worthy ends. He views himself as being confronted with difficult circumstances and power structures as he sought to better himself and the academic units for which he provided leadership. During this journey, his first struggles were rooted in tough economic lessons learned from the Great Depression and the difficulties of becoming a conscientious objector during World War II. Other of his formative experiences included working as a social worker and dealing with obstacles associated with translating his own modest socioeconomic background into success within an academic world emphasizing elitism and exclusivity. Dr. Sussman views his career as one in which many boundaries were crossed to challenge the bureaucratic rigidity of universities and the conservative norms of academia. The purposes of this struggle were to build better academic programs for students, productive research programs by faculty, and benchmark scholarly projects that synthesized our current knowledge about families.

Hamilton McCubbin's essay provides insights into the challenges faced by someone of Hawaiian ancestry whose early years were dominated by circumstances associated with being a minority in his own native land. With a stroke of a pen, he finds himself to be a citizen of the 50th state, but at the same time, realizes that maintaining his ethnic heritage is strongly discouraged. His decision to attend law school was changed as a result of a job working with disturbed youth that he performed for the period between his undergraduate graduation in January and the beginning of law school in September. This was a turning point in his career. Although he met many challenges and became a noted scholar and administrator on the U.S. mainland, he finally decided to fulfill his mother's wish and return to his homeland–to lead the school where he was once a student.

Viktor Gecas, born in a small town in Lithuania during World War II, reports early memories of fleeing by horse and wagon in the middle of the night with other relatives. Eventually, his family settled in Chicago where he became a member of a law abiding, non-violent, neighborhood gang, the "Jesters." Here, he was socialized into Chicago's inner-city culture and was provided a sense of solidarity and identity. During his first year at Beloit, a small, private liberal arts college, his gang jacket initially gave him a sense of identity but was eventually replaced by a preppie letter jacket and fraternity membership–the Chicago identity becoming less visible. His academic career has been at Washington State University at Pullman, where he is still located. Much of his subsequent work has focused on dimensions of the self (or identity), with special attention paid to the family's role in socializing the developing self-perceptions of youthful family members.

Born into a small family of the nobility with their own coat of arms, but no land, Helena Znaniecka Lopata's family believed in *noblesse oblige*. Her father received his Ph.D. but was unable to secure an academic position in Poland because of his political activity. His early publication of manuscripts on Poles who settled in America resulted in his meeting W. I. Thomas and his subsequent immigration to the U.S. After WWI, her father returned to Poland where Helena was born. Her family was part of Europe's and America's intelligentsia, a social circumstance from which Helena benefited. However, she faced many obstacles during her early life, from osteomyelitis, to time in a Nazi concentration camp, to adjusting to U.S. suburban life. Subsequently, she returned to college for a graduate education, largely due to the realization that more than motherhood and marriage was needed for fulfillment.

The son of a doctor, Gerhard Neubeck became a member of the working class when his family fled Nazi Germany and settled in New York. After completing an undergraduate degree in personnel and guidance and a Master's degree in psychology, he began his career as a marriage counselor and instructor in family life (an area for which he had no preparation) at the University of Minnesota. Following the completion of his doctorate from Columbia (he gained admission because he had met and admired Ernest Osborne), he ran a therapy group for married couples at the Margaret Sanger Clinic. Based on that experience, and contrary to the then-dominant concepts of psychoanalytic theory, he published the first article in 1954, which provided evidence that therapeutic work could be conducted with couples, not just individuals. Over the years, his scholarly work dealt with the areas of sexuality, sex education, and extramarital relations.

Unlike other scholars in this section who fled their country during a time of war, Michael Lamb's decision to do so was motivated by different reasons. He began his education in law and notes that he "had little doubt that I would be one of the politicians leading South Africa toward the post-colonial multiracialism." He soon realized, however, that the political climate in his country was not conducive to ideas favoring civil rights, democracy, and economic equality and that he was not suited for political combat. Moreover, he came to realize that he truly enjoyed economic and psychological theory. However, his radical activity during his lectureship at the University of Durban, which culminated in confrontation with the government in the spring of 1973, sealed his fate. Subsequently, he left South Africa for Johns Hopkins in the

U.S. to study with Mary Ainsworth, one of the foremost originators of attachment theory.

All of these leading family scholars, therefore, have crossed real and metaphorical boundaries on various pathways toward making fundamental scholarly and academic contributions. Their life stories reveal much about why they approached their chosen topics as they did and why we think about families the way we do today.

A Hero's Journey: The Lifeways of a Modern Day Asclepius

Marvin B. Sussman

KEYWORDS. Augobiography, faculty research, childhood, career

This is a turn around. For some 20 years as editor of the journal *Marriage & Family Review* I have invited countless scholars to tell their stories relating their scholarly work to their deeper selves. The posed question is: What in the lifeways of a scholar influences a selection of a field of study and generates the passion required to be a successful educator?

This is indeed a turn around for me, to tell my story, at least a partial history of my journey; its trials and tribulations, joys and successes. Thus, in this paper, I will relate episodes in my life through the process called "The Hero's Journey." My urge to do this has both inner and outer manifestations. My inner self is screeching to be heard, to tell my story, to explain what I have done and perhaps to obtain a new understanding of myself. Undoubtedly, I seek some catharsis in seeing the patterning of behaviors that have their bases in this deep unconscious level.

My other or horizontal self says, "Hey, wait a minute! Is it proper according to conventional, vis-à-vis professional norms to reveal one's most inner thoughts, feelings and experiences?" Such, if not held against you, at least will convey the image of weakness and even flakiness in some quarters. However, if there has been a lack in my training and career, it has been the neglect in paying attention to my inner being. To many, I have been an enigma. The time for revelation of self is here. My approach is to give a non-sociological treatise of my journey by dealing with issues, those which evoke both concern and passion, during my career.

Reflecting upon my life course and from discussions with others, I recently became aware that much of my behavior as an academic and as a person in serving others is rooted in past experiences and beliefs.

For example, while at Case Western Reserve University, I became involved in major studies on the natural history of diabetes and on childhood diabetes. The first study took five years to complete and was a longitudinal study examining the medical, social, physical, and psychological consequences for the diabetic individual (Sussman & Weil, 1960, 1961; Crain, Sussman, & Weil, 1966a; Crain, Sussman, & Weil 1966b; Weil, Sussman, & Crain, 1967). The study of diabetic children was similar to objectives that were stipulated for the adult population, but with greater emphasis upon childhood development and consequences for other family members. My interest in this research was quickened by the fact that my daughter on her 16th birthday was diagnosed as a diabetic.

I have no doubt that such experiences, which create for us a new reality, give us the energy and passion to become involved in finding creative solutions for individual, group, and societal problems. My experiences with the depression, the events which occurred in the post depression period, and the beginnings of World War II increased my yearning to serve others. It undoubtedly influenced my decision to become a Conscientious Objector to seek solutions to problems using non-violent techniques and to find alternative service to a military role as well as to write in this area (Sussman, 1964; Marciano & Sussman, 1986).

Some of these experiences are family and culturally rooted and, like oracles, tell us what is permissible and what is taboo. While I was a nonconformist in my family, the blood ties and early family experiences provided guidelines and subsequent forces which influenced my work in life. Before I discuss specific events and feelings that have influenced my life's work, I present the model from the works of myth. It is this mythic journey that we take time and time again that provides a framework for presenting and understanding the rationales and explanations that we either adopt or not to live out our lives.

Homer's *The Odyssey,* a tale of great proportions and adventures, deals with the life of Odysseus, King of Ithaca, who was exiled for 10 years and then strode with perilous delight from Troy back to Ithaca to the bosom of his family, friends, colleagues, and enemies. The journey provided Odysseus with very few options, and there were severe risks associated with each of the choices he had to make. Whatever he chose would cause woundings, pain, anguish, fear, loss of physical strength, and high levels of stress. For example, when Odysseus' ship came into the Straits of Messina, it had to pass between Charybdis, who created a whirlpool, and Scylla, whose plaintive wailing attracted ships to her from which she plucked sailors for her meals to satisfy the demands of her six-headed body. Odysseus and his sailors survived but were severely wounded. One foci of this essay is on the wounding syndrome, those situations and events that create stress or depression, or, in some circumstances, act as incentive to change. There are components of the wounding which are self-imposed and those which are imposed by the society. We will get into the swirling waters frequently being caught between Charybdis and Scylla.

The epic of a hero's journey, whether it is a story of Odysseus or Parsifal in search of the Holy Grail, is usually presented in linear fashion. One moves from one episode and experience to another. The individual's life course transitions are dramatically described, where obviously what preceded before influences what occurs later on. It is a building up of experiences and processes and knowledge and feelings, all of which create the resistances that ultimately are overcome with the use of allies and that lead to the triumphant march home.

It is only in great myths and epics that such lineal progression occurs. In everyday life, the universe provides to the contrary. We are whirled about with highs and lows, obstacles and easy passages, and at times, we are unexpectedly thrust into the belly of the whale. There are marked transitions developed by the cultures in which we live and by our own aging and maturing processes. Yet these provide, at best, the structure within which extreme highs and lows occur regarding one's ability to cope, survive, engage in behaviors, and react with feelings that are conducive to experiencing some quality of life. The events that you will now hear are part of a passage that everyone makes over and over again.

I will now relate to you my own experiences as a wounded person as well as a fighter struggling to neutralize the power of large-scale bureaucracies and to create new options for families and their members. Perhaps in this story of self-revelation you may see the journey that you have experienced time and time again.

My first wounding occurred during the Great Depression. My father and grandfather's business was wiped out by the great crash. People just didn't have money to buy the things they sold. Resources were quickly dissipated. My parents and grandparents were inexperienced in the ways of welfare and other charitable organizations. In fact, it wasn't in their consciousness, let alone mine as a young child. Yet things became so desperate that they had to have some food in the house. Through contact with a charitable organization they received a piece of paper or card (I forget which, since I was very young at the time) which entitled them to get a bag of food.

They were so prideful and ashamed that they dumped this responsibility upon me to walk two miles to the welfare agency to get the bag and come back with the food. After all, I was the oldest child, having lost what would have been my older brother at the age of a year-and-a-half, when he was snatched from us as my mother walked me in a carriage and held him in her hand. One of Mr. Henry Ford's early products jumped the gully in the road and killed my brother Daniel. What else could I do but go? And so I did. My recollection of the experience is vague. I have tried many times to recapture what my feelings were. I felt sorry for my parents and other members of the family and perhaps was a bit angry, but I was more bewildered and resentful of what was happening which I could not understand was impacting our family in such a Draconian way. The trip was relatively uneventful. I soon discovered that I was not the only son of a family who was given this task. I had no problems with the functionaries of this charitable care-giving organization. My greatest difficulties were carrying the bag home intact and hiding my embarrassment.

The wounding was more to my psyche. Even today, when I consider myself to be a self-educated academic scholar as well as entrepreneur who could well afford to leave all the lights on in the house, I still go around turning them off. I have done this all my life, much to the chagrin of my four children. I am constantly looking for ways to save resources and to effectively manipulate the system. I look for bargains and coupons in my purchasing habits and may foolishly go long distances to shop for a good price on an item. This is a wounding I received at this very early age.

This experience unfolded a deeply felt concern to convert a societal depression and its attendant dysfunction to economically stable conditions for families and communities. Ultimately, I went into the field of social work and received a Masters of Science in group work education from George Williams College.

However, my group work experience has found an outlet in my research on group processes (Sussman, 1956a, 1956b), health (Sussman, 1989), maternal health and child care (Boek, Lawson, Yankauer, & Sussman, 1957; 1958), delivery of services (Cogswell & Sussman, 1972; Haug & Sussman, 1969, 1973), private housing for minorities (Sussman, 1957), employed mothers (Sussman, 1961; Gross & Sussman, 1997), poverty (Sussman & Chilman, 1964, 1969a), and disability and rehabilitation (Sussman, 1966a, 1966b, 1969a, 1972; Haug & Sussman, 1972; Haug & Sussman, 1973). In terms of early experiences, even my first career, watch repair, was researched (Strodtbeck & Sussman, 1956).

More details of this experience will be presented later in this paper. In 1948, I entered Yale to take a doctorate in sociology with the belief that through teaching and research I could evoke, catalyze, and provide knowledge for effective community and societal change. I was carrying out what was embedded deeply in my psyche, to serve others and to be the giver of the pure gift. Now back to the chronology of my life.

At an early age, while I could not understand the societal forces that were creating depressions and suicides that I read about or heard on the radio, I realized that something was wrong and that I was a part of it. I also realized that I would have to do things in order to protect myself. It was not something that I liked, but it was something that I recognized, at this very tender age, I would have to deal with. The best I could do at this time was to excel in school. I did well and even skipped a grade in primary school, which I am not sure did me much good.

I later found the power of Miss Steadman, who was my teacher in either the seventh or eighth grade and who still used the hickory stick and ruler to maintain order in the classroom. I remember her giving me 10 whacks of the ruler on the palm of my hand and putting me in the corner like a dunce. As I remember, this was because I didn't respond to what she was saying and what she had put on the board. At that time, neither she nor I realized that I was in need of glasses. Instead, I was located in the back of the classroom because she seated us in alphabetical order. My humiliation was further increased when, after I got glasses and she recognized what was the problem, she put me in the front row to be looked at and ostracized by classmates for being "four-eyed"-another wounding!

Within the matrix of the family, I found that the happiest moments of my childhood were when my father and I would go off to the mountains. He liked to do this and I guess I was his chaperon. I also spent a good bit of time with my grandmother on the maternal side; in fact, I lived with her for a year while I was in high school. Even though I had to commute several miles either by walking or by trolley, I remember those days. And one might say that I didn't get on too well with my mother. I can't say that my childhood was exceedingly happy, and, when I graduated from high school, I decided to leave our home in Connecticut and go to New York to work my way through college. This action was not applauded by the family, particularly my parents. And so, during college, I did all sorts of odd jobs in New York to make money and to have a roof over my head. We were coming out of the depression and gearing up for World War II.

Initially, I enrolled in night classes at New York University in Washington Square, and, subsequently, earned enough money and was able to float a college loan to go full time while still holding down several part time jobs. I moved more into the human service area and worked at Judson Baptist Memorial Church in the Village, at Labor Temple on 14th Street and 2nd Avenue, and at the famous Henry Street Settlement in New York City. I became active in college organizations, and particularly was moving in the direction of taking a position on the War, largely on moral and religious grounds. I was conflicted by the various positions as expressed through propaganda and, if I had known then what I know now, I might not have taken a pacifist position. My role models were Frank Olmstead and A. J. Muste, who were very active in the pacifist movement.

Upon graduation from college, I volunteered to work with the American Friends Service Committee and went to Mexico for a year to help rebuild the

Village of Tuxpan in the state Jalisco, not too far from Guadalajara. In those days, you had to pay money to volunteer so I took the $50.00 I received from my parents as a graduation gift and gave it to the cause and off we went in used station wagons, making the long trip to Mexico. Working in an earthquake stricken town, without water and other facilities, wasn't an easy job. It was a well-intended project, but as I look back on the experience, I cannot say it was well planned. Almost all of us were illiterate in the Spanish language, and although we developed some abilities to communicate, it was not sufficient to relate to and identify with the population in this village. I soon became aware of class differentiation and how what we were doing was largely controlled by the middle and upper classes, who considered themselves to be Spanish. In contrast, the poor people, the Toltec Indians, suffered the most from the earthquake damage when their adobe huts were razed to the ground. Although we accomplished some rebuilding of adobe houses and rebuilt the school, the interaction did not cut across class lines.

The Friends Service Committee Project had its own bureaucracy created by the emergence of individuals from our own group into hierarchical positions. I did not realize at the time, which I learned later on by working with the social psychologist Musafer Sherif, that individuals who best met the needs of the group would automatically become leaders in an emergent bureaucratic structure. This occurs in voluntary and spontaneously formed groups. Those who were adept in speaking Spanish soon became the natural leaders and subsequently enjoyed some of the available resources, such as social interaction with the village elite and setting agendas for everyday activities. Some layers of my idealism were peeling, and I was becoming more of a pragmatist who was aware of organizational realities. I recognized that I would have to find ways to deal with these circumstances while still maintaining my ideals and commitment to serve others.

After my stint with the America Friends Service Committee in Mexico, I found myself in the windy city of Chicago. I paid for my passage by driving a station wagon load of returnees and thus saved a few dollars which would be needed to take care of my primary needs until I became settled. A Quaker family, members of the 57th Street Meeting of Friends, took me in and I received a room and other privileges for doing work around the house. I then decided to go back to school and applied for admission to the famous University of Chicago School of Social Administration, which, at that time, was run by two maiden sisters whose family name was Breckenridge. I remember having an interview with them and not doing too well since I could not answer their specific questions about what social workers do. I presented a general frame of reference for wanting to be of service–and my application was denied. While I was exploring admission to the University of Chicago, I was also, in turn, exploring the possibilities of going into a group work program at George Williams College, located also on the south side of Chicago.

George Williams was an outgrowth of a traditional YMCA college but had gone through cataclysmic growth, both in philosophy and program. The new emphasis was on group work and its application in various group and institutional settings and was not primarily to train young men to be YMCA secretaries. I also had discovered that George Williams provided work placements for its students so that they could not only make their living, but also pay the modest tuition for their graduate education. It was more of a doing experience than a receiving one, which would have been the case if I had gone to the University of Chicago.

In terms of credentials, I was worse off attending George Williams rather than the University of Chicago, but then I didn't have too many options. However, an important learning experience for me was to mollify the hurt of rejection by the University of Chicago by finding an almost equally viable option. Thus, one stance I adopted was to seek multiple options that I could fall back on, ones which may work when others failed. This may be a component of multitracking, keeping a number of balls bouncing in the air simultaneously. Early on, I developed this posture of engaging in multiple projects in order to mitigate the stress of a single failure. Performing significant activities simultaneously proved to be a highly successful procedure. Obtaining an outcome which makes one feel good is a significant component of the healing process when one is wounded.

Before I was drafted, I had three fascinating work experiences while I achieved the Master's of Group work from George Williams College. One was working in the west side of Chicago at a Presbyterian settlement house in a Catholic area where the main interest of the Board of Directors was to have the staff convert the Catholics to Presbyterianism. A second experience was being assistant director of Old Town Boys Club, which was in a changing neighborhood where Chicanos and Blacks were in continuous conflict with one another. Here I experienced a dumping phenomenon where the director, who lived in a top floor apartment of this Boys Club, was preoccupied with personal matters; thus, he willingly gave me the administration of the program. This resulted in 12-hour-long days–from 12 noon until 12 midnight–doing my classes in the morning, and making long trolley rides from the south side of Chicago to the near west side.

My third experience was at the Hyde Park Neighborhood House, which was closer to my digs and run by an eccentric director who was considered to be ahead of his time. In all these three experiences, I found that documentation was critical for survival of these service organizations. As miniature bureaucracies, they constantly had to demonstrate the accomplishment of worthwhile things in order to command financial and other supports. Their balance sheets were constantly being audited, with the bottom line being profitable service and getting the biggest bang for the buck. I was drafted about the time I graduated. The consequence was that I moved abruptly from a setting of volunteerism to another of conscription and of dealing with more formidable and more impersonal bureaucracies.

I had registered as a Conscientious Objector (C.O.) and, when drafted in 1943, decided not to go to the privatized work camps organized by such religious groups as the Society of Friends, Mennonites, or the Church of the Brethren. Instead, I chose the government sponsored camp in Mancos, Colorado located in an arid region suited more for cactus than for human beings. The task in Mancos was to build a dam for a few ranchers in the valley.

I decided at the time to surrender to the system, which I did by attending this camp, a long way from home. I soon became aware that what I was doing was not helping humankind. Consequently, I gave some thought to seeking a release from this conscientious objector camp and enlisting in the army in a noncombatant service like the Ambulance Corps. As I was mulling over these possibilities, an opportunity arose for a person in the infirmary to work with the frail and disabled camp physician who came up the mountain each day from the town of Mancos, Colorado. The infirmarian whom I replaced became sick enough to obtain a psychiatric discharge. Before he left, however, I received a quick course in what to do and took the position of resident infirmarian.

I was soon conflicted by what I had observed. Among the camp population, on the one hand, were malingerers who took on the C.O. role in order to escape army service. There were also those, in turn, who had strong moral, humanistic, and religious convictions about what they were doing, coupled with the desire to serve the larger society. Our segregation in isolated Colorado was part of a larger public policy to keep us out of the sights and minds of our fellow citizens. Government bureaucrats probably thought this would be in our best interest and for our protection since those classified as 4E or 4F were not highly regarded by both those fighting in the armed forces as well as supporters at home.

Yet the need for human service providers was so extensive that a new policy emerged. Through what was called detached service, C.O.'s began to leave the camp to work in human service organizations. After a stint in the infirmary, I volunteered for such service and, following the usual bureaucratic delays, was transferred to Middletown, Connecticut (not too far from home), where I was assigned to work in the Middletown State Hospital. Here, we received $25.00 a month, plus room and board. Before I was discharged, I was in charge of a 500-bed unit, largely a geriatric population. I remember specifically the woundings and the verbal abuse we received in the hospital from patriotic Americans who felt we were traitors to our country. The modus operandi we adopted was to do our jobs and to do them well, with commitment and humaneness. We went the extra mile–by being open, empathic, and concerned human beings. We worked long hours and the night shifts, which for me were often harrowing as the processes of death and dying were experienced.

After three years of alternative service, I returned home very uncertain as to what I wanted to do with my life. I had been wounded, and this, of course, is my reflection based upon recall. The wounding was my discovery of the great dichotomy between what people preach and what they practice. My ideals were shattered.

Before I returned home, I had one other adventure which exacerbated the wounding. I was invited to help develop a new form of community by refurbishing the property and land of a well-intended human being who was dependent upon her brother who operated a series of radio stations in three large mid-western cities. As part of the operation, we opened a youth hostel. The volume of business, my unfamiliarity with the workings of a farm, and the discovery that I could not live on idealism alone quickened my exit from this undertaking, and I returned home.

I decided to go back into the family business and had a bench built for me. I took on the role of being a watchmaker, a trade in which all of us in the family were trained. My two brothers, who were younger and had been in the service, joined my Dad in this enterprise. After the depression and up through the early years of World War II, my father opened a chain of watch repair shops throughout parts of New York State, Connecticut, and Massachusetts. The paucity of help during the war and the unavailability of his sons to help meant the closing of this chain of shops. The headquarters shop in Bridgeport, Connecticut became the mainstay of the family's income. It was a good change for me to move from a role of service to one of dealing with inanimate objects where I could see the results of my efforts. The human service work I did in the old days and, I suspect, the work done now are not readily conducive to witnessing changes in human beings and human created institutions.

My hunger for knowledge and to use the intellect I possessed created stirrings in my innermost being. For such reasons and others of a personal kind, I decided to get on with my education and become a college teacher. My woundings had led me down the path of not going into the service and of helping others in the field to which I had been trained, namely group work. I had visions, in addition, of becoming a college teacher and effecting massive changes in the society. To begin such involvement, it became important for me to acquire training as a social scientist. What was evolving for me is exemplified in the maxim, "To engage in action without research is folly; and to engage in research without action is stupidity." I decided to try to get into

Yale, which was only 12 or 13 miles from where I was living in the countryside outside of Bridgeport, Connecticut.

Using the C.O. network, I discovered that a colleague who worked with me in the hospital had taken a position at Yale as an instructor in mathematics. The following anecdote exemplifies Sussman's law of fortuitous circumstances. Indeed, I wanted to go back to the university for a doctorate, but I hadn't identified the field in which I would do doctoral work. As an undergraduate at New York University, I excelled in history and was a member of the Honor Society. It was the one subject for which I had a passion, whereas I had very little sociology as an undergraduate. I remember having only one course on that subject. During my master's degree training at George Williams, on the other hand, I had taken more social behavioral type courses, obviously taught in such a way as to extrapolate their application to the problems of humankind. So after talking to Paul, I said, "Why not see if you could set me up with appointments with the chairs of History and Sociology Departments and see what you can do?" He said, "Well, I'll do that, and that's about all I can do because I am a mathematician and I know very little about these fields. Why don't you set aside Tuesday of next week and come up and we will have lunch, and I will set up these appointments for you? If you don't hear from me it means that everything is OK."

So the following week, on Tuesday, I met Paul for lunch in New Haven. He told me that the chair of the history department was suddenly called out of town, but he was able to make an appointment with the Chair of Sociology, Maurice Davie. I remember vividly my meeting with Professor Davie because we took almost five hours discussing a whole range of topics. He was particularly interested in the position I had taken in relation to war and peace and service. As I talk about it, I am experiencing being back with him. He has gone on another journey. He finally said at the end of our discussion, "Why don't you apply to Yale immediately and come in February, since this is the last time that Yale will admit people midyear?" This was the summer of 1947. I had a strong feeling that he wanted me in and would recommend that I be admitted to his department, which still had a heavy emphasis on anthropology.

I drove back to Stepney, Connecticut, where we lived, completely unglued since this was going to be such a radical change from what I was doing. My family was not insistent that I reject this opportunity to go back to school. It became apparent after a year or so of working together that there wasn't enough volume of business to support four nuclear families. Ruth, my spouse, was very understanding of what I was trying to do and could see that attending Yale would provide autonomy and independence for both herself and our children. Ruth and I married in 1942 and became the parents of four children. She was pregnant with our second child by the time I entered Yale.

Her brother, Arthur Strahler, was a few years younger than I, and he was becoming a nationally known Geomorphologist, who was located at a highly ranked university. By word and example, he became a role model for me. He, Ruth, and I felt that I would do well in academia.

By this time you may be wondering what this has to do with the fortuitous law of circumstance. Well, if the history chair was in his office that day, I may have become a starving historian rather than an affluent social scientist!

I had very little time in which to prepare to get into Yale and would have to take the GRE exams within two months. I was also flabbergasted because I had been out of school for five years and hadn't done much reading in the interim. I thought I might get credit for my graduate work at George Williams College. However, the gatekeepers of the Yale bureaucracy said, "If you want us to even consider the work you did at George Williams (and they did this with a mighty shift of the nose), we want you to satisfactorily pass the two language examination requirements prior to your matriculation–then we will consider your George Williams work for credit."

I remember a particular guardian of the threshold. In fact, as I write this, I can see him sitting at his desk giving me this message. I had enough to do in getting brushed up on the basics, using the College Outline series as a primary source. I had to work the system, although I knew that much of what I had to do in 1947 may not be related to what I would be doing afterward. At the GRE exams, I met an individual who later became a colleague and is today an outstanding medical sociologist. He was a Yale undergraduate and told me about the language exams. The department gave such a tough exam by having people read and translate sociology written in classical German so as to make certain that few students would pass the exam the first time. Such an assessment of realities determined what action I would take and so I withdrew my request to have my work at George Williams College evaluated.

My decision was to apply immediately for admission to Yale and to delay moving the family for at least six months. I needed to obtain sufficient income and work out arrangements so that I would be able to go to school and support my family with little dependence on my extended family for their financial assistance. I was admitted to Yale and took one course in the February semester of 1947. I commuted one day a week. I was winding down my work with the family business and set up a watch repair shop in our home. I then subcontracted work from my father and brothers and with a few other jewelry stores in town.

A year later, I had a master's in sociology and anthropology, and two years after that a doctorate in sociology. During this period, I held two other part time academic positions and continued repairing watches at home.

Not all of my experiences at Yale were pleasant. I envied some of my colleagues who had resources so that they could live a true academic life, which I labeled "the leisure of the theory class." They did not have to teach at the neighboring college and did not need to be a research assistant to a professor. Moreover, they did not need to fix any watches, work in a diner, or travel for business purposes from Bridgeport to New Haven and back. In summary, they did not need to work 18-20 hours a day to complete a doctorate in three years–the timeframe I gave myself and achieved at some cost.

The greatest wounding I received came in the form of a betrayal. While on a Sterling Fellowship, which paid my tuition and a small stipend during the second year of study, I became associated with a young assistant professor who was interested in some of the work I had planned to do for my dissertation. I began to work for him and to view him as my mentor. In fact, I gave up my Sterling Fellowship to become his assistant.

The handshake deal involved freeing him up from all responsibilities for his courses, except for lecturing, so he could complete a book that was critical for his impending promotion and tenure consideration. He was a fellow in one of the colleges and, therefore, had a suite. In return for my assistance, I was given an office in the suite, and I began to feel Ivy League for the first time since I was at Yale. I worked passionately for him with the expected reciprocation of support. He was astounded by my persistence and aggressiveness in pursuing the work for the degree and in handling so many of his affairs, particularly the students that came to his door with problems.

I was nearing the completion of my work for the doctorate in which I was studying intergenerational relationships within urban environments. This dissertation turned out to be a landmark one. It disturbed existing theories and created a plethora of research on the subject that has filled the journals of social and behavioral science for many years.

I entered the job market, which, during those years, was very sparse in terms of opportunities. Job markets run in cycles just like life cycles with their ups and downs. At that time, the field of sociology had a plethora of professors who were "novitiates" in the sense of having just finished their degrees either before or during the war. Almost a year previous to my search for a job, I had turned down a position at the University of Connecticut at Hartford because they wanted me to come and teach without finishing my dissertation. I thought this would be unwise to do because, once I became part of a university bureaucracy, I would be in a position of extreme stress, pressured to finish the degree, and I did not look forward to being an "ABD" (all but the dissertation) persona.

Continuing this survival regimen, I worked on my degree and tried to find a position for the fall of 1951. A letter was received from the chair at the University of Michigan indicating that there was an opening for a person to teach general courses and one particular course on the family. This was my specialty area and I went to my mentor for whom I served as an assistant and asked if he would write a letter of recommendation for me. He agreed to do this. Similar to other professional fields, the sponsorship or recommendation of key persons is a more salient measure of your qualifications and potential for placement than anything else, especially when you are a novitiate.

My mentor knew the faculty at the University of Michigan, a choice position placement at an outstanding university, even as it would be today with its prominent Department of Sociology. I thought I had a good chance of getting that job. But I was betrayed. I discovered that he wrote a letter recommending three of us and ranked us in order of quality. The first person was someone with whom he had very little association, nothing like the fiduciary relationship to which we had committed ourselves. This person had been a Yale undergraduate, had done well, and was given one of a few department fellowships that allowed him to spend all his time on his studies. Given this fellowship, he was held up to be a person of great promise and great expectations. I was ranked second and as doing well beyond his initial expectations. I was described as being aggressive, determined, and hard working, but obviously not as good as his number one candidate. The third ranking was given to a colleague of mine who has turned out to be one of the most outstanding social and behavioral scientists working in the cancer field.

As it turned out, the candidate ranked first never completed his Ph.D. Although he was offered the job on the condition that he would complete his thesis on time, he never did and never got the job. Maybe the gods in the heavens were playing games. My mentor later became embroiled in a conflict with a colleague in an American Studies program in which both served. This colleague of my mentor later became president of Yale, and my mentor never received a promotion or tenure. Eventually, he moved to a mid-west university where he was given a full professorship.

What I learned from this wounding was that one has to make things happen for oneself. That spring, I landed a position at Union College in Schenectady, New York, and spent the summer in New Haven, Connecticut, laying out the redevelopment areas for the newly formed Redevelopment Agency. I used to do a fair amount of community and urban research in my earlier days, and when I arrived at Union College in Schenectady, I became heavily involved in urban research. Consequently, I was instrumental in laying out the census track for the Census Bureau in the Schenectady, Troy, and Albany areas.

I had some amusing experiences during my three years at Union, beginning on the day I arrived for a two-day visit with members of the faculty. It was as if they were interviewing for a new president. I arrived on a Sunday afternoon at the president's house and had to make my way through the kitchen door to find him in the kitchen cooking. And while he cooked, he talked and found out a lot of things about me. He was interested in my background and experience during the war and my work as a watchmaker. Moreover, he was interested in the fact that, when I was in Chicago, I worked in the clock department of Marshall Fields Department Store and things of that order–topics of great import and obvious scholarly interest! During this interview, he noted that he was prepared to offer me the job at a salary of $3,600, provided I passed muster with his faculty. He informed me that $3,600 was $100 more than he was offering for a beginning assistant professor in 1951. What is amusing is that he hired a young historian from Harvard and paid him only $3,500 or $100 less than what I received because he did not have his Ph.D. So, what all this means is that going to Yale and getting a doctorate is worth $100 more than going to Harvard and coming out without a doctorate! This historian eventually got his doctorate and later became Dean of Union College.

These are not devastating experiences, but still they are woundings or impositions on the psyche. Another of these woundings, which may appear to be humorous at first blush, had profound impact upon my behavior. At the first faculty meeting of the college in the fall of 1951, the president introduced all the new faculty members. When he came to me, he gave a little spiel about me and pointed out that I came from a long line of watchmakers and had experience fixing clocks. He further indicated that I certainly would be a consultant to those who had any such problems. As it turned out, unfortunately, there were four or five faculty members who were collectors of antique clocks. All of them were higher in the power structure and one of them was Dean of the College, and it was obvious that this power system operated to the advantage of those in control. Consequently, I accommodated, just like all minorities have accommodated to the majorities from time immemorial.

It was a difficult situation to be in. I had my workbench with me because I still had to continue my repair business. I was also teaching night courses, performing my responsibilities as a full time member of the faculty at Union, and could not completely deny the expressed interest of my colleagues regarding their clocks. I was able to do some quickie repairs that did not take extensive rebuilding, but stopped short where clocks needed major works, such as new bushings for the gears. I indicated quite clearly that I was not prepared to undertake those repairs, since I did not have the set up for doing such basic renovations. My skill in this area undoubtedly enhanced my status, particularly with the Dean of the College, who was an avid collector. However, my interest was much more in getting them to recognize a new urban institute that I had created with a grant of $50.00 and a couple of ambitious undergraduate students.

Here I am only up to the beginnings of my career and there is so much to tell about the middle and later stage with little clock time. All this is necessary, however, to give you a complete picture of a modern day Asclepius with Don Quixotic tendencies.

I returned to the University of Chicago in 1954, but not to the Social Service School. I received an internship in General Education from the Carnegie foundation in 1954 and chose to spend the year at the University of Chicago rather than going to Harvard or Columbia. I arrived at the end period of a meteoric rise of non-traditional education initiated by Robert Hutchins at the University of Chicago. His one-page manifesto, just a few years before, did a traditionectomy on university education. The impact of his innovations in interdisciplinary education and learner-based education is still being felt. In 1955, the University of Chicago leadership under then-President Kempton and the departments were revealing their bureaucratic muscle. More formalism was being introduced, resistances to a return to the old ways were being beaten down, and the publish or perish motif was being reinstituted. The woundings were occurring, and a sadness overcame me as I moved on in 1955.

I spent over 22 years of the most productive part of my academic career at Western Reserve (which later joined with Case to become Case Western Reserve University) in Cleveland, Ohio. When I arrived I was part of a five-person sociology department that had a budget of about $45,000 a year, of which, except for the Chair, I was the highest paid faculty member. I also was the youngest person in chronological age and functioned in a very traditional bureaucracy. Consequently, it was difficult to get things done because one had to "work through channels." The attitude I perceived is found in so many non-academic organizations where your colleagues basically say to you, "You are free to do what you want, but don't bother us, and if you start pushing us around, you are going to be in real trouble."

A few incidents provided the experience for me to adopt patterns of action that would modify or turn around the hurts and wounds I and others had experienced in the University. The task was to have more creative and positive actions. Near the end of my first year at Case Western Reserve University, the Chair asked me to stop by his office. During the course of the conversation, he expressed that he and other senior members of the faculty were pleased with my enthusiasm and the work I was doing. Of particular note, he said, were my efforts to activate both Master's and Doctoral programs, which had been approved many years ago by the Faculty Senate and Administration, but were not in operation.

I was very pleased by the stroking and also thought it was a situation in which I could ask for something from him. I hesitated to ask for a salary increase, although I had two children and a third on the way. Moreover, I was hustling with overload teaching because I was not repairing watches any longer. I thought it inappropriate to come out directly for a salary increase and instead indicated a need for some supplies because I was getting involved in national work.

I had already published a half-dozen articles beginning in 1950 (Sussman, 1950) and was creating the first-ever printed *Sourcebook on Marriage and the Family* (Sussman, 1957, 1963, 1968). I was increasingly being invited to present at different professional meetings in various parts of the country and had begun developing a social network of colleagues. So I asked him if he could furnish me with postage stamps to do some mailings. He looked at me and asked me what the stamps would be used for, and I explained, as best I could, that the purpose was scholarly communication. He got into his desk and took out a sheet of 5-cent stamps. That's what it cost to mail a letter in those days. He tore off 15, and gave them to me and said, "Is this enough?" I said yes, that it was enough. The lesson I learned from this experience was a vow I made that afternoon or evening, talking to myself out loud and to the gods who would listen. I pledged that I would never go to him again to ask for anything, not even a paper clip. If I was going to be able to do what I wanted to do, I'd have to go out and do it myself.

I had an opportunity some years later to take over the chair's position and was given a mandate from a new Dean to develop sociology (to which I added anthropology) and to become one of the top departments in the country. Although I received very little financial aid from the Dean, I did, however, receive his tolerance and support for what I set out to accomplish. I inherited a budget in 1962 of about $60,000 ($10.00 was allotted for postage and mailing), but within five years had a departmental operation with a budget of a million dollars a year. The department grew to a total of six pre-doctoral training programs and a faculty approaching 25 in number with multiple sources of funding for research. This rapid development was not all due simply to my abilities or to those of my colleagues. The Universe was right, I had connections, and some of them provided me with resources to test the ideas I espoused. "Interdisciplinarity" became a basic tenet in our research program. We worked, for example, with Systems Development and Engineering faculty and students. Moreover, ample funding was available for the social sciences as a consequence of Sputnik and other policy changes on the federal level. We experienced "birthquaking" growth and eventually took possession of a magnificent historic building on campus.

Coupled with the search for self-reliance and efforts to reduce the frustrations, hurt, and past woundings, was the development of skills to deal with bureaucracies. A priority in my repertoire was skill in social relationships with other functionaries of the system.

Another case illustration of this is needed. During the heyday of my tenure as chair of the Sociology department, I would have regular meetings with the Dean about every two weeks. These would be scheduled for one to two hours, and each with a lengthy agenda. I soon learned from these meetings and other experiences that you do not go to authority when you have problems, but you solve them the best you can. When you do go, in turn, somebody has to seek a solution. That is, you are forcing a solution and, more often than not, it is not going to be in your favor. Running to the boss or running to the guru or running to the charismatic leader is a waste of time and energy and simply perpetuates the scars of the wounds one receives in the course of life.

In any event, I would go to these meetings with a prepared agenda and different options for him to consider. I tried to work the relationship with him to where he would have trust in me and confidence in my judgments and to where he still had the power to say "No" (which he did on occasion). I fitted his type of operation and was aware that a birthquake of activity was occurring in all departments throughout the University (he was in charge of 26 Arts and Sciences departments). He did not have the support staff (bureaucratic structure) to supervise carefully the activities of each of these units, so he instituted a more decentralized structure of working with each individual chairperson. Thus, when I came in with a twenty-item agenda, it became obvious that we had to make quick decisions when the issues were raised, rather than put them off for a later time. We did not spend a lot of time pondering whether it was the right decision, but we made mostly good decisions. I remember one day when we had a heavy session, with much negotiating, giving and taking, where he won some and I won some. At the end of the meeting, he said, "Marvin, we did an awful lot today and I don't know who conned who, but go ahead and go after those hires and support staff. It looks good. These new Ph.D.'s in sociology are doing well."

What was occurring was that the success we were having required the institution to recognize it and to begin to allocate resources to sustain and maintain this high level of performance. You move bureaucracies and those who control them, which I have called functionaries, not by preaching or by the most rational arguments, but by the results. Are you reaching the objectives using the most humane, considerate, and respected methods and procedures? To use a street phrase, "Are you for real?" If you can answer yes, then this will be reflected in your relationships with others in the development of trust. Even those who are parts of impersonal bureaucracies can extend to you that component which is in all of humankind.

Now let me turn to a couple of adventures in academia. The first resonates the medical sociology-rehabilitation nexus and the second, the publication of the *Handbook of Marriage and the Family* (1987).

In 1964, I received a call from the Office of Vocational Rehabilitation (OVR) asking if I would be interested in reviewing grant applications for them. The connection was made by an OVR staff member who had read my

Presidential Address to the *Society for the Study of Social Problems* in 1962, where I postulated and argued vehemently for reorganizing the multiple roles of the sociologist: the roles of educator, researcher, administrator, clinician, evocator, and social artist (Sussman, 1962). It turned out that the staff, many of whom were trained in psychology, were looking for more than a reviewer. Specifically, they needed someone who would help them relate rehabilitation concepts and processes which were not limited in their explanatory power by a medical model.

After a series of meetings in which the agency rehabilitation staff and I had intellectual exchanges, clarifying terms, concepts, goals, and procedures, a $50,000 grant was made. The intention was to introduce sociologists to the rehabilitation field and to catalyze research programs, linking rehabilitation with the fresh approaches of family and medical sociologists. The form was to be a high level conference at Carmel, California, with commissioned papers to be completed prior to the conference. Critiques and discussion were to be followed by the publication of 25,000 copies of this collection's papers for which we received a second grant for free distribution to all ASA members. This grant also funded free distribution of 3,000 copies to rehabilitation professionals and administrators as well as libraries and institutes nationwide (Sussman, 1965a). The ASA was the sponsoring agency and was eager to participate in the newest of ventures of a "non-pure" sociologic activity. The politics of attrition failed in Council, and ASA staff, few by today's numbers, made it work with zest and empathy.

It was one of the more inspiring and satisfying activities I ever accomplished, an illustration of forging disciplinary and professional linkages as well as the dissemination and utilization of information for practice and further research. Little did I realize at that time, my inner self was responding to what later was to become my archetype, Asclepius, the man/god of healing, integration, holistic well-being, the breaking down of barriers, tunnel vision, and parochialism. The rhythm was wounding–healing, wounding–healing.

This is but one example of social artistry where there is integration of the aims of the practitioner with those of the consultant or catalyst. Being a social artist, and I consider myself to be one, involves skills of timing, experimentation, advising but not controlling, hard work, and a passion to complete the work with compassion. Such criteria and action were employed successfully with six other governmental agencies.

In reviewing the approximately 240 articles, books, and monographs that I have written or edited solely or with colleagues, I have become intrigued with the question: Why did I expend so much energy, time, and funds on particular programs of research, training, social action and consultation? Did I make conscious choices or was the subconscious guiding the trajectory of my academic career? Also what characteristics of self influenced such choices? Were there instances of no choice where the activity was mandated?

To answer these questions, I begin with reflections which complement what has already been presented. I am a multi-model person with varied scientific interests. While I am identified with numerous substantive sociological areas, I go for the challenging problem or issue. I am sometimes viewed by others as being outside my area of interest. I am also an opportunist who has a sense of sociological trends and who is able to move quickly in conceptualizing the problem or issue. I was able to write proposals for research funding and to influence colleagues into "jump time" to get into the fray early in an area's development. What I am suggesting is both a logical and intuitive process whereby I am able to deduce what will occur and to time my moves in a manner that comes from the deep unconscious.

I have often been asked how and why I decided to study intergenerational family relationships beginning in 1948. The simple answer is I don't know. It is possible that this work in family connectedness, which was my dissertation (Sussman, 1953a, 1954b, 1955a, 1959, 1960), was the consequence of my own family experience. Could it be that my subconscious mind was saying, "Your family was not the best example of generational commitment over historic time. Maybe you need the proof of family continuity in urban society. Go for it"? This interest was one that continued throughout my career (Sussman, 1960; Sussman & Burchinal, 1962a, 1962b; Pfeifer & Sussman, 1991; Sussman, 1991; Sussman, & Romeis, 1982).

It is only recently that I have begun to realize that the kind of research I chose to do had both rational and non-rational bases. I also underestimated the influence I had on others in the various fields in which I made theoretical and empirical contributions. William C. Goode pointed this out to me when speaking at the 1988 celebration day gathering in honor of my "retiring." He said in relation to the 240 publications:

> The sheer quantity is also expressed in extensity, in the variety of topics, the range of explorations, often looking at social problems little noticed at the time and thus a fruitful research agenda for others to follow. It is not possible to make a complete list, and no matter how long I make it, some of you will be able to add a few topics to my summary. However, let me tell those of you who have thought but little about the whole enterprise, that it includes fertility, the care of the elderly, social intervention, generational links–one of his earliest and most influential inquiries–rehabilitation, child rearing, childhood romances, pets, the care of diabetics, deafness, obesity, watchmaking, microcomputers, wills and testaments, inheritance–and now I stop arbitrarily, not because the list is complete.

> Let me take note of one of those inquiries, notable because of its intellectual importance, which I assert has an impact on sheer size. For one of the typical consequences of a fruitful line of investigation is that it generates other studies, leads to thoughtful applications in real life, enables graduate students to understand social life more precisely, and helps them to develop good projects of their own. Marvin's study of relations between generations, and of course among kin generally, was such a line of investigation. It was seen as an attack on Talcott Parsons' view of the isolation of the nuclear family. Very soon, and in many countries, it was ascertained that family life in even the most highly industrialized countries is embedded in a bubbling network of kin relations. This line of thought also led to suggested applications, an example of which is the possibility of developing a rehabilitation of medical care strategy that actively uses kinfolk. This would especially make use of the younger generation by eliminating some of the existing bureaucratic costs and inconveniences that prevent its use.

In addition to believing and following the lyric that "action without research is wasteful and research with out application is stupidity," I found myself selecting substantive sociological topics both by dialoguing with myself as well as from events and situations over which I had no control.

EARLY INTERNATIONAL RESEARCH

In the late 1950s and the early 1960s, I received invitations from the Committee on Family Research of the International Sociological Association to participate in a family sociology meeting in Japan. This was my first international meeting in which I presented a paper that was subsequently published. It was entitled "The Urban Kin Network in the Formulation of Family Theory," and it appeared in R. Hill & R. Koenig (1970) *Families in East and West: Socialization Processes and Kinship Ties.* This foundational paper provided the conceptual rootedness for my subsequent research on family linkages and continuity over generational time.

In the late 1960s, while doing research on family connectedness and generational continuity, I wrote a number of articles which questioned the viability of continuing to use the traditional definition of families. In 1970, I co-chaired, with Beatrice Paolucci, forum 14 of the White House Conference on Children. Our forum explicated the concept of varied family forms and became the bell weather forum for all the other forums (Sussman & Paolucci, 1971). Our conclusions regarding the emerging development of varied family forms were used by the sixteen other Forums in establishing desired and needed policies and practices on behalf of children.

A plethora of articles, including some I authored (Sussman, 1971, 1975), ensued as a result of the White House Conference. In 1978, I commissioned James Ramey to do an article entitled "Experimental Family Forms–The Family of the Future." His article was in volume no. 1, 1978, *Marriage & Family Review.* Currently, families of all shapes and forms are varied in their membership. The intact family of husband and wife and children may symbolically represent the American Family, but the incidence and prevalence of this form is radically diminishing. This has been reflected in my research on divorce (Kitson & Sussman, 1982; Kitson, Holmes, & Sussman, 1983), single moms (Hanson, Heims, Julian, & Sussman, 1995), and homosexuality (Bozett & Sussman, 1989).

In 1973, a substantial grant in excess of $200,000 was received from the National Institute of Child Health and Human Development, as it was called at that time, to ascertain the status of family research in 10 different societies. A secondary objective was to simulate the research in these and other cultures.

Research across cultures became a basic component of my writing and research. The urge to learn how other cultures are organized and function became a dominant part of my being. Under the aegis of the Groves Conference on Marriage and the Family, I spent almost three years, not full time of course, in organizing an international conference on gender roles held in 1975 at Dubrovnik, Yugoslavia, which was attended by 300 scholars from all over the world. This built on my interest in cross national research (Sussman, 1966 1969b; Sussman & Romeis, 1982) and continued in 1996 with two volumes on intercultural variation in family research that I published with Roma Stovall Hanks (Sussman & Hanks, 1996a; 1996b). This collection, involving scholars in 23 societies, contained reviews on the development of family theory and research in their respective societies.

It was at the Dubrovnik conference of family researchers that I presented for the first time a paper on Marriage Contracts. This was a fun project supported with a grant from the Russell Sage Foundation. Primary aims were to ascertain the desirability of such agreements before marriage. The major assumption was that, if marital partners could agree on day to day as well as long-term goals, then they would have more joyful time to spend with each other, with the expectation that agreements about gender roles would be honored.

Prenuptial agreements have existed from time immemorial, with the upper classes being more likely to formulate such contracts. Our work focused more on middle class youth who were married or soon would be. The topic of marriage contracts is still in the public eye, as a recent issue of *Time* magazine (April 24, 2000), in which a full page was given to the current development of postnuptial agreements, indicates. These agreements, which are being discussed in the courts, are primarily contracts relating to the distribution of assets if any divorce occurs in the future. Thus they are really *post* rather than *pre*nuptial agreements and are fertile ground for sociological research.

My earliest experience as an academician was exposure to the concept and practice of interdisciplinarity. A simple but adequate definition of "multidisciplinarity" is that one looks at issues and problems from a perspective largely devoid of the tunnel vision of one discipline or profession. One needs to take into account and use theories and practices of other fields to make sense of what is being observed. For example, the rebuilding of a community requires the use of knowledge from various fields, such as engineering, architecture, landscaping, history, sociology, psychology, and many more. Smitten by the concept of multidisciplinarity, I accepted a Carnegie Foundation internship in 1954 to essentially study interdisciplinary departments in interaction at the University of Chicago. In the subsequent years at Case Western University, I was able to develop with colleagues in engineering, education, nursing, and psychology programs, as well as in the medical school, seven integrative doctoral training programs.

In publishing the first edition of *Sourcebook in Marriage and the Family* (Sussman, 1955), I proceeded to invite established and beginning scholars from the different social science and humanistic fields to be authors. Their varied perspectives on substantive issues such as child rearing enabled readers to obtain a more comprehensive description of what is involved in child rearing. This practice continued in subsequent editions of the *Sourcebook* (Sussman, 1963, 1968, 1974).

Many years later, this same interdisciplinary perspective was maintained in the publication of the *Handbook of Marriage and the Family,* in 1987 and the second edition in 1999. The motivation for such activity is my own inability to accept what I perceive to be the truth from a single perspective. Such tunnel vision allowed perception without knowing, and I could not continue to do research from the narrow confines of one discipline.

In 1970, I published with Judith Cates and Davis Smith a book called *The Family and Inheritance*. This was the first empirical study on linking family with legal systems. The study is concerned with what happens in a family at death and why? The findings represented a sampling of over two million cases and made use of interviews with family members, others named in wills, and those who would have inherited in the absence of wills. Sociologists, lawyers, historians, and anthropologists made up the interdisciplinary team. The principal linkage was between lawyers and sociologists. They dialogued on concepts and procedures as well as hypotheses to be tested. We learned more fully how families felt and reacted to the death of their loved ones and the meaning of the legacy left to the survivors. Such meaning was more symbolic than economic. Our interdisciplinary perspective gave richness to the data. I later addressed this topic in 1981 in my Burgess Award address (Sussman, 1983).

The Call to Adventure. There are two processes involved in receiving the call. The first is blunder and the second is herald. Where blunder is a factor in the call to adventure, the individuals join with forces that are not understood. The individual might be in the right place at the right time; this is Sussman's law of fortuitous circumstance, or in other terminology there appears to be a critical mass that is present. What the ingredients are is difficult to fathom. They are likened to ripples on the surface of life being produced by unsuspected springs. Conditions in the environment are appropriate for something to occur; the blunder may amount to the opening of the destiny.

In 1986, I completed with Suzanne Steinmetz a monumental work which I began about 10 years previously, the *Handbook of Marriage and the Family* (Sussman & Steinmetz, 1987). Completion would not have occurred without Dr. Steinmetz's participation. I found that the 10-year experience in developing the handbook fitted the life course of a hero's journey.

In 1964, I heeded the call to become editor of the National Council on Family Relations' flagship publication, *The Journal of Marriage and the Family.* It was a herald to follow in the footsteps of previous great editors, Harold Christensen, Ivan Nye, Ernest Burgess, and Meyer Nimkoff.

In 1978, I blundered into what turned out to be a 20-year relationship with The Haworth Press to create the journal *Marriage & Family Review* and to edit it for 20 years. I have had the privilege and honor to turn over the editorship to two sterling scholars, Suzanne K. Steinmetz and Gary W. Peterson.

Returning to the *Handbook* story, I happened to be at a national professional meeting, bored to tears with the ad nauseam presentations, and retired quietly to the lounge where I found a corner to have coffee and to read once again an "invent the wheel" type of paper which I was discussing on the following day. A fellow sufferer at a nearby table, unbeknownst to me, observed what I was doing and entered into a friendly conversation. He was a relatively new editor of a staid publishing house that wanted to get into the soft field of family science. His house had a great reputation for producing Handbooks and once he found out who I was, he became elated and very seductive. He presented an antidote to what I was experiencing. My being rose to mythic proportions and I thought what I might be able to do was to set the field right. I thought to myself, you will collect the best stars in the constellation of family social science and with your own creative powers produce a document that will receive world acclaim. I had indeed blundered into this call for adventure.

The herald, which did not occur as the call for the *Handbook* adventure, is a summons. It may be a summons from a person you regard very highly who indicates that it is about time you did this or that. It may be the wakening of yourself where you see the light, the ahahs, where you put things together and now can take the next step by answering the call to adventure.

The next stage is the *Refusal of the Call.* The rationales I presented for refusing were the disturbances of my own routines: the lack of time and energy; the fear of failure; the impingements and constraints of the academic enterprise of which I was a part; and the priorities that I had established to have a life. Refusal of such a summons may convert the potential adventure into a negative experience. Think of how many times you have refused the call to adventure and what you perceive as a flowering world simply became a wasteland of dry stones whose greening is yet to come.

In my own experience with the *Handbook,* I almost refused the call. I sat on the contract for many months. I had very good reasons and rationales for this behavior. I had just experienced a life course and marital transformation as well as taking a new position after being based at an institution for over 22 years. Perhaps, most importantly, I was reluctant to give up those things that I felt would provide me with security and structure. In refusing the call, one goes back to one's local self where the ego functions in a protected environment of self-interest. However, I answered the call because service to others is a definite component of taking up the call. As I reflect back on my history in the educational field, I have seldom refused the call to adventure. My commitment to serve all others has been a dominant value in my life.

For those who have not refused the call, the first encounter of the hero's journey is with a protective figure, which provides one with amulets against the dragon forces one is about to encounter. The form of supernatural aid I received was the memory of the late Dr. Meyer Nimkoff, who 25 years earlier had launched my publishing career. He had catalyzed my adventure at that time to develop and create the first sourcebook in the United States on marriage and the family. I never studied with Meyer Nimkoff. We had an almost extra-sensory perceptual relationship in which he was my protector. His presence has been felt over the years, and he is one of those ageless guardians who will come to the floor of my consciousness when needed.

Once I took up the call, I seemed to be riding the great rhythm of a historical process. I was doing something that nobody had done since an older colleague, Harold Christiansen, had done his classical work back in 1964. And while the analogy may be inappropriate and misinterpreted, I felt very much like Napoleon did at the opening of his Russian campaign when he said, "I feel myself driven toward an end that I do not know. As soon as I shall have reached, as soon as I shall have become unnecessary, an atom will suffice to shatter me. Till then, not all the forces of mankind can do anything against me." I possessed that feeling when I took up the call. Once the commitment was made, the forces in the universe appeared to be in order, and with support, both supernatural and in this life, the work began.

Crossing of the Threshold was the next stage of the journey. One has to pass the guardians of the gates, the ogres, other persons, and our own ogre-like behavior. Familiar chants of ogres are: "I don't want to do that"; "That's not my problem, that's your problem"; "I know it's tough, but I don't want to be involved"; "I don't want to do this, it is not in my best interest"; "I told you so." Such guardians and ogres may not be harmful and the task is how to outwit them. In academia, especially in undertaking an editorship of a volume or a journal, or in authoring a book, the threshold guardians will not recognize the importance of such callings and will engage in covert and overt behavior, which attempt to thwart the process of a successful outcome. The Handbook was no exception to the rule, with the major guardians being top administrators at my university. While I commanded some authority and power by the nature of my position and had some control over resources, I was kidded about this undertaking. These critics saw it as making very little contribution to the well-being of two institutions that were providing me with means for my life's work. I should point out that these institutions were the Union Institute, where I was a core faculty member, and as Unidel professor of human behavior at the University of Delaware, from where I continued to work after my retirement from 1988 until 1998. Thus, my strategy to outwit these ogres was to work hard enough to be sufficiently successful in the undertakings that they were deemed to be important to the position I held. Thus, I could neutralize any overt action, which would further slow down the pace of development of the project.

The next stage of the hero's and heroine's journey is *Being Swallowed into the Unknown,* with the appearance of having died but to be born again (i.e., to have undergone a metamorphosis). This is called being in the *belly of the whale.* I cannot claim that the *Handbook* experience was a religious one, but it did have some qualities close to my own resurrection after having died with the project. I became more sanguine and understanding of the foibles of humankind, and I figuratively died with the project because of consternation and frustration, but experienced a rebirth after making a wise decision to invite Dr. Suzanne Steinmetz to be a collaborator. Sue was a former student, for whom I was her major professor when she was working on her Ph.D. at Case Western Reserve University. She had come to my rescue some years earlier when I had experienced a betrayal which resulted in the elimination of the Department of Marital Health from an eastern medical school. She was instrumental in my coming to the University of Delaware as a Unidel professor, one of the major chairs at the university.

The seventh stage of the hero's and heroine's journey is the *Road of Trials,* a perilous path of victories and defeats. The role of trials relating to the *Handbook* project consisted of external barriers presented not only by administrators of hierarchical structures but also by the more human failures of colleagues. Some made commitments and accepted responsibilities but evidently did not give the production of a creative synthesized chapter their highest priority. Other trials and tribulations were such experiences as the expected or unexpected birth of a child, a divorce, or a mental breakdown, which probably originated in discriminatory practices on the job, unresolved fears, and authors' internal conflicts.

The picture was even more clouded by rapid change in Plenum House editors to work in the development of the project. The initial editor, who was my lounge companion mentioned previously, had decided to pick up his gear and move on to better fields for publishing heroes by creating his own firm. Consequently, there was a succession of editors until the present one, who has had the longest period of stability and is an understanding, friendly, and down-to-earth human being who developed a working relationship with myself and my colleague beginning in 1983. Dr. Steinmetz, who joined me in this project some five years into the mission, experienced some of the trials and tribulations concerning our authors. She encouraged them to heroic efforts, and her dogged persistence and perseverance greatly facilitated the achievement of the final product. Her knowledge of the field enabled selection of persons for whom expectations of greatness are reasonably certain, but not assured. Thus, we had a combination of highly established and experienced investigators and young stars in the constellation of family sociology.

Sue, more than most, enabled me to move into the next stage of the hero's journey, *Recognition of Self as Hero*. In this stage, as is true with all of us who experience this journey, I became more aware of how I have changed, became far more knowledgeable about myself. My perceptions of reality broke from a tunnel vision pattern. I became more aware of the reality of the work and research I had been doing and the reality of the field of endeavor in which all of us had been laboring so diligently. My colleague's energy and motivation helped me leave the *belly of the whale,* in so far as the *Handbook* was concerned, and to move the project along where one requirement was to make some very hard decisions regarding quality and appropriateness of different contributions. In some instances, we changed chapter authors; in other cases, we were quite frank about the product and took it upon ourselves to do radicalectomies of submitted material. In other cases, we reformulated the focus and content of articles to reflect what we thought were new areas of marriage and family studies. These behaviors suggested an element of risk taking, which is part of the recognition of one being a hero.

Being catapulted into a process of introspection, examining one's inner self where the effort was to penetrate to the basic source of one's deep consciousness, such musings were influenced by the *Handbook* experience. This process of introspection I attribute to Jean Houston, a prophetic and eclectic teacher, an evocator of the spirit, human capacities, and potentials.

The experience of sailing in uncharted waters of the deep psyche created a reluctance to ***Return to the World of Everyday Life,*** which is essentially the ninth stage of the hero's and heroine's journey.

In this stage of return as a hero or heroine, at least a mythical one, it is appropriate to relate newly discovered knowledge and skills to everyday life. The experience of doing this *Handbook* created for me a new sense of awareness of the complexities and differentiation of persons, the personalities, perceptions of reality, and the suppressed desires and conflicts of individuals who take on a commitment and attendant responsibilities and perform either brilliantly or problematically. I learned that groping and being in the belly of the whale, and experiencing betrayal and other trials and tribulations, is part of the growth process. It is part of life. It is part of becoming more aware of the connections of the cosmic nature of life on this planet. I have also become more aware of what I would have done if I were to do such a project once again, or if I could set back the years to 1975 and commence once again.

I am a slow learner and was enamored by the success of the *Handbook*, so I succumbed to the overtures of Plenum's editor and agreed to undertake a second edition. This undertaking was 9 years in the making and finally appeared in print in 1999. We faced the same issues and problems that plagued us with the first edition. It was most fortunate that we were able to add a third editor, Professor Gary W. Peterson, a motivated and eclectic Sociologist. Both my co-editors completed heroic journeys almost as long and cataclysmic as those experienced by Odysseus on his ten-year return journey to Ithaca.

The final stage is the *Master of Two Worlds.* This is the world of inner space, inner being, and the outer world, the so-called world of reality, its interpersonal relationships and human created institutions, systems, and social structures. The *Handbook,* which is an example of the positivistic natural science mode and attendant phenomena, has not suffered one iota because of the cosmic dance I have been relating to you. In taking the freedom of passing back and forth across the world divisions of inner and outer being, I have not rested heavily in a single spot, but have gaily and lightly leaped from one position to another.

Finally, the *Handbook* is only as good as the work of the contributors, whose diligence and patience must be recognized. This is our expression of recognition and empowerment. The story of the hero's and heroine's journey, told in myths and stories of past ages, has its relevance to current myths, which pervade our practices in academia and in publishing. I find those of the journey a more appropriate context for the realities of the everyday world than those which we have created in our professional setting, such as publish or perish, and publish, for God's sake, in refereed journals. I find these old paradigms increasingly more academic and creating a vast wasteland in need of greening.

My concerns with the inner being, the feelings of reflective human beings, the deep yearnings and unspoken desires, should be examined as my visions and behaviors. My journey is my own doing. Great persons and perhaps ordinary souls must leave the path of tradition and obedient subordination. They must trust the supreme and indefinable power, strike out on a new trackless course where experience is no guide (paraphrased from Magister Ludi).

What does all this mean? At this point I am not certain or completely uncertain. Some catbird seat views are:

1. Work to create multiple options so that wounding, betrayal, rejection, and related negatives can be neutralized and beginnings can be made on a transformed path.
2. Learn to live with the fracture between idealism and reality. The differences you experience between these two conditions is a normal consequence. It is not worth succumbing to the wounding of one's psyche.
3. Perceive wounding in the context of grappling, influencing, and combating bureaucratic forms of organization. Recognize the hard work in doing this and its endemic stress and the need to normalize and control such encounters.
4. Entertain the notion that many woundings are self-inflicted and persist because of derived psychic and other benefits. As a family consists of persons in intimate interaction and is ruled by its sickest member, a learning group is most likely to be controlled by its most wounded member. Such groups curse the "system" and do little else.
5. Recognize that betrayal is a normal event. Evidence for this belief is our litigious and divorcing society.
6. Be aware that hunger of the spirit, body, and mind is the antidote to woundings and betrayals. Let the woundings, betrayals, and endemic mind states and behaviors occur for the transformation that follows. Metaphorically, let the spears sink deep into your gut for this is the way you get iron in your blood.
7. Work at cutting the ego as you would drop poor performing stock or an unworkable human relationship. Ego reduction is correlated with finding and living a good life. The more you reduce, the more you live with meaning and joy.

In closing this journey, I need to note that my family has enriched my life in these later years. My four children are married. Stuart is a corporate financial officer, and he and his wife Carol, an accountant, have 4-year-old twin daughters Sarah and Megan. Marty, an herbalist, and her husband Jefferson, director of managed health care at Ohio State University, have two grown children: Jessica, a forensic chemist with the FDA, and Luke, who is with a fast food chain developing and managing new outlets. My own love of painting and design appears to be present in the job choices of two of my children. Kenneth is a landscape architect and is married to Joanne, an art teacher. Nancy is an architect; she and her husband Michael have a toddler, Thomas. I will soon become a Great Grandfather! I do not feel that old! So be it!

EDITORS' NOTE

The editors were responsible for inserting citations and creating a major portion of the bibliography from material supplied by the author.

REFERENCES

Boek, W. E., Sussman, M. B., Yankauer, A. (1957). Social class, maternal health and child care; an interviewing study of mothers with three-to-six month old babies. New York: New York State Department of Health.

Boek, W. E., Sussman, M. B., & Yankauer, A. (1958). Social class and child care practices. *Marriage and Family Living, 20*, 4, 326-333.

Bozett, F. W. & Sussman, M. B. (1989). Homosexuality and family relations: Views and research issues. *Marriage & Family Review, 14*, 3-4, 1-8.

Cates, J. N. & Sussman, M. B. (1982). Family systems and inheritance. *Marriage & Family Review, 5*, 3, 1-24.

Cogswell, B. E. & Sussman, M. B. (1972). Changing Family and Marriage Forms: Complications for Human Service Systems. *Family Coordinator, 21*, 4, 505-516.

Crain, A. J., Sussman, M. B., & Weil, W. B., Jr. (1966a). Effects of a diabetic child on marital integration and related measures of family functioning. *Journal of Health and Human Behavior, 7*, 2, 122-127.

Crain, A. J., Sussman, M. B., & Weil, W. B., Jr. (1966b). Family interaction, diabetes, and sibling relationships. *International Journal of Social Psychiatry, 12*, 1, 35-43.

Gross, H. E. & Sussman, M. B. (1997). Needed research on the employed mother. *Marriage & Family Review, 25*, 1-2, 1-6.

Hanson, S. M. H. Heims, M. L., Julian, D. J., & Sussman, M. B. (1995). Single parent families: Present and future perspectives. *Marriage & Family Review, 20*, 1-2, 1-26.

Haug, M. R. & Sussman, M. B. (1969). Professional autonomy and the revolt of the client. *Social Problems, 17*, 2, 153-161.

Haug, M. R. & Sussman, M. B. (1973). Rehabilitation counseling in perspective: A reply to the critics. *Rehabilitation Counseling Bulletin, 16*, 4, 226-238.

Hill, R. & Koenig, R. (Eds.) (1970). *Families in East and West: Socialization Processes and Kinship Ties* (pp. 481-503). Paris, France: Mouton.

Haug, M. R. & Sussman, M. B. (1972). *Agents of social control: Issues in rehabilitation manpower.*

Kitson, G. C. & Sussman, M. B. (1982). Marital complaints, demographic characteristics, and symptoms of mental distress in divorce. *Journal of Marriage and the Family, 44,* 1, 87-101.

Kitson, G. C., Holmes, W. M., & Sussman, M. B. (1983). Withdrawing divorce petitions: A predictive test of the exchange model of divorce. *Journal of Divorce, 7,* 1, 51-66.

Marciano, T. D. & Sussman, M. B. (1986). The Threat of a Nuclear Holocaust: A Planetary Perspective. *Marriage & Family Review, 10,* 2, 1-8.

Pfeifer, S. K. & Sussman, M. B. (Eds.) (1991). Families: intergenerational and generational connections. NY: The Haworth Press, Inc.

Ramey, J. (1978). Experimental family forms: The family of the future. *Marriage & Family Review, 1,* 1, 1-9.

Strodtbeck, F. L. & Sussman, M. B. (1956). Of time, the city, and the "one-year guaranty": the relations between watch owners and repairers. *American Journal of Sociology, 61,* XX, 602-609.

Sussman, M. B. (1950). Mate selection among Negro and white college students. *Sociology and Social Research, 35,* 1, 46-49.

Sussman, M. B. (1953a). The help pattern in the middle class family. *American Sociological Review, 18,* 1, 22-28.

Sussman, M. B. (1953b). Parental participation in mate selection and its effects upon family continuity. *Social Forces, 32,*1, 76-81.

Sussman, M. B. (1954). Family continuity: selective factors which affect relationships between families at generational levels. *Marriage and Family Living, 16,* 2, 112-120.

Sussman, M. B. (1955a). Activity patterns of post-parental couples and their relationship to family continunity. *Marriage and Family Living, 17,* 4, 338-341.

Sussman, M. B. (1955b). *Sourcebook in Marriage and the Family.* NY: Houghton-Mifflin Publishers. Second edition, 1963; third edition, 1968; fourth edition, 1974.

Sussman, M. B. (1956a). "The calorie collectors": a study of spontaneous group formation, collapse, and reconstruction. *Social Forces, 34,* 4, 351-356.

Sussman, M. B. (1956b). Psycho-social correlates of obesity; failure of "calorie collectors." *American Dietetic Association, 32,* 423-428.

Sussman, M. B. (1957). The role of neighborhood associations in private housing for racial minorities. *Journal of Social Issues, 13,* 4, 31-37.

Sussman, M. B. (1959). The isolated nuclear family: Fact or fiction. *Social Problems, 6,* 3, 333-340. Reprinted in S. K. Steinmetz. (Ed). (1988). *Family and support systems across the life span.* (pp. 1-10). NY: Plenum Press.

Sussman, M. B. (1960). Intergenerational family relationships and social role changes in middle age. *Journal of Gerontology, 15,* 1, 71-75.

Sussman, M. B. (1961). Needed research on the employed mother. *Marriage and Family Living, 23,* 4, 368-373.

Sussman, M. B. (1964). The social problems of the Sociologist. *Social Problems, 11,* 2, 215-225.

Sussman, M. B. (Ed.) (1965a). Sociology and Rehabilitation. Washington, DC: American Sociological Association in Cooperation with the Vocational Rehabilitation Administration, US Department of Health, Education & Welfare.

Sussman, M. B. (1965b). Outcomes and Outlooks. In M. B. Sussman (Ed.) *Sociology and rehabilitation* (pp. 179-262). Washington, DC: American Sociological Association in Cooperation with the Vocational Rehabilitation Administration, US Department of Health, Education & Welfare.

Sussman, M. B. (1969a). Dependent disabled and dependent poor: Similarity of conceptual issues and research needs. *Social Service Review, 43,* 4, 383-395.

Sussman, M. B. (1969b). Cross-cultural family research: One view from the "catbird seat." *Journal of Marriage and the Family, 31,* 2, 203-209.

Sussman, M. B. (1970). The urban kin network in the formulation of family theory. In R. Hill & R. Koenig (Eds.) *Families in East and West: Socialization Processes and Kinship Ties.* Netherlands: Mouton.

Sussman, M. B. (1971). Family Systems in the 1970s: Analysis, Policies, and Programs. *Annals of the American Academy of Political and Social Science, 396,* July, 40-56.

Sussman, M. B. (1972). A Policy Perspective on the United States Rehabilitation System. *Journal of Health and Social Behavior, 13,* 2, 152-161.

Sussman, M.B. (1975). The four f's of variant family forms and marriage styles. *Family Coordinator, 24,* 4, 563-576.

Sussman, M. B. (1983). 1981 Burgess address: Law and legal systems: The family connection. *Journal of Marriage and the Family, 45,* 1, 9-21. Reprinted in S. K. Steinmetz (Eds.) (1988). Family and support systems across the life span. (pp. 11-34). NY: Plenum Press.

Sussman, M. B. (1989). Epilogue–AIDS: Opportunity for humanity. *Marriage & Family Review, 13,* 1-2, 229-239.

Sussman, M. B. (1991). Reflections on intergenerational and kin connections. *Marriage & Family Review. 16,* 1-2, 3-9.

Sussman, M. B. & Burchinal, L. (1962a). Parental aid to married children: Implication for family functioning. *Marriage and Family Living, 24,* 4, 320-332.

Sussman, M. B. & Burchinal, L. (1962b). Kin family network: Unheralded structure in current conceptualizations of family functioning. *Marriage and Family Living, 24,* 3, 231-240.

Sussman, M. B., Cates, J., & Smith. (1970). *The family and inheritance.* NY: Russell Sage Foundation.

Sussman, M. B. & Cogswell, B. E. (1972). The Meaning of Variant and Experimental Marriage Styles and Family Forms in the 1970's. *Family Coordinator, 21,* 4, 375-381.

Sussman, M. B. & Haug, M. R. (1968). Rehabilitation counselor recruits. *Journal of Counseling Psychology, 15,* 3, 250-256.

Sussman, M. B. & Hanks (1996a). *Intercultural Variation in Family Research and Theory: Implications for Cross-National Studies Part I.* NY: The Haworth Press, Inc.

Sussman, M. B. & Hanks (1996b). *Intercultural Variation in Family Research and Theory: Implications for Cross-National Studies Part 2.* NY: The Haworth Press, Inc.

Sussman, M. B. & Paolucci, B. (1970). Changing families in a changing society.

Report to the President: White House Conference on Children. Washington: GPO, 1971, pp. 227-238.

Sussman, M. B. & Romeis, J. C. (1982). Willingness to Assist One's Elderly Parents: Responses from United States and Japanese Families. *Human Organization, 41*, 3, 256-259.

Sussman, M. B. & Steinmetz, S. K. (1987). *Handbook of marriage and the family.* NY: Plenum Press.

Sussman, M. B., Steinmetz, S. K., & Peterson, G. W. (1999). *Handbook of marriage and the family* (2nd Edition). NY: Plenum Press.

Weil, W. B., Jr., Sussman, M. B., & Crain, A. & J. (1967). Social patterns and diabetic glucosuria. *American Journal of Diseases of Children, 113*, 4, 454-460.

My Autobiography

Gerhard Neubeck

KEYWORDS. Autobiography, therapist, faculty, childhood, career

Life may begin in utero, but real life begins in the delivery room–and a bloody one it is. Until later in life, I had never seen evidence of this, though my father, a doctor, had often referred to it. But 22 years later, after I had made my entry into the world, I was confronted with this bloody mess. Not as my son, the doctor, was born, but as a porter in a hospital, though I was a well-protected son of a physician. You see, refugees had no choice about many things. We took any job that provided us with a living, and being a porter in a hospital gave me room, board, and $50 or so in cash–not for the week, of course, but for the month. And the delivery room clean-up was the first real job I ever had. The real getting my hands dirty, using Bon Ami to scrub the tiles down on my hands and knees, mopping up after mother and baby had left for their rooms. A brand new mother and a baby to prove it. As Gene Fowler expressed so well, "Prudish old senses forbid it; Reformers adroitly have hit it; Though each person on earth arrived here by birth, to testify two people did it."

That was my entrance into the family field. Not that I was conscious of it–conscious that this was family in the sense that we are conscious of it now. After all, we're talking about the year 1940. But in retrospect, that's what it was. Evidence that a man and a woman had mated (had intercourse or made love–had screwed, if you please) whatever the act involved–duty, pleasure, love, who knows? The sperm of the man with whom the woman had been together found an ovum of hers all right, and the result was this bloody mess that I had to clean up. Little did I realize that these activities between men and women would become central to my professional life. It would give me enormous satisfaction in the pursuit of my career as well as pay me a salary in and out for the rest of my life.

As I said, I was a refugee. I'd come here from Germany, and I made my abiturium, which is the high school examination plus two years of college in Germany. My family and I were fleeing from the Nazis, and I had no career ideas whatsoever. I enrolled at NYU in New York and received a B.S. degree in personnel and guidance work in two years. This was followed by a master's degree in psychology at Northwestern University. Subsequently, in 1948, I became an instructor at the University of Minnesota in a field that I had originally not even thought of, namely, family life.

I got this instructorship as sort of a fluke, because I had really very little preparation for teaching family study, having taken only one sociology course during my undergraduate days. But it worked out, and I later also obtained a job as a marriage counselor for the Student Counseling Bureau at the University of Minnesota. I was now faced with the fact, in turn, that if I wanted to be promoted, I needed to get a doctoral degree. I chose Teachers College Columbia because I'd known Ernest Osborne who appealed to me as a person from whom I could learn a great deal. Subsequently, he became my mentor, and I am forever grateful for his guidance and caring.

I obtained an Ed.D. and became a kind of a pioneer because it was the first time that someone worked with couples. At the Margaret Singer Clinic in New York, I ran a therapy group for married people that sought to help them with their marital problems. In 1954, I published a paper based on this work in *Marriage and Family Living* (Neubeck, 1954). This became the first article ever to provide evidence for the possibility of working with couples–which psychoanalytic theory at that time had claimed was impossible–not just individuals. This was the first outcome of what I believe were pioneering efforts on my part.

The next chapter in these pioneering efforts was my work on extra-marital relations. I published articles in 1962 and 1967 (Neubeck, 1962, 1969a), edited a book, and wrote several chapters for the book, *Extra-Marital Relations* (1969b), which was the first of its kind on this subject. It is, of course, the area of sexuality in which I seemed to have made a splash. Having always devoted considerable time in my marriage course to sexuality, I thought it only fair that students be provided a full time course on sexuality.

Under the aegis of the Family Study Center at the University of Minnesota, and with the help of Reuben Hill, I made a proposal to the faculty curriculum committee to offer a course on human sexuality. I'd done my homework by soliciting responses from departments throughout the university about courses dealing with sexuality. I had learned that there were no such courses, and there were hardly any courses that included any references to sexuality. Thus, I was able to convince the curriculum committee to give me the go ahead. Subsequently, in the fall of 1967, I began teaching a course entitled "Human Sexual Behavior," which was written up in *Look* magazine in (April 1) 1969 in an article entitled "Sex Goes to College." It gave me a certain degree of fame, and it seemed that every publisher in the country was now after me to publish.

There's a cute anecdote connected with that experience. Several pictures were published in *Look* magazine, and I was very proud to be featured. My wife and I went to the supermarket, and I, that day, took one of the magazines and opened it up to the page with my picture. When we went to the cashier, I turned to her and said, "Do you recognize this person?" She looked at it and said, "Yeah, everybody has a double, right?" My wife chuckled and said, "That served you right for being so vain."

Ruth, my wife, has always been a great supporter of my career, and she certainly was the heroine in my presidential address to the NCFR in 1978, which I entitled "In Praise of Marriage." During all the earlier years, Ruth helped me with tuition because she always had jobs taking care of mothers and their newborn babies after they left the hospital. So we were a good team.

Besides the human sexuality course, I later developed a course on adolescent sexuality, which I believe was also a first in higher education in the United States. In 1964, again with the great support of Reuben Hill and the Family Studies Center, I began to direct an NIH-supported post-doctoral, post-MSW training program on marriage counseling training. For 5 years, we provided the theoretical courses for six to ten people per year who then took their clinical training in various agencies located in the Twin Cities.

We had a very good run for five years and were actually renewed, but NIH ran short of money, a fact that led to the end of the program in 1969. Richard Haye was my second in command; he had been a fellow student at Teachers College, and I was happy to have him at my side. The list of postdoctoral students in the program included people like Carl Broderick, David Olsen, Mike Sporakowski, to name only a few. We were a really good group and, I hope, made a contribution to the field of marriage counseling.

One other innovation needs to be mentioned. For a number of years, I taught a sexuality course in the Minnesota Correctional System. This course caused quite a sensation, being offered, as it was, in a prison with a medium security system that made me go through closed and locked doors. But it did work, it did work! One other thing, after my retirement, I also went to do some volunteer teaching and taught a sex course for junior high school kids, probably the toughest teaching I've ever done in my life. Junior high school kids are all hormones and gum, and their attention span is zilch. After I finished this task, I thought I'd done a really bad job, having been very frustrated by those kids in my attempt to get and retain their attention as well as make any headway in teaching some of the basics of sexuality. Despite such feelings, at the end of the course, I got a note from one of the boys who wrote that "if I achieved nothing else, he would be able to do a better job with his own kids than his parents had done with him." Based on this, I felt that I had made a contribution.

After I had received my doctorate degree at Teachers College, I went back to my position at the University of Minnesota and started what I also believe was a first, namely, teaching a functional course in marriage. This was a departure from the typical sociology of the family course in that I related findings from research to the actual living experiences of young people in terms of their own dating, premarital, and marital relationships. This had been the direct result of taking courses in teaching at Teachers College and proved to be a great boon for student learning experience at the university. This did not mean, however, that it was easy to convince my superiors to let me try this kind of teaching. Although there was a lot of opposition to this, I was able to prevail. My background at Teachers College, with a lot of encouragement from Osborne, had taught me that it was possible to both be a teacher and be caring and loving at the same time. There again, Ruth was in the picture, too, because Osborne had hired her to help with his newspaper column–so the Osbornes and the Neubecks became good friends.

Later, the Family Studies Center, under which I'd done my teaching, suffered budgetary problems and could no longer support me. So I moved into the newly developed Family Social Science Department in the College of Home Economics of the University. Here I found a supportive home and felt honored to be among a faculty that for many years claimed the number one rank among "family programs" in the United States' university system. However, the Family Studies Center also had been a wonderful home and Reuben Hill an unbelievable positive supporter.

I had an interesting experience with Osborne. In 1950, I'd gone to the NCFR conference in Denver to interview with a number of people about entering graduate school–Osborne was one of them. The following year when I went to the next NCFR convention, I found a note from Osborne in my box asking me to be part of a committee to evaluate the conference. I had not even been a graduate student of his but he remembered me and gave me substantial support.

I also have an anecdote about Reuben Hill. After I had published my first paper on counseling couples, Reuben wrote me a note saying that he wanted to tell me how much he valued my article and that, from now on, all his graduate students would be assigned that article as required reading. Support from colleagues like this doesn't make a career, but certainly helped to shape my feelings toward students in terms of wanting always to be very supportive and stand behind them in any way I could. I think I succeeded with that.

My experience working for the Student Counseling Bureau at the University of Minnesota was also worth mentioning. In 1948, that agency was the only one in the country that provided full-time marriage counselors. In many other counseling settings, some of the counselors devoted time to marriage counseling, but it was uniquely at the University of Minnesota where greater emphasis was placed on this approach as an important part of the university's responsibility to students. This was particularly true for returning veterans, who were having difficult times in their marriages after returning from service in the United States armed forces.

When I was in New York doing graduate work, I was able to develop a small private practice, which I later developed to a much larger degree. Believe it or not, back in 1952-53, the fee I charged for counseling was $5.00 per session. Later, at the university where I did my marriage counseling, students were not charged any fees at all. During the early '50s, therefore, even the fees for private practice were very low. Sometimes I even exchanged fees for vegetables and corn from farmers around the area. Those were the days!

I am proud that I was president not only of what was then the American Association of Marriage Counselors, but also of the National Council on Family Relations. Thus I was one of a very few people who have been president of both major organizations in the family field. I was also active in the American Psychological Association's attempt to bring papers on family counseling or therapy to the attention of psychologists. This effort eventually paid off in the sense that now there's a full-blown division on family therapy in APA. I was also one of the earlier supporters of Masters and Johnson and arranged their appearances at the University of Minnesota Medical School. Last but not least, I partook of the so-called SARS, the sexual awareness seminars that began here at the University in the early '70s. This enterprise is now a nationwide effort and part of many medical schools' curricula.

I'd like to interject a note here. I grew up in Germany and went to the Gymnasium, which is a high school including education that is equivalent to two years of undergraduate work in the United States' educational system. I received a classical education that included Greek and Latin, or really a bit of elitist education. However, if elitism was part of my upbringing, it surely changed after I came to the U.S. in dire circumstances. Being both penniless and an underdog made me view the world in a different manner, and I became the champion of the underdog in more ways than one. I'd grown up in a protected family with my father being a physician, whereas I had to begin here in the U.S. from the very bottom by doing manual labor and with no protection whatsoever. However, my Gymnasium education did pay off, and I was able to have to a career that has been very satisfying.

Certainly, I was also helped by being at the right place at the right time. That is not unusual during careers, and it certainly paid off for me–as the two following examples illustrate (and may also make you chuckle). I was at a convention of the American Psychological Association in Los Angeles, going down an escalator, when I saw two people I knew at a table nearby, Sidney Jourard, a well known psychologist, and Herbert Otto, a writer of books in our field (either books he wrote by himself or the editor of books that featured papers by other writers). We waved at each other, and I sat down next to them as they were discussing another book that Otto was planning. Otto was discussing the various chapters, and he said to Jourard, "I really need somebody to write a chapter on sexuality." "Oh," I piped up, "maybe that's something I can do." Well, that was the origin of my chapter entitled "Sex and Awareness" (1968) in Otto and Mann's book, *Ways of Growth*, which I would never have offered if I had not accidentally spied these two at the APA convention. And so it goes. Moreover, I may never have ended up in our field had it not been for accidentally riding with Dorothy Dyer, a former president of NCFR, when she mentioned the intent to leave her current job at the Young Women's Christian Association for a new position at the University of Minnesota in St. Paul. Her goal was to establish a family life program for which she needed instructors–I, of course, was ready for the bidding.

I want to emphasize, however, that my career has been helped by my earlier educational experiences in Germany and the intellectual curiosity that I derived from that education. And of course, my own family strength has helped, my wife Ruth having been greatly supportive of me–in addition I have admired her attitudes toward children all these years. One thing that I have admired always was that she treated children as real human beings rather than as puppets. From children's earliest ages, Ruth always spoke to them as if they understood every word that she was saying–and she never spoke to them in baby-talk. This has been true of children for whom she was hired to take care of when she came to the U.S. as well as for our own kids as they grew up. This has been a wonderful experience to witness.

One of the things I'm most proud of is that I learned to write in a second language, though I wasn't always sure that would be the case. Early in my undergraduate work, I flunked a course in English and was desperate in my attempt to learn this new language. But I persisted in my efforts and mastered my second language in more ways than one. Not only have I written professionally for academic sources, but I've published, and continue to publish, poetry (including one book of poetry with University of Minnesota faculty, *The Broken Glass Factory*, 1974) and have written a novel, *Mixed Doubles*, which was never published, though was under contract with Bantam at one time.

Well, I've been interested in many areas of our field, but mostly have been motivated to explore areas which have not received much attention. With my colleague, Vivian Hewer, I published the results of studies on university students' attitudes toward the employment of as well as the occupational roles of fathers and mothers (Neubeck & Hewer, 1959). This was my first empirical research, and from then on, I was always torn between continuing to do empirical versus theoretical topics. Later, I gave up both of these areas to concentrate on essays.

Other research projects that I should mention are my early work in the area of extramarital relations. I think my article that appeared in *Marriage and Family*

Living was the first article ever published in this area (Neubeck & Schletzer, 1962). This led me then to concentrate on that topic both in my own writing (Neubeck, 1967a; Neubeck, 1969a) and as editor of the book *Extra-Marital Relations* (1969). I was also interested in what appeared to be the more aloof attitudes of Scandinavians towards affection, a focus which resulted in a comparative United States-Scandinavian study on this topic (Neubeck, 1967b).

Later in my life, when I became a diabetic, I also became interested in the effects that diabetes has on male sexuality. Out of that came a piece of research (Neubeck, 1985) ascertaining the difficulties that this problem created within the marital and family unit. While such projects are worth mentioning, I began later to do a lot more essay writing, though I continued my former approaches to some degree as well. This continuing pattern included, in turn, a paper on the theory of marriage counseling called "A Humanistic Approach." Among the essay papers worth mentioning are the following: "The Myriad Motives of Sex" (1972), "In Praise of Marriage" (1979), "In Praise of Sex" (1983), "In Praise of Parenthood" (1981), and a chapter, "Sexuality: Developing Togetherness" in a book edited by McCubbin and Figley (1983).

Let me finally be allowed some musings about our profession. I have witnessed an evolution over the years that has finally resulted in the liberation of the family field from sociology. This means that "family" is now a discipline in its own right, and many departments have not only been labeled family science, family social science, or derivations on this theme, but have established themselves as legitimate and well-respected departments at major universities. When I took my graduate work at the Teachers College, the Education for Marriage and Family Department was the only one of its kind in existence; what a great change has occurred since then! And perhaps, to some degree, I've been responsible, or partially responsible, for some of this change.

EDITORS' NOTE

Professor Neubeck was honored on April 8, 2000 as one of the 100 most influential people in the field at the Centennial Celebration of the College of Human Ecology, University of Minnesota.

REFERENCES

Neubeck, G. (1954). Factors affecting group psychotherapy with married couples. *Marriage and Family Living, 16,* 2, 216-220.

Neubeck, G. (1967a). The Dimensions of the extra in extra-marital relations. In H. L. Silverman (Ed.), *Marital counseling: Psychology, ideology. science* (pp. 136-147). Springfield, Illinois: The Charles C Thomas Publishing Co.

Neubeck, G. (1967b). Patterns of affection. *International Journal of Comparative Sociology, 8,* 1, 20-25.

Neubeck, G. (1968). Sex and awareness. In H. Otto and J. Mann (Eds.) *Ways of growth* (pp. 69-76). New York, Grossman Publishers.

Neubeck, G. (1969a). Moderator-editor of roundtable: The significance of extramarital sex relations. *Human Sexuality, 3,* 10, XX.

Neubeck, G. (Ed.) (1969b). *Extra-marital relations.* Prentice-Hall, Inc., Englewood Cliffs, New Jersey.

Neubeck, G. (1972). The myriad motives for sex. *Sexual Behavior, 2,* 7, 50-56.

Neubeck, G. (Ed.). (1974). *The broken glass factory.* Poetry book with University of Minnesota Faculty.

Neubeck, G. (1979). In praise of marriage. *The Family Coordinator, 28,* 1, 115-117.

Neubeck, G. (1983). Perspective: In praise of sex. *Family Relations, 32,* 3, 297-300.

Neubeck, G. & Hewer, V. (March, 1959). Occupations of fathers and mothers of entering University of Minnesota freshmen, Fall, 1959. *Personnel Guidance Journal, 40,* 7, 622-627.

Neubeck, G. & Schletzer, V. M. (1962). A study of extra-marital relationships. *Marriage and Family Living, 24,* 3, 279-281.

Schmitt, G. S. & Neubeck, G. (1985). Diabetes, sexuality and family functioning. *Family Relations, 34,* 1, 109-113.

Zuengler, K.L., & Neubeck, G. (1983). Sexuality: Developing togetherness. In H. I. McCubbin & C. R. Figley (Eds.) *Stress and the family,* Vol. 1 (pp. 41-53). Brunner/Mazel, Inc., New York, 1983.

In Search of Resiliency in Families: Vision Quest of a Native Hawaiian Family Scholar

Hamilton McCubbin

KEYWORDS. Autobiography, faculty, Hawaiian, administration, childhood, career

HAWAIIAN HISTORY AND MY HAWAIIAN ROOTS

The island of Molokai, one of the eight islands in the State of Hawaii, is still referred to as the place of "lepers and Father Damien." To the people of Native Hawaiian ancestry, Molokai will always be viewed with respect and reverence as the home of Kalaupapa, the community of Native Hawaiians stricken with leprosy or Hansen's Disease. For me, Kalaupapa has very personal and special meaning. This part of my family's history was a whispered secret that I uncovered quite by accident, although my friends who read the book *The Celestine Prophecy* (Redfield, 1997) would be quick to point out that such "accidents" are part of a mystical plan with a purpose and not due to chance. At the invitation of good friends, a psychiatrist and social worker who are both of Hawaiian ancestry and also community leaders, I spent a weekend at Kalaupapa with their families. This rare opportunity to reside at Kalaupapa was open only to very few and only with the permission of the small number of remaining members of the former leper colony still in residence on the island.

This infamous community sits at the foot of the steep Molokai cliffs. Approaching the narrow landing strip in an aircraft, there does not appear to be sufficient room between the mountain and the ocean for the plane to touch the ground. This speck of land separating the cliffs from the windy shores is Kalaupapa–a community isolated, remote, seemingly inaccessible and selected exactly for these characteristics.

The community and its few residents received us with open arms, the traditional Hawaiian way with hugs accompanied by genuineness and trust.

These remaining members of the colony who greeted and cared for us showed obvious physical deterioration in their fingers and face–a shocking reminder of the tragedy which affected so many Hawaiians and their families. In the Aboriginal tradition, we spent the few precious days and nights there singing, laughing, learning about the community and the people of Kalaupapa and its history, and talking stories. Unexpectedly, our "talking stories" revealed a long held secret: my family's history was woven into the fabric of Molokai, the leper colony, and Kalaupapa.

"What did you say your last name was?" asked one of the members of the colony. "McCubbin?" "We had a McCubbin here," he responded. "I recall two persons named McCubbin. Did you have relatives here? Willy McCubbin was one of them; they were brothers, I recall. Willy died soon after they closed Kalaupapa. There was another McCubbin here, Hamilton was his name, I think, but I don't remember him. I am sure he died and is buried here on the island. Were they part of your family?" He inquired. His sharp recall and penetrating look into my eyes gave me a feeling that he knew I was about to learn something about my past. "Could Willy and Hamilton be related to me?" I asked myself. The members of the colony spoke warmly and caringly about Willy, as though he was family, part of their family. While I felt a special bond with them, I was anxious about the prospect of discovery of my family history that only my mother would be able to clarify. He seemed to respect the fact that I did not have an answer for he did not bring the matter to my attention again. He knew I was searching for answers.

When I returned to Honolulu and "talked stories" with my mother, my feelings that *family* was an integral part of my Molokai experience were confirmed. Hamilton and Willy McCubbin, my father's brothers, both contracted leprosy and were sent to Kalaupapa. My Uncle Hamilton died there at a young age. Uncle Willy lived into his 40s. The story my mother told revealed many touching and special dynamics of my family's history. I came to know my family on my father's side and my mother in a new way. I marveled at my family's dedication and abilities to face and overcome adversity. By their behaviors, as my mother described in great detail, they gave new meaning to family functioning, adaptation, and coping. My father's older brother and sister moved to Kalaupapa to work as cooks, to feed the members of the community. My father visited and worked there as a volunteer every weekend he could. My mother's "stories" revealed her decision to work at Kalaupapa as a nurse even before she married my father. My mother's stories were filled with a sense of pride that the family gave of themselves so Uncle Willy and Uncle Hamilton would continue to have "family" there. It was a family thing to do. Although the members in the leper colony were not allowed to physically touch family members who visited, as seen through my mother's eyes, the family's presence held great meaning for Willy and Hamilton; they were still a family and not outcasts of society.

What is it about families that motivates them to rise above adversity, and in their own ways make both big and small contributions to, and sacrifices for, each other in the midst of chaos and unpredictability? How is it that my father's family and my mother found meaning in a life of added hardships when tragedy drained from them the dreams and expectations of the "good life" for Willy and Hamilton? Where did they find the courage, the wisdom, and the conviction to act as they did? My father's family was fragmented by diseases over which they had no control, yet the family, although separated physically, remained connected in meaningful and inspirational ways, transcending the most indescribable of circumstances. Family members chose to live in a community in which visual contact was the only direct human connection. Nurturance was offered by preparing foods. Commitment was expressed through courage to risk personal well-being by living in and visiting the colony. And love was expressed by glances, words, and tears and through sharing by whatever means was possible. Are these indices of resiliency in families? Are culture and ethnicity integral parts of resiliency?

The Molokai weekend encouraged me to see family life and behavior as having new dimensions and processes. Alternative family paradigms emerged as to how families respond to trauma and catastrophic conditions. Is boundary ambiguity always dysfunctional or can it be a motivator for resiliency? Would laboratory studies have revealed these dynamic family processes of adaptation designed to fit the circumstances over time? Have we, through our research, really captured what families do under stress in response to crises such as this? Our linear models of family behavior do not do justice to the dynamic strategies families adopt to forge a meaningful adaptation in the face of unusual situations. Under what circumstances and in what ways do culture and ethnic heritage play a role in family coping and adaptation?

Family adaptation in crisis situations calls for changes in the ways families function and also change in the community context as the situation unfolds and presents new challenges. Adaptation appears to involve a more dynamic process than has been described and depicted in earlier research and writings. The concept of family, particularly for ethnic groups such as the Hawaiians, has been broader and more flexible, allowing for persons not related by blood or marriage to be included. Culture and ethnicity appeared to have a profound positive moderating and, in some cases, mediating influence on the meanings families attach to trauma and change and on the behavioral responses family members display in response to the situation. The Hawaiian words and concepts of *koa* or courage, *malama* or caring, and *aloha* or love guided our family's behaviors and gave meaning to the way we lived and survived. Understanding, valuing and affirming my ethnicity, seeing myself as a person of color, as a Native American of Aboriginal Hawaiian ancestry, once relegated to my distant past, was now an integral part of my future and development as a family scholar.

THE OHANA (FAMILY): THE ROOTS OF MY QUEST

I realized early on that I came from a family with a long history of adversities and crises but also accompanied by endurance and survivability. I recall most of all the good fortune of being born of Hawaiian and Japanese ancestry to the Ohana or family of Jonathan Kuihe and Betsy Chisayo McCubbin in Honolulu, Hawaii, in 1941. On December 7th, five months after my birth, the Japanese attacked my homeland, forced the United States into World War II, and drove my family to relocate me and my two sisters to the "big" island of Hawaii to live with my grandparents. This traumatic situation demanded a positive adaptation to the stigma of being part Japanese, and opened up a new world of understandable distrust of Japanese Americans. My family was also very fearful of being sent to internment camps. My Ohana, the extended family, made us all feel loved, appreciated, and secure. As circumstances would dictate, our grandparents, Yonekichi (Oji-chan or grandfather) and Toyo (Ob a-ban or grandmother), became the center of our young lives. The love they, both parents and grandparents, gave my two older sisters, Carol and Jonnette, and myself was special. Their adult behaviors and open sharing of affection made us feel secure when the world was filled with threats. Family acts of encouragement made us look to the future with hope when the future appeared tentative. Discipline, rules, high expectations, and persistence, which were parts of their heritage and which we resisted at times, were nonetheless parts of their teaching and thus part of our learning.

As I look back on these early years, remembering the windows painted black so the attacking Japanese airplanes could not see our home at night, I also recall the good times when family and friends found enjoyment and caring in our home. For many of my father and mother's friends, our home was the only place they could come. Following our return to Honolulu, as the immediate threat of another invasion was lessened and our internment an unlikely scenario, our family was reunited. My family became a large one with a household that included four aunts, four uncles, and all of my cousins on my mother's side, a total of thirteen people in addition to our family of five. Yet our home never seemed crowded! This was the Hawaiian family and the Hawaiian way. My father's worldview was to be inclusive and accepting. He had a big heart and made a concerted effort to make everyone feel welcomed.

I loved that Hawaiianness about him. Although my father died at the early age of 45, as his father did, my dad always sought and emphasized the goodness and best qualities in people. This, too, was the Hawaiian way and his philosophy of life: to recognize, value, and build on people's strengths and capabilities. Out of my extended family, I felt a sense of well-being rising as though a foundation of internal security for my future was laid as a valuable reference point and resource I could call upon by remembering. By their actions, my parents and extended family passed on values of hope, caring, respect for all and particularly our elders, support, sharing, loyalty, and commitment which prepared me to face the challenges of growing up Hawaiian in America.

CULTURE LOSS: GROWING UP HAWAIIAN

It was in the spring of 1959, with statehood for Hawaii approved by the Congress of the United States, that we, the students of Hawaiian ancestry and of the Kamehameha Schools, marched proudly in the parade celebrating our transition from being a territory of the United States to becoming the 50th State of the Union.

Statehood was viewed as a new beginning for the Hawaiians, or so we were socialized to believe. Following my self discovery at Kalaupapa and with a revived sense of ethnic identity, I look back upon this event with a new backdrop of history and renewed appreciation for our great Hawaiian leaders, in particular Queen Liliuokalani, who governed Hawaii from the same Iolani Palace grounds on which we were assembled. I now realize how blind we were to what was happening; how uninformed we were of our own Hawaiian history, and how we were taught to see the world through history books and lessons which excluded us and our Aboriginal and Native American heritage. Somewhere along the way, and over time, our roots and rich heritage were relegated to insignificance and in their place, America's worldview, by mandate, became our worldview.

We marched in unison down Kalaukaua Avenue to Kawaiahao Church for the Statehood ceremonies, dressed in the military uniforms which were patterned after those worn by cadets at the United States Military Academy at West Point, reflecting our deep commitment to the values of the United States. I never once asked why. Why were we not allowed nor encouraged to develop our native language? Why were we not allowed to develop and enrich our lives by developing our culture and heritage, our ethnic identity? Why were men and women of Hawaiian ancestry not allowed to learn and practice the traditional chants and dances of our ancestors? Why were we subjected to a humiliating process of ridding ourselves of any remnants of our language and made to demonstrate our cleansing through "tests" before a public forum of teachers from the mainland United States? We were led to believe that we were less than others; that only a few of us would be successful and that only a handful were "college qualified," but we needed to accept this limitation of life. We were better suited for the vocational arts, the military, and for the hotel and entertainment industry in support of tourism, we were told. I celebrated Statehood along with everyone else, never once asking why and how I felt about this situation from the perspective of being a Native Hawaiian.

The illegal overthrow of the Hawaiian Monarchy over one hundred years ago is now in the consciousness of the people of Hawaii and the United States as a whole. How are we, the brown people of Hawaiian ancestry and of America, faring in the first decade of the 21st century, with discrimination against us more evident and open, and with the renaissance of the Hawaiian culture and people gaining momentum in search of regaining their sovereignty through self governance? The abuses of discrimination, racism, and the economic injustices upon the oppressed people of Hawaiian ancestry have now been brought to light. The Hawaiians, the *Kanaka Maoli,* the people of the lands of Hawaii, are now seeking remedies. They realize that the harm already done to generations of Native American Hawaiians can be corrected for future generations; there does not need to be continuing acceptance of past acts. We know now that hatred, bigotry, and exploitation of the Hawaiians cannot and should not be tolerated.

As I grew up in Hawaii, we were told that Hawaii was a "melting pot" of cultures and that we were part of the "mixture," a special characteristic of Island people. But we were also socialized to believe that we were less than the "Orientals," the Japanese and Chinese people in Hawaii, and certainly less than the "Haoles," or Caucasian people of the Islands. We had come to believe that it was best that we accept *this fact of life* and our social station in life. Yes, there would be exceptional Hawaiians, particularly those who attended the Military Academies (West Point, Annapolis, Merchant Marine Academy, and the Air Force Academy), but for the majority of Hawaiians, it would not be in the cards; equal opportunity was not intended for Hawaiians.

Hawaiians needed to be thankful for what we had or what we were given; to ask for more and to demand more would have been inappropriate, because we were not worthy of more. We were and still are expected to be "grateful people." Even if we rise in professional circles or on the job and achieve roles of importance and related responsibilities, we are asked not to take our achievements seriously. We are reminded that what is given can be taken away and only those in power control their destiny. People of color receive opportunities as gifts; we have only earned the right to be eligible for more gifts. "Be grateful and submissive and you shall be rewarded." Heaven forbid if people of color were to act as leaders, scholars, and administrators or to present themselves as accomplished. We are warned and punished if we deviate from these societal expectations. We don't really expect you to exercise your rights and responsibilities as a person of influence is the real message. Once implemented, this cycle of control and submission and of denigration and oppression is designed to be self-perpetuating.

It is a disquieting thought that these beliefs were and still are being passed on. It appears the many children of Hawaiian ancestry feel this way about their futures, much as I felt on the day Statehood was celebrated in Hawaii. Painfully, I confronted the truth about socialization: not only was I taught to believe all of this, but also I accepted it all. I believed I had no real future, as I was not among the "chosen" in my class. Whatever happened in my life beyond high school was to be a lucky opportunity, an adventure, an experiment, but which would likely lead to nowhere.

My upbringing and life experiences at home and in my educational experiences, which offered me self confidence, a willingness to venture into the unknown, and love of reading and of education, what we might call protective factors, allowed me to challenge and to call these stereotypic life scripts into question. I remembered that my father lived a life of exploring opportunities, none of which offered guarantees of success. As a labor foreman and supervisor of construction, he worked in Kwajelin, Guam, and the Philippine Islands. A voracious reader and storyteller, he shared his experiences through stories, many of which were life threatening (to him) and scary to me. I liked the part of his memories in which he overcame the odds. He lived a life of challenges much like his father lived. Grandpa, also named Hamilton, who was an engineer and adventurer of sorts, died unexpectedly and accidentally in the Philippine Islands when my dad was a young man.

Much to my dismay, and leaving me with a destabilizing emotional void, my father also died when I was young; I was 14 years of age. I did not idolize my father, but his death motivated me to take on challenges and to find ways to endure. I remember the boxing matches we used to attend together on Friday evenings–live and up close. For some reason, he seemed to root for the underdog, the fighter who was not doing as well. He would cheer them on. When the underdog fighter won or put up a better struggle even though he may have lost the fight on the judges' points, my father made it a special point to tell me how the fighter rallied from near defeat. My father valued the fighter when he put up a good showing and endured with class even when he was losing the fight. "Never give up," he would always say! Maybe boxing was his metaphor for his life of struggles. The very principles and values that my father lived by and showed by his behavior were passed on to me. I embraced them then as I do now.

Given this early family confrontation with the vicissitudes of war and family loss, I have often asked myself if my interest in family stress, coping, and the study of resiliency are natural outgrowths of these early experiences? Probably, I would respond to my Freudian oriented inquirers, but be quick to add that there was more to the emergence of my life's scholarly work. In recognition of my father's, mother's and extended family's contributions to my development, particularly my values, I have come to embrace and believe in the words found in *Jonathan Livingston Seagull*: "We teach best what we need most to learn."

WOMEN LEADERS: THE MENTORS AND COLLEAGUES OF HOPE

As I look back on my experiences, certain people and events emerge with clarity as central reference points for my motivations, inspirations, and hope for the future. Five prominent women, Queen Liliuokalani, Princess Bernice Pauahi Bishop, Betsy Chisayo McCubbin, Dr. Marilyn Ann McCubbin and Dr. Anne I. Thompson, set the stage for my work. They emerged over my life course as special mentors, colleagues, and friends. The first two women, who emanated from the royal families of Hawaii, are but pictures in my mind put there by my education. The third is my mother, Betsy, who nurtured me as a person and shaped my ideology and the perspective of life. The fourth is Dr. Marilyn McCubbin, my spouse, friend, mentor, and collaborator (e.g., M. McCubbin, & H. McCubbin, 1989, 1993; H. McCubbin & M. McCubbin, 1988, 1993, 1997; H. McCubbin, M. McCubbin, Thompson, Hans, & Allen, 1997; H. McCubbin, M. McCubbin, A. Thompson, & E. Thompson, 1998), whose commitment to our children, Todd, Wendy, and Laurie, and to academic scholarship and professionalism continues to have a profound influence upon my professional and personal outlook and scholarship. The fifth is Dr. Anne Thompson, my colleague who joined my commitment to share research and writing opportunities with colleagues and students.

Queen Liliuokalani was the last reigning member of the monarchy to rule the Hawaiian Islands. She wove together the fabric of Hawaii, provided the islands with very strong leadership, and created a sense of unity. This remarkable woman became the symbol of the plight of the native Hawaiian people. On March 16, 1893, the United States government and military overthrew Queen Liliuokalani. The "story telling" of my kupunas, or elders, portrayed our Queen as standing proud and defiant of this injustice. In the confines of her palace where the United States Government held her captive, Queen Liliuokalani wrote passionately and eloquently in stating her views. She communicated her views in the form of writings and also in music. Today we find courage and inspiration in her behavior and writings. The dominant power of the United States relegated Hawaii to the status of a territory and brought with it a hammer that crushed the history and worldview of the Hawaiian people. The resulting changes in our homeland were dramatic and traumatic.

Our cultural interests in the family, or the "*ohana,*" were defined by a broad network of close relationships linked by blood, marriage, and community and were created by the overarching philosophy of everyone contributing to the benefit of the whole. These traditional ideals were replaced by individualism, entrepreneurship, domination, power, and emphasis on success pursued for the purposes of recognition, stature, land, and money. In contrast, the Hawaiian culture was characterized by emphasis upon the collective "we" as a group or community. A Western emphasis on the "I" and individual success replaced these values, clearly at the expense of the common good. Personal sacrifice for the well-being of all was replaced by an ideology that emphasized self-fulfillment. Historically, as Hawaiians, we had been taught to learn from each other as a network or team and as friends. This was replaced with formal learning and competition, thus relegating to insignificance the sharing and transmission of knowledge across generations by story telling. Teamwork was replaced by self-achievement. As was true for the Native American Indians, the Native Aboriginal Hawaiians faced the loss of their land, and thus the loss of the power and spirit of the Hawaiian people and its harmonious relationship in the balance of nature and man.

In the seventh grade, after being raised under the influence of Buddhist teachings and educated through the sixth grade in a Catholic School, I transferred to a Protestant high school, into a program open only to children of Hawaiian ancestry called the Kamehameha Schools. The underpinning of my identity as Hawaiian took shape and was nurtured by this school. The Kamehameha Schools was established through the wisdom of Bernice Pauahi Bishop, the last royal descendent of King Kamehameha I. This unique preschool through high school program, through a well designed and orchestrated educational program, was intended to shape the lives of many Hawaiians like myself in an effort to fulfill the wishes of its benefactor Bernice Pauahi Bishop. Her last will and testament gave birth to the School's mission–to mold and shape children of Aboriginal ancestry into industrious men and women. Over the years of her relatively short life, she accumulated great wealth from her aunts, who gave her sizable parcels of land of great financial value located throughout the Islands. She had the vision to establish the Bishop Estate with a singular mission to educate the children of Aboriginal Hawaiian ancestry. Furthermore, she saw education as the cornerstone for the preservation of the Hawaiian race and the cultivation of the Hawaiian people. She believed that her investment would cultivate the strengths and capabilities of men and women of Hawaiian ancestry, so that ultimately they, in turn, would make a contribution to the Hawaiian people. This vision of hope for the Hawaiian people became my vision of a more promising future.

My mother made me attend the Kamehameha Schools. She said it was for my own good. My mother, Betsy Chisayo Yamamoto McCubbin, raised three teenagers as a single parent, working full time and sometimes working two shifts as a private duty nurse. This was no small undertaking. She accepted the challenge in the typical Japanese manner: with courage, commitment, in silence but with determination. There was never any doubt she would do it and do it well. I am certain that from her perspective, raising us was like riding a roller coaster. It was always unstable, seemingly with more downs than ups, and, once started, there was no getting off until it was all over. She was there when I needed her with her firmness, clear statements of expectations, and unwavering dedication to our well-being. There were times, numerous times, when we did not see eye to eye, but she never backed down from what she believed in and what she felt was right. I blamed her for "making" me complete my work to become an Eagle Scout. I blamed her for encouraging Mr. Allen Bailey, the principal, to "make" me a boarding student for greater discipline and to encourage me to focus on my studies in high school in preparation for college. I blamed her for being kind to my English teacher, Ms. Elizabeth Kellam, who, in turn, made me diagram sentences, write stories and who pushed me to have one published. I blamed her for joining Mr. Jack Nielson, my biology teacher and a Wisconsin graduate, in encouraging me to apply to the University of Wisconsin. I blamed my mother for finding something good in myself, anything which I valued, such as reading and writing, which she encouraged and fostered. She seemed to enjoy being blamed! With each fulfilled expectation came affirmation and encouragement, and I came to understand and appreciate her efforts on my behalf. I blamed her for believing in me and for making me believe in myself.

With my final semester of undergraduate study at Wisconsin in progress and the fulfillment of my dream and personal promise to my mother to become the first college graduate in my family just a few months away, I asked Marilyn Behrens to join me in marriage. We wanted to begin a new generation, a new Ohana. With her consent, her Nebraska based parents' blessings, and my family's encouragement, we married and shared dreams filled with hope. Already established as a distinguished graduate of the University of Nebraska School of Nursing and my boss at the University Hospital where I worked part time as a hospital orderly, Marilyn encouraged me to explore options. She encouraged me to take on challenges, to develop myself, and to shape my choices on the basis of my experiences. She never once doubted my abilities even when I questioned them. She also accepted me, my weaknesses and vulnerabilities as well as my ethnic heritage, and the fact that our interracial marriage would bring on unexpected challenges and hardships. She embraced and was in turn loved by my Wisconsin *Ohana,* Mr. and Mrs. Wesley and Nina Farnsworth. Marilyn shared my deep appreciation of the many people who supported me during my transition from Hawaii and undergraduate studies. These lifelong friends included Mrs. George McCue,

John and Susie McCue, Lowell (Ole) and Peggy Elver and their daughter Kelly, Dean and Audrey Elver as well as Neale and Rodney Katz. These Wisconsin families created opportunities for me to work, to obtain scholarships, and to learn to wear boots, gloves, cap, and warm coat in the winter. They wanted me to have a family life away from my Hawaii family. They also became part of my Wisconsin Ohana.

Following the completion of her public health nursing masters and her doctorate from the University of Minnesota, Marilyn has become a collaborator of a special type; an individual committed to Nursing and Community Health Nursing in particular but with the added commitment to the study of families. She integrated family and resiliency theory into her own work with families of children faced with chronic and life threatening illnesses and, in so doing, contributed to the advancement of theory and practice. Not only was Marilyn a distinguished scholar in Nursing and a tenured Full Professor at the University of Wisconsin-Madison, but she was also selected as a Fellow in the American Academy of Nursing (FAAN), and as the recipient of the distinguished research scholar award from the Midwest Nursing Research Society. I marvel at her accomplishments and value her contributions.

The fifth special colleague is also a friend, Dr. Anne Thompson at the University of Wisconsin-Madison. She saw her special mission as that of contributing to the well-being and success of the School of Human Ecology, the students and faculty we served. It was fortuitous that I would find a friend and colleague at this stage in my career that would be a collaborator for fourteen years and who shared in the belief that we would create a working environment designed to create opportunities for students and colleagues to share in the experience of conducting research, writing, and other scholarly work. Anne made no claims to and was reluctant to accept recognition for her contributions, although she was affirmed for them. She saw collaboration and sharing as being of the highest priority and the greatest reward. Her values and beliefs were consistent with my personal perspectives and goals. As a team member, Assistant Dean, and Associate Director of Research, together, we had accomplished much, shared through collaboration with others, and contributed to the education of others as well as to the advancement of knowledge and the development of outreach to the community. It was a privilege to work with a colleague who adopted a worldview emphasizing the importance of "we" and "Lokahi" or "sharing." Such a partnership and friendship I have come to appreciate as, indeed, unique and to be cherished. Some would argue that such professional partnership comes but once in a lifetime.

EDUCATION, SCHOLARSHIP, AND LEADERSHIP ROLES

Opportunities, Choices, and Mentors

The legendary story that behavioral scientists follow a linear path leading to their career goals as professors, and with a focused academic and research agenda, certainly doesn't apply in my case. During my sophomore year at Wisconsin, I was honored to receive a congressional nomination to the United States Naval Academy. After considerable discussion with my Wisconsin family and Marilyn, I declined the appointment and chose to remain at the University to complete my studies. Upon graduating from the University of Wisconsin-Madison with a major in political science and being officially commissioned as an Officer in the United States Army, I was also admitted to law school. The delay between graduation (January) and the beginning of law school (September) was filled with my employment at a unique center for emotionally disturbed children.

This "chance" opportunity changed the course of my professional life. This "center for children" was also an experimental laboratory, designed to introduce and determine the effectiveness of different therapeutic strategies, psychoanalytic interventions, group process interventions, and behavior modification, for children with emotional or behavioral problems and their families. Given the experimental nature of the center, research was evident throughout with direct observation, as well as videotaped and external observer-recorded measures used in a planned and systematic fashion. All of this was new to me and, as one might anticipate, piqued my interest even though my pre-law training was not helpful in this context.

We worked in teams, creating a collaborative environment characterized by mutual respect channeled toward achievement of common goals. I will always remember the pure sense of excitement we shared about what we were doing for the good of the children and their families. The esteemed Dr. Martin Fliegel, who headed the behavioral and medical team at the Center, sensed my interest and encouraged my involvement. I was allowed to design my own quasi-experimental study on team development (under their supervision) and was assigned to join the newly established family therapy team. They felt I could work with families even though I was "destined" to be a lawyer. Sadly, my first research experiment did not produce statistically significant results. My project was a failure, but I was hooked on research and wanted to do more! My initial family therapy encounter with Dr. Carl Whitaker, the noted family therapist and a consultant to the Children's Treatment Center, was equally impressive and set the stage for my enlightenment. In a family therapy session, I accidentally bumped the renowned family therapist, who served as my co-therapist for the session, as I squirmed to find a comfortable position in my chair by crossing my legs. I apologized to him quietly.

His open response and seemingly loud retort startled me: "Some physical contact is better than none." Personally embarrassed, I thought to myself: was he talking to me or to the parents across the table who were struggling to achieve intimacy? The educational and therapeutic moment for both the novice therapist and family was bundled in one statement! The learning of the art and science of family therapy meant new discoveries about others and myself.

With a scholarship, traineeship, and a late admission to graduate school in hand, negotiated on my behalf by the inspiring psychiatrist Dr. Martin Fliegel, and psychologists Drs. Donald Stover and John Geibink, who were my mentors at the Center, I changed my career and abandoned becoming a lawyer. I also successfully renegotiated my contract with the Department of the Army, allowing me to pursue graduate study in social work and educational psychology/behavioral disabilities instead. With the military's blessing and encouragement, I was fortunate to pursue and complete my Master's and Doctoral studies uninterrupted by the Vietnam War.

The Vietnam War and the University of Wisconsin-Madison were never meant for each other. In the late 1960s and early 1970s, the University became the magnet and setting for peace demonstrations. Faculty and students launched their own war on the federal government and the Department of Defense, demanding an end to an unjust war. The foment on campus was national news, with tear-gassed students and disrupted classes becoming the norm of university life. The photographs I took of the disturbance on the Wisconsin campus bring back memories. My son Todd is able to recall the strangeness of the campus with military vehicles filling an entire intramural football field–which is now the parking lot in front of the School of Veterinary Medicine. The military vehicles brought National Guard troops to restore order to the chaotic campus. In 1969, with both my Master's and Doctoral studies completed, I put on the uniform of an Army Officer, with the rank of Captain, and entered active duty to fulfill my responsibilities and prepared myself and my family for my expected departure for Vietnam. Before leaving Madison, Wisconsin, we had the wonderful addition of our second child by adoption, Wendy Ann McCubbin. Upon Wendy's arrival to the McCubbin household when she was a few months old, we departed for Fort Riley, Kansas, via Fort Sam Houston in San Antonio, Texas, expecting that war, once again, would become an uninvited part of my family life.

The military had other plans for me. The Vietnam War exposed cracks in the social structure and fabric of the military. The military was plagued by a lack of personal and personnel commitment to the fulfillment of the military's stated purpose of defending the *Constitution* and the United States. Some soldiers deserted in the face of combat and others deserted to avoid being sent to Vietnam. These soldiers became absent members of the community that took pride in unity and its *esprit de corps.* The numbers of such "deviant soldiers" kept growing. The military was challenged to find solutions to the increasing national concern that the military would be flooding the country with individuals who received less than honorable discharges, people marked for life with the stigma of being unreliable and of questionable character. These individuals were destined for the welfare rolls, unemployment, and the criminal life, so the public believed. My assignment as a new doctoral-prepared social scientist was to serve as director of research and evaluation for a program designed to rehabilitate these wayward soldiers at the U.S. Army Correctional Facility (CTF) located in Fort Riley, Kansas. This was the beginning of my involvement in action research. There, clinical practice, social policy, and research converged with a common purpose: to return these soldiers to duty or to a meaningful role in society and, in so doing, contribute to society's common good. Given my Hawaiian heritage and its emphasis on doing the most for the common good, this blending of public service and the military for a common purpose was inspirational. In the two-year period of this assignment, we conducted a wide variety of studies on social deviance in the military for the Department of Defense. Through evaluation research, we confirmed the value and effectiveness of the Army's effort to rehabilitate and provide a "second chance" for these wayward soldiers. The research team prepared publications for future military leaders on the prevention of deviance. This was the beginning of my experience in the conduct of large-scale studies involving total populations.

After two years, my official obligations to the military were now complete, and we looked to the prospects of a new beginning. With the birth of our third child Laurie Dawn, we explored the option of going to San Francisco and Letterman Army Medical Center, which included offers of further training in family therapy, clinical practice, and additional education. Postdoctoral study in drug and alcohol treatment at Yale University was an additional incentive and thus became my initial training ground for San Francisco. It was fortuitous, for within a few months of my arrival in the Bay area, I was assigned the task to design and serve as the Director of the Army's Drug and Alcohol Program at the hospital. Concomitantly, my responsibilities included the task to develop drug and alcohol training programs for all commanders and clinical staff assigned to military bases throughout the 6th U.S. Army (Western–Colorado to Hawaii) Region. As we all came to learn, the substance abuse problem among military personnel returning from Vietnam presented another challenge for the military, struggling to answer the national concern that the military was dumping drug abusers and users into society without giving them much-needed assistance. Once again, the Army took on the responsibility of designing rehabilitation and prevention programs for society's common good. Within a year, the Army returned me to

Yale University for additional postdoctoral training in the prevention of substance abuse. My second visit to New Haven was equally exciting and valuable. But I did not have the opportunity to apply this rich experience. The Department of Defense had other plans for my family and me.

In 1972, the Department of Defense, involving all three branches of the Armed Services, assembled a team of scholars and assigned them to an interdisciplinary research laboratory in San Diego, California, known then as the Navy Neuropsychiatric Research Institute (later renamed the Naval Health Research Center). Captain Ransom Arthur, a distinguished research psychiatrist and pediatrician, led the Institute. Psychologists, psychiatrists, epidemiologists, social workers, and family scientists were drawn to this single laboratory to study the long term effects of war on family life and children, the dynamics of survival for military personnel held in captivity, coping with extreme stress, and the short and long terms effects of stress upon the physical and psychological well-being of military personnel. Unique to the Institute/Center was the added mission to conduct family research and to design research-based programs to address the difficulties experienced by families of the missing or captured soldiers, pilots, state department personnel, and members of the Central Intelligence Agency. Motivating the creation of the Center for Prisoner of War Studies was the families' united voice of anguish that had reached such a pitch and level of influence that both the Pentagon and Congress were compelled to act responsibly. For the first time in military history, family research was encouraged and supported and findings were used to guide the development of Department of Defense policies and practices.

The Center for Prisoner of War Studies, headed by a distinguished psychologist named John Plag, became my home for four years. It was a unique assignment which led not only to my lifelong commitment to understanding families under stress, their capabilities, the design of programs, and policies to address family needs, but also to our current work on resiliency in families. The scientific foundation for my research and theory building was established here.

To just say the Center was a special laboratory would be a major understatement. Our research was comprehensive, involving the compilation, analysis, and cataloging of all data available on prior Wars: World War II, Korea, Vietnam, and other conflicts that were not widely known. Data on prisoners of war, hostages, and their survival in adverse circumstances were compiled and examined. The most comprehensive library of research conducted on families under stress was established and made available for scholars. International collaboration was commonplace. Travels took me to France to negotiate a collaborative exchange of information on families collected by social workers and psychiatrists following the French Indochina War. Our trips to Israel to understand the effects of war on families and children also became an important focus for collaboration.

We had a solid team of scientists working to advance the family research agenda. The team included Dr. Edna Hunter, Dr. Philip Metres, Dr. Richard Rahe, Dr. Raymond Spaulding, Dr. Steven Nice, Dr. Philip Ballard, Gary Lester, Marilyn Robertson, Dorothy Benson, and Inez Dunning. Barbara Dahl, a developmental psychologist, became my valued collaborator in research and writing, and this partnership continued through the publication of books on families and children well after my departure from the Center in 1976. Dr. Pauline Boss also worked collaboratively with the Center for Prisoner of War Studies. Her conceptualizations and theory on psychological father presence piqued my interest at the St. Louis meeting of the National Council on Family Relations, and I invited Pauline Boss, who was then a doctoral student at the University of Wisconsin-Madison, to consider applying her theory to the study of families of missing military members. This invitation resulted in Dr. Boss's dissertation and contributed to her subsequent writings on the concept of boundary ambiguity.

Following the end of the Vietnam Conflict and the return of American Prisoners of war in 1973, our research made appropriate shifts to focus on prevention and the determination of what could be done to reduce the risk for families faced with prolonged separation. The studies also focused on what protective factors could be enhanced in family functioning to promote their adjustment and adaptation to the hardships of military life. Prospective and longitudinal studies on family life and functioning under stress were launched. Such costly and intensive studies were unprecedented in the history of military family research. We interviewed families preparing for separations, faced with the separations, and after family reunions. We interviewed the military members at sea in the Pacific and the Indian Ocean. The Philippine Islands became a base for family research. We conducted interviews with Navy pilots aboard the aircraft carrier USS *Ranger* while they were deployed on a military mission in the Philippine Islands and the Indian Ocean. For the first time, we learned about family problem solving communication processes and the dynamics of family hardships from another point of view–that of the military member at sea.

The research team's landmark work, from 1972 through 1976, which was guided by the consultative services of Dr. David Olson (University of Minnesota), Dr. Charles Figley (then of Purdue University), and Dr. Robert Beavers (then of the Timberlawn Foundation), served as a solid foundation upon which to base recommendations for improving services to military families throughout the world and across all branches of the armed services. The Navy established a uniform social work program in support of families. Congress changed policies, as did the Department of Defense, to be more supportive of family life in the military. Military family research became an important agenda for all branches of the armed services. For the first time, we developed policies and programs designed to facilitate the transfer of both civilian and military personnel from hostage and captivity situations; programs that were needed to facilitate the individual's and family's adaptation after being separated, released, and now reunited. We studied and monitored these programs with the return of American prisoners of war, the return of American hostages from Iran, and other less known and unpublicized returns of American personnel. We were proud parties of this policy and programmatic developments and changes in the Department of Defense. For one of the few times in military history, family research changed and shaped military policy. Social science research had an impact and what became known as "action research" had a beginning in the military.

In the context of family research and the advancement of family sciences, the San Diego laboratory fostered the revitalization of interest in family stress theory and the classic writings and research of Reuben Hill. His landmark work from World War II became the reference point and foundation for the creation of alternative and new constructs, family level measures, theory construction, and emerging propositions and hypotheses to describe and explain family behavior in response to stress and post-crisis adaptation. This laboratory and research mission of the Center for Prisoner of War Studies brought about our efforts to revisit his World War II studies on family separation and reunion.

In serving as the head of the Family Studies branch of the Center, I visited with and invited then-Regents Professor Reuben Hill to become a consultant to the Center. Initially, Reuben Hill was extremely uncomfortable with the invitation to be part of military research. He did not have fond memories of the military and was reluctant to work with an organization which dealt with "classified" data. All publications were screened and assessed. The Navy Neuropsychiatric Research Institute/Naval Health Research Center fortunately had an international reputation for superior scholarship. Censorship was a "foreign" concept. Journal and book publications were the norm. Ultimately, after several visits to the Center to gain first-hand knowledge of how the military conducted social, behavioral, and medical research, Reuben consented to join the team.

We both became frequent visitors to each other's communities–he to San Diego, California, and I to Minneapolis, Minnesota. But most significantly, a special friendship evolved out of this collaborative effort. For those who knew Reuben, it is not surprising that my mailbox was flooded with articles and research manuscripts, including dissertations, designed to give me "baseline" information and to "get me up to speed." Collaboration for Reuben meant that we shared a common knowledge base, so that new ideas could emerge with full respect given to preexisting ideas and constructs.

The Double ABCX Model of family stress theory (McCubbin & Patterson, 1983) emerged from this body of research and had its origins over dinner and dessert, with Reuben exploring our observations and educating the research team as to the limitations of his original ABCX formulations. His original formulations did not, in his opinion, capture the complex processes involved in the family's efforts to overcome adversity and recover from family crises. For example, his C factor, he reminded us, was conceptualized as the family's definition of the stressor. In the case of chronic stress or catastrophic conditions, the family's appraisal was far more complex, demanding that the pile-up of co-occurring life events be considered, the family resources and capabilities be appraised, and the family's patterns of functioning in context of all of these capabilities be taken into account. These additional aspects of appraisal (C Factor) called for a reframing and redefining of the original construct to be more inclusive of appraisal processes involved in post-crisis adaptation. For example, creating a "family meaning" to the crisis situation appeared to facilitate the family's ability to change its patterns of functioning and legitimate the changes in family patterns needed to adapt to the situation created by the crisis. Were family meanings part of the original "C" factor that Reuben began with, or were we talking about new formulations? Reuben argued then that the C factor was specifically operationalized to emphasize the family's definition of the stressor and related hardship and not the changes in family patterns of functioning which appeared to follow the crisis. Reuben argued that his focus was on pre-crisis and not on post-crisis adaptation and recovery.

One of the more salient observations that emerged from our after-dinner discussions was a realization that in the face of family crisis producing situations, families move through at least two phases but not necessarily in a linear fashion. A pre-crisis phase appeared to capture the ABCX components of Reuben's original work, which focused on why some families, with certain protective factors operating in the family and in the community, in the face of a stressor made smoother and easier *adjustments* than others to achieve harmony and stability. Observations from the families of prisoners of war and those missing in action revealed a family post-crisis phase, with an outcome of family adaptation. In these families, the crisis situation created a family scenario which demanded more systemic changes in the way the families operated and functioned in order to achieve stability and harmony. The POW and MIA family investigations revealed the emergence of a complementary set of variables and factors, a combination of restructured or rebuilt protective factors and the addition of recovery factors that appeared to shape the course and the outcomes of family adaptation.

Reuben encouraged these lines of questioning and theory building formulations that led to different perspectives on family stress theory. He was always present to support these advances, all of which he challenged as a conscientious scientist. He encouraged changes in theory; concepts and propositions even to his most closely held and personal conceptualizations. Reuben argued that it was inevitable that changes would be made in his formulations and that these changes in stress theory would be based upon direct observations of families in highly stressful, if not catastrophic, circumstances. He welcomed and encouraged inductive theory building and research. With that twinkle in his eye that we all remember so well, he challenged our research team by pointing to our need to conduct in-depth interviews, to supplement and guide our major survey efforts, and to instrument development. These were the tools for the advancement of theory, he would repeat time and time again.

Our interdisciplinary research team was also challenged to find a more common language for all to use to describe the phenomenon we were observing over time. Reuben Hill bristled with our psychologizing of the family. One of his "sensitivities" was laziness and our reluctance, if not hesitancy, to introduce family group-level variables, which better described the phenomena we observed. He used the concept of "cognitive" to make his point. I recall Reuben Hill speaking to us and luring us into his "teaching trap" which created his "teaching moment." The research team had "no trouble" embracing the concept of cognitive coping. We joined the discussion with passionate expression of how valuable the concept of "family cognition" could be and carried our enthusiasm to the point of linking this concept to Reuben's "C," or appraisal, factor in the ABCX model. We bought the hook, and he reeled us in. Having us where he wanted, Reuben was quick to remind us that "families don't think," "families don't perceive," and "families don't cognate." Families may create and have shared or divergent definitions, appraisals, and meanings, but they do not have a mind of their own. His point was well made! We learned that passively agreeing with his arguments was never sufficient in a meaningful dialogue in family science. He expected the research team to move beyond his arguments, to present our data to support our viewpoints even if we allegedly agreed with him. He demanded we take ownership of our viewpoints and was persistent in demanding an independent argument from the research team if we sided with him because he was the senior scholar. He called such passive arguments both patronizing and signs of lazy scholarship. Needless to say, we were forced to argue whatever viewpoint we offered, a learning process we have come to appreciate and value. The mentoring process with Reuben Hill was a personal and rewarding experience we had all come to cherish.

As he was to many of us in the family field, Reuben Hill was more than an academic scholar. He was a genuine friend who saw his role as a nurturer of ideas, a facilitator of critical thinking, and a mentor and motivator of developing social and behavioral scientists. His visits to our home in San Diego, and later in Minneapolis and our shared meals and partnerships in travel gave new meaning to the words friend and mentor. Due to Reuben's influence and his encouragement, the Center for Prisoner of War Studies in San Diego became a unique setting in which family stress, coping, social support, problem solving, appraisal, and adaptation became commonplace words. In the process, family crisis theory was modified to take into account unique family observations and findings and to allow the introduction and examination of competing and emerging paradigms. Reuben was a visionary. He encouraged and monitored the evolution of new research paradigms and affirmed the need to question the old, even those to which he was most wedded. For those of us at the Center, his efforts propelled family-based scientific inquiry into a new era.

TRANSITIONS: MILITARY RESEARCH TO UNIVERSITY SCHOLARSHIP

It was inevitable, some would say, that we would eventually move to the University of Minnesota. Our gradually evolving attachments to the University through Reuben Hill and his family made everything seem right when the opportunity emerged for me to accept a position in Social Work and Sociology as an Associate Professor with tenure. The Army's acceleration of my promotion to the rank of Major, assignment to their advanced course in Health Care Administration, and offer of a professorship at the U.S. Air Force Academy did not outweigh my ties to Reuben Hill and the added Minnesota incentive for my wife to pursue her graduate studies in public health nursing. Regent's Professor Hill and his wonderful wife Marion were there to guide our decision-making and to facilitate my family's transition. They gave Marilyn and the children a home while I finished my research in the Philippines. As I flew from Asia to my new home in Minnesota, I could not help but reflect on the coincidence that my work in the Philippines represented the third generation of McCubbins to work in the Philippine Islands. I happened to be at Subic Bay, the Navy Base my father helped to construct twenty-five years earlier.

My work with the military did not end with my transition to Minnesota, for parts of the research at the Center for Prisoner of War Studies were transferred to Minnesota (McCubbin, Dahl, & Hunter, 1976). Under the title of the Family Stress Coping and Health Project, many investigations were conducted which were supported by the School of Social Work, the Department of Sociology, the Graduate School, the Agricultural Experiment Station, the Minnesota Family Study Center, the Family Impact and Analysis training grant, and the Department of Defense. Additionally, in my initial year at Minnesota, I was awarded a Bush Foundation Fellowship to participate in the post-doctoral program in early childhood education. It was the result of this fellowship and training that I became an active faculty member with the Institute of Child Development and particularly the nationally recognized program at Minnesota in Early Childhood Education.

In our new home in academia, there were many opportunities for collaboration. Dr. David Olson created a partnership to conduct a national study of family functioning and strengths, resulting in a book entitled *Families: What Makes Them* Work (Olson, McCubbin, Barnes, Larsen, Muxen, & Wilson, 1984). The resulting family measures are now used throughout the world and are translated into seven languages. Dr. Charles Figley formed a partnership to advance theory and clinical interventions for traumatized families, resulting in two book volumes on *Family Stress and Coping* (Figley & McCubbin, 1983; McCubbin & Figley, 1983), and Dr. Marvin Sussman created a partnership to advance theory and research, resulting in a book entitled *Social Stress and the Family: Advances in Family Stress Theory and Research* (McCubbin, Patterson, & Sussman, 1983). With a history of research linking family science to individual health outcomes, Dr. William Doherty and I collaborated to create the Family and Health Section within the National Council on Family Relations and co-edited *Family Systems and Health* (Doherty & McCubbin, 1987) to promote this line of scientific inquiry.

This was also the beginning of my collaborative work with my spouse Marilyn, who cultivated my interest in the study of families of children with chronic illness as a vital step in advancing and testing the new concepts and propositions of family stress theory. With her public health interests and encouragement, research on children with cystic fibrosis and spina bifida became the focus of my attention. While Marilyn never sought credit nor accepted recognition for her substantive contributions and the hours upon hours spent discussing my observations and ideas and reviewing and editing my articles, chapters, and books, her influence upon my research and writings was constant. It was not until Marilyn pursued and completed her doctoral studies in family science, and with her permission, that the full impact of her contributions was made evident and received recognition (McCubbin, M. & McCubbin, H., 1988, 1989).

Over a period of twenty years, guided by continuous research and building upon past research and inductive theory building, and through the process of collaboration, I and my much-appreciated colleagues and collaborators have made a concerted effort to advance the development and testing of family stress theory (McCubbin, 1979). We created a clear and focused emphasis upon the identification, definition, and measurement of factors that come into play and the processes involved in a family's response to and recovery from crisis situations. Initially, in collaboration with Dr. Joan Patterson, who was then a doctoral student, our theory building efforts (McCubbin, Cauble, & Patterson, 1982) emphasized the specific components of family adjustment and adaptation and led to the advancement of the Double ABCX Model of Family Adjustment and Adaptation (McCubbin & Patterson, 1983). This framework evolved into the Family Adjustment and Adaptation Response Model (FAAR Model) (McCubbin & Patterson, 1983) with the added delineation of *the general processes involved* in both adjustment and adaptation. These important efforts were followed and influenced by the research and theory building of Dr. Marilyn McCubbin, which focus on family post-crisis response to family trauma with a sharper delineation of the critical factors and processes involved in family adaptation. The emergent modification of the FAAR model resulted in the "T"-Double ABCX Model (McCubbin, M. & McCubbin, H., 1989) that attempted to capture the importance of family change in response to crises. This evolution of the family stress framework emphasized the importance of family typologies (referring to the "T") and the role of established patterns of family functioning and the newly instituted patterns of family functioning in the family processes of family adaptation. With an added emphasis on clarifying the components of family adaptation and the gradual shaping of the framework (Double ABCX, FAAR, T-Double ABCX) to study families of different ethnic backgrounds and cultures, the most recent evolution of the family stress framework has been named the *Resiliency Model of Family Stress Adjustment and Adaptation* (McCubbin, M. & McCubbin, H., 1993; McCubbin, H., McCubbin, M., Thompson, E. & Thompson, A., 1998). This framework clearly emphasizes the importance of the family's ability to bounce back from adversity, guided by the family's hardiness, problem-solving abilities, and appraisal processes of family schemas, paradigms, and coherence. In the current formulations of resiliency theory, risk, protective, and recovery factors and family processes of adaptation became the dominant constructs under investigation. In this most recent conceptualization of family stress theory, namely this resiliency framework, my origins as a Native American Hawaiian and my interest in the variable of ethnicity had finally found a fit (McCubbin, H. & McCubbin, L., 1997), particularly with the added emphasis on family schema, paradigms, and adaptation (McCubbin, H. & Thompson, A., 1988). It comes as no surprise to anyone that my collaborative work would have ethnic and cultural underpinnings as some of its important building blocks in explaining and predicting family behavior under stress and in the recovery process following a family crisis.

Reflecting back on my beginnings and the current renaissance of Polynesian cultures, including the Hawaiians, my past experiences and present work as a family scholar were now congruent and in harmony. This confluence of past and present, ethnicity and family, personal stress and family stress, is not accidental. Several other historic events came to play a powerful role in shaping this emerging research agenda. After I joined Reuben Hill, the Minnesota Family Study Center, and the Department of Family Social Science as their department head, the Department of Defense "called" me back to active military duty to design and direct a major study of 1000 Army families located in Western Europe. These families were located on the then East German and Czechoslovakian borders. The military wanted to understand the risk, protective, and recovery factors involved in families faced with the prospects of war. Of greatest importance, the military wanted to determine how families could be supported to maximize the prospects that their military members would be ready for combat should the need arise.

In preparation for this research, I was offered and accepted a Mellon fellowship for postdoctoral studies at Stanford University at the Center for Advanced Studies in the Behavioral Sciences. My Stanford University experience, involving twenty-two scholars from throughout the United States, focused on theory and research in the study of stigma, racism, and discrimination. It was at Stanford and in the study of ethnic issues that the concepts of family schema and paradigms, which were integrated into our later developments of family resiliency theory, had their beginnings. These themes and my heightened sensitivity to ethnic issues, resulting from this rich experience at the Center for Advanced Studies, had a profound influence upon my Europe-based studies and all of my future work (McCubbin, H., Thompson, A., Thompson, E., Elver, K., McCubbin, M., 1998; McCubbin, H., Fleming, W., Thompson, A., Neitman, P., Elver, K., & Savas, S., 1998).

Interestingly, this unique opportunity at Stanford University was preceded by a few months by a W.T. Grant Foundation invitation to join scholars at the Center for Advanced Studies in the Behavioral Sciences to discuss current and future research on resiliency in children. It was in this context of discussions with Dr. Norman Garmezy, Dr. Michael Rutter, Dr. Emmy Werner, Dr. Mavis Hetherington, Dr. Barry Pless, and Dr. Robert Haggerty that the foundation for the study and conceptualization of family and schema resiliency took shape (McCubbin, H., Thompson, A., & Thompson, E., 1998). Was the convergence of meetings at Stanford University on resiliency, a post doctoral fellowship at Stanford and the Center for Advanced Study on stigma and discrimination, and my recall to active military duty to direct the study of military families in Europe coincidental, accidental, or part of another mystical plan? I have often wondered.

It was in the conduct of this comprehensive study of Army families (McCubbin, 1998), particularly families of enlisted personnel, and involving a representative sample of families of color, that I also experienced for the first time the might and power of censorship in the conduct of family research. The research team's discovery of patterns of racism and discrimination quite unexpectedly set in motion the wrath of civilian social and behavioral scientists at the most senior levels of organizational leadership all acting in concert to suppress the information. It was a tragic, unnecessary, and unfortunate response, for the additional information about the strengths and resiliency of these families of color never found a forum for discussion. I have admired and will always admire the military for taking the initiative to understand the families affected by their policies. The military leaders I have been exposed to had always sought to know the truth in order that they as leaders could address the problems raised. I found the behavior of civilian scientists affiliated with the Army research laboratory at the time to be unprofessional and troublesome. Their role as self-proclaimed and misguided guardians of the military's image appeared to outweigh their integrity as scientists and appeared to overshadow their need to act responsibly as social and behavioral scientists in support of military leadership and the military mission. There was no question in my mind that my being a person of color shaped the nature and intensity of this adverse response. This unfortunate experience, however, deepened my commitment to the study of the plight of ethnic families, strengthened my resolve to stand up against racism and discrimination, and brought me full circle to linking my heritage and ethnic identity to my research on families under stress. My experiences at Stanford University and a revisiting of the vicissitudes of families and the risk of war once again shaped the course of my research.

In 1985, I transitioned from the University of Minnesota and from being the Department Head of Family Social Science for 7 years with a sense of pride in the department's *numero uno* national ranking. Such rankings are always the result of outstanding faculty and academic programs, but one can take pride in making a contribution to the advancement of scholarship and the administration of such a fine program. The invitation to join the administration and the faculty at the University of Wisconsin-Madison and to assume the deanship of the School of Family Resources and Consumer Sciences, which was renamed the School of Human Ecology, at my alma mater was compelling and special. I was honored by the chance to make a contribution to the revitalization of an academic program which had faltered in the eyes of senior administrators. Chancellor Irving Shain indicated the needed leadership to build a solid foundation and supportive climate for faculty research, promote the mentoring and tenuring of faculty, integrate the Cooperative Extension mission into the School, and do all of this with limited resources. I accepted this exciting new opportunity and the challenges that accompanied it.

The Family Stress, Coping and Health Project transitioned with me and became a distinct but integral part of the endowed Center for Excellence in Family Studies at the University of Wisconsin-Madison. Additionally, the

Family Stress, Coping and Health Project was integrated into the endowed Institute for the Study of Resiliency in Families. In this rich environment, guided by the *Mana* or spirit of mutual respect and shared vision, my collaboration with Associate Director Dr. Anne Thompson, Dr. Marilyn McCubbin, developing scholar Dr. Elizabeth Thompson, research associate Kelly Elver, and doctoral student Laurie McCubbin (McCubbin, H., & McCubbin, L., 1997) took shape as a unique partnership designed to contribute to the advancement of both theory and research. A series of books and articles on family assessment and measurement of family functioning, resiliency, coherence, family development, and ethnicity (McCubbin, H. & Dahl, 1985; McCubbin, H., Thompson, A., & McCubbin, M., 1996; McCubbin, H., Thompson, E., Thompson, A., & Fromer, 1988; 1998; McCubbin, H., Thompson, E., Thompson, A., & Futrell, 1998, 1999; McCubbin, H., Thompson, Futrell, McCubbin, M., 2000; McCubbin, H., Thompson, A., Pirner, P., & McCubbin, M., 1988) reflects the viability of this partnership and our continued investment in family science. These authored and edited volumes reflect the Project, Center, and Institute's commitment to the advancement of this line of scientific inquiry. Family stress, coping, and resiliency research had found a home at the University of Wisconsin-Madison.

It was fortuitous that Ruth Dickey, a faculty emeritus in Dietetics of the School, took a special interest in families and their central importance to the field of Home Economics. It was through her initial gift that we invited the renowned Israeli scholar Aaron Antonovsky and other scholars to the University of Wisconsin-Madison to advance our understanding of Professor Antonovsky's concept of Sense of Coherence, which had gained prominence throughout the world as important to our understanding of and explaining the variability in how and why some individuals and families are better able to adapt in crisis situations. Ms. Dickey attended all of the sessions, and it was the result of her excitement, interest, and endowment to the University and the School of Human Ecology that led to the creation of the Institute for the Study of Resiliency in Families. Soon after she passed away, the Institute published its first book on *Sense of Coherence and Resiliency* that was based on her conference (McCubbin, H., Thompson, E., Thompson, A., & Fromer, 1998b). The book was dedicated to her to honor her wisdom and support of this important development in family science. Sadly, just before the book was released, Dr. Aaron Antonovsky passed away. Both Ms. Dickey and Dr. Antonovsky would have been pleased with the resulting book series on family resiliency published by Sage Publishing Company.

With fourteen years of my deanship completed, I was pleased with the evolution and development of the School of Human Ecology, which was now ranked among the top 4 programs in the United States and had a nationally prominent faculty of outstanding scholars and particularly exemplary integrated faculty (Cooperative Extension Service). The School had shaped a strong program and climate for the advancement of research with a minimal infrastructure of administration, a superior record of mentoring and tenuring faculty, and a faculty with a shared vision and strategy for continued improvement. Having had the good fortune to be an administrator and to continue to contribute to the development of family stress and resiliency theory through research, I have gained a sense of affirmation that my decision of many years back to return home to Wisconsin was indeed a wise and rewarding one. It was also a very challenging one for a person of color in a leadership role. Of equal importance, at this juncture in my career, I also chose to leave the academic deanship after a total of 26 years in administration to return to my role as a teacher and social scientist.

Was this again a matter of timing or was this all a coincidence that five unique opportunities emerged at this same time? First, the Department of Defense reactivated the research on families of prisoners of war from the Vietnam Conflict and awarded us three grants. Secondly, children of families of men missing in action in Vietnam were now seeking guidance and support as they conducted their own studies of family and adaptation, and we agreed to assist them. Third, the National Institute of Drug Abuse had awarded our research team a grant to study strategies to promote resiliency in ethnic minority families and children in high-risk communities. Fourth, I now had the opportunity and support to conduct a follow-up study of Native Hawaiian Children who were given a unique educational opportunity in their early years; we needed to know what happened to them. Fifth, our 15-year longitudinal research on risk, protective, and recovery factors in children in the juvenile justice system in the State of Michigan had matured to the point where outcomes and predictors of outcomes could now be examined. The transition to being a full time scholar was rapid and already filled with new and exciting challenges.

BLENDING SCHOLARSHIP AND LEADERSHIP: TURBULENT WATERS FOR PERSONS OF COLOR

Many colleagues have inquired about my planned choice to seek and accept leadership positions calling for a combination of responsibilities of administration and scholarship, particularly research to coexist as viable partners in my professional roles. In total, I had been in these dual roles for 28 (of 30) years since completing my doctoral studies. I had been in research and clinical directorships (7 years), University administrative roles as a Department Head (6 years), and Academic Dean (15 years). The answer is simple but may be surprising to many. The challenges of leadership with the objective of moving the research, teaching, or outreach agenda of an academic unit to improved levels of collective achievement presented exciting opportunities, so I believed. I had been mentored in administration and worked in some of the finest behavioral science research laboratories with individuals who believed in and were exemplars of leadership and scholarship combined. For them, and for myself, the two roles complemented each other. It was both challenging and rewarding to nurture and support scholars to be excellent at what they wanted to be. Their successes brought success to the group as a whole; and they in turn nurtured others. It was the creation and maintenance of an environment that cultivated this cycle of support that I sought to develop through administration. My mentors also taught leadership by example; by demonstrating their own sustained commitment to research and writing as they promoted the competence of others. Scholarship, in turn, brought satisfaction and meaning to the world of administration, which was oftentimes mired down in politics and conflicts. It goes without saying, because there were so few persons of color in these leadership roles, I was encouraged to fulfill these roles as a representative example of emerging opportunities for other persons of color.

I look upon these years in these combined roles with a much deeper appreciation for the plight of persons of color who choose and are fortunate to have the opportunity to take on these senior leadership roles. While I loved the challenges of academic administration, I was also cognizant of the costs to me personally; at times I struggled with the fact that the cost seemed much too high a price to pay. I recognized the trials and tribulations created by harassment, racism, and discrimination, which were unfortunately alive and well, but so much subtler and punishing than I ever imagined. Flashbacks wrench me to recall a few glaring incidents that I try painfully to ignore and suppress. I recall an administrator's planned destruction of longitudinal research data that I had spent years collecting and that is now lost forever. I recall deliberate efforts of my colleagues to confiscate and claim copyrighted research instruments representing my work as their own. I try to forget the blatant acts of discrimination and harassment against men and women of color which I exposed and for which I sought guidance and mentoring. In all incidents, however, I was dismayed by the demand of senior leadership that the matters be suppressed and swept under the rug for the "benefit of the organization or the University." Even today, I am reminded of the direct attacks upon me for trying to address the issues of discrimination. Deliberate acts to discredit me and my reputation accompanied me with each administrative role that I assumed. Discrimination, racism, and cruel racially insensitive acts against me, however, were never so blatant and harmful as it was in my Deanship at the University. While I tolerated repeated abusive behavior from senior leadership during the last 6 years of my Deanship, my memories continue to focus on the strength of the University of Wisconsin-Madison, the encouragement and support others afforded me when I was a student there, the wisdom and guidance I did receive as Dean from Chancellor Irving Shain, and the wonderful faculty and staff I was privileged to work with.

Central to the success for any university in attracting and maintaining persons of color at the undergraduate, graduate, faculty, and leadership levels of the university community, is the degree to which a safe, accepting, and supportive climate is created throughout the campus environment. Academic leaders extolling the virtues of diversity on the University campus often display mixed reactions to dealing with bigotry and racism. Unfortunately, some have chosen to look the other way when racially motivated injustices occur for fear of a backlash from the majority community for addressing the flagrant violations. I am perplexed by the negligence of senior administration in addressing these issues. Why would a Provost choose to suppress a blatant case of sexual harassment with a white male chairperson of a search committee propositioning a black female scholar interviewing on campus for a faculty position? Why would a Chancellor choose to dismiss the manipulation (e.g., inaccurate and negative presentation of faculty academic records, contrary to the data) of the academic record of a black female faculty candidate being considered for tenure? Why would a Chancellor and Provost deliberately ignore repeated requests by an Asian faculty member to help mediate harassing acts by an interim dean? Why would these senior administrators ignore the discriminatory and racist behavior of the interim dean towards other ethnic minorities? Why would a Provost, after negotiating the relocation of an outstanding ethnic minority female scholar to another College because of confirmed harassment and discrimination, and in so doing negotiate a detailed written and signed agreement (by all deans involved), then refuse to support the specifics of the letter of agreement? In my experience, the processes designed to correct the injustices created by racist and discriminatory acts did not reflect an institutional commitment to diversity and the creation of a climate of fairness and equal opportunity.

On the other hand, I have also had the good fortune of working with outstanding military and civilian as well as academic leaders whose display of sensitivities and affirmation of the meaning of diversity were truly exceptional. There were a select few of the senior leaders in academic administration who provided me with opportunities for development and advancement, stood by me when I made difficult and unpopular decisions, and treated me with fairness; they had the courage and the conviction to treat me with respect. Personal interest and kindness emerged with clarity and meaning. Chancellor Irving Shain and Vice Chancellor Bernard Cohen took a bold step forward in support of diversity in appointing me as the University of Wisconsin's first academic dean of color, and they were publicly supportive of my decisions; they stood by me and mentored me in my role. My mother recalls experiencing special affirmation of my administrative role, strange as this may sound. After finishing her welcoming remarks to a warm and enthusiastic audience, Chancellor Donna Shalala, who became the United States Secretary of Health and Human Services, walked immediately from the podium to the second floor of the auditorium to greet and welcome my mother personally. My mother was truly touched and felt affirmed by the Chancellor's public behavior that my leadership role in the University had meaning and purpose. I was part of the Chancellor's team.

It was this very act of support and kindness that also gave my mother reason to understand and accept why I would eventually choose to accept, then to decline an offer by the University of Hawaii Board of Regents to become the first Native Hawaiian to serve as Senior Vice President of the University of Hawaii. With this offer, my mother believed her son would now return home and give back to his culture and affirm her pride in my accomplishments. The pain was lessened, however, when I explained that Chancellor Shalala and a renowned scholar of academic leadership, Dr. Joseph Kaufmann, served as counsel to me and, after careful thought, recommended that I decline the Senior Vice Presidency for reasons best left unstated and out of the public eye. Because of her personal anguish, I have questioned the wisdom of my decision from time to time. My mother was especially kind, as mothers are, in noting her acceptance: "I am still very proud of you, son." While I always remember the cruelty and insensitivity of the Provost on the day of my mother's burial and the unnecessary pain he inflicted on me and my children, I also remember Chancellor David Ward calling me in Hawaii to express his condolences in noting my mother's passing; he and his wife were kind to my mother.

I also wonder at times if the anger I feel and suppress is demanding a voice, crying out for justice, or at least a confrontation for the injustices done. I did then, as I do now, suppress layer upon layer of rage during these troubled periods–most of which was and is provoked by individuals who deny us opportunities, treat us unfairly, and hold us inferior because we are not of the majority. In the final analysis, I continue to choose to focus my energy on proving them wrong. The energy I would like to expend to sustain my animosity towards these tormentors would be, I believe, wasted otherwise.

These unfortunate and sometimes distasteful professional experiences and personal challenges must also be placed in a broader context of other priorities. As I look upon my life, I also see good fortune and opportunities that were beyond my wildest dreams. I have been blessed, I told myself. Trite as this may sound to many, when considered along with my Hawaiian and Japanese family history as well as my children and our grandchildren, my professional hardships can be put into a perspective which gives my life meaning and purpose. Together, Marilyn and I started our family with our first child Todd. He was with me through graduate school and, as the oldest child, shouldered the family responsibilities as I traveled far and wide to conduct research. He graduated from the University of Wisconsin-Madison in Engineering, became an Air Force Pilot, Instructor Pilot, and an exchange pilot with the Canadian Air Force. He is currently a field grade office (Major) and a command pilot for a C5A Squadron at Dover Air Force Base. He married Jennifer Whitesell, also a graduate of the University of Wisconsin-Madison in Journalism, who earned a master's degree in education and is currently a teacher. Together Todd and Jennifer became the proud parents of two lovely girls, Jessica and Rachel, our first grandchildren.

Wendy, our joyful and outgoing daughter, currently in computer marketing and sales, graduated from the University of Wisconsin-Stout with a teaching certificate and a major in marketing and marketing education. She met and married a college friend Todd Frantz, who also graduated from the University of Wisconsin-Stout. Residing in Savage, Minnesota, this wonderful couple added a son, Hunter Michael, who became our first grandson.

Laurie, the youngest of our three children, attended St. Olaf College and finished her undergraduate degrees in psychology and art history at the University of Wisconsin-Madison. With learning opportunities in London, England; Florence, Italy, and Costa Rica and working for a corporate executive training institute, Laurie worked on her Master's in International Business at the University of St. Thomas in St. Paul, Minnesota. Laurie entered and completed her master's degree in counseling psychology at Boston College and is completing her Doctoral studies in Counseling Psychology at the University of Wisconsin-Madison.

We have come face to face with the long-term hardships of different forms of cancers that have threatened my wife and thus our futures. We have shared the loss of a "to be" son-in-law to a heart attack a few months before the wedding. We have coped with Marilyn's parents' struggle with Alzheimer's and a tumor, followed by my mother's sudden and unexpected passing, which left me with a major void. We have found meaning in the unexpected loss of my godson, Ainsley, to AIDS. In the grand scheme of things important, I feel I have more important elements in my life, which I believe transcends the hassles and insults created by harassment, racist acts, and discrimination.

We are proud of our children and grandchildren and take special comfort in knowing that our children share the same common values and beliefs. The children, Todd, Wendy, and Laurie, are comfortable hugging each other and us in the public context. They share a common valuing of elderly persons. They are committed to the well-being of their families. We marvel with pleasure at the development and display of their warmth and caring for others. So I have reason to be positive and upbeat about the future and continue to press forward with hope and a positive outlook even with the full realization of the injustices I experienced.

CYCLES IN OUR PROFESSIONAL LIVES: FATE OR UNIQUE OPPORTUNITIES

Being of Hawaiian ancestry, I find myself pulled to the concerns of Polynesia. Raised to see the strengths of people and families, I find myself pulled to the study of resiliency in individuals and families. Being of many cultures, I find myself committed to the study of cross cultural issues. Trained to study families and war, I find myself pulled to the concerns of families at risk. Educated at the Kamehameha Schools for Hawaiian Children, I find myself pulled to the needs of the children of Hawaiian ancestry. Are these the centripetal forces of the cycles of life, I ask? For the past eight years I have been privileged to be a part of the Pacific Basin meetings held on the island of Maui at Kapalua Bay. Sponsored by the East West Center and the Maui Economic Development Board and supported, in part, with federal funds, the international meetings emphasize the involvement of representatives from the governments of all the Pacific Island Nations, including Western Samoa, Micronesia, Tahiti, Cook Islands, Papua New Guinea, and Fiji, to name a few. These island nations, through their governmental representatives or heads of state, meet to address the issues of westernization, technological development, and economic development and how they could work together as a Federation to improve upon the development of each island nation.

War and its impact on families once again called to me and sent me into Kuwait. Immediately following Operation Desert Storm, the American code name for the war against Iraq, to regain independence and freedom for the people of Kuwait, the Kuwaiti government created a Scientific Advisory Board to assist the government in the rebuilding of the country and in meeting the needs of their people. Appointed to this Scientific Board, I and my research team made several trips to Kuwait to understand the plight of the Kuwaiti people and to work with the team to develop social policies and programs to assist and support families and to guide future policies to serve the people of Kuwait. The visits revealed the importance of culture and the people's Islamic beliefs in the nation's survival and rebuilding.

The social and educational developments in the Middle East also lured us to the United Arab Emirates University (UAE) in El Ain. Under the auspices of Sheikh Zayed bin Sultan al-Nahyan, the Chancellor of UAE University in Al Ain, and the country's leader, we were asked to redesign an existing family science program at the University; the Sheikh also asked me to form a team of family scholars to assist him and his appointed Vice President to create a College of Family Sciences and help to create two new Universities, to be named Zayed University for women with campuses in Abu Dhabi and in Dubai, the major cities in the Emirates. The development of Zayed University for National Women had been rapid; students were admitted within a year of the University's founding. Students were admitted into the Family Science major one year later.

These developments in the Pacific and Middle East share a common principle that the family as society's social unit is a solid and important foundation upon which to build the future and stability of a nation, as each undertakes change as a natural and predictable part of social and economic development in the 21st century. How resilient families are in responding and adapting to change on a global basis is a line of questioning which must and should be pursued. As a participant in these developments, I am inspired and affirmed by the feelings and concerns of nations as they square off to face the future. With the family at center stage, nurtured and protected in the midst of change, I am motivated to seek greater understanding of how and why families throughout the world endure, survive, and adapt in the midst of what appears to be massive social and economic change. Sensing that culture, beliefs, and ethnicity will receive much-deserved attention as nations make social change and economic development priority agendas, I am also motivated to continue my line of inquiry. How and in what ways culture and ethnic identity will shape the course of a nation and its development begs for deeper understanding and clarification. In this global context, I find comfort knowing that my professional interests are very much in congruence with international and global concerns.

Just as I came to settle into my faculty role and embrace the international view of resiliency and the importance of culture, my life took a series of unexpected turns. I accepted the role of the Interim Dean of Zayed University in the United Arab Emirates to foster the development of the College of Family Sciences. After 6 months, I also decided to pursue my lifelong dream to study resiliency in children of Hawaiian Ancestry. In the process of setting up the project with the Kamehameha Schools and Bishop Estate, the 7 billion dollar Trust committed to the education of Children of Hawaiian Ancestry, I was offered and accepted the challenge of becoming the first Chief Executive Officer of the Trust, now renamed the Kamehameha Schools. With the blessings of Sheik Nahayan, I embraced my Hawaiian culture and heritage, retired from the University of Wisconsin-Madison, returned to my roots, and to my family of origin, to spend the remainder of my professional life giving back to the culture and people who have given so much to me. I know my mother, along with my family, is pleased, for she always wanted me to return home. I am truly blessed by this opportunity to give of my self to the benefit of Hawaiian children. Without intending to be melancholy, in my reflective moments in Hawaii, I find myself accepting the belief that my life course, even with the events of racism and discrimination, had a purpose, maybe even a cultural and divine purpose to prepare myself to return and to give back. I have been fortunate to be part of four returning cycles: Being prepared for military life and having the opportunity to give to the well-being of military families; being prepared to study families and having the opportunity to study with Reuben Hill and to give to promoting resiliency in families; being prepared in administration and scholarship and returning to the University of Wisconsin-Madison to serve as an Academic Dean; and being prepared, as a person of color and educator, to return home to give back to the Hawaiian people as a leader and educator. What a blessing. Maybe I can believe that I had the opportunity to be there at the right time, right place, and with the correct assignment.

I look forward to making a contribution toward the advancement of knowledge in this arena, however limited it may be. For one of the few times in my professional life, I feel a sense of what the Hawaiians call *Lokahi,* a sense of harmony about family, culture, profession, heritage, and who I am as a family scholar. My vision quest has been achieved, and now a new vision emerges on the horizon.

REFERENCES

Doherty, W., & McCubbin, H. (Eds.) (1987). *Family systems and health,* Minneapolis: National Council on Family Relations.

Figley, C., & McCubbin, H. (Eds.) (1983). *Stress and the family: Coping with catastrophes, Volume II.* New York: Brunner/Mazel.

McCubbin, H. (1979). Integrating coping behavior in family stress theory. *Journal of Marriage and the Family,* 41 (2) 237-244.

McCubbin, H. (1998). *Resiliency in African-American families: Military families in foreign environments.* In H. McCubbin, E. Thompson, A. Thompson, & J. Futrell (Eds.). *Resiliency in ethnic minority families: African-American families, Volume 2.* (pp. 67-97). Thousand Oaks, CA: Sage.

McCubbin, H., Cauble, A., & Patterson, J. (Eds.) (1982). *Family stress, coping and social support.* Springfield, IL: C.C. Thomas.

McCubbin, H., & Dahl, B. (1985). *Marriage and family: Individuals and life cycles.* New York: John Wiley.

McCubbin, H., Dahl, B., & Hunter, E. (Eds.) (1976). *Families in the military system.* Beverly Hills: Sage.

McCubbin, H., & Figley, C. (Eds.) (1983). *Stress and the family: Coping with normative transitions, Volume I.* New York: Brunner/Mazel.

McCubbin, H., Fleming, W.M., Thompson, A., Neitman, P., Elver, K., & Savas S.A. (1998). Resiliency and coping in "at-risk" African-American youth and their families. In H. McCubbin, E. Thompson, A. Thompson, & J. Futrell (Eds.), *Resiliency in ethnic minority families: African-American families, Volume 2.* (pp. 287-328). Thousand Oaks, CA: Sage.

McCubbin, H., & McCubbin, L. (1997). Hawaiian American families. In DeGenova, M.K. (Ed.), *Families in a cultural context.* Mountain View, CA: Mayfield Publishing.

McCubbin, H., & McCubbin, M. (1988). Typologies of resilient families: Emerging roles of social class and ethnicity. *Family Relations,* 37(3) 247-264.

McCubbin, H., McCubbin, M.A., Thompson, A.I., Han, S., & Allen, C. (1997). Families under stress: What makes them resilient. *Journal of Family and Consumer Sciences,* November, Fall, 3-15.

McCubbin, H., McCubbin, M., Thompson, A., & Thompson, E. (1998). Resiliency in ethnic families: A conceptual model for predicting family adjustment and adaptation. In H. McCubbin, E. Thompson, A. Thompson, & J. Fromer (Eds.), *Resiliency in ethnic minority families: Native and immigrant American families, Volume 1.* (pp. 3-48). Thousand Oaks, CA: Sage.

McCubbin, H., & Patterson, J.M. (1983). The Family Stress Process: The Double ABCX Model of adjustment and adaptation. *Marriage & Family Review, 6*(1-2) 7-37.

McCubbin, H., & Patterson, J. (1983). Family transition: Adaptation to stress. In H. McCubbin & C. Figley (Eds.), *Stress and the family: Coping with normative crises, Volume 1* (pp. 5-25). New York: Brunner/Mazel.

McCubbin, H., Patterson, J., & Sussman, M.B. (1983). Social Stress and the family: Advances in family stress theory and research. New York, The Haworth Press, Inc.

McCubbin, H., & Thompson, A. (1988). *Resilient families in rural communities: Trapped in the wake of the farm crisis.* Madison: University of Wisconsin, Research Monograph.

McCubbin, H., Thompson, A., Futrell, J., & McCubbin, L. (Eds.) (2000). *Promoting resiliency in families and children at risk: Interdisciplinary perspectives.* Thousand Oaks, CA: Sage.

McCubbin, H., Thompson, A., & McCubbin, M. (1996). *Family assessment: Resiliency, coping and adaptation–Inventories for research and practice.* Madison: University of Wisconsin System.

McCubbin, H., Thompson, A., Pirner, P., & McCubbin, M. (1988). *Family types and strengths: A life cycle and ecological perspective.* Edina, MN: Burgess International.

McCubbin, H., Thompson, E., Thompson, A., & Fromer, J. (Eds.) (1998a). *Resiliency in ethnic minority families: Native and immigrant American families.* Thousand Oaks, CA: Sage.

McCubbin, H., Thompson, E., Thompson, A., & Fromer, J. (Eds.) (1998b). *Sense of coherence and resiliency: Stress, coping & health.* Thousand Oaks, CA: Sage.

McCubbin, H., Thompson, A., Thompson, E., Elver, K., & McCubbin, M. (1998). Ethnicity, schema, and coherence: Appraisal processes for families in crisis. In H. McCubbin, E. Thompson, A. Thompson, & J. Fromer (Eds.), *Sense of coherence and resiliency: Stress, coping and health.* (pp. 41-67). Thousand Oaks, CA: Sage.

McCubbin, H., Thompson, E., Thompson, A., & Futrell, J. (Eds.) (1998). *Resiliency in ethnic minority families: African-American families, Volume 2.* Thousand Oaks, CA: Sage.

McCubbin, H., Thompson, E., Thompson, A., & Futrell, J. (Eds.) (1999). *The dynamics of resilient families.* Thousand Oaks, CA: Sage.
McCubbin, M., & McCubbin, H. (1989). The typology model of family adjustment and adaptation. In Figley, C. (Ed.), *Family stress and coping, Volume III.* New York: Brunner/Mazel.
McCubbin, M., & McCubbin, H. (1993). Family coping with health crises: The Resiliency Model of Family Stress, Adjustment and Adaptation. In C. Danielson, B. Hamel-Bissell, & P. Winstead-Fry (Eds.), *Families, health and illness.* New York: Mosby.
Olson, D., McCubbin, H., Barnes, H., Larsen, A., Muxen, A., & Wilson, M. (1984). *Families: What makes them work.* Beverly Hills: Sage.
Redfield, J. (1997). *The Celestine Prophecy.* New York: Warner.

Life as a Sociologist

Helena Znaniecka Lopata

KEYWORDS. Autobiography, faculty, widowhood, childhood, career

I have decided to write this life story, rather than speaking it onto a tape [as suggested by M. Sussman]. I am basically a writer and prefer to read than to hear. The second decision is not to write it in one fell swoop–life is so complicated and memory so dependent upon current construction of reality that a single stretch at this computer (this marvelous invention) would tend to flatten life unavoidably into limited themes. Coming here to write after different situational experiences will help broaden my ability to express my different selves (obviously, the symbolic interactionist nature of my thought has come out). I will also allow myself to use indications or symbols of sub-thoughts ( ) and variations–, even unfinished sentences. As Dick, my husband, points out, I have a habit of unfinished sentences as I wander off to new ideas. So here goes.

My identities and feelings are deeply lodged in not only my family history, but also that of two countries. My father, Florian Witold Znaniecki, grew up in Poland, a son to a "shlachta" or small nobility family with a coat of arms and strong feelings of "noblesse oblige" but with no land. His grandfather, father, and uncles had been inducted into the Prussian armed forces during the Franco-Prussian War and lost their estate from the costa under Bismarck's Germanization policy. Poland was partitioned by Prussia, Russia, and Austria for 125 years, and they lived in the Prussian part, so there was no choice. His father managed somebody else's estate, and father and his two sisters grew up in rural surroundings, being educated by governesses and what he called self-education until he was ready for gymnasium, when he was sent to Warsaw to live with relatives. His life story is important to tell here because of its strong influence on my life. In short, the gentry felt strongly a moral obligation to maintain and develop Polish culture in opposition to the three political states which occupied Poland from 1794 until after World War I. All three, but particularly Prussia, tried to impose their cultures upon the conquered population. The fact that the Polish culture did survive for 124 years is evidence of the strength of this determination on the part of the gentry, which had previously developed a democratic government, with elected king and a "liberum veto" allowing all members of the parliament the right to veto any bill. This was a democracy in 18th century terms which excluded women and propertyless men, so was limited to the gentry–even those families which no longer held major property. It was also a major reason for the loss of political freedom–as the parliament was frozen by the refusal of each of the status-competitive Poles to allow the passage of bills introduced by others.

Anyway, father grew up in this nationalistic atmosphere, got into trouble with the Russian authorities in the gymnasium for political activity and went off to the Sorbonne in Paris and Universities in Switzerland to continue his education. About this time, he fell in love with the wife of a friend, faked a suicide in Lake Geneva, and joined the French Foreign Legion. He managed to get an honorable discharge after shooting himself "accidentally" in the shoulder and shooting thumb. He returned to Switzerland and France for more courses and finally ended up getting a PhD at the Jagiellonian University in Crakow. Still unable to get a position in Poland because of his political activity, he took a job at the Society for the Protection of Emigrants, where he published manuscripts about Poles who had immigrated to America and two philosophical books on Social Values. It was there that he met W. I. Thomas, a University of Chicago sociologist who was in Poland to collect information on the immigrants. The contact resulted in father coming to Chicago to help Thomas. He brought with him on the last train before World War I his first wife, a Pole who had been fellow student in Switzerland, but left behind with her sisters a son, Juliusz Znaniecki.

Father's first wife died in Chicago in an accident, and he later met and married my mother, Eileen Markley, a lawyer with Legal Aid. She had obtained her law degree in 1915 from the University of Chicago, having finished a BA at Smith College and an MA at Columbia University (Columbia would not admit her into its law school, Chicago did). Mother quit her job and helped daddy with the *Polish Peasant [PP] in Europe and America* (Znaniecki & Thomas, 1927), which he was writing with W. I., and with *Cultural Reality* (Znaniecki, 1919), which contained the ideas he could not get into the *PP* (daddy knew English–along with 7 other languages–and had already published a philosophical article in that language). W. I. got kicked out of the University of Chicago in a big scandal, World War I ended, and Wilson helped Poland regain its independence. Daddy got an offer of a professorial chair in philosophy at the Adam Mickiewicz University in Poznan. Seeing little hope for a career in America and being very turned off by the anti-intellectualism of this country (he even wrote an article published anonymously in the *Atlantic Monthly* on this subject), Daddy asked for the chair to be changed to sociology and returned to Poland. Mother went along, giving up her law career, gaining the disapproval of her family, and not knowing a word of Polish.

So, I was born in 1925 in Poznan, Poland, under the name of Helena Beatrice (mother's sister) Lubicz (coat of arms name) Znaniecka. I was really raised as an only child since my half-brother, who was 17 years older, did not spend much time in our home. The aunts who kept him while Daddy was in America refused to allow mother–an uncultured American, as all Americans obviously were in their eyes–to raise a Znaniecki. Both daddy and mother taught at the University and surrounded themselves with couples of a similar secular intelligentsia lifestyle. The atmosphere of intellectual noblesse oblige, a humanistic desire to build a better world and contribute to both national and international cultures, dominated the home. We had an apartment in the city and later one in a suburb and spent summers and winter vacations in the mountains. Mother was aged 39 and Daddy 44 when I was born, but their closest friends, Daddy's distant cousins (still considered family in Poland) had two children approximately my age, and we spent most of our free time with them. The mother, Aniela Dietl, spoke English and was a head of a library (all the women in their circle were professional). The father, Bronislaw Dietl, had been a governor of a province (or its equivalent) and lost his position in a fight with Pilsudski, the dictatorial head of the Polish government. He then stayed home, not being willing to take a position that was lower in status. He was marvelous, teaching his daughter Basia, two years older than I, and son Jerzy, a year younger, to play bridge, and reading all the great Polish classics to us. Basia became a biochemist. Jerzy, a professor of economics at Lodz University, was a senator in the first non-communist parliament in the 1990s. We (Dick and I) still see them, especially Jerzy, periodically in both countries.

The intelligentsia community in Europe and America has always traveled extensively, and we often had guests from abroad. I remember W. I. Thomas, Ted Abel, L. von Wiese. . . . Daddy was invited to Columbia University as visiting professor in 1932-1934. We lived on Morningside Drive, and I went to Horace Mann school, learning English without any difficulty. However, the next summer I spent on Martha's Vineyard with mother's sister, Beatrice, and her three older sons–and promptly forgot my Polish. Horrified, my parents sent me the next summer back to Poland with the Abels to relearn Polish. They returned home in the fall.

Another experience that had a profound effect on my life was osteomyelitis. I developed it at the age of 10, having an emergency operation on my leg, just below the knee, on Easter day. To make a long story short, I almost died, could not walk for a year, and had repeated attacks for many years. While off my feet I started a stamp collection, read Zane Gray in Polish translation, was tutored, and spent a great deal of time by myself.

I remember a very pleasant childhood in spite of the illness–children learn to adjust to a great variety of things as long as the atmosphere surrounding them is happy. Then the Nazis entered Poland on September 1, 1939. There are many memories from that time until we got out in March, 1940, memories that started coming back after the first return in 1966, but only one set fits this story. Daddy had gone to New York to lecture again at Columbia University in the summer of 1939, but Mother decided to stay in Poland to supervise the building of a house in the mountains. When war broke out, Daddy was on the Atlantic on his way back. The ship, *Batory*, was stopped in England and its passengers finally sent back to America. Immediately upon landing, he was offered a professorship at the University of Illinois, which he accepted. He then, with the help of mother's family, tried to find out where we were and get us out. They sent money to ports surrounding Germany, including Genoa, Italy. Nothing could be done about getting us out.

We returned to Poznan just before the invasion, and Mother decided to stay rather than escaping, because she did not know where Daddy was. This turned out to be a bad idea, since our name was on both the Nazi and the communist blacklists (sociologists and their families are dangerous!!). We were picked up one December night during curfew by bus and taken to a concentration camp with other members of the intelligentsia and Polish leaders. The camp was on the outskirts of the city and served a single function: to fill it with Poles, bring in cattle cars, pack people in and drive them around until they froze; then they dumped the bodies in another part of Poland. The Nazis had incorporated our section into Germany and wanted to get rid of our kinds of people, as well as of Jews, to resettle the area with Germans. (The Nazis had several types of camps: extermination, concentration for removal, labor, prisoner of war–a memorial stone in the place where our camp was located states that 110,000 women, children, and men had gone through it. All in all, the Germans killed 6,000,000 Poles, of whom 3,000,000 had been Polish Jews; the remaining were Poles of other identities.)

None of the Poles had really believed rumors as to such camps, but mother realized their truth when the cattle cars came into the camp. Knowing that we could not survive, especially I with osteomyelitis, she marched to the commander and demanded to be let out as an American citizen (this was December, 1939, and the United States was not yet involved in the war). She claimed to be an American citizen (which she was not because of marriage to a foreigner before the 1924 law that allowed women to keep their citizenship in spite of such a marriage) visiting her sister in Poland when the Germans had come and not to understand Polish or what was going on. She demanded that I, her Polish orphaned niece, also be allowed out. The commander was petrified that her "important connections" would create a problem and let us out immediately (don't forget–mother had won a battle to be a woman lawyer in America).

The story of our getting out of Poland is also long and complicated and not part of what I want to tell you. Anyway, we finally escaped with the help of the Polish underground and "outweiss" papers belonging to a daughter of a Warsaw family.

Arrival in Champaign-Urbana, in the Midwest of America, where people were not even aware of the war and did not believe any of our tales, was traumatic. I started high school in April, ahead of the other sophomores because of having learned much more in the Polish system. I had been a lousy student in Poland, competing with my best friend for the worst grades, but I made the National Honor Society in America. Magically, I was a very good student and loved it. However, my co-students made my life miserable, most not wanting to have anything to do with anyone as weird as I was–a foreigner. Mother and I went around the neighboring states making speeches about the horrors of the war and collecting money for medicine and clothing. Mother packaged these items and sent them to Poland, Siberia, and wherever else they were needed. The speeches probably helped me get over some of the trauma and provided the opportunity for me to develop some self confidence to offset the other stigmatic encounters. *[Written May 3, 1992, Polish Independence day, after spending a day and a half at the University of Chicago's centennial celebration of the Sociology Department–which are obviously some of the situational influences upon my memory.]*

BECOMING A SOCIOLOGIST

Smith College offered me a scholarship as the daughter of an alumna, but Mother thought I had better not take it because that would take money away from helping Poles during and after World War II. I was to go to the University of Illinois, where Daddy was on the faculty. Daddy suggested that I join a sorority. (This suggestion went against all his democratic/socialist inclinations.) However, he was right. My sorority "sisters" took me in hand, and, by the end of the pledge year, I was sufficiently Americanized to enjoy college and life.

I had been fascinated by physics in high school and started in that direction at the University of Illinois, but found chemistry no great pleasure and shifted to psychology. That subject was full of rats, so I moved to philosophy, with a sociology double major. It was not until my MA work that a kind philosopher pointed out that I really belonged in sociology since my paper on social values was not appropriate for his course. So, finally, I ended up happily in sociology–not surprising because that is all I heard at home.

I met Richard Lopata, a disabled Marine veteran and president of the veteran's association at the University of Illinois, and we married February 8, 1946. The ceremony was totally free of religion, the first time anyone around there had witnessed such a lovely event. I did not attend graduation, choosing the honeymoon instead. My parents offered us two rooms, a bedroom and study, in their house and dinners for the great sum of $25 a month, as long as we got out of the house by 8:00 since things had to be quiet when Daddy was writing.

Dick graduated the next year in economics and both of us obtained our Master's degrees at U of I. We then wandered off to Massachusetts to sell the house at Martha's Vineyard. Dick obtained a job teaching at U of Massachusetts and I at the Pioneer Valley Association working out of Northhampton. I loved the East and was offered a job teaching at Smith College by Gladys Bryson. Coming home (a proctor's apartment in an all-male dormitory full of veterans) one day, I found Dick playing solitaire and stating that he was fed up with the East and with academia, so we were going back to Chicago. I told him to go back–I was staying–and here I have remained, in Chicago from 1949 to the present. Actually, it worked out very well, because I entered THE UNIVERSITY (U of Chicago, of course) at absolutely the right time. There was a student body of 210, mainly male veterans, and a faculty that had had much smaller numbers before. So, we formed study groups, and these are the people with whom I continued friendships for all these years. We did not live near campus; I was a woman married to a businessman and did not apply for fellowships. Thus, I was not in the inner sanctum of people surrounding the main faculty members, especially Hughes and Wirth. However, my birth name was of sufficient interest to the faculty so that my dissertation committee consisted of Wirth, Blumer, and Hughes. That was not so good, since Wirth died and Blumer went to California (luckily not until he gave me honors in social psychology–which I thought however was to make up for his criticism of the *Polish Peasant*). I did not do as well in theory, having learned at Illinois only the theories of the men whose courses I took.

Dick was called into the Air Force (having joined the reserves a few weeks before) during the Korean war, so we ended up at Langley Air Force Base in Virginia after my first year at University of Chicago. That was an experience in itself, since I had never been in the South (I hope the Virginians forgive me for calling them Southerners) or among Americans outside of academia. I finished my prelims the summer and fall of 1950, staying with Bernard and Rhoda Goldstein or the Londons–not necessarily a pleasant experience for them since I was pregnant and experiencing not-just-morning sickness (what woman wouldn't under those complications).

I had planned a theoretical dissertation upon entrance to University of Chicago–but the department had other ideas and sent me to Polonia (the Polish American community) to determine why it had not dissolved, as predicted by Thomas and Znaniecki (1927). I knew nothing about Polonia except that Dick was second generation Polish American and his mother was involved in many associations. The family helped me not to make some dumb mistakes by believing all the literature about the community. Hal Orbach recently discovered (as presented in Trento, Italy at a conference on Znaniecki, organized by Luigi Tomasi) that the *Polish Peasant* volume(s) were intended as only part of a trilogy, the other two studies focusing on the intelligentsia and the bourgeoisie. The more rounded picture of all three classes was never done. However, the disorganized image of Polonia in the *PP* stuck while the melting pot theory of American society focused sociological and historial attention on the assimilation of individuals. Thus, there was relatively little interest in the community as a complex and competitive, many-layered community. Dick's family, especially his mother, kept breaking the stereotypes with her stories of life in Polonia.

Most of my work on Polish Americans was actually accomplished at Hampton Institute in Virginia through interlibrary loan, since I traced the development of the community historically and used many resources from the Polish Roman Catholic Union library. Hampton Institute is, or was then, a totally black university and the neighbors and officers of Langley were really freaked-out seeing a white, increasingly pregnant woman entering its gates daily. My life again became completely marginalized as it had been at Champaign and Urbana high schools (we moved while I attended these). I identified with academia, represented by my parents (daddy was teaching at Wayne State University and I stayed with them prior to going to U of C for the prelims) and by all my friends at U of C. I missed the study groups in theory, race relations, and social psychology and I missed being with Rhoda (Blumberg) Goldstein and Gladys Lang–the only women I knew going through the same combination of getting a PhD and having a baby at the same time. Then I was also the wife of an Air Force Officer in Virginia and nothing I did, thought, or said (except for being good at poker and bingo) was acceptable to all those involved. Our daughter, Teddy, was born in July, 1951 at Dixie Hospital. I ended up back in the hospital with a bad attack of osteo, and my background to the dissertation was not finished (the osteo started giving me trouble again after the stint in Poland under the Nazis, and I was not supposed to have children–but at that age who listens!!). When I returned from the hospital, the dear old colonel's wife called to say that I must appear at the club at least twice a month. I chose bridge (ruined my bidding, but won all our baby sitting money) and started a book club (15 people out of hundreds).

Anyway, I learned a lot about American society those years at Langley. Dick hated the armed service; we finally got out, and he rejoined his marketing management firm in Chicago. Apartments, however, were hard to find, and we ended up in Berwyn, not much help to a person with my characteristics and a small baby. The U of C faculty sent me out to Polonia to actually talk to people (my MA thesis had been on international cooperation in medicine, and I did not need to leave the library for that) and attend organizational meetings. Mom Burns (Dick's mother) helped again, this time with babysitting, and I finally finished the dissertation (and moved to Skokie to a ticky-tacky but very nice little house).

OCCUPATION: HOUSEWIFE

By the time I got my PhD in 1954, I had been fighting so long to remain a sociologist and the kind of person I thought I was that I finally gave up and dropped out. I became a proper, very proper, suburban homemaker. I learned to cook, buy antiques at the Salvation Army and church rummage sales, reupholster and finish them, and I took care of home, husband, child, and dog. We then had another child, Stefan, in 1955, and I ended up having a major operation, with 7 weeks in the hospital and months of not walking again (however, that operation did it, and I have had no outbreak since).

Daddy once asked when visiting and observing my Skokie life why was I not doing anything with my sociology, and I wisely replied that I was completely out of contact with that environment. I had assumed that my dissertation was no good because I had so few criticisms (Hughes suggested that I better get someone who knew English to correct it because "of course" is not spelled "off course"). I did not even have the nerve to summarize it for a chapter in Burgess and Bogue's *Contributions to Urban Sociology* (1965). They had someone else do it for me.

However, my learning got the better of me and, following mother's advice to study what I know, I started research on suburban housewives, who were all around me and with whom I had my only adult contact (businessmen avoided me, not just because I was a housewife but also when they found out I was a sociology PhD). I learned about their views of their roles and those of their husbands, of the intergenerational contrast in these roles, and of neighboring and perceptions of urban and suburban life.

Daddy died in 1958, having become quite frail even when hosting the American Sociological Society's meetings on the U of I campus when he was president. Two years later, my brother Julek committed suicide. We had stayed with him and his wife and son in Warsaw after getting out of the camp during the winter of 1939. He was caught by the Germans during the Warsaw uprising and sent to Dachau. He was later released by the American armed forces. He had tuberculosis and missing teeth, but managed to get better and finally to come to America. He wrote and transmitted at the Voice of America. He had been a poet and novelist in Poland, but could not write in English nor forget his experiences. No one wanted to read about such horrors in those years, and he became increasingly depressed.

MOVEMENT BACK INTO SOCIOLOGY

Mother asked me to prepare my father's unfinished magnum opus for publication as *Social Relations and Social Roles* (Znaniecki, 1965). The experience was very useful, and I have since then worked with modification, the concept of social role as a set of social relations rather than in the Lintonian focus on one person alone. (I realize that I use the term "Daddy" when talking about him in interpersonal relations with me, "father" when writing about him as a sociologist.)

The study of the housewives expanded, with the help of a grant from *The Chicago Tribune,* to include 300 women in 12 socioeconomically and otherwise diverse suburbs of Chicago. I started teaching part-time, meaning one course a semester in the evening at De Paul and then at Roosevelt Universities, never as yet seeing myself again as a sociologist. I was an American housewife, who almost dabbled at being a sociologist. I tried to publish articles from the study in women's magazines and rejection slips from them joined those from departments of sociology when I was looking for a job after completing my MA.

What really pushed me back into serious involvement in the life of a scholar and transformed my self-concept was a very painful experience. I had wanted to return to Poland for a visit as long as I could remember, being very homesick and feeling that there was my real home. The Polish government finally gave me a visa in 1966, and Dick, Teddy, Stefan and I drove there from countries west, hitting Poznan first. There, and later in Warsaw, I was faced with a shock–the realization that I had deserted the obligation of the intelligentsia to contribute to world culture. How could I live just for myself and my family? The young woman whose papers got me out of Poland died because she could not leave the city when typhus hit. Should I not pay back all the people of the underground who helped us and contribute what those who had died could not? This was a terrible burden. My children were quite taken aback with Poland, with everyone talking a language they did not understand, and crying. Many showed the effects of the war and, especially, of Nazism and tried to explain the horrors of communism (which had actually let up somewhat in 1956). It took a long time before my 16-year-old daughter again identified with me.

We traveled from Poland through Yugoslavia, a lively Italy, France, and England, and the children became happier. They all went back to America and I to the International Sociological Association's meetings in Evian, France. Jan Szczepanski, a former student of Daddy's, was president of the

ISA in those difficult years for Poland, and I finally awoke to the realization of how different I had become, how focused on such a limited world of American suburbia.

Upon return to America and our lovely home in prestigious Highland Park, I tried to make some use of my homemaker studies; I moved into full time teaching at Roosevelt U (actually, the students petitioned to have me gain that position because they assumed that sexism kept me at the instructor level). I cried through most of the writing of *Occupation: Housewife* (Ann Oakley made fun of my admissions in the preface in her review of the book) and suffered with the rejections from publishers. No one wanted to read about housewives. Just as my male friends from University of Chicago that I saw at meetings have never recognized, I was doing real sociology in which basic "sensitizing" concepts were applied to studies of women.

However, I really can't complain about all of the U of C colleagues. I finally sent the *Occupation: Housewife* (Lopata, 1971) manuscript to Howie Becker, who recommended it to Irving Louis Horowitz, who recommended it to Oxford University Press. The salesmen of the press were not exactly enthusiastic, but the book has become a classic. Other papers came from that research and from the portion of *Social Relations and Social Roles* (Znaneicki, 1965) to which I had added my theories, but which Chandler consultants did not want to include. Irving Goffman gave good advice to convert that portion of role theory into articles. Joseph Gusfield liked my study of the ballroom dance studio, and it found a place in *Transaction* (Lopata & Noel, 1967). All my painful self-examination and self-reconstruction paid off, and I began to believe in myself as a competent person in this area of choice.

This does not mean that these transformations met with the total approval of anyone but my mother and my daughter. My son deeply resented my becoming a "public figure," with television appearances, when friends and conversation at parties at home turned to sociology and focused on my work. Although Stefan was 10 by the time all this began to happen, he thinks of me as always teaching and being a strange mother. The principal at Elm Place School (recently determined to be the best grade school in the United States) told me that Stefan could not eat lunch at school the three days I was gone in 1965 because such arrangements were made only for mothers who *had* to work. And, I was the only "career mother" among all our suburban acquaintances except for one who ran a model agency!!! As late as high school, our son asked me why I had to be a scientist–when I asked what he would prefer me to be, he replied, "real estate is nice for mothers." The only other "working mother" he knew at Lake Forest Academy inherited a real estate firm from her father.

Business associates of Dick's and some of his male relatives thought I should remain his back-up and that my career was interfering with his. He was warned not to allow me to teach at Roosevelt University, since knowledge of that might hurt his relations with clients. And there were many times he was irritated as I met my own demands and turned my attention to my own work. We had a real fight at an ASA annual meeting to which he came and took over, all the men focused their attention to him, while I was turned into a wife. That is not what I wanted out of meetings, which still form a major source of revitalization of ideas. Dick has never learned how to be a wife, so I go to conferences by myself. However, Dick did take a lot of sociology and has learned to understand my work and, for a wife, the strange schedule that goes with it. He is not a typical businessman. *[May 4, 1992. I now start concentrating on a updated revision of* The Polish Americans: Status Competition in an Ethnic Community *(Prentice-Hall, 1976; new contract with Transaction Publishers).]*

LIFE AS A SOCIOLOGIST

The transition from being an American suburban housewife to being a sociologist with both national and international interests and involvements, painful as it was, has become a real source of satisfaction. This is especially true now that I can allow myself to do the kind of studies and write the kind of stuff that I wish. I published my first article at the age of 40, having, however, never given up wanting to write since I was asked by the editor of our Poznan newspaper if I wanted him to sue another "poet" in another paper for plagiarizing one of my poems (I was about 12 at the time and the local paper had a children's section). An English lit professor at the University of Illinois encouraged me to write non-fiction, since I could not master American speech patterns, and I have persevered in writing sociology. The only time writing was not a real pleasure occurred in conjunction with my attempt at large-scale surveys, in spite of all my socialization into qualitative work. I ventured into highly funded quantitative survey work while trying to establish myself as a sociologist in the 1960s. This also occurred during the time when I still had some vision of myself as Joan of Arc, having to save the world, or at least paying back some debt for my life. After much internal debate concerning ways of meeting these goals, I hit upon the idea of studying death and widowhood. By that time, Daddy was long dead (1958), and Mother was a widow, but I did not think of her that way. The impetus came from the 1966 trip to Poland. I even taught courses in dying, death, and bereavement. I had a post-doctoral fellowship from the Midwest Council of Social Research on Aging to complete analysis of the homemakers (Warren Peterson and the MCSRA council were liberal in their definition of aging). With their help, I applied to the Administration on Aging for a grant to study role modifications of older widows (at that time I thought the elderly included ages 50-64 and 65+). I got the grant, NORC drew a sample and interviewed, put the data on IBM cards, and I had to learn some statistics and computer usage. That grant resulted in several papers and a book as well as in a large contract with the Social Security Administration, which wanted to learn more about its current and former beneficiaries. Their statisticians drew a five-layered sample, and I was stuck with having to manage a vast amount of data. I found that I greatly disliked writing from statistical tables. What saved my sanity in this and the next study was my excellent background in what became called "grounded theory," so that I could develop a theoretically consistent interview and knew what I wanted out of the results. I certainly could not have written or used the software to get what I wanted had I not moved to Loyola University of Chicago in 1969 with the role modification study. That study resulted in *Widowhood in an American City* (Lopata, 1973), for which I had a great deal of help with the SSA support systems study of widowhood in the form of graduate assistants and my project officer, Henry Brehm, a PhD in sociology with a specialization in methodology. A book, *Women as Widows: Support Systems* (Lopata, 1979), and articles resulted from this study.

The support systems study had the added advantage of access to the Public Law 480 funds in several countries. The funds are a result of the United States government's sale of wheat and other items to countries whose currency it does not want. The currency stays in the buyer's country to be used for embassies, research, and other activity that the governments approve. Henry Brehm obtained permission to use these funds in Egypt, Poland, and Yugoslavia, and we organized teams in these countries to study widowhood. It is at the conferences with these teams that I hit upon the concept of support systems (social role as a set of relations between a social person and a social circle was too complex a concept to use cross-culturally so I broke it, or at least part of it, into sets of in- and out-flow of supports which had meaning in the other societies). Unfortunately, the anthropologist working at the American University in Cairo quit her position and nothing came from the study, although it had been conducted and would have been fascinating. The Yugoslav department of war, to which the project was sent, forbad it (too many war widows?), and the Polish government withdrew its permission at the last minute. Fortunately, Jackie Touba of the University of Tehran obtained money from the Shah's wife's budget and conducted the study in that city, even carrying the data with her when she left the country after the revolution. The interview, or major parts of it, has also been conducted in Korea and Australia, the theoretical framework used in other countries, such as the Philippines, Israel, Turkey and parts of North America (see *Widows: The*

Middle East, Asia and the Pacific [1987a] and *Widows: North America* [1987b]. See also Lopata & Brehm, 1986).

The two widowhood studies created another source of frustration besides having to deal with statistical data. As far as I could tell, the lengthy reports that I sent to the governmental agencies which funded the studies had never even been examined. The representatives were simply pleased to have reports, and good ones if I may say. They informed me that many grants do not produce any results. The frustration of not having the knowledge known and distributed pushed me into a whole round of speeches at universities, area agencies for the elderly, etc. The process was exhausting, and I began to worry about my heart, having frequent pains which resembled angina and suffering from pain in the neck (literally, not just figuratively). I admit that I overworked–but how can you make a dent on the world from the ivory tower alone?

In the meantime, I finally had enough courage about my work to go back to Polonia and my dissertation to see if it could see the light of day. Prentice-Hall was interested and so I wrote *Polish Americans: Status Competition in an Ethnic Community* (Lopata, 1976). As usual, the book was much too long and the publisher wanted it to fit into a series including Jewish, Japanese, Greek, and other Americans, so much of it was cut. I stuck to the theory but let go of many details of the community and its relations with Poland and with the United States. But this track of thought and analysis has remained interesting to me. My dissertation was written in the early 1950s, the book appeared in 1976, and I am again returning to the community in the 1990s. There is another interesting aspect to all this. People often claim that the rut they get into during their dissertations is never left–they stay within the same area of research and writing most of their lives. What probably kept me from staying in the race and ethnic or community relations field was that long sojourn in American suburbia among homemakers. I had taken only one course in the family (summer in U of Colorado-Boulder, with hardly any studying but lots of fun) and considered myself a symbolic interactionist with an occupations and professions field specialization. I do spend a lot of time doing and thinking in these ways, but I have certainly done much in family sociology!

I did get back to occupations and professions in two ways. Rita Simon was an over-all editor for the sociology series for JAI Press and asked me to edit a series on sex roles. I replied that there is no such thing as a sex role (pervasive identity, yes, but not a role; gender not sex as content), but that I would edit a series on social roles. I named the series *Research on the Interweave of Social Roles* and edited *Women and Men* with Judith Wittner and Nona Glazer (Lopata, Glazer, & Wittner 1980), *Friendship* (Lopata & Maines, 1981), and *Families and Jobs* (Lopata & Pleck, 1983). However, no one seemed to know what the series title meant, so I finally got practical and changed it to *Current Research on Occupations and Professions.* I edited volumes 4 (1987a) and 5 (1990a), got tired of working as editor, and asked Judith Levy, Gale Miller, and Muriel Cantor to edit the next ones. Anne Figert and I edited volume 9, subtitled "Getting Down to Business" (Lopata & Figert, 1996), and I edited volume 10 on "Settings and Circles" (1998). Kevin Henson agreed to co-edit volume 11 on unusual occupations or unusual organization of usual occupations (Lopata & Henson, 1999).

The other return to the area that showed the influence of E. Hughes (I wrote to him about this, and he said I never left it) came with my final large survey. This study was first designed for the new Department of Education, but finally, it was located again in the Social Security Administration, on changing commitments of American urban women to work and family roles. The first stage of the study was to involve a sample of Chicago area women aged 25-54, to be expanded then into several American cities. The Chicago stage was funded, very well in fact, but federal research funds were being cut back by the time we were ready for the second stage. This time, I again had the help of Henry Brehm as the project officer and a very good team of co-researchers at what I had established in 1972, the Center for the Comparative Study of Social Roles at Loyola University-Chicago (LUC). The study was fun to do. Kathy Norr and I sent two major reports to SSA. She then left LUC, but two graduate students, Cheryl Allyn Miller and Debra Barnewolt, and I decided to further develop one of the major themes of the study: a focus on the actual occupations of the respondents. We divided the sample (of 1,877 women, weighted), by occupational category and sub-category by complexity (for example, service workers were divided into cleaning, food, health, and personal/protective). I again over-wrote the introduction, which became a separate volume entitled *City Women: Work, Jobs, Occupations, Careers: America* (Lopata, Miller, & Barnewolt, 1984). The second volume, focusing on Chicago (Lopata, Barnewolt, & Miller, 1985), was a joint venture. Cheryl examined the background of the sampled women in her dissertation, including family background but especially their schooling, job training, and patterns of labor force entry and exit. I then analyzed the women's perceptions of the job, its complexity, importance to beneficiaries, and so forth, while Debbie took the role cluster (her dissertation was on this subject).

Cheryl accepted a post-doc at Johns Hopkins but developed cancer and died in 1984 at the age of 32. Loyola University and the Sociologists for Women in Society, with the help of the Miller family and other contributors, have established a Cheryl Allyn Miller symposium. The purpose here is to bring a feminist sociologist to the university for a major speech, to be repeated with invited speeches at 2-3 small colleges. SWS has taken over the award which, therefore, continues to contribute to feminism.

I am fortunate in my academic location, in view of the fact that I am not geographically and so professionally mobile. Dick is a management consultant, now partially retired, who has always wanted to remain in Chicago. I have taught at Guelph College (1987), Boston College (1982), University of Minnesota (1980), and University of Southern California (1975) for periods of less than an academic year. The Loyola location is good for several reasons, the most important being the sociology department. The University in general is very cooperative and has treated me well in terms of salary, help in the establishment of the Center, and with internal grants. It is located in two very nice places, on Lake Michigan 65 blocks north of the loop and at the Water Tower center of the "Magnificent Mile" of Michigan Avenue. We live in a condo right on a lovely beach of Lake Michigan, only seven blocks from the north shore campus. In addition, we have a house at Delavan Lake, Wisconsin, where we go every weekend (when we are not traveling or I attending meetings). The house is 80 miles from the apartment. The Menascos, daughter Teddy, son-in-law Dennis, and granddaughter Allisa, live 3 miles away. Son Stefan, daughter-in-law Peggy (pure Irish like my mother), and two small granddaughters Caitlin and Colleen are about 40 miles away.

We sold the big house directly on the lake where we had lived for 20 years and built a house in the woods on the same land. The old house afforded much pleasure as the children grew up, sailing and boating, swimming and visiting. I belong to the garden club and both of us continue membership in the Delavan Lake Yacht club where Allisa sails, Teddy is membership chair and treasurer, and Dennis has been commodore. It is a little lake so all these titles do not represent the kind of status that Lake Geneva enjoys. It is also quieter. The only people we meet are connected with these two groups, which is a small and insular circle. Dick would like to spend most of his time here. He has breakfast with the old World War II buddies, the retired judge, publisher of the local paper, realtor, doctor, management consultant, and so forth.

Delavan presents a problem to me, much as I love the area. The problem lies in the characteristics of the lake population. It is 100 percent white, with a western European background. Most go to church or at least identify as Protestants or Catholic (a large Irish contingent of former Chicagoans of our generation has moved here permanently). Jewish weekend and vacation families have bought up here recently, although the only resort on the lake used to be "for Gentiles only" not that long ago. (I believe there is one Jewish family living in town year round.) Some Mexicans, who used to be migratory workers, have now settled in town, to mixed reactions. There is now a dog track which brings different kinds of people, but without the "terrible consequences" anticipated by the lake people who fought its development. The town has suffered economically in recent years, so its residents have been much more in favor of the track. There is a town-lake tension. The lake people are conservative and those whom I know consider me such a flaming liberal and feminist that they treat me gingerly. I am fully stereotyped in their minds. The topics which can be discussed are very limited, and I would simply die on the vine if I had to live here all the time. Summers and weekends are okay because I work–the computer is here and I can lug up books and other resources. We import members of the department and other folks like that for weekends (no one wanted to come this winter since there was no snow and just icky weather).

In addition to the work and the university, I maintain my pervasive identity as a sociologist by going to meetings with others of my ilk. I love meetings–if they are not too long or too close together. I can talk with people interested in my areas, and in a whole lot of other things (I am more likely to agree with sociologists on basic values than with the Delavan crowd), eat, drink, and have fun. I find the Midwest Sociological Society a great pleasure and do not even mind the ASA meetings. I have become much more involved in the international world of sociology in recent years, not surprising in view of my strange background. Teddy used to travel with me, but is now fully settled down and owns a landscaping and snow plowing business. (She finally got a teaching degree in social sciences but could not find a job in the area, so became an entrepreneur.)

I believe that it would be a mistake for me to retire from the university. I am of an age in which this will not be necessary, and I enjoy the relations and the resources too much. The active sociologists whom I have known who did retire, without the advantages provided by some universities, have phased out of total involvement in this social world. I would hate that. In fact, I have started, with the help of several Midwest Council for Social Research on Aging colleagues, a study of the "phasing out and hanging in" processes of academics. That's to do after the Polish Americans and an overall widowhood book. It looks like a full and pleasant future. By the way, while I was at Boston College, I was almost headed for bypass surgery, but an angiogram preceding it discovered two aneurysms, which make my system not too efficient, but appear not to be too dangerous. Getting rid of anxiety is great.

[May 9, 1992. Back to the Polish Americans. We leave for Taiwan next week for a conference of the Family Research Committee of the ISA. I give a paper there and at a local university, and Dick promises to stay away until that is over. We then go to China for a vacation tour.]

[May 22, 1999]

All the above was written seven years ago, and I have not seen it since, having mailed the disk to Marvin Sussman, as directed by him. It was a pleasure to hear from Sue Steinmetz with the news that she and Gary Peterson have taken over editing *Marriage & Family Review* and will include our autobiographies in a forthcoming volume.

Much has happened in these years, the most important event being Dick's illness and death. I finally experienced the grief work and identity reconstruction about which I had been studying and writing since 1968. Several people have asked me what I find unexpected about this, and I guess my answer is the extent of emotionality involved in the process. A major reason for the extent and breadth of the emotions and sentiments was the way in which Dick took his illness and death. He had not been to a doctor in years but seemed to suspect that something was wrong, so finally went to his Delavan doctor in 1992 and was sent to Lakeland hospital for tests. I had stayed in Chicago to attend a "work in progress" of the sociology department, held at Kirsten Gronbjerg and Gerry Suttles' home. On the way out, I twisted my foot. Upon arrival in Delavan, I learned that Dick had been in the hospital undertaking tests for the past two days. The memories are vague for both Teddy and me, but when I got to the hospital, he told me that they had found diabetes and probably prostate cancer. He then sent me to the emergency room to have my foot examined–they found a small broken bone and put me in one of those boots that serve as a cast. We came home and then started the long process of convincing ourselves that the diagnosis was true. Dick was convinced that he had osteoarthritis, which was the cause of his back pain. Dr. Deraza got cancer specialists to look at the tests and talk to Dick both at Lakeland and at Beloit hospital. The University of Wisconsin at Madison had cancer specialists who came occasionally to see patients in Beloit. The decision was finally made for radiation. Dick told the children at Christmas when all came to our new house. I had to finish the fall semester teaching, so I took Dick to Beloit on Mondays and Fridays, and Teddy took him Tuesdays, Wednesdays and Thursdays. He regaled her with his stories on the way there, so she gave him a tape recorder to preserve these stories for Christmas. He unexpectedly got furious that we were trying to bury him and would not use the recorder. After the treatment, he would sleep on the way home. That summer we went to Budapest for the International Gerontological Congress. Dick accompanied me with all his diabetes equipment. I gave a scientific paper and was so full of myself that I did not pay attention to my purse, which slid back when we were getting on a streetcar, and someone stole my wallet with the passport. That was a special problem since I am a naturalized citizen, and the American embassy had to cable Washington to verify my citizenship. I had another speech so Dick had to return to the embassy to get it. The embassy was filled with other people with the same pin (the congress gave us all pins to travel freely around Budapiest–a giveaway that we were foreigners). Dick managed tourism in that city, and we even took boats and trains to Vienna and Prague. We had never been to Prague, and we were enchanted.

I went to the Gerontological Society of America meetings that November and found Dick crying when I returned. He was convinced that as soon as he died, I would find another man who would waste all that we had collected in almost 50 years of marriage. From that time until his death on July 13, 1994, he was very depressed. He even stopped playing solitaire, which he had done by the hour. We went to a psychiatrist to see if he could regain emotional balance, but he had begun reliving his father's accidental death and being sent to a military school by his mother. She did not want him living in the tough neighborhood in which she had a grocery store and so she went to Marshall Fields for advice about a school for him, paid for with the insurance money. The school was in a small town west of Chicago in Illinois, and she left him there for six years. Even during the summer, she would visit him, but not take him back home. He felt completely deserted, especially since she had boyfriends.

Dick actually did not have much pain, at least he said so, but we finally asked the Lakeland hospice program to help us with his health and care. The head of the program and Teddy even carried a hospital bed from the hospital to our home when Dick finally felt that he could not climb the stairs to the bedroom any more. The bed was enormously heavy and I am still in wonder about the ability of these two women to move it. The hospice people were great, and, for the final days, I had a fulltime nurse stay here. Dick died gradually, his system shutting down until death. The nurse told me that he would not die for a few days, so I rushed down to the university to tie up loose ends. Subsequently, however, I was reached by Wanda, Dick's sister, who came to be with him those last days, who said that he died peacefully without gaining consciousness. Stefan came and stayed with me that first week. Poor Teddy had a double shock because Dennis collapsed the day Dick died, and they found that he has Parkinson's disease. Finally, new medication is making him feel better, and he has a good job and has been commodore of our Delavan Lake Yacht Club.

Dick wanted to be cremated, so we had a "celebration of life" reception at home, and then Teddy scattered his ashes in the lake. We planted a river willow at the Yacht Club. It is doing well.

I had been asked by David Klein and Bert Adams to put together all I knew from my studies and those that followed about widowhood for their *Understanding Families* series of books for Sage (Lopata, 1996). I was in the middle of this effort when Dick was diagnosed and died. It was possibly a good thing for me to have to work through the grief and associated emotions by writing, as I had always used this as a means of catharsis. The whole experience made me realize how dependent I had actually been upon Dick and being married, in spite of my great independence and identity as a sociologist. Self-concepts and identities had to be reconstructed, a process that is still taking place and probably will the rest of my life.

My friends at Loyola, especially Kathy McCourt, Peter Whalley, and Judy Wittner, convinced me to delay retirement so as not to lose too much at the same time. Last May (1999), I finally became a senior scholar or emerita. This means that I teach one course a year, the spring semester, and have office space and the use of university facilities. That has been great. The retirement party was tremendous, with people coming from as far as Britain. People ask me how am I enjoying retirement–and I must explain that one does not retire from being a scholar. I still write books, articles, chapters, and edit my own and others' works. I attend seminars and conferences with my papers, correspond (thanks to e-mail often too much) with a variety of people.

My main focus at present is on *The Cosmopolitan Community of Scholars,* which gives me an excuse to go everywhere, talk and read about everything. Not bad for a 73-year-old woman with many identities and complexities of the self-concept.

In the meantime, I have been spending more time at Delavan and have developed friendships with two groups of women. We eat, play crazy games, go to movies and talk. It is good to have friends in both places.

EDITORS' NOTE

During the 1990s, Lopata also edited *Friendship in Context* (1991) and authored *Polish Americans* (1994), *Circles and setting: Role changes of American women* (1994), and *Current widowhood: Myths and realities* (1996).

REFERENCES

Lopata, H. Z. (1965). The Function of Voluntary Associations in an Ethnic Community: Polonia. In E. Burgess & D. Brogue (Eds.) *Contributions to Urban Sociology* (pp. 203-223). Chicago: University of Chicago Press.

Lopata, H. Z. (1971). *Occupation: Housewife.* New York: Oxford University Press.

Lopata, H. Z. (1973). *Widowhood in an American city* Cambridge, MA: Schenkman.

Lopata, H. Z. (1976). *Polish Americans: Status competition in an ethnic community.* Englewood Cliffs, NJ: Prentice-Hall.

Lopata, H. Z. (1979). *Women as widows: Support systems.* New York: Elsevier-North Holland.

Lopata, H. Z. (Ed.) (1987a). *Widows: The Middle East, Asia and the Pacific.* Durham, NC: Duke University Press. Volume I.

Lopata, H. Z. (Ed.) (1987b). *Widows: North America.* Durham, NC: Duke University Press volume II

Lopata, H. Z. (Ed.) (1990a). *Current research on occupations and professions: Societal influences.* (Volume 5). Greenwich CT: JAI Press.

Lopata, H. Z. (Eds.) (1991). *Friendship in context.* Greenwich, CT: JAI Press.
Lopata, H. Z. (1994a). *Polish Americans.* New Brunswick, NJ: Transaction. Second Revised Edition with chapter by Mary Patrice Erdmans.
Lopata, H. Z. (1994b). *Circles and settings: Role changes of American women.* Albany: State University of New York.
Lopata, H. Z. (1996). *Current widowhood: Myths and realities.* Newbury Park, CA: Sage. with chapter by Annette Prosterman.
Lopata, H. Z. (Ed.) (1998). *Current research on occupations and professions: Settings and Circles* (Volume 10). Greenwich, CT: JAI Press.
Lopata, H. Z., Barnewolt, D., & Miller, C. A. (1985). *City women: Work, jobs, occupations, careers: Chicago* (Volume II). New York: Praeger.
Lopata, H. Z., Barnewolt, D., & Harrison, K. (Eds.) (1987). *Current research on occupations and professions: A research annual* (Volume 4) Greenwich, CT: JAI Press.
Lopata, H. Z., & Brehm, H. (1986). *Widows and dependent wives: From social problem to federal policy.* New York: Praeger.
Lopata, H. Z., & Figert, A. (Eds.) (1996). *Current research on occupations and professions: Getting down to business* (Volume 9). Greenwich, CT: JAI Press.
Lopata, H. Z, Glazer, N., & Wittner, J. (Eds.) (1980). *Research on the interweave of social roles: Women and men.* (Volume I). Greenwich, CT: JAI Press.
Lopata, H. Z., & Henson, K. (Eds.). (1999). *Current research on occupations and professions: Unusual occupations and unusually organized occupations.* (Volume 2). Greenwich, CT: JAI Press.
Lopata, H. Z., & Maines, D. (Eds.). (1981). *Research on the interweave of social roles: Friendship.* (Volume 2). Greenwich, CT: JAI Press.
Lopata, H. Z., Miller, C. A., & Barnewolt, D. (1984). *City Women: Work, Jobs, Occupations, Careers: America* (Vol 1). New York: Praeger.
Lopata, H. Z., & Noel, J. R. (1967). The Dance Studio: Style Without Sex. *Transaction/Society* 4(3), 10-17. Reprinted in G. Stone, (Ed.) *Sports, Games and Power.* New Brunswick, NJ: E. P. Dutton.
Lopata, H. Z., & Pleck, J. (Eds.) (1983). *Research on the interweave of social roles: Families and jobs.* (Volume 3) Greenwich, CT: JAI Press.
Thomas, W. I., & Znaniecki, F. (1927). *The Polish peasant in Europe and America (2 vols.)* (2nd ed.). NY: Knopf (Original, 1919).
Znaniecki, F. W. (1919). *Cultural Reality.* Chicago: University of Chicago Press.
Znaniecki, F. W. (1965). *Social Relations and Social Roles.* San Francisco: Chandler Publishing Co.

My Biographical Self: A Brief Sketch

Viktor Gecas

KEYWORDS. Autobiography, childhood, career, identity, faculty

ORIGINS

I have been interested in matters of self and identity, of who we are and how we came to be this way, for a very long time. Some of this interest is probably due to the turbulent social and historical conditions in which I was born and some to my propensity to reflect on the past in trying to make sense of self and society.

I was born in the spring of 1942 in a small town in Lithuania. World War II was raging in Europe, and Lithuania was caught up in the conflict and chaos, a pawn (along with its Baltic neighbors, Latvia and Estonia) in the politics and conflict between Germany and Russia. From 1939 to 1945, Lithuania was occupied first by the Russians, as part of the deal Russia got in the German-Soviet Nonaggression Pact; then by the Germans when they broke the treaty and attacked Russia; then by the Russians again as they pushed the German army westward. The year 1942 was a pivotal year in the war. The tide was starting to turn against Germany, with defeats in Russia and North Africa. But the outcome was still very much in doubt. Three years later, World War II was over, Europe was in ruins, and there were millions of refugees, including my family.

My earliest memories are of the night we left Lithuania. I'm not sure if they are strictly my memories or those of my mother, who has recounted the story of our exodus to me many times. In any case, they are vivid and dramatic in my mind. I was 2 1/2 years old in late October of 1944 when my family left our home in Taurage, Lithuania, fleeing the advancing Russian army moving west. That night the war was all around us, with bombs and artillery shells exploding everywhere. My mother grabbed me from my crib and ran out of the house for fear the house would be bombed. She jumped into a nearby ditch for safety. From there I looked up and saw warplanes–some were dropping bombs, some were strafing the ground. One flew low to the ground and almost hit a house. It was spectacular! My father got a horse and wagon from the barn and loaded it with provisions. Decisions of great consequence had to be made immediately: who would leave, perhaps forever, and who would stay. The old folks (my maternal grandparents who owned the small farm) stayed behind with some of their children. The young adults with their young children (two families) and those without children (two aunts and an uncle) left in the wagons that night, and became part of the mass of refugees on the crowded roads heading west.

We spent almost a year on the road, occasionally stopping to work for local farmers in exchange for food and shelter, and continually seeking safe haven from the war. It was during one of these stops at a German farm somewhere in Bavaria that my sister, Irene, was born under very difficult circumstances. Amazingly, she and my mother survived. I am still amazed at the courage, fortitude, and resourcefulness of my parents during the war years. We were also very lucky. For example, we stopped in Dresden for a while with many other refugees, but left the city for better prospects two weeks before the allied firebombing that leveled the city. From my mother's account, there were many such close calls and lucky escapes.

So much of life is based on luck. I was very lucky to have the parents I got. They were excellent parents and wonderful people. My father was actually born in America, in Chicago, of Lithuanian parents. At the age of eleven, he and his family emigrated to Lithuania. There he settled, went to school, and (lucky for me) met and married my mother. As a young man, my father was a church organist and a parish scribe, recording births, deaths, etc., in the parish records. When we came to America, there was not much need for these talents. He found work as a machinist in a large factory and worked at that job until his retirement.

The phrase "salt of the earth" applies well to my father. He was a hard worker, forthright and steadfast, a rock of dependability and responsibility, stubborn but caring. He was of the old school of manliness: strong and stoic, but also kind and caring. He didn't talk about his troubles. For that matter, he didn't talk much at all. He was a hard man to know, but he was always there when needed. He wasn't overly strict, but his word was law in the family. My sisters and I respected and obeyed him.

My mother was the emotional anchor in the family, the center of love and affection. To me and my sisters, she was the primary nurturer, teacher, and socializer. She was kind and generous, sentimental and expressive, and wise. It was easy to know and to love my mother. She was used to caring for others. Within her family of origin, she was the second oldest in a family of nine brothers and sisters. During much of her childhood, she had the major responsibility for caring for her younger siblings.

Although my mother only had a high school education, she was widely read and greatly valued education. She would read me Lithuanian stories and folktales, most of which involved some type of moral lesson, as well as classics from other languages which had been translated into Lithuanian. Most of what I know of Lithuania, of the war years, and of my extended kin, I learned from my mother.

At the end of the war, we settled in a refugee camp in the Bavarian region of southern Germany. The camp (fortunately located in the American sector) was a converted medieval castle, Shoenfield Castle, housing several hundred refugees, mostly Lithuanians. The castle had rather primitive living quarters, but it was much better than what we were used to, and for the kids in the camp, it was a great place to live. We could play in the huge courtyard and the surrounding countryside, explore the dungeons, and pretend we were knights of old. We lived in the castle for four years, longer than many of the other refugees. This was due to the difficulties involved in obtaining permission to emigrate to the United States and to my bad health. I was a sickly child, contracting not only most of the common childhood illnesses, but also becoming sick with tuberculosis. But eventually I recovered, and, in 1949, we got permission to emigrate to America.

We crossed the Atlantic in an old converted German battleship. The journey took ten days or so. For me it was a great experience being on a huge ship on the ocean, seeing dolphins and whales for the first time, eating ice cream. Even the stormy weather was exciting. For my mother, it was a miserable trip. She was four months pregnant with my youngest sister, Violet, and had morning sickness and sea sickness the whole time. Violet was born five months later in Chicago, a healthy, happy baby.

GROWING UP IN CHICAGO

We arrived in America in October of 1949 and settled in Chicago because that is where my father's godmother lived. She was our sponsor. Without sponsorship (i.e., someone guaranteeing housing and support for you) immigration to the United States would have been denied. In that case, we would have gone either to Canada or to Australia (as did our refugee relatives and friends), which had much more lenient immigration policies. Chicago had, and still has, a substantial Lithuanian population, perhaps the largest outside of Lithuania. Although we did not live in a Lithuanian neighborhood, having a Lithuanian community in the city helped us in adjusting to this new country.

Chicago in the 1950s was a good place and time to grow up. My childhood and adolescence in Chicago were quite stable and ordinary, compared to the turbulent and difficult early years. We settled in a blue collar neighborhood on the south side, 56th and Racine. It was an ethnically mixed neighborhood composed mostly of 2nd and 3rd generation Irish, Polish, Italian, and other European stock, who were mostly Catholic.

Within the first week or two of settling into the neighborhood, my parents enrolled me in the local public school, Oliver Wendell Holmes Elementary. I spoke no English and no one else spoke Lithuanian at the school, and the customs and routines were strange to me. When the recess bell rang that first day, I thought it was time to go home, so I headed out. But I didn't know where home was and got lost. Fortunately, a friendly policeman found me and somehow got me back to the school. I was miserable those first few weeks and begged my parents to send me to a school where at least some of the teachers spoke Lithuanian. But we didn't live near any such schools. My mother consoled me by saying, "You're a smart boy, Viktoras, and you will learn English fast. And when you do you will like school." She was right. After a few weeks, I started feeling comfortable in school. After a few months, I could speak English as well as the other kids. By the end of the school year, I was one of the best students in my grade.

My first friend in the neighborhood was a boy named Roger. He lived two houses from me and was a year older. Our initial interaction consisted of playing catch with a ball. We didn't talk to each other at first, since I spoke no English. He would throw a ball to me and I would throw it back. We became best friends. He taught me much about American ways. I think he took me on as his socialization project, expanding the English proficiency I was learning at school with the more colorful vernacular used in the neighborhood. He also brought me into his network of friends, six or seven other neighborhood boys. We were a close group throughout grade school and high school, spending almost all of our free time together–playing games and sports, going to the movies, and hanging out. We formed a neighborhood gang, the Jesters, as a symbol of solidarity and identity. Chicago was known for its youth gangs. But ours was not one of the "known" gangs. We were generally law-abiding, non-violent, and we were few in number (seven). We managed to avoid confrontations with other, more notorious gangs. But we did have our gang jackets (maroon and gray), and we wore them proudly wherever we went.

My neighborhood friends and my school friends were two separate and non-overlapping groups. All of my neighborhood friends were Roman Catholic and went to Catholic schools. My family was also Catholic, but I went to public schools because it was cheaper. The differences between my neighborhood and school friends became more evident in high school. My school, Lindblom High School, was a large inner-city school, similar to other city schools and to the Catholic high schools in the area. However, it had a special curriculum for those students identified as "college prospects." Thirty of us were part of this college-bound program. We took the same classes together in all of the core subjects, and we had the best teachers. All of us went on to college. None of my neighborhood friends went to college, except for Roger, who tried college for one year, dropped out, and joined the army.

I liked school. I liked learning, and I liked the other activities associated with school: sports, school-yard play, and, especially, art. I loved to draw and paint. By the fifth grade, I was considered the school artist. My paintings and murals covered the walls of our school. For every major holiday I would do large thematic paintings. My fifth grade teacher, Mrs. Janis, was especially instrumental in developing my artistic interests and talents. She nominated me for a fine arts program at the Art Institute of Chicago for public school kids. The Art Institute conducted classes on Saturday afternoons in painting and composition, figure drawing, and art history. I started going to these Saturday classes when I was in sixth grade and continued through high school. Every Saturday during the school year I would take the "El" (elevated) train to downtown. The art classes would last an hour to an hour and a half. Afterwards, I would spend several hours downtown–going to the Field Museum (my favorite natural history museum), checking out the book stores on Wabash, wandering through Marshall Field and the shops on State Street, or seeing the new exhibits at the Art Institute. I loved my Saturday afternoons.

Throughout grade school and high school, I thought of myself as an artist and considered some type of artistic career as my eventual destination. These thoughts continued into the college years, where I took a number of classes in painting, sculpture, and figure drawing. But my interest began to change sometime in my sophomore year. I started thinking that it would be hard to make a living as an artist, that many serious artists go hungry. Also, I was becoming interested in the social sciences and an intellectual career became increasingly appealing. So for me, art slipped from the status of career goal to a life-long avocation. As it turns out, my oldest son, Erik, is an artist. He has an MFA degree in sculpture and has ambitions to be another Piccaso. In the meantime, he's driving a UPS truck to pay the rent. But he lives for his art. I'm proud of my son who, unlike me, is willing to risk hunger and to live a minimalist lifestyle for a career in art.

THE COLLEGE YEARS

By the time I graduated from high school, I was ready and eager to leave home and go to college. I'm not sure why I picked Beloit College, a small liberal arts college in Wisconsin, rather than go to the University of Illinois downstate, where most of my high school friends went. I had a scholarship to

Beloit that covered my tuition. Savings from summer jobs covered most of the rest. Still, it would not have been any more expensive to go to the state school. Looking back, I think Beloit was a good choice. The classes were small, with lots of student-faculty interaction, lots of individualized instruction, many writing assignments, and good teachers. Also, I met my future wife there.

Most of the students at Beloit were from upper middle class backgrounds and came from the well-to-do suburbs of Chicago. Some, like my wife, came from small towns and suburbs in New England. Very few came from the inner city of Chicago. I liked being different in that respect. I even wore my gang jacket that first year to distinguish myself from the preppies from suburbia. But before long I became one of them. I joined a fraternity, partied with sorority girls, went out for college sports, and by the end of my second year replaced my gang jacket from Chicago with a letter jacket from Beloit. The Chicago identity was still there, but much less visible.

I loved college–the freedom from parental constraints, the social life, the sports, and even the academics (in that order). If I could extend the duration of one period of my life, it would be the college years. Sports were a big part of my college experience. I've always liked athletics and was a pretty good athlete in our neighborhood pick-up games of baseball, basketball, and touch football, but I didn't have the time for sports in high school. But I did in college. Even though I was a pretty good athlete, I would not have been able to compete in the big time, high pressure athletic programs of most universities. But little Beloit College was just right for my level of talent and dedication to athletics. There were no athletic scholarships at Beloit. And as an athlete, you were still expected to be a good student. You were a student first and foremost, and an athlete second.

I went out for football, track, and wrestling. I was bad at football, not having played it in high school and pretty much ignorant of the basics. I was better at track (the 100 meter dash and the shot put), but it wasn't much fun and the Wisconsin weather in the spring was lousy. My best sport turned out to be wrestling. I was strong and quick, had good balance and stamina. I liked the elemental one-on-one contest matching your strength, stamina, and competence against an opponent's. Wrestling is an individual sport. Other members on the team cheer you on during your match, and there is a strong sense of camaraderie, but the basic contest is one-on-one. I liked that. I was on the wrestling team for four years, wrestling at the 167 pound weight class. About the only thing I didn't like about wrestling was making weight. My normal weight at the time was about 175. So during the wrestling season, I was always hungry.

In my sophomore year, I met Sally Young, my wife-to-be (although it did not seem so at the time). She was the girlfriend of a fraternity brother, so she was off limits. But I was attracted to her. She was tall, attractive, smart, and independent (still is!). As it happened, this fraternity brother had another girlfriend as well. This strained his relationship with Sally and made her fair game. Sally and I started dating at the beginning of my junior and her sophomore year. My social life improved substantially. We continued to go steady until I graduated the following year.

While I was interested in a wide range of academic subjects, I was particularly attracted to the social and behavioral sciences: sociology, psychology, political science, and anthropology. These seemed to deal most directly with my interests in understanding self, society, and the human condition (which was second only to my interest in girls). But I also found courses in biology, geology, philosophy, history, and English literature interesting. And of course, I still liked fine arts. My problem was that I found too many fields interesting and worth studying. Also, most of my professors at Beloit were dedicated teachers with a passion for their subject, which they conveyed to their students. So I had trouble deciding on a field of concentration. At one time or another, I majored in each of the social sciences.

Eventually, it was the influence and inspiration of a sociology professor, Don Summers, that prevailed and commenced my intellectual development as a sociologist. Don Summers was as much a philosopher as a sociologist. He had an incredible intellectual range of interests and used a Socratic style of teaching that required student participation. Each of his classes was an intense seminar on an eminent social thinker. We had seminars on Freud, Sartre, Weber, Mead, and Goffman, which we read in the original (or the English translation) and discussed at great length. I lived in fear of not being prepared when Professor Summers would call on me in class with a question about the readings: "What are the psychological implications of the Oedipus Complex?" "Do you see any problems with Sartre's position on authenticity?" "What is the importance of role-taking in Mead's account of the development of the self?" I did a lot of reading for Don Summer's classes, motivated as much by fear of disappointing my professor as by interest in the subject matter. I don't think I studied as hard in graduate school as I did for Don Summers' classes. By my senior year in college, I had decided I wanted to be a sociology professor like Don Summers.

GRADUATE SCHOOL: UNIVERSITY OF MINNESOTA

In the fall of 1964, I entered graduate school in the Sociology Department at the University of Minnesota. I had applied to several other universities with strong programs in social psychology (Illinois, Iowa, Wisconsin, and Michigan), but the best offer came from Minnesota–an NIMH fellowship in family sociology. Although I was puzzled to be offered a fellowship in family sociology, since I had not expressed any interest in family studies at the time, I eagerly accepted the fellowship.

My first year of graduate school was miserable. I had no friends and was living alone in a strange city. My girlfriend was back in Beloit and neither of us was sure about marriage. I was back at the bottom of the pecking order in school. There was very little effort by faculty or students to integrate the new students into the department. The relationship between graduate students was very competitive, and the new students had to endure a certain amount of intellectual hazing. I wondered if I had made a mistake in coming to Minnesota. The bad weather didn't help either.

Somehow I survived that first year of graduate school, an accomplishment due less to strength of character than to lack of alternatives. In fact, the alternatives were quite grim. The Vietnam war was heating up in 1965 and I was at risk of being drafted if I were not in graduate school. I was so opposed to the war that if drafted, my options would have been either escape to Canada or go to jail. I don't know which I would have chosen. Fortunately, I didn't have to make that decision–although I came close in 1967 when my student deferment was canceled and U.S. mobilization for the war was at its peak.

But 1965 was a major improvement over the previous year, both in my personal life and in graduate school. In June of that year, Sally and I got married, overcoming a year of ambivalence and vacillation between being engaged and being unengaged. It was the right decision, and after 34 years of marriage and five grown children, we wonder why it was such a difficult decision. Being married to Sally made life in Minnesota so much better. We rented a cheery little apartment near campus. She started teaching third grade in the Minneapolis school system while I continued my graduate studies. We discovered that Minneapolis and the surrounding area were full of recreational opportunities: canoeing, fishing, camping, cross-country skiing, and lots of city things to do. Our honeymoon lasted about six years, until we started having kids (more on that later).

Life in graduate school also improved substantially in my second year. That fall, a new and fairly large group of students was admitted to the Family Studies Program. It was a remarkable cohort which included Darwin Thomas, Andy Weigert, Elizabeth Rooney, and Mark Hutter. We became close friends, partly because of the interesting mix of personalities, and also because all the NIMH fellows were housed together in Clay School, an old elementary school located next to the Social Science Building. Old Clay School was a dilapidated building; plaster was falling off the walls, the windows were permanently dirty, and the drinking fountains were about a foot off the ground, and you had to kneel to get a drink. But it was a great place for us. One of the large classrooms in the school served as our common office, where each of us had a little enclave consisting of a desk and bookcase. There was a large table in the middle of the room where we would have lunch together and talk sociology and many other things under the sun. For example, Andy Weigert, with his classical education in the Jesuits, would give us Thomas Aquinas's perspective on the human condition and the moral order. Darwin Thomas would argue for the remarkable compatibility between the new philosophies of science and Mormon theology. Mark Hutter, a native of New York City and a fan of Erving Goffman, was suspicious of people who smiled a lot. David Franks, whom we adopted from the NIMH Deviance program, saw epistemological problems wherever he looked and would point them out to us. Elizabeth Rooney thought San Francisco was the apex of western civilization and wanted the Clay School group to relocate there.

Ecology can be a major factor in the development of social bonds. We spent a lot of time together at the office, in classes, at each other's homes. We talked at great length about what we learned in class, what we recently read, and about the sociology profession, and the peculiarities of individual faculty members. We even organized study groups in preparation for prelim exams. Our Clay School group was an exceptionally rich, stimulating, and supportive environment–so much so that I didn't want it to end. I tried to talk the others into staying on an extra year after the prelim exams while we were working on our dissertations. Four of us were doing dissertations in the area of family socialization, and we included some common measures in each of our studies. We had talked about combining parts of our dissertations into a book on socialization. One more year together at Minnesota, I argued, and we could complete the book. But the others (Darwin, Andy, and Elizabeth) were not as interested in extending their student status an extra year and left for permanent jobs at various universities. I stayed on one more year to finish my dissertation. We did eventually collaborate on a book from our dissertations, *Family Socialization and the Adolescent* (1974), which was published a number of years later.

The Sociology Department at Minnesota in the late 1960s had an impressive group of family scholars on the faculty: Reuben Hill, Murray Straus, Joan Aldous, and Irv Tallman. Reuben Hill was Director of the Family Studies Center. With his stature in the field, prodigious organizational skills, and extensive academic and political networks, Hill made Minnesota the top family studies center in the country. It was a lively place back then. There were always visiting scholars in residence from around the world, and a number of major research projects in progress. I benefited greatly from these faculty. Murray Straus served as chair of my master's thesis. I learned how to do sociological research under his guidance. Reuben Hill was my major professor for my dissertation. Like a wise parent, Hill knew when to push me and when to give me slack; when to criticize and when to give support. I learned much about being a professional sociologist and a mentor from Hill.

Joan Aldous and Irv Tallman provided enlightening and entertaining seminars on family theory and research.

I also benefited from the presence of other sociology faculty: Arnold Rose, Don Martindale, Ed Gross, and, especially, Greg Stone. Stone was the symbolic interactionist guru in the department. He was an intellectual descendant of G. H. Mead via Erving Goffman. Stone was an articulate advocate of symbolic interactionism and an impressive teacher, when he wanted to be (which was only during his lecture course in social psychology). Graduate students would transcribe and circulate collections of class notes from Stone's lecture course. Those of us who had any interest in social psychology were heavily influenced by Greg Stone and his brand of symbolic interactionism. I was fortunate to have experienced Stone when he was still near the peak of his intellectual abilities, before his demons and his life style destroyed him.

My interest in socialization and self-concept formation really began to take shape during my last two years at Minnesota, especially as I began to work on my dissertation. The title of my dissertation was: "Parent-Child Interaction and Adolescent Self-Evaluation." Through a questionnaire survey of about 600 high-school students, I examined the effects of parental control and support on various aspects of the adolescents' self-concept (e.g., self-esteem, self-efficacy, identities, and frames of reference). Not surprisingly, I found that parental behavior mattered for offspring's self-conceptions, that parental effects varied by sex and social class of parents and children and by dimensions of self-evaluation, and that parental effects diminished outside the family context. But like most sociological studies, mine raised more questions for me than it answered. And as it happens, I have spent much of my career as a sociologist pursuing some of the themes and questions initially formulated in my dissertation, such as the effectiveness of socialization attempts in the family, the differential antecedents and consequents of self-worth and self-efficacy within the self-concept, contextual variations in self-esteem, and the development of identities. I continue to find endless variations on these themes in my research and theorizing about self and socialization.

CAREER AS A PROFESSOR OF SOCIOLOGY

I left Minnesota in 1969 with a Ph.D. in sociology. The job market for sociologists was very favorable in the late '60s and early '70s. Sociology departments were expanding to meet the increasing interest in social issues generated by the social unrest and cultural upheavals of the times. I wanted to live in the northwest, probably because I thought it would be less crowded and more picturesque than other regions of the country, so I applied to only a few schools in Washington and Oregon. Washington State University made me an offer first. I accepted, and in the summer of 1969 I moved to Pullman, Washington.

While it was easy getting a university job in 1969, it was not easy being a professor then. It was a politically turbulent time on many campuses, including WSU. Student demonstrations against the Vietnam War, campus disruptions over issues of social justice, and challenges to authority at every level were almost daily occurrences. The previous year, while I was still at Minnesota, was certainly a volatile year as well with urban riots, political assassinations, the chaotic Democratic convention in Chicago, etc. But I was so busy writing my dissertation and teaching full time at a local college that I barely noticed. But the campus turbulence at WSU my first year was impossible to ignore. For example, a rumor circulated through campus that militant students from Seattle were coming to WSU to torch buildings. The rumor was taken seriously, since someone had torched the football stadium and attempted to set fire to the ROTC building the previous month. Security of university buildings was increased. This consisted mainly of recruiting professors to do nightly guard duty in the classroom and office buildings. I had the 3:00 to 5:00 a.m. shift on one of those nights. I wonder what I would have done if I had actually encountered a "terrorist" during my watch. Fortunately, nothing happened that night, nor that week. The rumor proved to be false. But those were indeed tense times on campus. Eventually, things settled down on campus. The Vietnam War ended and political protest on campus essentially disappeared. Students returned to more traditional pursuits: studies, football, and beer parties. I focused my energies on being a professor, and on becoming established in the profession.

Most of my early publications came out of my dissertation and dealt with parental effects on children's self-concepts. They were generally framed within symbolic interactionist ideas about the development of self-conceptions in social interaction and the importance of meanings in interpreting behavior and defining situations (Gecas, 1971; 1972). But I was also interested in examining how the larger social structural and cultural contexts affect these micro interaction processes (Gecas et al., 1970; 1972). My intellectual agenda was, and still is, to integrate symbolic interactionist ideas about self and socialization with mainstream sociological ideas about social structure, power, and culture.

In my second year at WSU, I accepted an offer to join the Department of Rural Sociology on a half-time research appointment. At the time, the Department of Rural Sociology was a small, primarily research, unit in which each of the five research faculty were on joint appointments with the Sociology Department. It was an advantageous appointment, since it reduced my teaching load by half, increased my salary from 9 months to 12, and provided state money for research projects. There were some costs involved, such as a more applied emphasis in the College of Agriculture where Rural Sociology was located, but the benefits outweighed the costs. Ivan Nye was Chair of Rural Sociology at the time. He wanted greater strength in the family area, so he offered the vacant position to me, and my research took a somewhat different turn, a more applied and problem-focused turn.

My first study, sponsored by the Agriculture Research Center at WSU, was a study of Hispanic farm workers in the Yakima Valley of Washington state. Half the sample were migrant farm workers who followed the crops; the rest of the sample were Hispanic farm workers who had settled in the small towns in the valley. I was interested in studying how poverty, culture, and migrant lifestyle affected family relations, socialization patterns, and self-conceptions. The study involved face-to-face interviews with four family members (father, mother, and two children) in about 200 families. Little did I know what I was getting into in doing this study. There were obstacles and vested interests at every turn. For starters, the campus Chicanos, especially the faculty of the Chicano Studies Program, took a dim view of an "Anglo" studying "their people." They threatened to sabotage the study unless they were brought in as consultants. In the summer of 1972, when I was conducting the study, the political climate in the Yakima valley was tense. Caesar Chavez was trying to unionize the farm workers in the valley, efforts which were strongly resisted by the farmers and farm corporations. I had hired about 20 local Hispanics through community colleges in the area as interviewers. In spite of considerable public relations work on my part, both sides in the labor dispute were suspicious of the research project. A number of the farmers and farm managers refused my interviewers access to the labor camps. Some of the families were reluctant to participate for fear of reprisals from the employers. Eventually, the study was completed. But it was a huge effort, and the scientific payoff was meager (Gecas, 1973, 1980). However, it was a valuable learning experience for me in the politics of minority research, especially when vested interests are perceived to be threatened.

Several other applied, state-supported research projects followed over the next decade or so: a large study of injured workers, sponsored by the Washington Department of Labor and Industries and a large study of welfare mothers in the state. Both studies were politically charged and involved a lot of public relations work to explain and justify the scientific effort. It was stressful and exhausting, and I became convinced that this was not how I wanted to spend my time. Life in the ivory tower pursuing primarily intellectual challenges was much more appealing. So I backed off from doing applied and problem-focused research. By then I was well established at the university and had greater flexibility in my choice of research topics. Besides, the Department and the College were supportive of just about any kind of research I might do in the family area. This led to a number of research projects on more general populations dealing with family role dynamics (Gecas, 1976; Nye & Gecas, 1976); the development of social competencies in children (Gecas & Schwable, 1986; Gecas & Seff, 1989); and socialization into marital roles, a longitudinal study of the first five years of marriage (Tallman, Burke, & Gecas, 1998). To be sure, these studies had some practical implications for family relations, socialization practices, and individual and family well-being. But the main purpose of these research projects was scientific, i.e., testing ideas about family interactions and individual outcomes derived from general sociological theories, particularly from symbolic interactionism and social exchange theories.

It is not always evident how one's personal life affects one's academic interests, although I'm sure it does. For example, favoring theories that have generally optimistic or pessimistic views of family relations may be a function of one's own happy or unhappy family circumstances. Family stresses and disruptions may heighten one's sensitivity to these aspects of family life, and to the theories that address them. Having children may alter one's perspective on life, on oneself, and on family relations. It did for me.

Sally and I had our first child, Erik, in 1971, and then four more at about two-year intervals. We didn't plan it this way (we only planned the first two as I recall), but we're happy with the outcome. We have four sons and a daughter: Erik, David, Joe, Ben, and Kathy. All very different and very interesting kids (young adults now). Erik is an artist, David a zoologist and also a good artist, Joe a college football player, Ben a banker and father, and Kathy a college student. Our youngest, Kathy, left for college this fall (1999), so the end of our active parenting years is in sight, and the heavy-duty aspects of it are over. None too soon, since we're exhausted. I liked being a father. It certainly was challenging, often stressful, but also very rewarding. I felt important and needed. Parenthood revealed aspects of my personality that I had not seen (e.g., patience, but also a temper) and also developed some aspects that had not been there (e.g., wisdom in adjudicating disputes). It also showed me aspects of my wife that I had not known–she is an excellent mother. Parenthood also affected my thinking about family dynamics, socialization, and self-concept formation. This effect was mostly humbling. I was much more of an "authority" on socialization before having children than after. That is, I lectured and wrote on socialization with greater confidence and certitude in my knowledge before becoming a parent. And my confidence in socialization theories and research seemed to decline as the kids got older. I became much more aware of the limits of parental influence and on the effects children have on parents (e.g., on my self-concept, self-efficacy, and self-esteem); on the importance of sibling relations in children's development; on the influence of peer groups; on how marital relations are affected by children; and on the ability of children to resist socialization attempts and assert their own will. Some of my publications reflect these new sensitivities, such as, "Beyond the looking-glass self" (Gecas & Schwalbe, 1983); "Birth order and self-concept in adolescence" (Gecas & Pasley, 1983); "The motivational significance of self-concept for socialization theory" (Gecas, 1986).

When I entered the "launching stage" of the family life course, which is now nearing its completion, my scholarly interests shifted from the primacy of the parent-child bond to the marital bond. Over much of the past decade, I have been involved, with Irv Tallman and Peter Burke, in a longitudinal study of marital relations: "Socialization into Marital Roles." We followed a sample (300) of newly married couples for five years, investigating (by means of extensive interviews, video-taped interaction, and daily diaries) how husbands and wives socialize each other into marital and gender roles, how self-conceptions stabilize and change, how processes of communication and conflict affect marital commitment and individual well-being. The data analysis for this project will continue for some time.

I continue to be interested in theoretical and empirical issues surrounding self and socialization: how parents and children affect each other (Gecas & Seff, 1990); how the larger structural and cultural contexts within which families live affect processes of socialization and self-concept formation (Gecas, 1979); and how the self as a source of motivation affects the process of its own socialization (Gecas & Burke, 1995).

Autobiographies typically are written at the end of a career. I don't think I am there yet. According to my pension plan, I still have about a decade to go. So this essay is more of a mid-term (or a little later) retrospective, a reflection on the road traveled so far. The road ahead does not look as long, but hopefully it will continue to be productive and fulfilling, and, with the kids finally off on their own, more peaceful.

REFERENCES

Gecas. V. (1971). Parental behavior and dimensions of adolescent self-evaluation. *Sociometry, 34,* 4, 466-482.

Gecas, V. (1972). Parental behavior and contextual variations in adolescent self-esteem. *Sociometry 35,* 2, 332-345.

Gecas, V. (1973). Self-conceptions of migrant and settled Mexican-Americans. *Social Science Quarterly, 54,* 3, 579-595.

Gecas, V. (1976). The child care and socialization roles. In F.I. Nye (Ed.), *Role structure and analysis in the family* (pp. 33-59). Beverly Hills: Sage Publications.

Gecas, V. (1979). The influence of social class on socialization. In W.R. Burr, R. Hill, I.L. Reiss, & F.I. Nye (Eds.), *Contemporary theories about the family,* Vol. 1 (pp. 365-404). New York: The Free Press.

Gecas, V. (1980). Family structural influences on the educational and occupational aspirations of migrant and settled Mexican-Americans. *Rural Sociology, 45,* 2, 272-289.

Gecas, V. (1986). The motivational significance of self-concept for socialization theory. In E. J. Lawler (Ed.), *Advances in group processes: Theory and research,* Vol. 3 (pp. 131-156). Greenwich, CT: JAI Press.

Gecas, V. & Burke, P. (1995). Self and Identity. In K. Cook, G.A. Fine, & J. House (Eds.), *Sociological perspectives in social psychology* (pp. 41-67). Boston: Allyn and Bacon.

Gecas, V. & Pasley, K. (1983). Birth order and self-conception in adolescence. *Journal of Youth and Adolescence, 12,* 6, 521-535.

Gecas, V. & Schwalbe, M. (1983). Beyond the looking-glass self: social structure and efficacy-based self-esteem. *Social Psychology Quarterly, 46,* 2, 77-78.

Gecas, V. & Schwalbe, M. (1986). Parental behavior and adolescent self-esteem. *Journal of Marriage and the Family, 48,* 1, 37-46.

Gecas, V. & Seff, M. (1989). Social class, occupational conditions and self-esteem. *Sociological Perspectives, 32,* 3, 353-364.

Gecas, V., Thomas, D., & Weigert, A. (1970). Perceived parent-child interaction and boys' self-esteem in two cultural contexts. *International Journal of Comparative Sociology, 11,* 4, 317-324.

Gecas, V., Thomas, D., & Weigert, A. (1973). Social identities in Anglo and Latin adolescents. *Social Forces, 51,* 4, 477-484.

Nye, F.I. & Gecas, V. (1976). The role concept: Review and delineation. In F.I. Nye (Ed.), *Role Structure and analysis in the family* (pp. 3-14). Beverly Hills: Sage Publications.

Tallman, I., Burke, P., & Gecas, V. (1998). Socialization into marital roles: Testing a contextual, developmental model of marital functioning. In T.N. Bradbury (Ed.), *The developmental course of marital dysfunction* (pp. 312-342). Cambridge University Press.

Thomas, D., Gecas, V., Weigert, A., & Rooney, E. (1974). *Family socialization and the adolescent: Determinants of self-concept, religiosity, conformity, and counter-culture values.* Lexington, MA: D.C. Heath and Co.

Exploring and Defining Early Social Ecologies and Their Impact: Mothers, Fathers, Families, and Cultures

Michael E. Lamb

KEYWORDS. Autobiography, researcher, career, child development, fatherhood

The great Danish philosopher Søren Kierkegaard wrote in 1843 that "Life must be understood backward [although] it must be lived forward." His perceptive observation challenges developmental psychologists like myself, who strive to understand, explain, and predict developmental trajectories, and is also apt in the present context. In the course of reviewing and explaining our own intellectual odysseys, it is difficult not to emphasize the bold lines that connect events and reveal the continuity that most of us perceive in our lives. Such reconstructions, of course, often give inadequate attention to key decision points at which alternate and equally defensible choices might have presaged much different trajectories. Furthermore, retrospective accounts often ignore the unexpected events that can play havoc with even the most careful planning. As another rebellious youth named John Lennon wrote six generations after Kierkegaard, "Life is what happens while you're busy making other plans." Readers should thus be forewarned that this essay is not the account I might have constructed contemporaneously in a diary, and emphasizes my career as a family social scientist, ignoring both my own family life and my research on other research topics (such as forensic interview techniques).

ACT I: YOUTHFUL IDEALISM

When I entered the University of Natal, Durban campus (UND) in 1970, shortly after my 16th birthday, I neither planned to become a social scientist nor even recognized the existence of such an option. At the time, I was passionately interested in politics and had little doubt that I would be one of the politicians leading South Africa toward the post-colonial multiracialism that I had observed in Northern Rhodesia/Zambia, the land of my birth. Despite this conviction, my approach to undergraduate study reflected the aversion to risk and the philosophical commitment to multi-determination and over-preparation that have marked the subsequent years of my life as well. Because most politicians and political leaders then (as now) were trained as lawyers, for example, I expected to study law and I was able to take enough legal courses as an undergraduate that my post-graduate law degree could be obtained in two rather than three years. In addition, I reasoned that competent political leaders needed to understand the behavior and motivations of their contemporaries; therefore, I selected psychology and economics as my majors.

As I carefully chose the disciplines needed to prepare me for a life in politics, ironically, I overlooked two of the most glaring reasons why my career choice was a poor one. For a start, South Africa offered a political climate that was quite inhospitable to a young man ideologically committed to civil rights, democracy, and economic equality. In addition, as I was to learn through bitter experience, I had absolutely no acumen for the realities of political combat. I saw politics as a rarefied conflict between grand ideas and ideals, with the best ideas likely to prevail following logical debate and analysis. The fact that ideology was often used merely to attain or maintain power completely escaped me. To make matters worse, my naiveté was readily apparent to my more politically astute colleagues and competitors, ensuring that I was regularly manipulated into positions that seemed superficially consistent with my grand ideals but had consequences completely at variance with my goals. Furthermore, the national election of 1970, which I expected to represent a turning point in the political evolution of South Africa, resulted in a national government that looked depressingly like the one that proceeded it.

Disillusionment led me to refocus my efforts towards the end of 1970, and, as I did so, I became intrigued by the psychological and economic theories I encountered. I was particularly excited in 1971 when John Bowlby's (1969) masterful integration of psychoanalytic thought, ethological theory, and control systems theory in his book, *Attachment*, and Piaget's (1952) *The Origins of Intelligence in Children* were chosen as the central readings for a unit on developmental psychology taught by the most engaging lecturer in the department, Veronica Albino. Bowlby and Piaget were "big" thinkers and Albino (a psychoanalyst by training) eloquently amplified their shared belief that early experiences helped shape the course of later development. More than that, babies seemed pure, as yet unsullied by the crassness that characterized "meaningful relationships" (read 'politics') among adults. I was hooked. Meanwhile, economic theorists such as Keynes, Marx, Samuelson, and Sen (those I remember best) painted on a big canvas too, and because most instructors shared my political values, the pictures they drew were more appealing than the gritty realities on which I had earlier focused.

It would be nice to claim that my newfound commitment to psychology and economics was motivated purely by intellectual zeal, but much of my interest in academic pursuits must in truth be attributed to the realization that my career plans needed revision. The disappointing election results of 1970 had left the few liberal South Africans feeling that political transformation would likely be achieved through violent means, which I abhorred. As a result, my reformist dreams shifted to the international arena. I could not study abroad without financial support, however, and I was fortunate to be selected as a finalist for a Rhodes Scholarship, then one of the most lucrative and prestigious awards available in South Africa. Not surprisingly, the other finalists had much more impressive credentials than I did, and I naively sealed my fate by offering an awkward critique of the selection criteria, particularly the exclusion of "future leaders" who were neither white nor male. Unfortunately, my persuasive powers, like my tact, were inadequate to the task!

To my surprise and delight, however, many universities, particularly in North America, offered financial support to foreign students, so opportunities for graduate study in both psychology and economics loomed. As luck would have it, furthermore, a junior lectureship in economics opened at the University of Durban (UD) as I completed my bachelor's degree, and I was enthusiastically recommended by the head of the economics department at UND, George Trotter, who perhaps still harbored hopes that I would switch my growing allegiance from psychology to economics.

The decision to take the position was not easy, however, because University of Durban (UD) was, as one of a handful of new, well-endowed universities, established by the government to provide "separate but equal" tertiary education for members of specific racial/ethnic groups. On the one hand, UD (located in a formerly Indian suburb of Durban) had been established for Indian South Africans, and acceptance of a position at the university involved further complicity with a political system that I despised. On the other hand, it promised an opportunity to become more familiar with non-white South Africans during the months between the end of the Southern academic year in October/November and the start of the Northern academic year in September. In truth, the students at UD were not much impressed by my limp expressions of solidarity, but I was able to earn some respect when my continuing naiveté forced me into an unexpectedly intense confrontation with the government in the spring of 1973. I was identified in the press as a UDW staff member who supported the nationwide student protests, and I quickly learned that it was illegal for UDW lectures to take public political stands. I was immediately asked by the chief administrator of the university to resign, and, although the ensuing publicity provided some protection against outright dismissal, repeated threats of restrictive actions took their toll. I resigned my position in late April and left South Africa hurriedly, further convinced that the prospects for peaceful change were minimal and that my future lay outside Southern Africa, rather than in it.

ACT II: INTELLECTUAL NIRVANA

On Memorial Day of 1973, I arrived in Baltimore, where I planned to study at Johns Hopkins University under the tutelage of Mary Ainsworth, the undisputed "mother of attachment theory" to whom I had been introduced by Veronica Albino. Ainsworth had been a close friend and collaborator of John Bowlby, whose integrative book had drawn my attention to developmental psychology two years before, and Ainsworth's nurturant, attentive, and stimulating care profoundly affected my career. In light of the tremendous impact that she was to have on me, however, it is worth noting that my final "decision" to study with her at Johns Hopkins was entirely fortuitous. I had applied to five or six graduate schools and had been warned against the risks of being apprenticed to a single well-known advisor, which made me hesitant about attending Hopkins. Nevertheless, Johns Hopkins not only sent its letter of acceptance earlier than all the other institutions, but it included a visa authorization form which allowed me to enter the United States. In fact, Johns Hopkins' was the only acceptance letter I received before leaving the country so precipitously, and I thus felt honor-bound to study there. It proved to be a life-transforming stroke of fate.

Compared to my peers, I was in some respects the best prepared and in most respects the least prepared candidate for graduate school. I benefited from an undergraduate education that demanded some familiarity with all areas of psychology whereas most of those entering graduate school with me had been able to study selectively and were thus familiar only with a very narrow range of topics. Although I had never read a scholarly journal and had no familiarity with recent advances in the field, I was able to excel in the required broad 'proseminars' focused on diverse aspects of psychology, and this allowed me to complement my work in developmental psychology with advanced study in neuropsychology, animal behavior, and social psychology. My willingness to tackle topics that most new students avoided gave me unfettered access to two remarkably tolerant and talented faculty members, David Olton and Elliott Blass. Under the guidance of these two men, I undertook, respectively, a never-published study on the role of the limbic system in maternal behavior, and a review of the literature on the physiological bases of maternal behavior in rats that was published, almost without revision, in the prestigious *Psychological Bulletin.* More importantly, these mentors taught me how to evaluate literature in disparate areas and convinced me that an inclusive understanding of phenomena as complex as human attachment had to be broadly based. I never lost interest in the biological bases of behavior, despite subsequent fluctuations in its popularity, and I became eager to explore the sociological and social-psychological contexts more fully as well. I was energetic, single, and impoverished–reading and studying were all I could afford to do–and I quickly mastered the scholarly literature on early social development of which I had been wholly unaware before my arrival in the United States.

Since the early 1960s, Ainsworth had devoted most of her energies to the longitudinal observational study that was to dominate her professional life and secure her standing in the field. With home visits of two to four hours every two to three weeks, Ainsworth compiled copiously detailed notes on early infant-mother interactions that were to keep students such as myself productively occupied for years thereafter. Spurred by the publication of Bowlby's *Attachment* (1969) and by the burgeoning professional awareness of Ainsworth's empirical approach to the validation of attachment theory, talented students had begun seeking the opportunity to work with Ainsworth. Robert Marvin, Barbara Wittig, and Sylvia Bell were thus followed by Mary Blehar, Inge Bretherton, Alicia Lieberman, Mary Main, Everett Waters, and Robert Woodson–most of whom went on to distinguished careers as clinicians or researchers. Thus Ainsworth's last years at Johns Hopkins, including the one I was fortunate enough to share, were marked by extraordinary intellectual excitement as her students coded and analyzed the observational transcripts and began publishing, with Ainsworth, the empirical papers that constituted some of her most enduring contributions to attachment theory.

Ainsworth focused on individual differences in the quality of infant-mother attachments and believed that individual differences in 'secure base' behavior, apparent in the "Strange Situation" procedure she developed, were largely a product of contrasting experiences in the preceding months of the infants' lives (Ainsworth, Blehar, Waters, & Wall, 1978). Infants whose mothers responded sensitively later behaved securely, she argued, whereas those whose mothers were insensitive and unresponsive behaved insecurely in the "Strange Situation." This conceptualization of the ways in which infants were shaped by their earliest social experiences became an integral part of attachment theory and a central component of basic texts on early development. In the hands of Ainsworth and her students, the psychoanalysts' speculation had been turned into empirical fact for the first time.

Fortunately, professional acclaim did not spoil Mary Ainworth's essential decency and commitment. She encouraged my exuberant enthusiasm for attachment theory, offered me the stipend I needed, and did not hesitate to welcome me into her home (and laboratory) when I arrived unexpectedly early in the US. Insightful, complicated, and (at least in my case) naive questions always elicited copiously detailed and meticulously typed responses, many of which I continue to treasure and have often shared with my students and associates.

It was exciting for graduate students such as myself to feel so integrally involved in the revolutionary ascent of attachment theory, although it was also somewhat disconcerting because the most important discoveries appeared to have been made and the next major empirical steps were already being undertaken by Ainsworth's more senior graduate students. To Alicia Lieberman and I, however, it appeared that one obvious question had been ignored: Did individual differences in security of attachment predict aspects of the children's adjustment as they moved into childhood?

Sylvia Bell had shown that differences in attachment security were associated with patterns of cognitive development (a topic I studied in my undergraduate "thesis" at UND), and both Mary Main and Inge Bretherton showed that individual differences in Strange Situation behavior were associated with differences in the patterns of interaction with strange adults. All three dissertations focused on near-contemporaneous associations, however, although Ainsworth, Bowlby, and their psychoanalytic forebears clearly expected the individual differences evident in infancy to have a major impact on the children's later development.

Nevertheless, when Lieberman and I approached Ainsworth to suggest that we jointly re-contact the infants in her longitudinal study, she strongly discouraged a follow-up study, reasoning that it would be too difficult and too risky. We might find no associations between infant experiences and the children's later adjustment, she feared, and such a finding would be misinterpreted, handicapping attachment theory at a vulnerable moment in its struggle for acceptance. I was initially both shocked and disappointed by this reaction, although in retrospect I understand Ainsworth's concerns much better. Her sample was indeed very small and was split into two small cohorts of children who could not (at 12 to 13 and 7 to 8 years of age) be assessed using the same measures. Already sparring with Bettye Caldwell, Jerome Kagan, and Michael Lewis, Ainsworth was decidedly unwilling to bring another controversy onto herself, and, given our dependence on her, Lieberman and I abandoned our nascent plans.

ACT III: UNANTICIPATED OPPORTUNITIES

During the 1973/1974 academic year, three prominent visitors proved especially significant to my own intellectual development. The first was John

Bowlby, Ainsworth's long-time associate, friend, and mentor, who had been attempting to integrate evolutionary theory, developmental psychology, research on animal behavior, psychoanalytic precepts, and control systems theory for two decades. Bowlby was much less scientifically critical than Ainsworth and appeared unaware that her empirical work, particularly on individual differences, had dramatically enhanced the visibility and acceptability of attachment theory. Bowlby's visit, nonetheless, consolidated my confidence in attachment theory, while confirming that Ainsworth's research group–of which I was now a part–had supplanted the Tavistock Unit in London as "the" forum for scholarly analyses of early social development. It is hard to convey the excitement and pride that evoked.

Another noteworthy visitor was Mel Konner, who had recently completed his Ph.D. in anthropology at Harvard University. As part of a large project directed by the distinguished anthropologists Irvin DeVore and Richard Lee, Konner had observed patterns of infant care among the !Kung Bushmen in Botswana. Konner's reports were extremely important to attachment theorists such as Bowlby and Ainsworth because the Bushmen appeared to model patterns of early care most like those believed to have characterized what Bowlby called "the environment of evolutionary adaptedness." Konner's observations revealed the patterns of highly responsive parenting, frequent breast-feeding, and near constant holding that attachment theory presumed and thus appeared to validate attachment theory. In addition, Konner, like Ainsworth, had demonstrated the tremendous value of painstaking observations in naturalistic contexts. This means of data gathering is now well established among students of children and families, but at the time it was rather novel. Through the 1950s and 1960s, it has been much more common to *ask* parents what they did than to *observe* what they did, and although animal behaviorists, particularly ethologists, had emphasized the importance of observation in naturalistic context, it was the example set by scholars such as Ainsworth and Konner that fostered the acceptance of these techniques among those who studied humans. Students like me joined the first generation of social scientists for whom observation was the preferred means of data gathering. Observational methodologies have since become central to empirical research on many aspects of family life, social psychology, and developmental psychology.

The recent and often-recounted experiences of the third distinguished visitor only strengthened my interest in observational techniques. Urie Bronfenbrenner, a developmental psychologist at Cornell University, was being courted by The Johns Hopkins University at the urging of its new President, Stephen Muller, who had recently moved from Cornell himself and wished to enhance the University's reputation in the social sciences. A Russian by birth, Bronfenbrenner had conducted many studies outside the United States and was more interested than many of his peers in the effects of culture and class on parent-child relationships. Bronfenbrenner was still very much a product of his era, however, and most of his studies had involved questionnaires, typically completed by parents. At the time, such studies dominated the scholarly literature on socialization, with little attention paid to the possible disadvantages of obtaining all data from a single potentially biased source. By the early 1970s, however, Bronfenbrenner had come to question this methodology. In sessions with the graduate students at Johns Hopkins in the spring of 1974, he also recounted how he had explained a network of correlations between indices of parental values, practices, and parent-child relationships in a featured address to the Eastern Psychological Association. Upon returning to Cornell, Bronfenbrenner found that the correlations had been reversed inadvertently; all the associations that appeared to be positive were in fact negative! The following year, therefore, Bronfenbrenner returned to the society's annual meeting and began explaining the correlations that he now believed to be valid before interrupting his analysis to challenge his audience. "How," he asked rhetorically, "can we be satisfied with a body of literature that allows us to explain contradictory patterns of association with equivalent confidence?" Something must be wrong with such a discipline, he reasoned, urging his peers to abandon their cherished research methods.

Bronfenbrenner was a spell-binding speaker, and he did not simply question popular research techniques. In a series of presentations, of which his talk at Johns Hopkins was but one of many, Bronfenbrenner argued that developmental psychology as it then existed was fundamentally flawed. "Much of contemporary developmental psychology," he said in one of many quotable turns of phrase, "is the *science of the strange behavior of children in strange situations with strange adults for the briefest possible periods of time*" (1976, p. 1-2; italics in original). Social scientists, he argued, needed to study children in the natural contexts in which they live out their lives if they wished to elucidate both the course of development and the processes by which socialization took place.

This defiant message resonated with those that I had been distilling from Ainsworth, Konner, and the ethologists, and I was further energized by Bronfenbrenner's enthusiastic reaction when I proposed observing infants with their mothers and fathers both at home and in semi-structured settings. Mary Ainsworth considered it foolish for me to study fathers (in part because Milton Kotelchuck, a former Hopkins undergraduate, had recently completed a dissertation at Harvard on this topic), but Bronfenbrenner's passionate critique of the establishment empowered me. As far as I could tell, attachment theory offered no rationale why infants should not form attachments to people other than their mothers. Indeed, as I understood the attachment formation processes explained by Bowlby, it seemed abundantly clear that infants *should* form attachments to all those adults who provided consistent, sensitive, regular, and warm patterns of care over time. My own experiences as a child involved warm, attentive, sensitive interactions with both of my parents and, although I knew little about American families, I assumed that at least some American infants must have comparable experiences. Ainsworth's criticisms of Kotelchuck's methodology–he employed a complex laboratory procedure to compare infant-mother and infant-father attachments–helped me formulate a simpler procedure that was attentive to Ainsworth's concerns, and Bronfenbrenner's embrace was enormously valuable. Arguing that my still sketchy proposal represented precisely the sort of "outside the box" thinking that he wished to promote, Bronfenbrenner announced that the Foundation for Child Development (FCD) had recently set aside funds to support new research within the ecological framework that he was advocating. He felt sure that my proposed study would be funded.

Of course, I first had to think through and compose the proposal, and while working on it, several major changes were taking place within the department of psychology at Johns Hopkins. Most importantly, the former chairman, James Deese, had become department chairman at the University of Virginia, and he offered a faculty position to his old friend, Mary Ainsworth. Ainsworth invited me to move with her to Charlottesville, but because her own long-term plans were still somewhat uncertain and her support of my proposed research on infants, mothers, and fathers was quite equivocal, I decided to re-open discussions with some of the other departments of psychology from which I had not received responses before leaving South Africa. David Feldman, the young faculty member responsible for recruiting graduate students to Yale, responded supportively, although the forbidding and aloof demeanor of many of the faculty members I met there and my near complete ignorance of their research programs made me doubt my suitability for the department while underscoring how much I had still to learn. Intriguingly, it seemed clear that I would be able to substitute the statistics courses I had taken at Johns Hopkins for the *only* required class at Yale, leaving me free to take whatever courses I found interesting and to focus on the research Bronfenbrenner had encouraged. Furthermore, I was impressed by Edward Zigler's commitment to socially relevant issues and by his long relationship with Urie Bronfenbrenner, and although Bill Kessen had focused primarily on infant perception, he was at the time studying both day care and language development. He expressed an interest in infant social development, moreover, and seemed to be one of the most broadly-read and erudite professors that I had ever met. On balance, the move to Yale appeared worth taking and so on Memorial Day 1974, exactly one year after arriving in Baltimore, I moved to New Haven. Fortunately, the closer supervision at Hopkins had given me some of the skills and self-confidence I needed to thrive in the diffident–even neglectful–environment at Yale. I was free to do whatever I wanted, and I did!

Although Bronfenbrenner had arranged funding, my efforts were greatly facilitated by Kessen's affiliation with both the psychology department and the Child Study Center, the psychoanalytic arm of Yale's medical school that shared a building with the psychology department. The existing circumstance between the psychology department and the Child Study Center was illustrative, however, of the continuing gulf between psychoanalysis and psychology in the sense that all doors between the two units were kept locked on every floor! The observation room I used actually belonged to the Child Study Center, however, and I thus became one of the first graduate students to have symbolic affiliations with both of these programs. Amply supplied and protected by negligence, I completed a study of infant-mother and infant-father attachment that was accepted as a Master's thesis before I officially enrolled at the university in the fall of 1974!

Impressed by the speed with which I had implemented, undertaken, and completed this project (while perhaps not recognizing that, unlike other grantees, I had nothing else to occupy my time), Bronfenbrenner arranged further funding for a longitudinal study focused on infant-mother and infant-father attachment in the naturalistic home environment. Like Ainsworth, I chose to rely on dictated transcripts although, having spent a year attempting to interpret and code her transcripts, I decided to dictate my observational records as the events unfolded before me rather than to recreate them after the fact as Ainsworth and her colleagues had done. This strategy, I reasoned, would allow me to preserve the sequence of behaviors and incorporate more information about qualitative features of interaction than the check-list procedures that were then becoming popular. (Videotaping was a novel and presumably intrusive technology which I did not embrace until some years later.) Prompted by Ainsworth, I hoped to focus on individual differences in patterns of interaction between infants and their parents, but Bronfenbrenner's distaste for the "Strange Situation" unfortunately led me to avoid it–in retrospect, it would have been an invaluable adjunct to my study. Instead, I observed infants in their homes repeatedly between 7 and 24 months of age, with the first four of the observational points providing data for the doctoral dissertation I completed and defended as a 21-year-old, although the University's residency requirements delayed my graduation for nearly a year.

ACT IV: SHARPENING CONCEPTIONS OF FATHERHOOD AND PARENT-CHILD RELATIONSHIPS

The first studies I conducted at Yale confirmed that most infants formed attachments to both their mothers and fathers. As Kotelchuck had reported earlier, one-year-olds obtained comfort and support from whichever parent was with them. Separation from either parent elicited little distress from most

American infants and toddlers provided that one parent remained with them, whereas separation from the two was regularly a source of concern and distress. Observations of infants during the first year further confirmed that most infants became attached to both of their parents at roughly the same time, in the middle of the first year of life. Although this conclusion appeared rather obvious to me, it was not so viewed by the majority of developmental psychologists, and I thus undertook a larger integrative effort to help reconceptualize early development in light of new research. Ever economical, I ensured that my review of research on the role of the father in child development served double duty as both the literature review that I was required to complete before submitting my dissertation and later as the introductory chapter of the first book I edited, *The Role of the Father in Child Development* (1976).

Skeptical responses to my research on infants and parents ensured that this first book had a simple message: It made the case that infants formed meaningful relationships to both of their parents and that students of socialization thus needed to recognize the extent to which both fathers and mothers influenced subsequent development. Disconcertingly, however, I was quickly designated as the "Father guy," although my interest was (and remains) recognition that infants are integrated into and socialized within a social system much more complex and comprehensive than social scientists–especially developmental psychologists–had hitherto acknowledged. Of course, family social scientists had long recognized that fathers shaped family dynamics in important ways, although they rarely noted that fathers had direct influences on children as well as indirect influences mediated by the closeness, richness, and supportiveness of the relationships with their wives, and they continued to view infancy as a special phase of infant-mother intimacy.

My efforts to broaden the ways in which researchers thought about early developmental processes and experiences were both helped and hindered by the belated awareness in the late 1970s that changing female roles had to be complemented by changing male roles. Those feminists advocating such social change believed that increased paternal involvement could be fostered by emphasizing the many ways in which fathers influenced their children's development. Ironically, therefore, despite having helped to "discover" fathers, I often found myself attempting to downplay the significance of father-child relationships. It was then and remains true that the average American father is much less important psychologically than he could be even though the benefits of greater involvement are increasingly clear.

My misleading identification with the importance of *father*-child relationships remained wide-spread even after I began conducting research on the impact of siblings, peers, and nonparental care environments. These studies helped to demonstrate the extent to which infants and young children were integrated into and shaped by a social environment much broader and more complex than the infant-mother or even infant-parent relationship. Inattention to the complexity of socialization processes fosters and parallels the continuing and misguided search for "silver bullets," those uniquely significant events that unalterably shape development.

Substantial progress had been made by scholars over the past 20 years, of course. Hundreds of studies have enriched the empirical literature, while theorists have elaborated and refined the conceptual frameworks brought to bear on the understanding of parental roles. When the first edition of my book was published in 1976, for example, social scientists in general, and developmental psychologists in particular, doubted that fathers had a significant role to play in shaping the experiences and development of their children, especially their daughters. As a result, the contributors made concerted and often explicit efforts to demonstrate that fathers indeed had a role to play in child development, were often salient in their children's lives, and affected the course of their children's development, for good as well as for ill. Though somewhat less defensive in tone, contributions to the second edition, published just five years later, emphasized the same conclusions (Lamb, 1981). By contrast, the chapters in the third edition (Lamb, 1997) all reflected the widespread acceptance of the notion that fathers are often affectively and formatively salient. This conclusion encouraged a focus on more nuanced issues and concerns, particularly the recognition that fathers play complex, multidimensional roles, with many patterns of influence being indirect. Moreover, the point was made that social constructions of fatherhood vary across historical epochs and subcultural contexts.

Fathers influence their children by interacting with them directly, of course, and much of the literature is concerned with the ways in which children are affected by caretaking, teaching, guidance, companionship, maltreatment, or neglect by their fathers. Recognition that indirect patterns of influence are pervasive represents one of the major conceptual revolutions marking the 20 years of scholarship that took place between the first and third editions of *The Role of the Father in Child Development,* however. Indeed, fathers, mothers, and children are now viewed as parts of complex social systems in which each person affects every other reciprocally, directly, and indirectly. From this vantage point, of course, appraising the father's impact is much more difficult, both conceptually and statistically, but the newer perspectives promise much greater validity and, ultimately, generalizability.

Equally important, social scientists no longer cling to the simplistic belief that fathers fill a single unidimensional role in their families and in their children's eyes. Instead, they recognize that fathers play a number of significant roles–companions, care providers, spouses, protectors, models, moral guides, teachers, breadwinners–whose relative importance varies across historical epochs and subcultural groups. Only by considering the father's performance of these various roles, and by taking into account their relative importance in the socioecological or subcultural context concerned, can we evaluate any individual father's impact on child development.

ACT V: WAS IT ALWAYS SO?

If social scientists have embraced a more realistic model of the socializing environment in contemporary North America, they have failed dismally in their inattentiveness to cultural and historical variations in socialization processes. Most social scientists implicitly speak of "universal" processes and practices where their models of parenthood and child development are reflective primarily of white North American families characteristic of the late 20th century.

Consider, for example, our frequent reference to "traditional" patterns of child care. Contrary to the claims of its contemporary defenders, the "traditional" family is of relatively recent origin. Although it is true that women have always and everywhere assumed primary responsibility for the care of very young children, this responsibility has seldom precluded either their major involvement in provisioning or a substantial reliance upon other caretakers (Lamb, 1998). Consider, for example, the !Kung Bushmen, whose habitat and hunting-and-gathering ways may constitute a modern facsimile of the ecological niche in which we evolved. Among the !Kung, gathering by women accounts for about 60% of the group's nutritional needs, and toddlers or preschool-aged children are frequently left in the care of older children, siblings, and other adults.

Although the strategies of provisioning, protection, and childcare are different in industrialized countries and even in those societies where pastoral or agricultural traditions have replaced nomadic hunting and gathering, similar choices must be and have always been made. Exclusive maternal care throughout the period of dependency was never an option in "the environment of evolutionary adaptedness," and there are no societies today in which it is the typical practice. Indeed, exclusive maternal care was seldom an option in any phase of human history; it emerged as a possibility for a small elite segment of society during one small portion of human history. It is testimony to the power of recent mythology and ignorance of the dominant human condition throughout history, that exclusive maternal care came to be labeled the traditional or natural form of human child care, with all deviations from this portrayed as unnatural and potentially dangerous. Such deviations abound, with the available options and individual choices determined by economic circumstances, local social demography, history, and cultural ideology. Of these, economic forces–particularly the need for women to work outside of the home in order to help support their families–play the major role in determining whether and what types of nonparental care arrangements are made (Lamb, Sternberg, Hwang, & Broberg 1992). There is no evidence that the traditional family constellation is normative and thus the most adaptive for parents and children, nor that "nontraditional" arrangements are deviant and are likely to have adverse effects–especially on young children growing up in them. Fortunately, some "deviant" forms of family organization or child care (such as maternal employment and extrafamilial child-care) have been in evidence long enough for researchers to reject the assumption that "nontraditional is necessarily harmful," whereas other "deviant" or "nontraditional" styles and practices are of such recent origin or have been studied so little that empirical research remains limited. In addition, evaluative judgments about traditional and nontraditional family forms abound, making it difficult to separate opinions from facts.

ACT VI: WHOSE WORLD IS IT, ANYWAY?

Of course, if one cannot identify universal patterns and processes by examining childrearing practices during one historical epoch, the same must surely apply to studies focused on single cultural contexts. Yet even in my first course on developmental psychology, I was amused by a textbook's flat assertion that "the average child" observed more than 20 hours of television per week. The finding had been well established and has since been widely replicated by researchers in the United States, of course, but I was then living in a country where there was no television, on a continent where television was only recently becoming available to tiny and unrepresentative portions of the population. The majority of infants and children in the world watch absolutely no television even today, and ethnocentric assertions about the "average child" based on narrow observations of children in one demographically small country remains patently absurd. Such an assertion is characteristic of a continuing tendency to ignore the unrepresentativeness of the culture on which most social scientists focus.

Bronfenbrenner fostered my desire to examine the social environments in which children were more inclusively socialized, and the fact that I was an immigrant to the United States has always been an asset. Studies of families and children in other countries often afford the opportunity to shine light on practices or issues that cannot be studied within the United States, either because the necessary variations are not available for study there or because cultural homogeneity on a particular point fosters an unthinking and unquestioning sense of what is 'normal' or even 'possible.' Thus, for example, when I wished to determine whether the relative formative importance of father-child relationships varied depending on the extent to which fathers were involved in day-to-day child care, I began to study families in Sweden, where proportionally more men were involved in the care of their children. Through that work, in turn, I developed a lifelong association with Philip Hwang, a remarkable psychologist, collaborator, and friend.

To an extent unequaled in any other species, our behavior is highly flexible. Relatively few of our behavior patterns appear to be innately and immutably organized, and the evolutionary success of our species is attributable to our enormous adaptability. Furthermore, even when biologically-based predispositions exist, they are usually tendencies that bias behavior in certain directions subject to environmental demands; seldom do we find humans biologically impelled to behave in one way or another.

Through no fault of his own, my conceptualization of human behavior flexibility was facilitated by a marvelously rewarding relationship with an evolutionary biologist named Eric Charnov, who became my closest collaborator during the seven years (1980-1987) I spent at the University of Utah. Charnov was a pioneer of behavioral ecology, a branch of population biology in which scientists sought to understand the ways in which species-typical tendencies were shaped by the constraints and opportunities provided by the environment or *ecology* in which individuals live out their lives. Although Charnov's own research had focused mostly on insects and fish, he became involved in applications to the study of humans around 1980 and was particularly involved in empirical tests of the "optimal foraging theory" that he had developed as a graduate student. Through Charnov, I became introduced to a larger group of evolutionary minded anthropologists and biologists, and two of the lessons I learned from them were to be invaluable.

First, Charnov guided me through a theoretical updating of the theory that had first drawn me to the study of early social development. Bowlby's conceptualization of attachment had been influenced by the evolutionary theory of his time, but extensive research in the decades that followed rendered obsolete some of the concepts on which he relied, such as the notion of group selection. Fortunately, we found that the more recent reconceptualizations of evolutionary biology did not alter the fundamental predictions of attachment theory, although they did point toward interesting new research directions.

Second, Charnov helped me develop a framework for viewing cultural variation and for understanding how members of a single species might develop such vastly different patterns of behavior in response to differences in the physical and social ecologies that they encountered. Amongst other things, this exercise forced attention on the fact that individual differences in the patterns of infant-adult attachments, as evident in the "Strange Situation," might simply reflect adaptations to different rearing ecologies that had equivalent value to the individuals concerned. By extension, cultural differences in the distribution across attachment categories might reflect similar adaptations rather than cultural differences in the relative prominence of sensitive parenting. Introduced in 1985 (Lamb, Thompson, Gardner, & Charnov, 1985), these ideas received little attention at the time, although they have more recently achieved wider acceptance following their reintroduction by Belsky, Steinberg, Draper (1991), and Chisholm (1996).

By the late 1980s, several colleagues and I began a loose collaboration focused on the risks of focusing narrowly on childrearing in affluent Western societies. We chose to observe the everyday experiences of young infants in discrete social niches, beginning with representatives of the white, affluent, urban, two-parent, North American families that continued to dominate research and theory in the social sciences. We then sought opportunities to gather equally detailed descriptive accounts of babies and parents living in different social circumstances. To date, we have been able to conduct extended observations in nearly 20 different socio-cultural contexts and have begun to show just how different the experiences of infants can be even as early as four months of age when, by all accounts, their biological imperatives and needs should exert a homogenizing influence, minimizing whatever differentiating cultural differences exist. Nevertheless, our data consistently and repeatedly illustrate that the cultural context in which infants are raised has a dramatic impact on their social experiences. Cultures differ with respect to the number of individuals who take a significant role in child care and they differ with respect to the amounts of time that children spend alone, being held by others, socializing with others, or exploring objects and things. Culture also determines the number of individuals infants see on a regular basis. Middle-class American mothers and infants are often isolated to an extreme degree experienced by infants in few other cultures. Likewise, culture affects the emphasis on temporal organization, with affluent North Americans more driven by the clock than parents and infants in any of the other cultures we have studied.

EPILOGUE: QUO VADIS?

My continuing attempts to place early development in cultural context and to apply a behavioral ecological approach to the study of early development further underscore that an adequate understanding of early development in the context of the family is a complex multi-disciplinary endeavor. This objective cannot be achieved without a thorough analysis not only of psychological processes, but also of issues, approaches, and findings pursued and compiled by sociologists, anthropologists, behavioral biologists, demographers, and other family social scientists as well. Without any formal training in these other disciplines, I have had to familiarize myself with their literatures and, in the process, have surely been excited by claimed views, perspectives, and findings that are considered everyday assumptions within these other disciplines! Unfortunately, my attempt to embrace a more inclusive view of the social sciences had also coincided with a period of increasingly narrow specialization. Indeed, each of the social sciences itself comprises disparate groups of scholars who often have neither respect for nor knowledge of one another's literatures. Thus, students of social development are often inattentive to the work being conducted by animal behaviorists or students of cognition, while cultural anthropologists despise and disparage the post-modern deconstructionists and the physical anthropologists in their departments. As a result, social scientists today find themselves at a crucial crossroads. Will the social scientists of the future embrace the broad multidisciplinary perspectives and frameworks that appear essential to further insight, or will they ensure their own irrelevance and demise in isolated ivory towers?

REFERENCES

Ainsworth, M.D.S., Blehar, M., Waters, E.C., & Wall, S. (1978). *Patterns of attachment.* Hillsdale, NJ: Erlbaum.

Belsky, J., Steinberg, L., & Draper, P. (1991). Childhood experience, interpersonal development, and reproductive strategy: An evolutionary theory of socialization. *Child Development, 62,* 4, 647-670.

Bowlby, J. (1969). *Attachment and loss.* Vol. 1. Attachment. New York: Basic Books.

Bronfenbrenner, U. (1976). The experimental ecology of human development. Unpublished manuscript, Department of Human Development and Family Studies, Cornell University.

Chisholm, J. S. (1996). The evolutionary ecology of attachment organization. *Human Nature, 7,* 1, 1-38.

Lamb, M.E. (Ed.). (1976). *The role of the father in child development.* New York: Wiley.

Lamb, M.E. (Ed.) (1981). *The role of the father in child development* (Revised edition). New York: Wiley.

Lamb, M.E. (Ed.) (1997). *The role of the father in child development* (Third edition). New York: Wiley.

Lamb, M.E. (1998). Nonparental child care: Context, quality, correlates, and consequences. In W. Damon, I.E. Sigel, & K.A. Renninger (Eds.), *Handbook of child psychology* (Fifth edition, Volume 4) (pp. 73-133). New York: Wiley.

Lamb, M.E., Sternberg, K.J., Hwang, C.P., & Broberg, A.G., (Eds.) (1992). *Child care in context.* Hillsdale, NJ: Erlbaum.

Lamb, M.E., Thompson, R.A., Gardner, W.P., & Charnov, E.L. (1985). *Infant-mother attachment.* Hillsdale, NJ: Erlbaum.

Piaget, J. (1952). *The origins of intelligence in children.* New York: International Universities Press.

PART II: OVERCOMING OBSTACLES

In Memoriam

Bernard Farber
(1922-2000)

Er der will der Dichter verstehen / Muss in dichters Lande gehen–Goethe
(He who wants to understand the poet must travel into the land of poetry)

Overcoming Obstacles–Challenges to Life and Scholarship

Suzanne K. Steinmetz
Gary W. Peterson

Many of the scholars represented in this collection have faced barriers or obstacles that they need to overcome. Some, especially scholars whose essays appeared in the previous section, faced barriers as a result of entering the United States as immigrants. Others faced barriers because their parents, first generation settlers in the United States, were unfamiliar with the language, customs, and social demands of their new country. The children of their parents, several of whom became scholars whose autobiographies appear in this issue, had to navigate the unfamiliar terrain and negotiate a sense of self within an often-hostile environment. Still other scholars faced obstacles when a parent or a spouse died and they had to make unexpected decisions. Finally, some scholars witnessed their life goals or academic careers change dramatically when genetics or disease altered their plans. Most were shaped, to some extent, either by events they could not control or by forces in the larger society that set parameters for the options available. As such, their essays illustrate how a person's life and work are, in part, intertwined with and products of many larger forces that define the essence of "cohort effects."

The group of scholars in this section, Bernard Farber, Irv Tallman, Joan Aldous, Greer Litton Fox, Phyllis Moen, and Marilyn Coleman, all overcame obstacles such as those noted above. In this respect, they share a commonality, that of overcoming adversity, at different points in their careers. They are also, however, quite different. Three of the scholars, Aldous, Farber, and Tallman, were invited by Marvin Sussman to participate in this project. Thus, they had considerable updating to do in order to capture the approximately eight years that had passed since they had prepared the initial drafts of their autobiographies. Since Sussman had not imposed any page limits, these essays tend to be somewhat longer. He also had not requested that authors insert references–both to their own work as well as to the works of others that they noted in their essays. The authors or editors remedied this. The second group, Fox, Moen, and Coleman, were authors invited by Steinmetz and Peterson so that a broader array of scholarly viewpoints from the respective fields of family studies could be represented. In recognition of the practicalities of publishing, however, we chose to include a greater number of individuals, but imposed more stringent page limits.

The two groups also represent different cohorts. Unlike Farber and Tallman, who write of their World War II experiences, or Aldous, who most likely had contemporaries in the war, Fox, Moen, and Coleman are chronologically younger and represent a different cohort–individuals whose birth occurred either during World War II or during the baby boom that followed. Thus, the social context of the experiences faced by these two groups differed.

We also have the sad task of dedicating this section to the memory of Bernard Farber. How prophetic that Bernie Farber should choose as a title for one of his last works: "Now Take My Life–Please!" When we received his revised autobiography, the title reflected a take-off of the famous Henny Youngman line "Take My Wife–Please!" The title conveyed not only Farber's sense of comedy, but also his early background of writing comic scripts.

In his essay, Farber illustrates how life's twists and turns affect how one interprets life as well as what one studies. He analyzes the effect of life and death decisions that individuals make, and places these observations in a theoretical framework that shapes not only his personal beliefs, but also his body of research. Farber's essay may illustrate the classic position proposed by Leplay (1879) that one's personal history can give impetus not only to one's selection of research topics, but also to how to interpret what the data mean. Based on research and his personal observations, Farber raises the question about whether one can define oneself as being ready to die. Given the tone and timing of his essay, and the short interval between discovering that he had cancer and his death, one wonders if he had not made that decision. In his typical unassuming manner, Bernie describes a life and work that had great significance, both for family sociology and for those around him.

In Joan Aldous's essay, "By the Book: An Academic Memoir," she reveals that her initial goal, to major in international relations at the University of Chicago and eventually enter the diplomatic service, was cut short when she contracted rheumatoid arthritis. Not only did she have to change to another university, but she also had to change career goals.

Academia seemed a logical choice. Aldous's paternal grandfather was President of both Utah State University and Oregon State University; her father, who died when she was 13, was a Professor of Agronomy at Kansas State University. After her father's death, her mother, who had a bachelor's degree in home economics, obtained a Master's Degree from Columbia University Teachers College in New York City. Subsequently, she returned to a position at Kansas State in the Department of Family and Child Development, College of Home Economics. Although rheumatoid arthritis left Aldous with many physical challenges, her love for international affairs continued and is demonstrated in her accounts of cross-cultural experiences, research, and publications. The scholarly values of her family and a perpetual environment of books provided a powerful basis for her life pursuits. Aldous's life, therefore, has readily discernible themes (Smith, 1994) that emerge as a function of her own commitment, effort, intellect, and determination to cope with challenges that would overwhelm most of us.

"Living the Literature: Keeping My Family in Family Sociology" is the title of Greer Litton Fox's autobiography. Fox's initial career plan, to become an airline stewardess, was sidelined when, by the seventh grade, she notes, "I was the fifth-tallest person in the entire junior high school." What this meant, of course, was that her stature surpassed the specified height regulations for stewardesses. This outcome of her teen growth spurt, however, was a minor challenge when compared with the struggles that she and her husband faced when attempting to find employment as part of a dual professional couple. The dilemma, of course, is that universities only have one faculty position, but both academic partners need jobs. Finally, as a new assistant professor, Fox faced the reality that, although she had devoted considerable time to teaching, mentoring, and numerous service activities, she was advised that such endeavors would not result in promotion and tenure.

Fox notes that two of her independent undergraduate research projects at Randolph-Macon, studies of federal correctional institutions and the social contexts of racial prejudice, continue to be research interests. Likewise, feminism and women's role in society, an interest ignited during her undergraduate years, continues to be an important part of her teaching and research agenda.

Irv Tallman, in an essay entitled "Aspirations and Possibilities: Coming to Terms with Other People's Reality," describes the challenges one faces when his or her particular theoretical perspective, methodology, or subject matter is contrary to those that are popular at the time. The challenge of having different perspectives was possibly, according to Tallman, the result of two factors: (1) growing up without any close ties or identification with any religious or ethnic community, and (2) constantly moving to such locales as New York, Seattle, Los Angeles, and the San Francisco Bay Area. By the midst of adolescence, he had attended 15 different elementary schools and eight junior high schools, while in the Bay Area.

Thus, Tallman saw the world as being in a state of constant flux. For him, adequate explanations of effective social systems are those that maintain stability under conditions of change–a positivist perspective during a time when Marxist-type explanations were gaining favor. Moreover, he favored experiments and observational techniques when sociology was enamored with large sample surveys and computer-generated statistical analysis. In a manner similar to that of Farber, Tallman ponders whether we have really added to our body of sociological knowledge. An underlying concern here is that the advance of recent sociological knowledge has been hindered by the continued existence of multiple theories that plague systematic theory testing.

"Constructing a Life Course" by Phyllis Moen provides insights into the challenges faced by a full-time mother of two small children, living on a farm in Northern Minnesota, when she is informed that her husband has only a few months to live. Married at 18, Moen became a full-time housewife and mother, but continued to take correspondence courses and an occasional night course. She notes that, when she returned to school, she benefited from the new educational opportunities open to women in the 1970s.

Moen reports that her childhood was filled with ups and downs. Some of the "downs" came when her mother returned to work after she was divorced during wartime, and her biological father never saw her after he returned from the war. In contrast, her "ups" came from excellent day care, and a stepfather who, as a professional in the Army, caused her to live abroad and spared her from the drugs and feelings of disillusionment common to the Baby Boomer generation. Moen reports that, during her childhood, notions of *cultural relativity* and the *flexible self* developed as her southern background was challenged by living in Germany, Japan, and San Francisco. The idea of linked lives, women and work, and generational continuity are themes in both her personal life and her research.

Marilyn Coleman's autobiography has the most unique title: "Following a Non-Linear Career Path: Dietetics + Child Development + Special Education = Family Studies." In this essay, Coleman's life illustrates the old saying, "If life gives you lemons, make lemonade." Known for her work in Family Studies, she reports that not only does she not have a degree in family studies but that she also has very limited course work in this area. In college, her general ineptitude in sewing and interior design, and her dislike for the child development classes, resulted in her obtaining a degree in dietetics–in spite of a series of catastrophes in her undergraduate foods and chemistry classes.

Since there were no jobs for dieticians, she completed a postgraduate year in education. After teaching for a few years, she obtained a master's degree in Child Development and pursued doctoral work while employed as a Child Development Specialist. Because Coleman had taken or taught all the available courses in Child Development, a doctorate in Special Education was the closest related field. Eventually, Coleman and her husband, Larry Ganong, collaborated to examine all facets of divorce and its aftermath–stepparenting, custody, relations with grandparents, inheritance, child support, and remarriage.

A general idea conveyed in these essays, therefore, is that the very act of writing about themselves often forces a kind of self-examination that assists these scholars in understanding what their lives and work have meant (Smith, 1994). These essays also help us to understand that the scientific study of families is truly a human endeavor, shaped by individuals who bring their own developmental experiences into the scholarly process. Through their hard work and insights, knowledge is gained about families that falls somewhere between subjective and objective constructions–but the versions of "reality" they have provided are intriguing enough so that we keep trying to make sense of it all.

REFERENCES

LePlay, F. (1879). *Les ouvriers europeens* (2nd ed.). Tours: Alfred Mame.

Smith, L. (1994). Biographical method. In N. K. Denzin & Y. S. Lincoln (Eds.). *Handbook of qualitative research* (pp. 286-305). Sage Publications: Thousand Oaks, CA.

Now Take My Life–Please!

Bernard Farber

KEYWORDS. Autobiography, research, scholar, kinship

INTRODUCTION

When I was a graduate student half a century ago, the concept of projective systems was popular among social scientists. Based upon psychoanalytic thought, this concept refers to the act of taking significant experiences in one's own development and unconsciously sublimating those experiences in formulating ideas about society and social relations. If one would take a universal experience (such as timing of toilet training), then one could use this experience (e.g., early and rigorous training) as a way of explaining why the norms in a particular society about governmental authority or matters of "inner directedness" were prevalent in that society. These norms thereby represent the projection of a mode of personal experience upon the society. Of course, one cannot rigorously test this interpretation. Yet, the idea of transforming personal experiences into general ideas seems an interesting approach to suggesting how one's autobiography may reveal insights into (a) the theories and conceptual frameworks one has either formulated or introjected from others and (b) areas of research interests. (I return to this theme in the Conclusion section.)

Lives are too complex to be encapsulated into a single theme. Although the presentation may focus upon matters related to the production of a projective system, other areas of concern are included as well. Information about my family background and career development is presented below. Succeeding sections deal with concerns about good and evil, defining moments in my life, my research on family and kinship, my children and their lives, and a brief concluding section on my framework of analysis as a projective system.

BACKGROUND AND LIFE TO ADULTHOOD

I was born in Chicago in 1922 to parents who were Russian Jewish immigrants. There was one brother, David, three years older than I, and six years later a younger brother, Irving, was born. My parents each traveled alone in 1914, barely out of adolescence: my father at age twenty and my mother at seventeen. Like most immigrants, they had no knowledge of English. Both of my parents had been raised in working-class families. My mother was from a ghetto in Polotsk, which had been the jumping-off point into Poland in earlier centuries. My father was from a small shtetl near Gomel. (When my father took up painting after his retirement, he produced a landscape of his village in Russia; the houses were little more than hovels.)

As for other characteristics of my parents' families of orientation, my father had about a dozen brothers and sisters, and, because of attrition through miscarriages and stillbirths, my mother had only one brother, who was at least ten years older than she was. However, the extended families of both parents were large (but virtually all of them were killed when the Germans invaded Russia in World War II). My paternal grandfather was a roofer, and my paternal grandmother supplemented the family income by selling groceries out of the house. My maternal grandparents made a similar kind of accommodation. My maternal grandfather was a cabinetmaker, and my maternal grandmother taught young girls to read and write in Yiddish and Russian. (These patterns were significant as forerunners of my own parents' division of labor.)

In religion, my parents' families were Mitnagdim (i.e., against Chassidism). The Mitnagdim emphasized rationalism and Talmudic learning as a mode of adaptation to modernity and the Enlightenment. Their position was opposed to the Chassidic emphasis upon piety and mysticism of the followers of the Bal Shem Tov, the eighteenth-century religious leader. The Chassidim sought to shield themselves from the Enlightenment. In literal translation, the Mitnagdim comprise the middle cluster, and the Chassidim are the pious ones. In America, like most socialists, my parents tended toward a secularist outlook.

My father's motivation for migrating was to escape being drafted into the Tsarist army (a lifetime commitment). My mother's motivation was more unusual. For years, my maternal grandfather would have a weekly chess game with the local Greek Orthodox priest at the priest's home. One afternoon, quite unexpectedly, the priest suggested to my grandfather that his lovely daughter (my mother) could escape a lifetime of poverty by marrying the priest's son and converting to Christianity. Fearful of the consequences of rejecting this proposal, my grandfather delayed his response. That very night, the extended family pooled its funds and made arrangements for my mother's migration to America. (I don't know the details.) By morning, she was gone. (Upon my mother's arrival in Chicago, she lived with her brother, who had fled from Russia following the failed 1905 insurrection.)

My parents met in Chicago at a dance sponsored by the Young People's

Socialist League (YPSL). My father became an automobile painter; his specialty was decorative white swirls. However, after the automatic automobile paint sprayer was introduced, the manufacturers no longer had to rely upon subcontractors, and my father had to seek other employment. From that time onward, my father had a sequence of newspaper stands (except for a short period when he owned a service station).

Through the years, my parents' household was relatively quiet. Voices were not readily raised. Any arguments between my parents were carried on in Russian (since we children understood Yiddish well). Never was I spanked. In extreme instances, my father would threaten severe beatings–but we knew that he was too gentle to carry through his threats. So we played the game and became obedient. As for my mother, she told us that once she found herself actually stomping on my older brother. She was so ashamed that she never used physical force again. My parents may not have been religious, but they regarded the peace of the home as sacred.

In my preschool years, we moved several times–each time my father switched to a new job or newspaper stand. But my elementary school years were spent in a single neighborhood populated mainly by Italian and Irish families, with a sprinkling of Swedish families. My parents were serious about our schooling. When my older brother and I reached school age, the family switched languages, from Yiddish to English (except for much backsliding). This brother and I both skipped a grade in elementary school. Yet, when the school requested permission for us to skip additional grades, my mother refused on the grounds that we would be much younger than our classmates.

We moved again during the high school years and yet again when I started college. My first college experience was at a recently founded institution, the Theodore Herzl Junior College. At that time, the academic program of the Chicago junior college system was modeled on the Hutchins-Adler curriculum at the University of Chicago. In fact, most of our lecturers in the survey courses were from the University of Chicago, Northwestern, or one of the other major universities in the area. I recall lectures by Wirth on urban sociology, Bobrinskoi on Russian literature, etc. Since faculty jobs were scarce at the time, the college was able to attract people trained at Ivy League schools as well as major European universities. Most unusual!

The remainder of my undergraduate work was done at the Central YMCA College in downtown Chicago. My degree was in Sociology; however, I lacked only one course for a second major in English. The relationship between the College and the YMCA was a precarious one. A couple of years after I received my bachelor's degree, the faculty resigned in protest over the YMCA board's wish to impose restrictions on the number of Jews and blacks at the college. This was the occasion for the founding of Roosevelt University in Chicago.

During my entire undergraduate years, I worked at least half time at a variety of jobs–pumping gasoline at a service station evenings and weekends, library assistant, cloak room attendant (and then manager), janitor during a summer term, electrician's helper, and so on. If I had not continued to live with my parents during these years, I'm not sure how I would have completed the degree requirements in three and a half years. I dropped out for a semester to manage a small service station. After that hiatus, I could hardly wait to register again the following fall.

In order to avoid further disruption of my undergraduate work, I enlisted in an army program that would permit me to get my degree before going on active service. In the spring of 1943, after completing my undergraduate requirements, I received notice of my activation. After a few months (and going through basic training at least twice), I was assigned to the Army Specialized Training Program (ASTP) to study engineering at the University of Idaho. While waiting for shipment, I was an army postal clerk at the Salt Lake City installation. There I discovered why I was not receiving a newsletter (*In Fact*) to which I subscribed; it was on the army's proscribed list.

At the University of Idaho, the students in ASTP were isolated from the civilian students. I took courses in chemistry, calculus, drafting, English composition, etc. Although the program was supposed to take fifteen months to complete, after the Battle of the Bulge, our unit at Idaho was closed. The students in my section were reassigned to the infantry–at first with the idea of preparing us for the hills in the Pacific Theater of Operations–to tend mules, no less–at the Hearst estate in California. (I saw only the hills from my tent, not the castle.) Fortunately, somebody decided that Jeeps were more efficient than mules, and instead we were sent to Fort Benning for–what else–basic training again. I "volunteered" to be company clerk because I said I could type.

I discovered later that I would also have to serve as message carrier in combat areas. This task later gave me a special appreciation of the movie *The In-Laws*, where Peter Falk keeps yelling at his co-parent-in-law, "Serpentine! Serpentine!" It reminded me of the time I had to cross an open field (that seemed endless) alone with a sniper with an apparently limitless supply of bullets shooting at me. The snapping sound as they whizzed by me only spurred me on. With each "serpentine" movement, I had to keep from repeating my previous maneuver to keep the sniper guessing. The movie was fun!

As the previous paragraph implies, we went to Europe and into combat. We took the scenic route through the Black Forest and ended up at Steyr, Austria, at the Enns River, where we met the Russians. (Actually, my primary job was to write vignettes of heroic deeds that members of my company performed, in order to secure medals for them. While I did not lie or exaggerate, my stories were quite colorful.)

Later in this essay, I shall have other things to say about my European experiences. For now, I shall merely indicate that I was discharged at Camp McCoy, Wisconsin, and immediately boarded a southward bound train to Chicago. There I intended to enter the University of Chicago for graduate work. Which area of study? I had not decided.

After my release from the army, I was unsure about the direction my life should take, and I underwent treatment with a psychoanalyst. My analyst was a neo-Freudian, trained by Karen Horney. Our sessions involved more give and take than is true for most analysts. Among the problems we uncovered, the most important for this essay was my handling of Oedipal complexities (to be discussed in the Conclusion section). As a neo-Freudian, my analyst subtly focused upon the social implications involved. A year or so later, my analyst moved from Chicago, and I decided not to transfer to someone else.

GRADUATE SCHOOL AND BEYOND

As I said earlier, when I returned from military service in 1946, I decided to enter the Graduate School of the University of Chicago. The major reason for choosing Chicago was practical; the university was only two miles from home. Of course, the academic reputation of Chicago also influenced my choice. After spending one term in the School of Business (likely as an effort to please my parents), I transferred to the Department of Sociology. Here were the scholars whose work I had studied as an undergraduate: Ogburn, Burgess, Wirth, Blumer, and Hughes. And here I was taking courses with all of them. They each offered a different "spin" on Pragmatism. (Of course, Ogburn was not a Pragmatist.) Blumer claimed to have inherited the mantel of George Herbert Mead, a claim that was vigorously contested by other Mead students (e.g., Leonard S. Cottrell and philosopher Charles Morris). In addition, I found excitement in demography with Hauser and in psychoanalytic thought with Goldhammer. I took the last seminar offered by Ogburn before he retired: The Economic Factor (through the prism of psychoanalytic mechanisms).

I continued to take course work at Chicago through 1949, when my GI Bill entitlement expired. I had married in 1947, and we were expecting a child. I inquired of Professor Burgess, who was the Department Chair, whether he knew of anyone who needed a research assistant. He asked me to return the following day. When I returned, Burgess hired me to help with the statistical analysis associated with the marital prediction study he conducted aong with Paul Wallin of Stanford (see Burgess and Wallin, 1953).

As assistant to Burgess, I had no direct contact with Wallin. (Burgess had no grant at this point and was paying me from his own pocket.) My office was in the basement of the Social Science Building. The room was shared with (a) Evelyn Duvall, the Executive Secretary of the National Council on Family Relations, (b) the staff of NCFR, namely, Duvall's secretary–and whoever helped to send out mailings–and (c) the computational staff of the Cowles Commission (six graduate students who sat at a table at my elbow and pounded six antiquated calculators to perform complex analyses of economic data)–plus my own part-time assistant. I regarded the room (with its exposed pipes) as "the dungeon."

Burgess was a patient and kind man. Although we spent much time together in his office, never did he use profanity (not even in anger); at most there would be a bit of sarcasm. Burgess had a readily apparent speech defect, with midsentence hesitations. I often wanted to complete his sentences, but learned to be patient. His statistical knowledge was weak, and, to compensate for this, he readily sought expert advice (e.g., Harold Hotelling). I had wondered whether he wrote easily (since I found writing laborious). I found his handwritten initial drafts to be filled with colloquialisms and grammatical shortcuts, to be edited later. He wrote as he spoke. Burgess tried never to waste anything; his instructions to me were written on almost anything: old envelopes, backs of old letters, little scraps of paper on which ends of phrases appeared sideways in the margin. Most obviously, his desk was piled with papers. (One professor at Illinois told me that Burgess had once lost his dissertation amongst those piles.) When he asked me to clear his desk upon retirement, stuffed among the contents were old letters, at least ten years old, some of them personal. I shall never know whether he answered them.

Perhaps what impressed me most was a certain youthfulness about Burgess even in his late sixties. His friends on campus included Charles Merriam (the political scientist) and Anton J. Carlson (the physiologist). Merriam would telephone at lunchtime and ask for "that kid, Ernie." Burgess told me that Carlson's view was that, since one's life span is uncertain, one has to live as if one will live forever, and that was Burgess's own perspective as well. Indeed, whenever I later visited Burgess in a nursing home shortly before his death, he would be working on a manuscript.

After two years as an assistant, I was appointed as Research Associate with the rank of Instructor. Apart from working with Burgess, my duties included lecturing in the family course with Burgess, William Lloyd Warner, and Albert Reiss. Burgess had been awarded a grant by the Russell Sage Foundation to prepare a summary of his prediction results for use in premarital counseling, including parts of my dissertation. For my doctoral dissertation, I did an analysis and revision of a rating scale that Burgess and Wallen had developed (Burgess & Wallin, 1953). This scale had been devised to analyze open-ended interview responses of engaged couples in the Burgess and Wallen study. Several graduate students and others had applied the scale to the interview data collected by Burgess and Wallen for about two hundred couples. Until my dissertation, no attempt had been made to evaluate the efficacy of the scale for predicting marital adjustment. When I completed my dissertation, four students tested the efficacy of my revision as their Master's theses.

Upon the recommendation of Dr. Burgess, I was hired at Henderson State College in Arkadelphia, Arkansas–my first faculty position. This was a last-minute appointment after another university failed to receive funding for a new position. Arkansas had received a grant from the Ford Foundation to develop a five-year program in teacher education. The first four years were devoted to a liberal arts curriculum; the education courses were restricted to the fifth year. For the most part, the students were from small towns in the Ouachita mountains and foothills. However, the faculty members in the Ford program were drawn from reputable universities, and they made life in a small Southern town tolerable. Besides, Hot Springs was close by.

My main task at Henderson was to prepare a curriculum for a general family course, practical in nature, to be taken as part of the liberal arts program. In addition, I taught Introductory Sociology and Rural Sociology. For the Rural Sociology course, I made a deal with the students: I would teach them Urban Sociology and they could compare that to rural contexts. While I was at Henderson, a significant national event occurred: the *Brown v. Topeka* Supreme Court decision on school segregation. When we discussed the decision in class, surprisingly, there was a split–the students from the plains near the Mississippi River were vehemently opposed, those few from Alabama very vehemently opposed, but those from the hill countryside were willing to accept the decision. An exciting class that day!

I was unhappy about not being at a research-oriented university and decided to resign at the end of the year. My letter crossed in the mail with the president's letter firing me. Presumably, by firing the two highest-paid faculty members in the Ford program, he could hire three at a lower salary. (Still, I have often wondered whether it was a coincidence that the two who were fired were the only Jews on the college faculty.)

The Institute for Research on Exceptional Children at the University of Illinois, Urbana was seeking a sociologist to undertake an investigation to determine effects on family relations of having a severely mentally retarded child. Again with Dr. Burgess's backing (and the willingness of Samuel A. Kirk, the Institute's director, to take a chance on me), I was hired, with a joint appointment in Sociology. I stayed with the Institute from 1954 to 1968. I then shifted to a full-time appointment in Sociology and left the University in 1971 for Arizona State University. The reason for leaving was an informal agreement with my wife following our divorce in 1970. Our relationship had turned "sour" after the death of my father-in-law in 1965. My perspective is that my wife's perpetual anger toward her father was redirected toward me. But my own responses were also inappropriate, and, a constant friction developed between us. By now, we had four children ranging in age from 14 to 20, and the question in our minds was whether divorce would be preferable to a conflict-ridden home. (Marital counseling was not effective in finding a solution.)

My years at the Institute were quite productive. I published several monographs in the series *Monographs of the Society for Research in Child Development* (Farber, 1959, 1960a; Farber & Jenne, 1963b), as well as the inaugural piece in the research monograph series published by the Council on Exceptional Children (Farber, 1960c). In 1968, there was also a textbook on social aspects of mental retardation (Farber, 1968b). Some of the concepts framing my research at the Institute included (a) the retarded child as inducing an arrest in the family life cycle (Farber, 1959, 1960a, 1960b), (b) an application of game theory (noted as Farber, 1960), (c) the family as a set of mutually contingent careers (1961), and (d) the mentally retarded as part of a superfluous population in society (Farber, 1968b). During my Institute years, I chaired several conferences on family research dealing with the retarded, and, as I left Illinois, I was appointed to the Mental Retardation Research Committee of the National Institute of Child Health and Human Development. (My conference chairing was interrupted when the FBI found that I had belonged to a mildly leftish organization during my undergraduate days; although I could still apply for NIH or NSF grants, for a while I could not receive any Federal appointment.)

My move to Arizona State University was preceded by remarriage. About the time of my divorce, I was invited to make a workshop presentation at the University of Arizona in Tucson. On the flight to Tucson, my conversation with my seat-mate, an older man, was quite friendly. He was going to have dinner with friends, his daughter, and her children at a restaurant and, to my surprise, he invited me. (His daughter taught at the University.) This man knew nothing of my marital status. Of course, what I am leading to is that the daughter and I were taken with each other, and the man became my father-in-law.

I came to Arizona State University as chair of Sociology. Since coming to ASU, I have twice been a journal editor, first as editor of *Sociological Perspectives*, the journal of the Pacific Sociological Association, and presently as co-editor (with Sampson Blair) of *Sociological Inquiry*, the journal of Alpha Kappa Delta, the sociology honor society. Along the way, I was elected to the presidency of the Pacific Sociological Association. I have also had the pleasure of receiving a couple of awards: (a) the E.W. Burgess Award of the National Council on Family Relations for "continuous and meritorious contributions to theory and research in the family field" in 1975 and (b) the Graduate College award that provided me with a year off to undertake research and to bring in a distinguished colleague from another university to replace me. John Mogey of Boston University was my replacement for the year, and he and Doreen stayed on a while afterward. Becoming friends with John and Doreen is the most important consequence of that award. (My life in Arizona will be discussed in later sections of the essay.) Finally, shortly before my retirement in 1992, I acted again as chair of Sociology. I probably could not have survived either of my administrative stints without the late Fred Lindstrom's friendship and his commitment to the Department he founded.

GOOD AND EVIL WRAPPED IN EMBRACE

While I was at the University of Illinois, Louis Schneider and I became friends, and I was intrigued with his notions about ironies in social relations. A student of Robert Merton, Lou was interested in the ways in which prior actions produced ironic twists in their consequences. (See Schneider, 1975.) In this section, I describe a few of these ironic twists in my life, interpreted in terms of good and evil.

Early in life I learned about the difference between good and evil–we all do. Cooperation and equity are good; exploitation and inequity are evil. Peace and goodwill are good, and war and violence are evil. Love and altruism are good, and hate and selfishness are evil. That's easy.

But even as a child my trouble began with trying to apply these concepts. Somehow good and evil did not always refer to opposites. Things I thought of as good were also tied with things that people regarded as evil and vice versa. Socialism I was taught early was good, and yet I had to keep quiet about its goodness in school because teachers and other kids said it was evil–socialists were "Reds"; to me, being Jewish was good, but the kids at school talked about "kikes" and "dirty Jews."

These incongruities troubled me. As I grew older, the idea crystallized that good and evil hold each other in close embrace–that they are inherently entangled–and this idea has stayed with me. What impressed me was how evil uses this embrace to degrade the good and to hide itself–just as we are told God hides his/her face–from us (and in doing so, seems to mock us). In this, I have not been as much concerned with people who conspire to harm others as I am with people who want to do "the right thing."

Here, I want to present three stories to illustrate how the bond between good and evil is related to my personal history and to discuss them briefly afterward. They each tell a tale of personal goodness and social evil. In each tale, the evil relies upon personal decency and integrity in order to survive. The first story goes back to my childhood, the second is an event that took place in my college years, and the third occurred immediately after World War II. With each succeeding tale, the evil grows stronger and more profound.

The First Tale: Through a Child's Eyes

During most of my childhood, my father ran a newspaper stand. To do so, he had to pay a bribe in order to obtain a franchise from the city (Chicago) to have the exclusive right to sell newspapers at an intersection of heavily traveled streets (usually a stand on each of the four corners where streetcars intersected). This enterprise turned out to be a joint family endeavor. Although my father's working hours were from about 9 a.m. to 7 p.m., the entire family was involved. My mother would relieve him at lunchtime and provide him with breaks during the day; my older brother and I would occupy the less busy corners after school and on Saturdays. Evenings, after my brother and I finished our homework at the dining room table, we sat around the table with my father to roll coins in paper wrappers (for bank deposit). We took it for granted that this was simply a family duty.

However, there was another aspect to the family enterprise. Selling newspapers and magazines did not suffice to raise a family; and the family income was supplemented by taking horse-race bets. This was common practice. For a commission (and later in partnership), my father would take wagers (always written on "slips") and before each race for which he had bets, he would telephone "the bookie." "The bookie" symbolized the whole apparatus of the Mob. Of course, my father did not identify himself as a "bookie"; he merely did this as a necessary sideline in order to provide a decent living for his family.

The Mob was a reality for us. Just prior to city elections, the police at the nearby station would inform my father that a "downtown" squad would be arriving to arrest him for taking bets. My mother would be prepared to take over at the newspaper stand. Rarely did my father have to remain overnight in the lockup. Usually the bondsman for the Mob would miraculously be waiting at the station to post bond. Although a trial date would be set, my father would not have to attend–all had been arranged.

What was evil was not the taking of wagers. Honesty was a basic rule in relationships between my father and the bettor and between my father and the Mob organization. Without honesty in such dealings, the industry would have collapsed. Rather, the evil lay in the corruption of the city's infrastructure–police, the courts, politicians. Even members of the Mob were caught in this corruption. At one point, "the bookie" my father telephoned (who was known as Gentleman Jim) wanted to retire, but he was prevented from doing so because he "knew too much" about the workings of the Mob organization. He had to continue.

As long as off-track betting remained illegal, the Mob could sustain its monopoly. By itself, betting on horses could have been legalized, but the Mob would have lost control over the industry. This way, the Mob could maintain its position. But that required corruption as a way of life. Our family's private good could endure by entwining itself with a public evil.

The Second Tale: Who Is Evil and Who Is Good?

My second story provides a different perspective on the intertwining of good and evil–morality and immorality. It begins with my brother David taking the job of bookkeeper for the South Side branch of the Mob. With his accounting training, this was the best-paying job he could have hoped for. In the South Side branch, the primary business was in betting on horse races. (The store front for one of their betting parlors had an ironic sign in the window: Supreme Cleaners.) The family of the South Side leader was not what one would expect of a Mob member. One of his brothers was an alderman, and another was a radio and television network executive with a degree from the University of Chicago. The governing board of the South Side branch consisted of two groups. Members of one group identified themselves as businessmen. They had come into the Mob during the late Prohibition era and earned sufficient capital bootlegging to operate the betting parlors as well as legitimate businesses. (The businesses were also of the sort that readily permitted money laundering–cocktail lounges, restaurants, and so on.) One member owned a large enterprise that, by coincidence, supplied towels and other sanitary products for all of the city-run restrooms: city hall, parks, police stations, libraries, etc.

As opposed to the businessmen on the governing board, the second group was identified as "hoods" (or hoodlums). This group had closer ties to the central leadership of the Mob. For example, one of these was a hit-man, "Golf Bag Sam" Hunt (so named because that's where he carried his equipment). The distinction between businessmen and hoods becomes significant later in the story.

For a few years, everything went smoothly. The betting business was so successful that the headquarters moved from the second floor over the leader's cocktail lounge to a storefront location. Some time after the move, just before the office closed for the evening and before the day's intake was entered into the ledgers, there was an armed robbery. No one was hurt, but the Mob lost the entire "take" for the day. This would have serious repercussions for everyone concerned.

For weeks after the robbery, the leader of the South Side board visited my parents' home (while I was at my college classes). He had suspected from the outset that this had been an inside job and had required the cooperation of my brother. The leader spent hour upon hour talking with my parents and my brother. He could not understand how a "nice Jewish boy" with such decent parents could do this. The money was gone, and that was that. His primary concern was that someone on the board had to have planned and executed the robbery. His purpose in pursuing this ongoing, persistent questioning was to determine who it was.

Actually, my parents and I had had misgivings earlier when my brother began increasingly to accompany some members of the board in their trips to roadhouses and other recreational venues, particularly to those in Joliet (where there were many Mob connections). My brother (may he rest in peace) then confided in me that he had begun to bet heavily and had agreed to the robbery to cover up his losses. (This part he told to the leader and to my parents.) But he was afraid to name the instigator to them for fear of a "hit" by the "hood." When my brother told me who it was, it was clear that there definitely would have been retaliation. My own sense of guilt arose from my feeling powerless to help him.

Then, like a god from a machine in Greek drama, the draft board intervened, and my brother was drafted into the Army. He was still fearful that either the board or the instigator would exact revenge even after his entry into the service. But he never heard from either again. He served as a Finance Officer in the Air Corps until his death in a jeep accident in Karachi, India, on V-E Day.

The intertwining of Good and Evil in this story is highly complex. The only action with clearly evil intention was undertaken by the "hood" who instigated the robbery–like the snake in Eden. Otherwise the evil is shrouded in good.

The Third Tale: Responsibility for Evil

My third story deals with activities associated with the Holocaust. Following V-E Day, our infantry unit was moved back from Austria, where we had met the Russian army, to a medieval town in Germany, Dillingen-on-the-Danube. At the initiative of the battalion recreation officer, Kenneth Gardner (son-in-law of Guy Lombardo), we formed a chorus, and a colleague and I wrote a series of skits. (My colleague had been a newspaper editor in civilian life.) For the next nine months or so, our troupe toured the U.S. army camps in Bavaria.

In Dillingen, my colleague and I stayed at a Gasthaus (instead of the improvised barracks at a school with the rest of the troupe), ostensibly to write. There, I spent much time talking with other residents at the Gasthaus. The conversations were in English, but I understood enough German to catch the nuances of the discourse among the Germans themselves. It was in these conversations that the story I am about to tell emerged.

During the time we were there, the only other long-term residents were two families from Berlin; they were there before we arrived and remained there after we left. The husbands had been executives at I. G. Farben. The younger one had headed the export division and the older one led another, apparently even more important, division. They had of course left Berlin before the Russians arrived.

Both couples were sophisticated and well-read. They had a wide range of knowledge and regarded themselves as "highly cultured." They spoke high German and had an excellent command of English (and other languages as well). The wife of the older man had been raised in the United States and still considered herself "American" in outlook; the younger woman spent most of her time schooling her children.

From time to time, the conversation turned to the Nazi regime and its policies. Yes, they were aware of what had happened. They knew about the Jews, about slave labor, the education system, German culture, and such. Yes, it bothered them greatly that these things had occurred. It offended their moral sense. But no, they did nothing about it. It would not have helped anyone if they tried. It would only have jeopardized their own lives and their mode of living. They had felt powerless to act. Their only hope had been for the terror to end without disturbing their own lives.

My initial reaction was, "So this is how the so-called good Germans rationalized their role in living with Naziism." Yet, I kept asking myself, "Were I in their position, would I have done differently? *Could* I have done differently?"

Consistent with my previous experiences, I concluded the following: Modern society has become so complex that acting according to our moral sense may well (often unknowingly and certainly unwillingly) involve actions that support the endurance of evil. It is not merely, as Hannah Arendt suggests, that a terrifying evil of Nazi Germany lies in banality, routine duties in bureaucracies. Rather, the horror is more general; in modern society, evil co-opts the good.

I still hold to that conclusion–the more complex society becomes, the greater is the intertwining of good and evil. A simple example: those of us who invest in IRAs, pensions, mutual funds, and so on unwittingly become owners and have an interest in the well-being of companies that may engage in fraudulent practices, unfair exploitation of employees, illegal trade, siphoning off of funds by executives (through excessive bonuses, options, golden parachutes), providing support for terrorist groups, or other evils. There is no way of our knowing.

Moreover, each invention of new devices and/or techniques and social relations associated with the inventions also introduces new opportunities for both good and (especially) evil. The greater the complexity of social arrangements wrought by introducing these new devices and techniques, the greater is the chance of generating evil uses inadvertently. An apt example is the rapid development of the Internet. There is a hue and cry over misuse of the Internet; yet investment in Internet stock continues to soar regardless of degree or manner of unethical use. Truly, in modernity good and evil are inevitably locked in passionate embrace.

CHOOSING LIFE, CHOOSING DEATH

There are moments in the course of living out our lives that transform our outlook ever after. Often these moments are referred to as epiphanies–moments of sudden intuition, insight, understanding, or revelation. Yet, these insights may at times involve a shift in perspective that has little to do with the joy of enlightenment. Rather, they may evoke a sense of horror at the nature of this enlightenment. Perhaps some examples will facilitate communicating what I have in mind.

Before proceeding, I would like to present a vignette of a defining moment early in my life: When I was seven, my best friend at school was Charles Peterson, a Swedish boy in the predominately Italian and Irish student body–another outsider. During recess, we would play marbles together in the school yard. Each weekend I looked forward to resuming our game. But one Monday, Charles was absent, and the teacher explained what strep throat was and that Charles had died of it over the weekend. But we had played together on Friday! And now he was gone. I could understand an adult's dying (my aunt had), but a child my age? That wasn't supposed to happen. Suddenly, unexpectedly!

Next, fade out the school scene and fade in a scene sixteen years later in Germany: I am walking on a field after our first major gun battle. I see my friends lying there, ready for body bags. But I saw them and talked with them just hours, minutes ago. The fragility. It's only a matter of a short time before . . .

Choosing Life When Death Is the Norm

In World War II, as our rifle company moved through southern Germany and into Austria, we came across a concentration camp that had just been liberated. The sight of the near-corpses supporting each other as they staggered through the gates and out along the fence and the road still haunt me. (This happened over fifty years ago.) Tears still well up when I recall that scene. If I could feel such horror in the fleeting moments it took to observe them, what was it like to endure that existence day in and day out for years? The inmates may have accepted the normality of dying, but what will did they muster to want to survive concentration camp life? For me, my reaction to that scene defined the Holocaust more intensely than the horrific number of six million or recounting the many relatives I lost (but never met).

In the succeeding years, the memory of this event affected my approach to family research. In that research, I took seriously Louis Wirth's dictum, taken from Goethe (I cite from memory):

Er der will der Dichter verstehen / Muss in dichters Lande gehen

(He who wants to understand the poet must travel into the land of poetry)

For example, in my study of families with severely retarded children, my reaction to the camp liberation underscored my views about the families coping day in and day out with their handicapped children. I realized that when I completed my interviews or other contacts with the parents and reviewed my notes or the interview protocols, I could leave the misery and hardship suffered by the family and return to my daily routines and other interests. I only visited and empathized with them, but the parents and siblings had to endure their grief night and day. I admired their will to persist. Ultimately (after a few years), I found the whole project too depressing to continue.

I had a similar experience in my study of families living in Salem, Massachusetts, around the end of the eighteenth century (Farber, 1972, 1973b). Because Salem was a seaport and trade center, death haunted the community. Sailors died of exotic diseases, or when they returned home, their entire family was sometimes wiped out. Women died early in childbirth or of tuberculosis. There was a high incidence of alcoholism. Entries in diaries or letters indicated: "Old Joe died, worn out"; "Millie died, just wasted away"; "Maude's baby fell into the fireplace–Maude was too drunk to care"; "Sarah's babies thrive at first, then they all get sickly and die–all five of them," and so on. Ships went on long voyages–often a year or more–without any news, and sometimes they would not return at all.

The smell of death had to have affected the family ties of the Salemites. Philippe Aries, in his *Centuries of Childhood*, made the point that as long as the lives of children in premodern Europe remained precarious, parents limited their emotional and material investment in their children. This emotional distancing from children was abandoned only when the expectation of death subsided. In Salem, contact between parents and their children was limited through an apprenticeship system. Although it was silly to do so, I mourned for these people who had been dead for about two centuries. But simultaneously, I marveled at those exceptional people with the will to transcend the milieu of death.

Choosing Death When Life Is the Norm

At various times in my life, I have toyed with the idea of choosing death instead of striving to live. In response to the question of whether he believed in free will, Isaac Bashevis Singer remarked, "Yes. But then God gave people no choice but to have free will." But when all avenues for choice are closed (as they often were for the concentration camp inmates), the last remaining choice was whether to live at all. People who have survived the Nazi concentration camps often relate that they could identify those who had willed themselves to death. They did not merely accept death; they chose to die. These "suicides by will" would become lethargic automatons, walking around without a soul. When all other avenues of choice had been blocked off, only one choice remained–whether to live at all.

I offer two examples in which I was probably instrumental in someone's choice to commit suicide. In the first example, an incident took place when I was Department chair at Arizona State. One day, a young sociologist came to my office. He had been fired from a tenure-track faculty position at a major Canadian university for his radical political activities. He was now living with his parents in Sun City. He was looking for a teaching position, and considering the time of year, he would have been content with part-time work. He was personable and articulate, and his credentials were good. He had earned his PhD from a university with an excellent Sociology department.

Ordinarily, I would have leapt at the opportunity to hire him. However, at the time, the budget was very tight; we had tried to get additional funds from the dean of the College, but had been unsuccessful. In order to avoid giving the young man false hopes, I informed him of our situation. He left understandably disappointed. However, after a month or so passed, one of our adjunct lecturers left abruptly, and I telephoned the young sociologist's home to tell him the good news. Unfortunately, no one was home. Then a few days later, his father returned my call. About a week before, the despondent young man had taken his own life.

The second example pertains to my then-next-door neighbor–the patios of our houses were adjacent, with a high wall between them. First, it may be helpful to know about the relationship between my neighbor and me. We were each living alone. My neighbor, a woman about ten or so years younger than I, lived with flair: expensive sports cars, expensive clothes, etc. She was well-read and knowledgeable about many topics. She had owned a horse, whose death she mourned years afterward. Unfortunately, she was also anorexic, an alcoholic, and had numerous "relationships" with men of various degrees of friendship. I knew that she was seeing a psychiatrist. She frequently asked me over. (Often she would appear at my front door and invite herself in.) Knowing about her activities, I was determined not to become one of her "relationships." (Once, she actually pushed me into the swimming pool so that I would have to take my soggy clothes off.)

Unlike the young sociologist whose choices had been severely narrowed, my neighbor suffered from having a plethora of alternatives (much like the anomic suicides Durkheim posited among the nouveau riche). In fact, my neighbor seemed to thrive on defying ordinary customs. For example, she told me that she had always had two or three men "on the side" (even when she was married), and asked, "Would I not do the same with women." But then, she also had called the police at one time to tell them that she was going to shoot herself–she later told me that she had no access to a gun and had no intention of getting one. What did bother her was her mother presumably saying, "They ought to lock you up in a loony bin and throw away the key." Sometimes, I think that it was her estrangement that fascinated me.

One early Sunday morning, the telephone rang and I recognized the voice of my neighbor. She apologized and said that she had intended to call a friend for lunch. I tried calling back, but there was no answer. Still, she had sounded strange–of course, she often sounded strange. I thought nothing further about it. Then, for a few days, I neither saw her nor heard any sounds from her patio or pool (where she ordinarily spent much time). I telephoned several times without success. Finally, I used my key (we had exchanged keys for security purposes). I found her fully clothed, face down, in the bathtub. The police informed me that it was an obvious suicide.

My sense of guilt over my action (or inaction) in the case of the two suicides above was replayed in my failure to recognize the seriousness of Rosanna's (my second wife) symptoms on the morning of her death. This occurred in 1988. Upon awakening, she seemed somewhat disoriented and complained of chills. My impulse was to wait to see if the symptoms continued as the morning went on. When they appeared to worsen, I decided to take her to the hospital emergency room. But before we could leave, she had a grand mal seizure.

Within ten minutes of my call to 911, the ambulance and paramedics arrived and tried to stabilize her condition. But she continued to have seizures. They rushed her to the nearest hospital. Twenty minutes later, the hospital social worker informed me of her death. The pathologist was stymied as to the cause of death. Very likely, my delay had no effect on the outcome. Nevertheless, after eleven years, I accuse myself. If only, if only. . . .

Could Rosanna have willed herself to die? She had had severe asthma and more recently emphysema, a condition that began during her first marriage and limited her activities. Before moving to Arizona, Rosanna was hospitalized continually. Over and over again she would utter, "I want my health back. I want to be the way I was." In addition to her pulmonary specialist, she tried numerous alternative therapies: acupuncture, chiropractic, a Japanese pressure-point therapy, macrobiotics, and so on and so on, all to no avail–if anything, her condition worsened. Had she given up and accepted death–or had she even chosen it? I'll never know.

With Rosanna's death, effectively my career as a sociologist ended. I withdrew from my commitments to edit papers presented at a conference in Hungary, as well as from my editorship of *Sociological Perspectives*. I continued teaching classes and later became acting chair of Sociology at ASU. I even wrote some papers. But the fire had been extinguished.

WHICH AMERICAN FAMILY?

In this section, I focus upon the development of my ideas and research on family and kinship organization. The first part reviews the background of family sociology as I interpreted it in my early years. After that, I go on to the formation of the conceptual framework I devised for understanding the diversity and changes in contemporary American family life. The third part deals with my attempts to reconceptualize family and kinship structures in a more general way and to seek empirical evidence regarding my conceptualizations.

Background

Pre-World-War-II sociology mirrored American public policy. Public policy was based upon a presupposition that the great ethnic diversity of immigrants would be assimilated into the traditional institutions of American society. In a practical sense, the immigrants were encouraged to become "Americanized" in language, in defining values, and in adopting an American "way of life." This trend continued into the postwar period, into the 1960s.

During this period, the dominant family sociologists incorporated the Americanization assumptions into their theorizing and focused upon central tendencies in family life: what was happening to *the* American family? Family forms that departed significantly from this normative tendency were considered to be somehow deviant. They were seen as lagging in their adapting appropriately to the movement of American society from a rural society, based on tribalism, to the urban condition. In his work on major social trends, William Fielding Ogburn (1929) described the adaptation as a loss of family functions (so that the remaining family function was primarily social-emotional in content). Talcott Parsons (1955) saw *the* family as a subsystem of American society and identified it as "isolated" from broader kinship ties in *the* American kinship system. (Parsons regarded upper class and lower class kinship as deviant forms from the dominant system.) Ernest W. Burgess (1945) portrayed the trend of family adaptation as a transformation from institutional bonds to companionship bonds. For him, the family had become a group–a unity of interacting personalities.

In opposition to the conceptualizations cited above, other sociologists (like Pitirim Sorokin, 1962, and his disciple Carle Zimmerman) regarded changes in family life as following a cyclical pattern, moving between strong organizations dominating the structure of society to weak, fragile units (at the mercy of other institutions) and back again. However, like Burgess, Parsons, and the others, the cyclical position also focused upon central tendencies.

When I began teaching courses in family sociology at Illinois, it occurred to me that what the theories current at that time were missing was the underlying dynamics of the trends. These theories rested upon the notion of adaptation. The process of adaptation implies the idea of fitting in, with the elements of a system behaving in ways to reduce conflict between themselves. More inclusive systems (e.g., technology, the economy, government, or urban population aggregation) require less inclusive systems (such as family) to change to be consistent with the needs of the more inclusive systems. (Although societies are by no means perfect systems, the system metaphor seems to work for understanding the concept of adaptation.) Only when family is coterminous with economic and governmental structures is the Zimmerman (1935) strong family viable. The theories thus imply a notion of efficiency in system functioning: the reduction of the lag of less inclusive subsystems to adapt to the needs of more inclusive subsystems.

By focusing upon the concept of adaptation, the current theorists were able to gauge the gross adaptations of family life to modern life. However, by avoiding apparent contradictory tendencies pushing family life in opposing ways, the theorists avoided observing the dynamics involved. To identify some family forms as deviant because they do not conform to the modes of living consistent with needs (posited by the theorists) of the economic structures or urban population aggregations seems to detract from one's understanding of social processes.

Reconceptualizing American Family Life

It was at this point that my interest in Marxist analysis became pertinent. What for Burgess was a desirable, natural phenomenon–i.e., the emergence of the companionship family–could be interpreted as well as the commodification of family life. In the Burgess studies of predicting "marital success," the criterion of success is the degree of happiness and satisfaction reported by the husband and wife. Similarly, the criterion for the utility of a commodity is one's satisfaction with it. Inasmuch as one's satisfaction with a spouse can vary, given an ideal situation in which only the utility of a commodity is considered, one would always be free to dispose of the unwanted commodity and "purchase" a more desirable one. This similarity gave rise to my concept of "permanent availability" in *Family: Organization and Interaction* (Farber, 1964).

To carry the equation of spouse and commodity further, I visualized a market where one is simultaneously (a) a purchaser seeking to maximize utility and (b) a commodity to be "sold" to a new partner. I assumed also that this market was a completely free and open market, where everyone is available as a purchaser-commodity to everyone else–without regard to current marital status. One is then under obligation to make one's self as attractive as possible throughout adulthood in case one (or one's spouse) might want (or need) to change partners.

The condition of a free and open market (without regard to current marital status) implies also that such factors as religion, social status, ethnicity, parenthood, etc., of the spouse to be chosen or considered are only matters pertaining to satisfaction rather than to any moral or ideological commitment. This condition permits a maximum opportunity for introducing new cultural or ideological elements into one's family life. In this manner, the notion of permanent availability is associated with chances for extensive change in family life from one generation to the next. Consequently, I wanted a concept that would reveal a tendency in opposition to "permanent availability."

The concept that I used as a conflicting basis for family organization to "permanent availability" was "order replacement"; that is, the kind of family that would maximize the chances of replicating a mode of family organization from one generation to the next. Here, the marriage market would be highly restricted to persons from similar background and with norms and values similar to one's own. Moral commitment would operate instead of personal satisfaction as a criterion of family success. (Personal satisfaction would operate as a means rather than as an end.) Tradition would be inviolate.

The opposition between "permanent availability" and "orderly replacement" was the organizing principle of *Family: Organization and Interaction* (Farber, 1964). But these concepts seemed too limited for understanding the relationship between social structure and the family. To pursue this matter further, I needed to examine concepts that would expose the structural dynamics underlying that opposition.

Broadening the Conceptualization

The main source of tension affecting the direction family organization might take seems to lie in the conflict between the forces of centralization and decentralization in social structure. On the one hand, there is a need for families to form a network of relationships that would integrate (or hold together) the society at any given moment in time. On the other hand, there is the need for families to act for the benefit of generations of their descendants (i.e., for the endurance of spiritual and physical welfare, status, and property rights of succeeding generations).

In simpler societies, the social structure can emphasize one form of integration or the other. In a society stressing contemporaneous integration, the instruments of societal endurance lie in overarching institutions (such as the universal Church, government, or intertwined economic enterprises). For example, one intention of the writers of Canon Law in the Catholic Church in the Middle Ages was to "create a unity out of diversity" by tying families into an intermarrying network; this movement involved the Church in accumulating property and wealth that might otherwise remain within families as well as seeing to the welfare of people both on earth and in the hereafter. In a more decentralized and segmented society, the instruments of social endurance lie in the domain of the family. An example here would be the twelve tribes of the Hebrew Bible.

These opposing tasks described above require different forms of family organization. In one case, where the role of the family is one of contemporaneous integration (i.e., a spreading of interrelationships with other families throughout the society), there would be a strong centrifugal force to form these webs of relationships. Here kinship ties would be weak and intermarriage among groups would be encouraged. However, in the case of families structured for lineal endurance, there would be a strong centripetal force. Close kinship ties would be encouraged, with a preference for first-cousin marriage (e.g., the patriarch Jacob marrying his cousins Rachel and Leah) and the wealth passed down within the tribe from one generation to the next (Farber, 1975).

In simple societies, the entire social structure can be oriented in one direction or the other. However, when we come to more complex societies, the conflict is not so readily resolved. Different segments of the society tend toward different solutions. In my thinking, the concept of "permanent availability" is the logical outcome of the centrifugal tendencies in family organization, while "orderly replacement" represents the centripetal tendencies. The different solutions to the centrifugal versus centripetal forces in family organization provided the topic of several of my research projects.

Studies in Family and Kinship

In order to explore different contexts that might reveal ways in which my general framework might provide some interesting insights into the interaction between family and society, I undertook a series of studies. Some of these envelop entire societies and use family law as an instrument in the investigation; others are more microscopic and use such techniques as ethnography and survey research. The order in which these investigations appear below is (for the most part) chronological.

Comparative Kinship Systems. Although this book (Farber, 1968a) deals with various concerns of interest to anthropologists, its primary contribution is the introduction of a technique of analysis indicating the particular paths of kinship identity passed down through generations (as well as kinship identities transferred in marriage) according to different kinship structures. One of the findings relevant to my interests was a strong tendency in state laws regarding marriage: states that forbid first-cousin marriage tend to permit marriage between any in-laws in a subsequent marriage (and vice-versa). In terms of my framework: kinship systems that push members outward to extend webs of relationships with previously unrelated families do not count in-law ties as persisting beyond the initial marriage (while those systems favoring the endurance of ties between closely related families [first cousin marriage] also assume in-laws are like close relatives).

Kinship and Class: A Midwestern Study. This was an ethnographic investigation of slum families whose children were enrolled in an experimental preschool program (Faber, 1971). Families whose children had progressed significantly (according to measures of achievement and intelligence) were compared with families where the child showed little or no improvement. The field work was completed before the children's progress was assessed. As compared with the families whose children improved, the families of the non-improvers had the following characteristics:

1. A more diffuse view of role and status of particular kin. The parents were more concerned with the distinction between kin and nonkin than between rights and obligations regarding different kinship statuses. The need to maintain mutual assistance networks outweighed the niceties of formal status of particular kin. One woman reported, "I was married when my children were born, but my sister never married, and she has as many children as I do. So what's the difference?"
2. Less information of ordinary facts about their relatives. Instead, respondents would say, "I never met my grandfather, so what difference does it make?" or (about a sibling living nearby), "I just don't know what sort of work he's doing now."
3. Less differentiation between generations within the family. For example, the fourteen-year-old daughter who has been accused by her father of being promiscuous said, "And who knocked up [the next-door-neighbor]? You have no right to accuse me of anything!"
4. Less control over the lives of their children. A father of a nonachiever reported that because he couldn't take his son's noise any longer, he beat the boy so hard that blood flowed down his leg. But now the boy was quiet. In contrast, one mother of achieving children found play-

mates for her daughters outside the slum to avoid the neighborhood influence.

There was little difference between responses by race or ethnicity. However, the contrast in views on kinship and family ties did differentiate the parents of the potentially upwardly mobile families from those destined to remain in their current state of existence.

Guardians of Virtue: Salem Families in 1800. I also studied the kinship arrangements among families in Salem, Massachusetts, during the 1800s (Farber, 1972). Before its harbor became inadequate to accommodate the great sailing ships of the nineteenth century, Salem, Massachusetts, was a port town. The dominant class consisted mainly of merchants, who were often shipowners, and, to a lesser extent, artisans. Kinship patterns differed markedly by socioeconomic levels. The merchants and artisans sought out relatives (whom they could trust) for alliances in enterprise and marriage. These alliances were needed for capitalization. There would be several marriages between sibling groups (e.g., the Cabots and the Higginsons) as well as first-cousin marriages in order to cement these alliances and ensure their endurance. By way of contrast, the laboring classes (including common sailors) lived a precarious existence, and their need for mutual assistance networks and a consequent web of kinship ties showed much resemblance to what I reported in *Kinship and Class* (Farber, 1971).

Family and Kinship in Modern Society. In this book (Farber, 1973), I studied the tension deriving from a growing disinclination in law to treat the family institution as a protected domain in contemporary societies. This trend of course reflects a revision of cultural notions about the role of the family in society. The analysis covers a series of topics: shifts in laws governing marriage and divorce, support, illegitimacy and adoption, and family and estates. In each case, there is a conflict between the traditional model of the family as a "natural," basic institution whose endurance should be protected and an emerging view, a legal model which does not recognize any inherent property that must be sustained. (See Rosen [2000] for an extension of this analysis to the end of the Twentieth Century.)

A Shift in Methodology

Until now, the evidence examined provided a perspective on the basis of general attributes of social structure. The question remained: do people at different parts of the social structure actually conform to the imputed models of kinship in their own thinking?

To address this question, I devised a technique for ascertaining whether people's ideas about kinship priorities conformed to patterns that emphasized endurance of families–that is, line of descent–or maintenance of networks between families. These differences are expressed in laws of succession (in case of intestacy). Accordingly, the respondents were asked to pretend they were writing a law for distributing estates if there was no will. To simplify matters, the respondents were asked to choose priorities between nine pairs of relatives (that differentiated between kinship models). (Equal choice was a permissible response.) Respondents were then classified by model into which the majority of their responses fell. (There were actually four kinship models used in the analysis, but I shall simplify the discussion by mentioning only two.)

In this transitional phase, I studied a random sample of college students and found that those who fell into the category representing the centripetal kinship model were more often in the sciences and had relatively higher grade point averages as compared with those in the arts and other areas. My interpretation was that the same influences that determined one's kinship orientation were also responsible for the self-discipline associated with the high GPAs and choice of academic major (Farber, 1977).

Conceptions of Kinship. The last study in the series was an investigation of 716 residents (aged 18-45) in the Phoenix area in household interviews (Farber, 1981). The sample was selected by Morris Axelrod. Generally, the results of the study supported my expectations–(a) Jewish respondents, devout Mormons, and certain fundamentalist Protestant sectarians tended to fall into "centripetal" kinship category; (b) people at high socioeconomic levels also did, while those at the lower socioeconomic levels favored "centrifugal" choices; (c) as might be expected, older persons tended to favor "centripetal" responses. This tendency also occurred in a Kansas City study of a Jewish sample (Farber, 1979, 1981: p. 211); (d) for women especially, those in the "centripetal" category, *far less* than those in the "centrifugal" category, were inclined to agree with the statement that couples should live together before marriage.

Probably the most interesting finding in *Conceptions of Kinship* is a serendipitous one. Initially, there was a surprising number of cases that could not be classified as to kinship type. On examining the distribution of responses in these cases, I discovered that there was indeed a consistent pattern. The choices in priorities among kin were the opposite of those in the "centripetal" model; priority was given to line of *ascent* instead of line of *descent* (as would have occurred in the "centripetal" pattern).

One implication of the serendipitous model is that of the value of individualism in America. In assigning priorities, the person favors those who have been responsible for providing one with a place in society rather than seeing one's task as providing for the endurance of the family over generations. The evidence in the study supports this interpretation. Ancestors were more often American-born. The respondents in this category had by far the fewest children in the sample, and were overrepresented among college-educated groups. Although the serendipitous category was the modal response in the sample, it was underrepresented especially among racial minority groups, Jewish respondents, persons with foreign-born fathers, and poorly-educated persons at poverty levels. Because of the prevalence of the serendipitous model in the sample and its association with middle-class attributes and native-born parentage, I called this pattern the Standard American model.

Aftermath. After I completed *Conceptions of Kinship*, a former student of mine, David Baker (1991), was able to compare my findings with those for an extensive European sample. He found that the modal response on the Continent was the "centripetal" model, rather than the Standard American model. It would be interesting to determine what the connection between the emergence of Standard American kinship and the extensive changes of women's roles in family and society might be in the future. What will be the distribution of various kinship and family structures at the end of the Twenty-first Century? Will the Standard American form still dominate the society (with attendant consequences for birth rates and living arrangements)? What modifications will occur in family law?

FROM GENERATION TO GENERATION

My Family

As I look back at my own family life, it seems as though I have lived according to the contradiction I have studied in my academic existence. Emotionally, there is no problem. I have always felt strongly about my children–in the past some people have suggested too strongly. Each one has given me much "nakhos"–a sense of joy, pride, and fulfillment.

But as my first marriage ended, I felt that I had deprived my children of an important element in socialization. I had been raised and had regarded myself as a secular Jew (i.e., one who was aware of the historical conditions under which Jews lived but could not accept the traditional notions of Judaism as a religion). I considered the prescriptions in Jewish codes as a response of these historical conditions and hence readily disposable. And, of course, my wife and I raised our children to follow in our beliefs. What was needed to replace these codes, we felt, should be a universalistic value system of brotherhood and sisterhood (which in terms of family and kinship would emphasize centrifugal tendencies). Our friends were similarly inclined in their notions about family life and social values.

Then I faltered. Something bothered me about the self-identity of my children and that of our friends' children. Although the children may have regarded themselves as Jewish ethnically, there seemed to be an underlying uncertainty about their way of life. What struck me sharply was that daughters of two of these friends committed suicide. These suicides may have occurred under any circumstances. Yet, the ambiguities in self-identity–leading to searching for alternative ways of life–that I sensed in my children and those of my friends led me to believe that we had been derelict in providing our children with a firm identity of exactly who they were.

As a result of my concerns, when I remarried and we had a daughter, Tanya, we sent her to Orthodox Jewish schools, first in Phoenix and later to a high school in Providence, Rhode Island. Our thinking was that whatever Tanya decided in her later life, at least she would have solid knowledge upon which to base her decisions. As an aside, the close-knit Orthodox community in Providence was instrumental in helping Tanya through the crisis of her mother's death. Tanya now teaches at an Orthodox high school in New York.

Obviously, there are other influences upon socialization beyond family organization. But it is apparently not accidental that all of the children from my first marriage in one way or another have occupations (or at least training) related to sociology:

1. My oldest son, Daniel, is Professor of law and Associate Dean at the University of Minnesota. Early in his career he "clerked" for Justice Stevens at the U.S. Supreme Court, and recently he was elected to AAAS. (Daniel has a Master's degree in sociology.) His wife, Dianne, is a sculptor-ceramicist. There are three children: Joseph, Sonya, and Nora.
2. My second son, Michael, after a long stint as manager and troubleshooter for a mainframe computer company, returned to college and earned a degree in archaeology at the University of Illinois. He is now a computer consultant and lives in Urbana, Illinois.
3. The older of my twin daughters, Lisa, is a clinical psychologist and teaches courses in sociology and psychology at community colleges near Troy, Ohio. She is married to Ronald King (a truck mechanic) and has a step-daughter, Hillary.
4. The younger of my twin daughters, Jackie (Jacqueline), also a psychologist, works as a Resource Specialist at the University of Illinois. She is married to Richard Billingsley (a landscaper) and lives near Villa Grove, Illinois (about 30 miles south of Urbana).

My second family, in addition to Tanya, includes two daughters from Rosanna's first marriage. Whereas the children in my first marriage sought their degrees in the social sciences, Rosanna's daughters had an interest in the physical and biological sciences (by coincidence, consistent with my research findings in Farber, 1977):

1. Rosanna's older daughter, Erica, first sampled the physical sciences (performing well, but unwilling to commit herself to a career in them), and ultimately studied physiology and exercise science. A former software troubleshooter, Erica is married to Max Cidon (a graphic artist), has one preschooler (Natalie), and works at the University of California at Santa Cruz.
2. Rosanna's younger daughter, Julie, received her degree in speech and hearing and then a Master's in the teaching of the deaf. Like Erica, however, her current occupation is not related to her university training. Living in Oakland, California, Julie is married to Matthew Golde (a prosecuting attorney), has one preschooler (Daniel), and works for the local Jewish Federation.

I do not argue that one approach to socialization is "intrinsically" better than the other. They each have their virtues and their risks. The current political issue about family values versus family adaptations is, in one sense, a restatement of the opposition between family organization based on the centripetal principle versus that based on the centrifugal principle. The former is a strategic approach aimed at the endurance of family and kinship structures, while the latter is a tactical approach for adapting to current social and economic conditions. The strategic approach necessarily is vulnerable to long-range historical crises threatening the endurance of family structures; the tactical approach depends more upon the efficacy of short-run adaptations to accommodate blips in webs of family relationships. As for personal vulnerabilities, one approach risks personal reaction against constraints and the need for self-discipline necessary for the endurance of family structures, whereas the other approach risks the uncertainties of the freedom to destroy (or ignore) family ties and/or to form new webs of domestic relations.

CONCLUSION

At the opening of this essay, I briefly discussed the position that family theories and conceptual frameworks of analyses are projective systems of the sociologists who formulate them. Others who then find these congenial to their own ways of thinking introject these theories and integrate them into their own systems of thought. Let us now ask: what evidence is there that the conceptual schemes presented in the section "Which American Family?" make up my own projective system?

Perhaps the primary evidence for this is seen in juxtaposing the section "Choosing Life, Choosing Death" upon the section "Which American Family?" The focus of both sections is upon the fragility of existence and the problem of endurance (or survival). The personal experiences in "Choosing

Life, Choosing Death" are transformed into societal concerns in "American Family." Survival becomes the transgenerational endurance of family and kinship structures and modes of socialization.

When one adds to this concern that of contradictory principles of organization, the unresolved Oedipal problems come to the fore. Have I seen in my mother the proletariat of Marx and in my father the bourgeoisie? Translated into the concepts I used: my mother represents the centrifugal form of family and kinship organization–adapting to concurrent needs in ways that spread the web of ties in the society and, in doing so, emphasize tactical means for maintaining social ties. My father represents the centripetal form of family and kinship organization–concerned with strategies that give stability to family structures over generations. It is the combination of the unresolved Oedipal concern with the survival concern that sustains my projective system regarding the perpetual conflict in structural needs in family and kinship.

One can find pieces of evidence regarding the reinforcement of my framework of analysis. These would include the influence of growing up in a minority group and (consistent with my Oedipal problems) the Marxist thought of relatives and college classmates. Certainly, growing up when terrorism in Germany and the Holocaust took place affected the formulation of my conceptual apparatus.

Together, all of these influences converged to form a basis for rejecting the optimistic, functionalist position of Talcott Parsons (1955). His view was that society as an adaptive *system* would ultimately reallocate roles in ways that would resolve structural contradictions. For example, he posited a family system of dual leadership, with the wife offering a supportive, social emotional role to maintain social ties, while the husband would take care of the instrumental role oriented toward the future welfare of the family. However, changes in family life in the last half-century give evidence of the inadequacy of Parsons' conceptual framework–high divorce rates, the practice of intentional births outside marriage, the expectation that a large percentage of children will live part of their lives in single-parent families, late marriage and cohabitation of unmarried couples (heterosexual and homosexual), and so on. But although the Parsonian scheme falters in the light of these changes, my projective system accommodates them.

WHAT NOW?

Which way do I turn at this time of life? Suppose I were to write an ad for a singles column, what should I say about myself? Retired university professor of sociology, aged 77, widower, good health, full head of hair, kosher kitchen (vegetarian), intellectual interests (particularly Judaica at this time), domesticated, caring, willing to try anything (within reason). Loads of children (ages 26-49) coast to coast. References.

Except for family and friends, there is little more to say about my current existence. Without doubt, my brother Irving, my children, and my grandchildren constitute the most important people in my life. As for friends, I must mention a few who are sociologists: Morrie and Zelma Axelrod, Len and Rena Gordon, John and Doreen Mogey, Mike Lewis, Alezah Dworkin Weinberg, Jose Cobas, and the Lindstroms. And the students who gave me the most "nakhos"-Bill Jenne, David L. Harvey, Howard Altstein, Jerry M. Lewis, Karen S. Smith, Ione DeOllos, G. N. Ramu, David Baker, and the late Sung Ling Lin.

EDITORS' NOTE

Dr. Bernard Farber died on May 5, 2000, a few months after completing a revision of this essay. The editors were responsible for completing and inserting the citations that Farber noted into the essay.

REFERENCES

Baker, D. J. (1991). *Conceptions of collaterality in modern Europe: Kinship ideologies from companionship to trusteeship*. Unpublished doctoral dissertation, University of Illinois, Urbana-Champaign.

Burgess, E. W. & Locke, H. J. (1945). *The family: From institution to companionship*. New York: American Book Co.

Burgess, E. W. & Wallin, P. (1953). *Engagement and marriage*. Philadelphia: Lippincott.

Farber, B. (1959). Effects of a severely mentally retarded child on family integration. *Monographs of the Society for Research in Child Development*, No. 71.

Farber, B. (1960a). Family organization and crisis: Maintenance of integration in families with a severely mentally retarded child. *Monographs of the Society for Research in Child Development*, No. 75.

Farber, B. (1960b). The perception of crisis and related variables in the impact of a retarded child on the mother. *Journal of Health and Human Behavior*, *1*, 2, 108-118.

Farber, B. & Others (1960c). Family Crisis and the Decision to Institutionalize the Retarded Child. Council of Exceptional Research Monograph, Series A, Number 1. Washington, DC.

Farber, B. (1961). The family as a set of mutually contingent careers. In Nelson N. Foote (Ed.). *Household Decision-Making* (pp. 276-297). NY: New York University Press.

Farber, B. (1964). *Family: Organization and interaction*. San Francisco: Chandler.

Farber, B. (1968a). *Comparative kinship systems: A method of analysis*. New York: John Wiley & Sons.

Farber, B. (1968b). *Mental retardation: Its social context and social consequences*. Boston: Houghton Mifflin.
Farber, B. (1971). *Kinship and class: A Midwestern study*. New York: Basic Books.
Farber, B. (1972). *Guardians of virtue: Salem families in 1800*. New York: Basic Books.
Farber, B. (1973a). *Family and kinship in modern society*. Glenview, IL: Scott, Foresman.
Farber, B. (1973b). Women, marriage, and illness: Consumptives in Salem, Massachusetts, 1785-1819. *Journal of Comparative Family Studies*, *4*, 1, 36-48.
Farber, B. (1975). Bilateral kinship: Centripetal and centrifugal types of organization. *Journal of Marriage and the Family*, *37*, 4, 871-888.
Farber, B. (1977). Social context, kinship mapping, and family norms. *Journal of Marriage and the Family*, *39*, 2, 227-240.
Farber, B. (1979). Kinship mapping among Jews in a midwestern city. *Social Forces*, *57*, 4, 1107-1123.
Farber, B. (1981). *Conceptions of kinship*. New York: Elsevier.
Farber, B. & Jenne, W. C. (1963a). Family organization and parent-child communication: Parents and siblings of a retarded child. *Monographs of the Society for Research in Child Development*, *28*, 7.
Farber, B. & Jenne, W.C. (1963b). Interaction with retarded siblings and life goals of children. *Journal of Marriage and Family Living*, *25*, 1, 96-98.
Ogburn, W. F. (1929). The changing family. *Publications of the American Sociological Society*, 23, 124-133.
Parsons, T. & Bales, R. F. (1955). *The Family, socialization and interaction*. New York: Free Press.
Rosen, D. M (1999). American Families and American Law. In M. B. Sussman, S. K. Steinmetz, & G. W. Peterson (Eds.). *Handbook of Marriage and the Family*. (pp. 553-570). New York: Plenum Publisher.
Schneider, L. (1975). *The sociological way of looking at the world*. New York: McGraw-Hill.
Sorokin, P. A. (1962). *Society, culture and personality*. New York: Cooper Square.
Zimmerman, C. C. & Frampton, M. E. (1935). *Family and society*. Princeton, NJ: Van Nostrand.

By the Book: An Academic Memoir

Joan Aldous

KEYWORDS. Autobiography, family sociology, research, gender, careers

FOREWORD

I did not plan to become a professor when I was young, but perhaps it was inevitable. All my life my surroundings have included academicians and books. Certainly not by the book, however, is the spelling of my first name and its pronunciation. My first name, Joan, is pronounced as if it were spelled Joanne. However, I have never thought of changing my parents' spelling. The pronunciation of my first name is one means I have for separating the people who know me and I care about from those I don't. I also have no middle name, and that has given various bureaucratic organizations problems. When I applied to enter the University of Chicago as a freshman, for example, those folks were concerned enough to give me the middle initial N. They assured me that it stood for "no name." So truly, as far as I am concerned, what's in a name? But with respect to my living my life by the book, that is worth an examination.

EARLY DAYS

My Ancestors

My ancestors on my mother's side emigrated from England in 1635, and my father's grandparents also came from England in the 1850s. My grandmother Aldous, however, was an immigrant from Denmark. I know less about my father's side of the family, because of his early death. My mother's ancestors were soldiers in the Revolutionary War and the Civil War, in the latter mainly on the side of the Confederacy. Reportedly, my great-grandmother often spoke of General Robert E. Lee, but always in hushed tones. I should add that another ancestor supposedly fought beside Abraham Lincoln in the Black Hawk War. Unlike most wars, it only lasted one day. Would that all wars could be so short.

One of my mother's ancestors with the remarkable name of Karenhappuck Turner showed the strength and determination that characterized my female forebears. After the Battle of Guilford Courthouse, North Carolina, during the Revolution, she journeyed on horseback from Maryland to nurse her wounded son and grandson as well as others needing care. There is now a statue of her on the battlefield site commemorating her nursing which she did in a log cabin. I should add the remark a Park Service official made when I visited the battlefield memorial several years ago. While in the visitors' building, I alluded modestly to my kinship. "Oh," he said disgustedly. "Every visitor claims that." The relationship did get my mother into the Daughters of the American Revolution in Washington, D.C. in 1915 when she was newly married to my father, then employed in the U.S. Forestry Service. She resigned later after moving with him to Manhattan when he obtained a position at Kansas State. The DAR members there, she thought, were just too "fuddy-duddyish."

My ancestors had all journeyed west after the Civil War, attracted by the Mormons' settling in Utah. My grandfather, and many of my other relatives of his generation later left that denomination, but not before he had taken a second wife, my grandmother. Men's having more than one wife was a part of the Mormon belief system. It was one of the reasons Brigham Young took his followers west outside the jurisdiction of the United States. Because of this practice, Utah's admission to the U.S. did not come until 1896. The Utah state legislature had by then incorporated into the State Constitution a provision against plural marriages, a law the U.S. Congress passed in 1862. Grandmother's family had been much against the marriage, and it probably contributed to their leaving the Mormon faith. My grandmother eventually divorced Grandfather. The divorce gave my grandfather the accepted marital status that later enabled him to obtain important university positions. To support her two children after the divorce, as Grandfather had a number of children by his first wife, my grandmother became a respected grade school principal in Logan, Utah. My mother understandably was never close to her father, and her mother died shortly after my birth. Mother only told me tearfully of the troubled situation involving her genesis when I was a teenager.

My Parents

My father, Alfred Evan Aldous, was a Professor of Agronomy at Kansas State University-Manhattan (then Kansas State Agriculture College), and my mother, Coral Kerr Aldous, stayed home. My parents had a happy marriage. Mother always joked that they only argued on moving day, and we moved very seldomly. I had one sister, Lois, who was 6 1/2 years older than I. We were never very close. I was the pesky kid sister who would sneak into her bedroom when she was gone and unearth her diary from her bottom desk drawer to read.

As I talk with lifelong friends and think back on those growing-up years, I realize that my arrival within our family disrupted her long-established family arrangements. No longer was she the center of attention. Her jealousy of this upstart newcomer colored her relationships with me and my parents. It led to disagreeable behavior that separated her from my father and mother. I became the favorite child even though my parents tried to make Lois happy. They did this generally by buying her things she wanted and letting her do what she wished. In the long run, their hands-off strategy did little to ameliorate her general unhappiness.

In some ways, though, Lois served as a role model for me. From my earliest years, I was surrounded by books. Regular trips to Manhattan's Carnegie Free Public Library were part of my routine encouraged by my sister's example. Lois always had a book in her hands. This love even got her out of her kitchen chores. She would entertain my mother by reading a story to her from the latest *Saturday Evening Post*, while my mother did the work Lois was supposed to do. Mother did not object, I am sure, because she enjoyed seeing Lois satisfied. She also liked hearing the stories she knew her busy life as a faculty wife would keep her from reading. In addition, we generally had a live-in "student girl" to help out, who attended K-State and earned her room and board by doing housework for us. This was a common practice for women students in the hard times of the 1930s.

My father's area of expertise was pasture grasses for animal grazing. He developed new varieties of grasses. He is the only person I have ever known or heard of who had his doctoral thesis accepted *before* filling the required year of residency in the Department of Agronomy at the University of Nebraska-Lincoln. My first view of education in action came from my rides with him to the K-State Agronomy Farm, where he checked on the grass plots he was using to try out different strains. These excursions with Daddy were times to fill him in on my doings, and he would explain to me what he did as an agronomist. These were years of drought in the Great Plains as well as the Great Depression, so his experiments, I realized, were very important to Kansas farmers' well-being. His graduate students who came to the house for supper made their admiration for him and his research very clear. He and they were adding to the information found in today's agronomy books. One former student, Kling Anderson, who replaced my dad at K-State, later even named a strain of grass after him. Daddy and I also would take long walks together with me talking nonstop. My admiration and love for him made me truly a "Daddy's Girl," although Mother provided a special source of affection. Certainly, these times with him developed in me a respect for research.

In the mid-1930s, Hugh Bennett of the newly established U.S. Soil Conservation Service got my father to add part-time work for it to his K-State teaching and research responsibilities. Our family was quite well off compared to many in those depression years. My parents could even afford to be staunch Republicans, as were most of their faculty friends, at a time when most folks were voting for Franklin D. Roosevelt and his New Deal designed to help the many poor and needy. Daddy's position and paychecks were secure, because they depended on state monies. But his double workload which demanded a lot of driving back and forth to Western Kansas probably contributed to the heart attack that killed him when he was just 53 years old, and I was 13. This was a devastating blow to our family. My mother not only lost her beloved partner, but had to find a means of support for her family. Fortunately, she had a Bachelor's Degree (in Home Economics) from Utah State University, a college degree being an uncommon achievement then for anyone, especially a woman. She saw her future in academia due to her education and to the university surroundings, and went to New York City to obtain a Master's Degree from Columbia University Teachers College. To my and Lois's delight, she then obtained a position at K-State in the Department of Family and Child Development, College of Home Economics. Given the scarcity of jobs in that era, she was lucky to be employed in her chosen field in a university.

Books and Education

When I got to be a senior in high school, I had great ambitions. I decided I wanted to go to the University of Chicago, major in international relations and eventually enter the diplomatic service. Most of my friends were going to Kansas State, so to leave Manhattan was unusual and costly, especially for my mother, an underpaid woman faculty member. But I had heard of the renowned Robert Maynard Hutchins, and how he was remaking university education at Chicago. I wanted to be a part of it. I applied for a scholarship, and my grandfather on my mother's side, William Jasper Kerr, agreed to pay for expenses my mother could not afford.

Grandfather was another bookish person in my background, who had translated his interest into administration. He had been head of Brigham Young Academy, and then President of Utah State University and Oregon State University, in that order. He ended his career as the first Chancellor of the Oregon System of Higher Education. I remember when he would visit us, how impressed I was by his comments about the university presidents of his day, such as David Starr Jordan of Stanford and William Rainey Harper of the University of Chicago, whom he had known.

All worked out for me to attend the University of Chicago, as I did receive a scholarship there. The University of Chicago at that time proved as exciting as I had heard. It was alive with ideas and controversy concerning the revolutionary changes in staid academic procedures that Hutchins was instituting. Demanding teachers pushed students to go beyond obvious answers, and we talked intellectual issues in our dorms. The home of President Hutchins was right across the street from my dormitory, and my buddies called me "golden" when I passed him on the way to class. It was the only university in my academic life where students felt honored just to catch a glimpse of their university's president.

Alas, in the midst of this heady, intellectual atmosphere, I contracted rheumatoid arthritis. This is a crippling disease which attacks more young women than young men and has consequences for the rest of one's life. Certainly, it changed what happened to me. As a result of it, I had to leave Chicago, and, after spending four months in a Kansas City, Missouri, hospital being rehabilitated, I came back to Manhattan and enrolled at Kansas State. I changed my major from international relations, since there was no such thing then at K-State. Now, more than ever, I realized my future lay in books and probably academia. I had only known academicians and university life, so such a career made sense for someone like me who was what people now call "disabled." Sociology appealed to me more than the alternatives of psychology and economics, as I was hooked on the social sciences.

GRADUATE EDUCATION

My mother had a sabbatical coming, so after my graduation from K-State, she and I headed for the University of Texas-Austin. It had a mild climate, and they gave me a scholarship. I got my Master's degree there in sociology, writing a thesis on "The Sociological Significance of the United Nations Educational Scientific and Cultural Organization." I was still trying to maintain my international perspective, even though I realized the diplomatic service was no longer a possibility for me due to the aftereffects of the rheumatoid arthritis.

Perhaps the only thing that was interesting, and significant, about my graduate work at UT was an encounter I had with my advisor. Head of the Department of Sociology, he was a man who had received his own training at the University of Chicago many years before, had a well-known textbook, and was giving the same lectures to his students as those he gave when he first arrived at UT. After I had passed my orals for my Master's degree, I asked him, "What do you think about my going on for a PhD?" He said he didn't think I should. "Understand," he assured me, "it is nothing personal. I just don't think any woman should get a PhD." It says something about my background and my own self-esteem that his advice didn't faze me. I knew he was clearly wrong, and I wasn't afraid to think that I would eventually, if I wanted to, earn a PhD. However, my worsening health took me back to Manhattan, and again to a hospital in Kansas City.

The Pleasures of Research

My mother had a colleague in the Department of Family and Child Development, Professor Leone Kell, who received a research grant from the K-State Agricultural Experiment Station. It included a research assistantship. This was far-sighted of the Experiment Station to grant funds to a woman professor doing family research. In many land-grant universities, these funds were and are used primarily for agricultural projects.

Leone was a dear friend of my mother's, and had also been my former teacher when I had attended K-State's nursery school as a preschooler. In that era, middle-class mothers who were full-time homemakers sent their children to nursery schools to cultivate their social skills. The mother of twin friends of mine had been an exception. At enrollment times, she "helped out" the K-State registrar to supplement her husband's limited income. Her children were in nursery school partly because of her periodic absences from home to earn money. But they were an exception.

Leone was good enough to ask me if I'd like to help her with her research project. It concerned the child-rearing ideologies of mothers and their college student children's views of maternal control. I leapt at the opportunity, or as far as I could, given my then using crutches and full-leg-braces. This was a wonderful chance, because it enabled me to learn research from the ground up. I could go beyond the library research I did for my MA. I had just returned from my five-month hospital-stay, again being "rehabilitated." Thanks to this study of Leone's, I found that, despite my using crutches and braces, I could still be a useful person. It was tremendously important for my morale.

My responsibility, after Leone and I put together the interview schedule, was to do all the K-State student interviews. I would enter Calvin Hall, the home economics building, and go to a room on the ground floor–no steps. I would then sit down, set aside my crutches, insert the tape in a huge tape recorder, the best available in the 1950s, start it, and interview the student. The students were about the same age as I, and we got along famously. The only disaster came when I lost half of one of the most fascinating interviews due to my inexperience operating the tape recorder. While I was doing these interviews, Leone was traveling all around the state of Kansas to do the interviews with the students' mothers.

This experience was extremely valuable, because I had to review the relevant literature and analyze the data in addition to conducting the interviews. This resulted in several co-authored publications with Leone Kell, one in *Child Development* (Kell & Aldous, 1960a) and two others in *Marriage and Family Living* (presently the *Journal of Marriage and the Family*) (Aldous & Kell, 1961; Kell & Aldous, 1960b). Since Leone did not like to write up the study results, she was very happy for me to do it. This research assistantship only lasted a year, but I continued to work with her after the funding ended. Because it was hard for me to get around at the University due to my crutches and braces, she was a darling and came down to my house at least once a week to discuss our various projects.

While doing this research work, I also pursued my own activities. I produced an article, "The Relation of Evelyn Duvall's Role Conceptions to David Riesman's Character Types," in which I compared David Riesman's ideas from *The Lonely Crowd* and Evelyn Duvall's work on personality. The article was accepted by the *Journal of Home Economics* (Aldous, 1956), and it was all my own doing, including the idea. I felt triumphant. There was also a spinoff from my research with Leone Kell that I did alone (Aldous, 1961). It appeared in the *Family Life Coordinator* (*Family Relations* nowadays).

Broader Horizons

After eight very happy years of having weekly visits from a physical therapist and doing many daily exercises, I got rid of the braces, although I still had to use crutches. I was keeping up on the sociological literature as well as the psychological research concerning parent-child relations. Thanks to my mother and Leone Kell, who would order books I suggested either through the Department of Family and Child Development or the K-State library, I had no difficulty knowing who the creative researchers were in this area, especially in the field of sociology.

In 1958 my mother had been elected President of the Kansas Council on Family Relations. There was money for a speaker at their convention to be held that year at K-State. She asked Reuben Hill to come. He had recently moved from the University of North Carolina-Chapel Hill to the University of Minnesota to head the newly-created Family Study Center. Leone took me to the dinner where he was to give his presentation. Even though my mother gave his introduction at the banquet, I was too shy to go up afterwards to meet him. I do not remember what Reuben Hill said that night, but, after the talk, he had become more to me than a name on a popular textbook, *When You Marry*, written with Evelyn Duvall (Duvall & Hill, 1945).

About that same time, I had started thinking of obtaining a PhD. My mother was going to retire in 1958. I knew that if I wanted to earn a living, a PhD was essential. Because of the research I'd done on the family, I decided it only made good sense to work in this area, especially since I now had several publications on the subject. I wrote to William Goode about the PhD program in sociology at Columbia University. He was very sympathetic, but he said he had no money. He suggested that I get in touch with Reuben Hill, who did. My mother and I drove up to Minneapolis in the summer of 1959, and I talked with Reuben. Roy Rodgers, soon to be in the Department of Sociology at the University of Oregon, met me at the elevator and led me into the great man's office. Reuben made me feel good by telling me that he was familiar with my publications. He urged me to come to Minnesota and suggested that I apply for a National Institute of Mental Health graduate fellowship. I applied for such a fellowship and, much to my joy, I was awarded one.

Thus, my mother and I pulled up stakes in Manhattan and left for Minnesota. Although she had long-time friends in the Twin Cities, a couple where the husband had been Head of Dairy Husbandry at K-State before taking the same but much better paying position at Minnesota, our departure must have been a wrenching one for my mother. She had just resumed her bridge playing and other pleasures with friends, wives of my father's colleagues, that she did not have time to see while being a professor and fulfilling my health needs. But without complaint, she joined me in my northern exposure. She was a dear.

The graduate school experience was one I enjoyed. It was an era when scholars like Arnold Rose and Gregory Stone, in addition to Reuben Hill, were at the University of Minnesota in sociology. Don Martindale, who was well known at that time for his work on sociological theory, taught that course. Both Reuben and Marion Hill had graduated from Utah State University, as had my parents. Marion Hill had also been a member of the same sorority that my mother belonged to some 25 years earlier. For these reasons, I always felt close to my major professor, which eased the transition. Another plus was getting acquainted with my fellow graduate students. They are some of the people you get closest to in life, because they are going through the same trials and tribulations at the same time you are. The wintry climate also proved to be less hazardous to my health than I had feared. Clamp devices that I put on my crutches enabled me to get through the ice and the snow without falling.

My PhD thesis topic grew out of the previous research I had done with Leone Kell at KSU. Reuben Hill and Nelson Foote had collected data from three-generation families–grandparents, parents, and adult children–in the Minneapolis-St. Paul U.S. Census Statistical Area. He gave me access to these data, and I decided to look at the continuities and discontinuities over the three generations in years of education, religious affiliation, and occupations. However, I had difficulty getting to work on my thesis. Part of this "fooling around" period I spent turning one of my term papers on kin relations in Sub-Saharan Africa into a paper that was eventually published in *Social Forces* (Aldous, 1962). This article proved to be very well received and was frequently quoted. I also wrote a proposal that I submitted to the National Science Foundation and to the National Institute of Mental Health for observational research on creativity in children.

Summer came, and still no thesis. Reuben Hill had offered me a soft money job in the Department of Sociology for the upcoming academic year. The understanding was that I would have to have my thesis finished by the end of the summer. I had had a job interview at another university, but had not been very happy either with my own performance, or the opportunities there. With a nonnegotiable deadline facing me, I frantically wrote a chapter a week. My mother would then type it up on our trusty Royal portable, and I would take it to Reuben. He would go over it and was usually very positive. Only on the last chapter did he express his impatience. For a Mormon, he got pretty upset. He said, "Good Lord! How can you express yourself so poorly? I think you've run out of gas. You've got to do this entire chapter all over again." It was a humbling experience doing the thesis, but I got it done. I was now a full-fledged PhD.

Another good thing was that my attempts to get a research grant paid off. These were halcyon days, when the federal government had the dollars to encourage social science research. The NSF agreed to fund my creativity research, but cut the budget. The NIMH also liked it. They even sent people, whose names I have forgotten, for a site visit. They were at the University to review another research proposal, so they looked in on me. I really enjoyed their questions and comments. They also seemed to have fun at our meeting. We did a lot of laughing in the course of our conversation, so much so that Reuben Hill worried they would not take me seriously. The outcome, though, was their recommendation for full funding of my project. I happily accepted the NIMH grant with its higher funding. I was now set with respect to my research.

PROFESSOR

I did, however, have to face a major lack in my academic qualifications. I had never taught before. Thank goodness, my teaching assistant was Wesley R. Burr, who had been the teacher in many classes before he had come to Minnesota to get his PhD. He was very kind about offering counsel to me on how to handle myself as a teacher. One example of his help was his talk to me before I entered my first class. I was simply terrified and without Wes's pleasant but firm insistence, I might well have "chickened out." Remember, I was still on crutches and very self-conscious about people's reactions to me.

Research has always been my cup of tea, though, and I have never had difficulty in writing up my findings for publication. My first project after my doctoral thesis research was the one on how parents influenced children's creativity. For it and my next study of family problem-solving research, using a large multi-year NIMH-funded multi-year grant to myself, Reuben Hill, Murray Strauss, and Irving Tallman, I used observational research to collect my data. I brought families, both parents and one child, into a laboratory with a one-way vision window. My research assistant would code the behaviors and the speech that these people would display in response to vignettes that I presented to them. This is a very good method for getting at process, but it is most time consuming, both with respect to data collection and to getting the data ready for analysis. Very few people do this kind of research in sociology. But I think it gave me good experience, and I've never regretted these studies.

Academics and Academia

An interesting aspect of my time at the U of M was that Reuben Hill was my mentor both when I was a doctoral student and after I became a faculty member. There were great advantages to this situation, but there were a few disadvantages as well. On the plus side, I had someone who could watch out for me at a time when university faculty, even in sociology, still tended to look at women faculty as not quite belonging. I was the first woman professor in the Department of Sociology at Minnesota, and the Head, a crusty older man who had grown up in the gangster and bootlegging years of the 1920s in wide-open Kansas City, Missouri, had difficulty accepting me. He swore quite freely, and in faculty meetings would apologize profusely to me each time. I hated being ostentatiously set apart from the other faculty. Finally, colleague Ed Gross intervened. "For God's sake," I remember him saying, "Joan's heard 'hell' and 'damn' before." The apologies finally stopped, thank goodness.

Reuben also gave me the opportunity to administer an NIMH-funded graduate training program at Minnesota that he had won. Such sociologists as Stephen Jorgensen, Texas Tech; David Klein, Notre Dame; Viktor Gecas, Washington State; Brent Miller, Utah State; Darwin Thomas, Brigham Young University; the late Elizabeth Rooney, San Francisco State University; and Andrew Weigert, Notre Dame, all got their PhDs through it. Hill and I also co-authored an article on socialization for marriage and parenting in a *Handbook of Socialization, Theory and Research* (Hill & Aldous, 1969) edited by David Goslin, and I was able to meet and establish lasting friendships with such visiting scholars at the Family Study Center as Wilfried Dumon and Karel Dobbelaere of the Katholieke Universiteit-Leuven, Belgium, and Takeji Kamiko of Osaka City University, Japan. The downside was that others, not Reuben, expected me in departmental controversies always to side with him.

He also was a bit of a sexist, which I found increasingly difficult to accept without argument.

I remember a run-in I had with him when women's rights were becoming an issue. My secretary and I together decided to substitute "she" for "he" and "her" for "him" throughout his and my joint article on socialization. This was the era when masculine pronouns were used in speech and writing because they supposedly covered all humanity. Poor Reuben could not see the humor in the situation. His Freudian vocabulary took over. "What is this?" he roared. "Some kind of masculine protest?" But I had the last word. "Aren't you hitting below the belt?" I gently asked, as I left the room. Of course, he was a product of his era and his religious background. Also, he had informed me early on that I was the first woman to complete her PhD with him. Others had dropped out without completing their theses. I was followed by other woman students like Phyllis Moen, his last PhD, now at Cornell, who did complete their degrees. And over the years, he mellowed, and I believe he became more positive toward gender equity issues. Since I was no longer at Minnesota, I was unable to see what part he played in departmental decisions concerning women.

Creating Controversy

By and large, though, my tenure at Minnesota was a happy and productive period for me. Through skillful surgery by an orthopedist at the University Medical School, I was able to be free of my crutches. What a blessing! I even got to escape the winters. The University was on the quarter system then, and my mother and I would flee to Nashville, Tennessee from January until the middle of March, from 1964-1969. There, I was a visiting scholar, first in the Department of Social Work at the University of Tennessee-Nashville and then at the Demonstration and Research Center for Early Education, Kennedy Center for Research on Education and Human Development, at George Peabody College, now a part of Vanderbilt University. Those were the days of the War on Poverty, and with friends from DARCEE I did some research on children's perceptions of adult roles. I worked in a poverty-stricken delta county in Mississippi at Head Start Centers. To see the cost in human lives of segregation and wretched living conditions was an eye-opening experience for this middle-class intellectual.

For my research in Clarksdale, Holmes County, two research assistants, one White and one Black, had come with me to do some of the interviews. I had met the White Head of the Advisory Council of the Holmes County War on Poverty to explain the research and to gain official approval for it. He telephoned me one evening at our room in the desegregated Holiday Inn to ask me to dinner at his home. I explained that I would not want to leave my research assistants behind. "Bring them along," he urged. "It will be fine,

I'm sure." Knowing he was a wealthy plantation owner, whose wife's only sustained contacts with Blacks had probably been with her host of servants, I explained that one RA was Black. "Would that make a difference?" I inquired. He audibly gulped, and there was a pause. "Just a minute," he replied. When he picked up the phone again, he said both RAs would be welcome. So we desegregated his home. Although my Black RA understandably made light of the event, she did note that her mother had told her to flee to the bus station if anything nasty happened during our stay. The bus station was officially desegregated because interstate buses arrived and departed there. Another indicator of the times occurred when the Director of the Head Start program in Holmes County drove me to Memphis to catch my plane back to Nashville. We were both more than a little apprehensive that White Citizens Council vigilantes might stop the car with its Black male driver and White female passenger. There was no "Driving Miss Joan" here. Both of us were sitting together on the front seat as equals.

During these confrontation-filled days of the late 1960s, I set aside the book of protocol and with good friend and fellow sociologist then in the College of Education, Shirley M. Clark, organized the Committee on University Women's Progress (CUWP). Along with other uppity women professors and students at the University, we pressed for more women faculty and higher salaries for them. Our activities took us outside the Twin Cities to present our case before the few women who were members of the Board of Regents. We also approached the University President, Malcom Moos, in his office. As I remember it, he appeared quite terrified as two women, both full professors, invaded his office to urge gender equity. We had an appointment, but he was clearly ill at ease. However, the fact that the CUWP no longer exists at the University of Minnesota is a tribute to the changes he and his successor put into place. Despite these changes, some departments, such as the Department of History, continue to be largely male. Its faculty, though, is trying to change things. Eight of the last 10 hires have been women (Smetanka, April 3, 1999, A12). Interestingly, Shirley Clark is now Vice-Chancellor of the Oregon System of Higher Education, my grandfather's old bailiwick.

Getting tenure had not proved to be a worry and came my second year on faculty. By then, I was on a regular faculty appointment and had at the end of my first year received a 50 percent salary raise of $3,000. It was the largest raise any faculty member received for the academic year 1964-65 in the College of Liberal Arts. With the increase, my salary became a munificent $9,000 a year. This promotion and raise were probably due to my having received the NIMH grant, and to my growing record of publications drawn from my doctoral thesis. I was also getting the hang of teaching. After observing several of my lectures, which was my early teaching style, Penny Baron, a thoughtful TA, suggested that I did better leading discussions. I was glad to ditch the laborious process of putting together my remarks on paper for reading. The anonymous student evaluations were generally positive. I still remember one. "Good class," it read. "That aqua outfit you wear is really great!" And it was. I have forgotten the year I made full professor, but it was a relatively short time afterwards, somewhere around 1970.

Around the World

When it was time for my sabbatical, my plans went far beyond the horizon. I flew around the world to reach Leuven, Belgium, where I was to be Visiting Professor, second semester. My next door office neighbor at Minnesota, former President of the National Council on Family Relations, and head of the Family Social Science Department at the University, Richard Hey had filled me in on the Hawaiian Islands' wonders. My first stop, therefore, was Honolulu, with side trips to Maui and Kauai. Japan was next on my travel agenda, since I had an NIMH grant to do research with Kamiko-san. He had replicated my research in northern Honshu on children's perceptions of adult roles.

The four months in Japan really made me a sociologist. I was so out of place in this, the most sexist world I had ever entered. The women students–there were no women professors–would come to me after my lectures at the various universities around Japan where I was asked to talk. The women would tell me how for the first time, because I was a recognized woman scholar, they were encouraged to come to lectures of outside speakers. After my talks, I would be taken to dinner or to someone's home, where my companions would all be male. Even wives were barred from the get-togethers except to wait upon the men and me. The U.S. Information Agency also asked me to give more informal lectures at their libraries in Fukuoko, Muroran, Sapporo, Toyko, and, of course, Kyoto, which I made my headquarters. Thus, I got to see much of Japan, including a special pilgrimage to Hiroshima.

Kamiko-san lived in Kyoto, and I would taxi out to his home. It had one table and four chairs in an otherwise Japanese-style home. I only tried eating once on the tatami floor with a lower place to put one's feet, their customary dining area. It took a pile of pillows for me to slide down, and Mrs. Kamiko and the three adolescent children later to get me off the floor. It was interesting, to say the least, to see how Takeji just stood and watched during our collective struggle.

The situation today in Japan is somewhat better, I am glad to note, than in 1969. I have a student, Keiko Hirao, who got her PhD with me here at Notre Dame. She has obtained an Associate Professor position at Sophia University in the Department of Human Philosophy. However, for those who believe in gender equality, according to reliable reports, there continues to be much to do in Japan, as is the case here.

After Japan, I continued my around-the-world tour with stops in Bangkok, Thailand, where I visited the family of a former student of my mother, and in Delhi, India. Friends from the U.S. Information Service showed me the sights there. I also had the good fortune to visit Tehran and Sheraz in Iran, a destination no longer open to Americans. My time in Leuven, Belgium, was agreeable both for the intellectual and pleasurable occasions my colleagues there provided.

Upon my return home, I had to face the deteriorating health of my mother. She had spent the time I was gone in an assisted-living apartment in Salt Lake City, watched over by my cousin, Barbara Kerr, and with visits from my sister. Due to my inability to care for her at home, I had to make the painful decision to put her in a nursing home. It was supposed to be the best in the Twin Cities, but the lack of attention she received there, despite my daily telephone calls and visits each Saturday and Sunday, made me literally weep. When she died in 1973, I was ready to leave Minnesota.

NEW BEGINNINGS

Experiences in the Department of Sociology, Tulane University, as Visiting Favrot Professor, and later a joint appointment in the Departments of Child and Family Development and Sociology at the University of Georgia led to new friends like Tom and Virginia Ktsanes, Jim and Lynda Henley Walters, and Sharon Price, as well as to different ideas. However, I decided to return to the Universiteit Leuven in Belgium in 1975-76 to finish a book, *Family Careers*, and to take advantage of funding from the USIA to travel about Europe, including Turkey and Scandanavia, to make talks at their various Centers. I had much to think about that year abroad.

Shortly before leaving Georgia, the Head of the Department of Sociology at the University of Notre Dame had telephoned, asking me if I would stop by on my way to Europe. To say I was surprised does not sufficiently capture my emotion. Because I am always open to new experiences, I did visit. I told the then-Notre Dame Provost, James T. Burtchaell, a priest in a Brooks Brothers suit, that I was a WASP who stood for practically everything I understood the Catholic Bishops were against. "Oh, that's all right," he replied, "as long as you don't propagandize." I assured him that I never pushed my particular values, but, undoubtedly, they would be apparent to my students. This discussion did not appear to worry the Notre Dame administrators.

Shortly after I got to Leuven, Belgium, the Dean of the College of Arts and Letters at Notre Dame, Isabel Charles, a first for a woman that has not been repeated, telephoned and offered me a professorship. As Miriam Hey astutely put it, Isabel was nice enough also to include the offer of the William R. Kenan, Jr. endowed chair for me to sit down in. Despite this honor, I thought it only wise to specify that I would be just a Visiting Professor. The faculty might not approve of me, and I could also be unhappy. The Dean of Home Economics at Georgia, Emily Pew, the best I have ever had during my academic years, agreed to my being on leave another year. She did ask me if I could "commute" to Athens to offer classes. I allowed as how I thought the distance might be a bit too great.

Now, why did I agree to "try out" Notre Dame and eventually decide to stay? At that time, in the mid- and late 1970s, Catholicism was still enjoying the fresh air that had invigorated it when Pope John the 23rd had thrown open the windows of the Vatican to twentieth-century ideas. Notre Dame, under the leadership of Rev. Theodore Hesburgh, C.S.C., was leaving its parochial past and trying to become a real university. I represented a few firsts: first woman full professor; first woman faculty offered an endowed chair; first tenured woman in the Department of Sociology, etc., etc., and my position and accomplishments gave me special opportunities. Now, of course, the present Pope is busy slamming shut any windows still left open on this century and retreating back to the Middle Ages. The sexism and authoritarianism in Catholic dogma are apparent in current church actions despite the opposition of many lay people and priests. I can honestly report, though, that I have had complete freedom over the years to express my ideas in classes, publications, and research. Notre Dame administrators have also been cooperative in helping me fulfill my various projects.

Back to Belgium, where I had a most enjoyable and productive year. I was a USIA lecturer in such places as Istanbul, Turkey; Helsinki, Finland; and Rome, Italy. It was also an adventure to be in Madrid and Barcelona, Spain, and Lisbon, Portugal, shortly after the fall of dictators, Franco and Salazar respectively. I reveled in the new openness I found in both countries. Back in Leuven, I finished my book, *Family Careers* (Aldous, 1978), no small undertaking, since I am an article, not a book, author. The year was out of the ordinary in a number of other ways. I lived in a women's dormitory and got to know the students on my floor well. We'd talk about all sorts of things, including what they'd been reading that I knew about. I even ventured into reading, speaking, and publishing in French.

I returned to the U.S. and my trial year at Notre Dame with some trepidation. I feared it would all be so different. I need not have worried. All went swimmingly, beginning with my arrival at the airport, where my secretary-to-be met me with a bouquet of flowers. I liked my colleagues, my students, and the financial support for research the University offered. A former student at Minnesota, good friend, and fellow family sociologist, David Klein, also was new that year to share the academic happenings. Professor Wilfried Dumon of the Katholieke Universiteit Leuven, Belgium, stopped by in November, and I told him, and at his urging the Provost, that I would stay. The Dean, perhaps in celebration, brought in Dumon and his family second semester, so Wilfried and I could finish some joint research. And the Provost came over to my office to inquire if I needed anything. In all honesty, I could not think of a thing.

So I settled down at Notre Dame and lived happily ever after, aside from various years abroad once more at Leuven on sabbatical. There, I inaugurated the first gender studies class given at the University. I have also attended various committees on family research (International Sociological Association), and seminars in such exotic locations as Tampere, Finland; Ma'ale Hachamisha Kibbutz, Israel; and Strobl, Austria. I even got to Kashmir as a side trip after attending an International Sociological Association Conference in Delhi, India. These destinations were all quite a distance, both geographically and intellectually, from my starting-out address in Manhattan, Kansas.

Decisions, Decisions

David Klein and I set to work several years after our joint arrival to put together a study funded by the National Institute of Aging on how family size and other factors affect parent-child relations at parents' midlife. We had both been struck by the large size of our students' families. One sophomore, I remember, had a newly arrived brother, which made 13 siblings for him. It was also about then that the Dean wondered if I would be Head of the Department. Like other opportunities I have had since to apply for Deanships, I gave the offer careful consideration before saying, "No, thanks." I revel in my teaching and research and fear my impatience would make me a poor coordinator and overseer of other professors' doings.

I have never forgotten the story Peter Rossi once told me about when he was Chair of the Department of Sociology at Johns Hopkins. He had been fighting for a number of years to keep a man he felt was incompetent from being promoted to full professor. Peter had just returned from a meeting where he had been overruled in this judgment. At this point, the man in question came into Peter's office to complain about the quality of toilet paper in the University restrooms. Peter was so ticked off that he threw a chair at the man, but, alas, did not hit him. He then stalked off to the Dean's office and resigned as Department Chair. I admire most administrators, but also remember that "head" and "dean" are four-letter words.

Here, at the University of Notre Dame, too many people still tend to look askance at anyone, male or female, who declares herself/himself to be a feminist. In fact, some of the things I am happiest about have to do with my acting on my equal rights convictions. Thus, a woman professor of English, a nun theologian, and I organized a course concentration in Gender Studies. I continue firmly to believe that it is difficult to study women without studying men as well. As a consequence, I resisted the title "Women's Studies" for our concentration. A colleague and friend in American Studies, Kathleen Maas Weigert, and I were put in charge of getting initial funding for the undertaking. We obtained monies from the Lilly Foundation to hire a Director for the Program and got it off and running, much to our satisfaction. I also feel very good about a Seneca Falls lecture series I organized in the academic year 1998-99. It commemorated the 150th anniversary of the Conference, one of the first times people organized to speak out for women's rights. Barbara Bergmann, Professor Emerita of Economics at American University and the University of Maryland; Jacqueline Jones, Truman Professor of American Civilization at Brandeis University; and Elisabeth Schüssler Fiorenza, Krister Stendahl Professor of Divinity at Harvard University Divinity School, all gave talks at Notre Dame on the position of women today.

I have also pressed strongly for the appointment of women in my own and other departments as well as in higher administration. My department, sociology, has always been open to qualified women. Most of its members are convinced of the need for gender equity. Because of Catholic dogma, however, this is a continuing struggle at Notre Dame. In addition, as any good social scientist knows, not all women, as is true of men, have the qualifications to obtain faculty positions or, if they do, are willing to stand up for equal rights. For some, it goes against their religious training of conformity to persons in authority. For others, it is fear of reprisals from their male colleagues. And a number, as is true of men, are unwilling to exercise their citizenship responsibilities. After all, estimates are that only about 10 percent of the population at the time of the American Revolution were in favor of it. Because of my faculty position, I have never feared retaliation for my outspoken advocacy of women's rights. I have served with too many mentally-challenged men to be anything other than skeptical of their supposed greater perspicacity. Men who want women to stay in the home often fear women's competition outside it.

Professional Responsibilities

Before I arrived at Notre Dame, opportunities had begun opening up for me to help shape others' research endeavors. Service on the NIMH Population Research Review Section under the leadership of Jeffrey Evans was my first such experience. After that commitment, which ended in 1977, I felt I had done my share of reading research proposals. However, when the NSF asked me to serve on their Sociology Panel, the then-ND Provost, Timothy O'Meara, urged me to accept. He had had NSF grants and wanted ND represented. This service from 1979-1981 meant work in assessing proposals but also fun at our periodic meetings in Washington, D.C. Stanley Lieberson, Harvard University, and Peter Rossi, then of the University of Massachusetts, Amherst, managed to keep us laughing at the more boring projects as well as at ourselves. They often turned to Karen Cook, Duke University now, for help on the long-winded organization proposals. They knew she would have summarized them in good form, something they were less apt to have the patience to do. I was let off the hook on reviewing their assignments, since my family expertise kept me too busy with those submissions to help them out.

My joking relation with Stan continued when he was President of the American Sociological Association, and I was on the ASA Council. At one Sunday morning meeting of the ASA Council, I remember, he singled me out with the comment, "I know this meeting hour on Sunday is hard for Joan as a good Roman Catholic." I didn't miss a beat and replied, "Oh, you Southern Baptists are always so hard on us Roman Catholics."

These service activities did not prevent me from doing research and publishing the findings. David Klein and I had several on midlife parents based on our NIA-funded research. One I especially liked, probably because of my own family life, was on characteristics of parents' favorite children. My concerns as a political "junky" also were coming out in policy-oriented research, first with Wilfried Dumon comparing U.S. and European family measures, as well as an article on birth-control socialization. It was around this time that social scientists were beginning to consider seriously with the backing of the NIA the phenomenon of the aging population. Egged on by Vern Bengston and Maxi Szinovacz, I started paying particular attention to the not-always-greeting-card relations between grandparents and grandchildren (Aldous, 1983, 1985, 1996, 1998). And finally, thanks to the statistical and analytic skills of Rodney F. Ganey, now head of a company serving hospitals wanting to know what their patients think of their services, I put together two articles based on my observational data on family problem solving (Aldous & Ganey, 1989, 1999).

More agreeable is my work with graduate students. Through the research of graduate student Robert C. Tuttle, now a Professor of Sociology at Wilkes University, Wilkes-Barre, Pennsylvania, I became very aware of the problems unemployed persons face and what the federal government can do about them (Aldous & Tuttle, 1988). Robert M. Birkey, Professor at Goshen College, Goshen, Indiana, continued my education through his study of how position in the welfare hierarchy, ranging from client, through caseworker, up to supervisor and state commissioner, affected the holder's views of the program. It deservedly won an NSF doctoral research grant.

Another NSF grant winner was Keiko Hirao, as I noted earlier, now on the faculty at Sophia University, Tokyo. With funds from the Social Science Research Council and NSF, she collected interview data, as did Bob, for her project. Her subject was how number of years of education affected Japanese women's leaving the labor force after having a baby, the usual phenomenon. As with my other graduate students' projects, I learned a great deal. Both Bob and Keiko completed their doctoral programs while maintaining viable marriages and rearing children. Through their research, I expanded my "book learning." It is great to have Bob close by to give guest lectures at my Family Policy classes. Keiko is a bit far away for the talks at my comparative family class that she used to give.

My teaching goes well. I still am full of fear before every first class, but it takes less urging from kind outsiders to get me inside the classroom. I've even received the ND Graduate School Award for excellence in teaching and scholarship. And when the Lilly Foundation awarded Teaching Fellowships to Assistant Professors beginning their careers, two Award winners, Assistant Professors in Sociology here, asked me to be their mentor. This involved going to their classes to observe their pedagogical procedures, talking over problems with them, and surveying their students as to what they liked or didn't like about the Professors. I sharpened my own teaching skills by way of these experiences. I now ask a colleague to do this questioning of students in my classes at midterm while I am absent. Students' anonymous comments permit me to improve my teaching in the rest of the semester.

My constant reading and interest in books has carried over to my civic activities. I served a term on the St. Joseph County Public Library Board. Of the six members and the Director of the system, one other member and I were the only ones who actually read books. The meetings were generally routine, filled with bureaucratic minutiae. The exception occurred when Madonna's autobiography, *Madonna Live*, appeared. The petitions and colorful oratory we received against its being part of the collection demonstrated again how important and how constantly threatened are our First Amendment rights. We were lucky to have Notre Dame librarians testify to support the system's purchasing the book and so a free press. We did have to agree not to let anyone under 18 check it out, and persons wanting to do so had to go to the librarian for an okay. It was not on an open shelf. During my tenure on the Board, I did get the Board to approve a bookmobile to go to public schools and playgrounds in poorer neighborhoods. It is very inviting, as Jim Davis let us have Garfield invitingly displayed on the outside of the bookmobile.

Certainly not by the book was my experience as President of the National Council on Family Relations. Finding sites for national organizations to hold their periodic meetings requires much preplanning before the actual date. For NCFR, it is some two to three years. Ruth Jewson, the predecessor to Mary Jo Czaplewski as NCFR Director, had made the arrangements for us to meet in Dearborn, Michigan, for our annual convention, the upcoming year of my Presidency. Shortly after my tenure as President began, a member telephoned me to question the choice of Dearborn. He said it was a widely known racist community, and we should change the location. I immediately telephoned Mary Jo. She had heard no such reports, and also told me about how much money it would cost NCFR to break its lease agreements with the hotel, etc. I got back to the member, but he continued to be worried. He wrote and telephoned me several more times, each time with the same message, "Get NCFR out of Dearborn." After each call or letter, I'd talk to Mary Jo. The outcome was always the same. It was literally "no go." The cost to break NCFR's contracts was too high, and where could we go at this late date? Large conventions require blocks of hotel rooms and meeting rooms, not easily found on short notice. She also assured me Dearborn to her knowledge was not racist.

Consequently, we met in Dearborn, and rightly or wrongly, many members saw the city as racist. Black members, after much loud talk, met in Detroit. I became the innocent victim of harangues at our officer and section leader meetings. I have never been so rudely yelled at as at those meetings. No one listened to my explanations. To say I resented the criticism is an understatement. I still can't meet my successor as President, who joined in bad-mouthing me, without wanting to spit in his eye. And this feeling continues despite my upper-middle-class upbringing and faithful reading of Miss Manners' etiquette columns. Mary Jo, I should add, was a tower of strength.

Oh yes, to make the Convention even more memorable, after I gave the Presidential address, a "friend" leapt up on the platform and proceeded to give lengthy comments on it. She sheepishly apologized later, saying several people had criticized her for taking over the rostrum. I could but laugh, and in the time since maintain cerebral hygiene on this whole ghastly episode. Fortunately, dear friends Miriam and Dick Hey were staying with me in my penthouse suite, and they helped me to keep things in perspective. Even receiving the Ernest W. Burgess Award for "continuous and meritorious in theory and research in the family field" and being named among the first NCFR Fellows in the ensuing years has not removed the bad taste left from that NCFR convention for me. When folks talk about being victimized, I know just what they mean.

AFTERWORD

In looking over this memoir, I see that I have generally left out the disappointments–the submitted papers turned down by stupid journal editors, the misunderstandings, disagreements, and downright conflicts I've had with colleagues and students and the usual cares and preoccupations everyone faces. And that's the way it should be. I have thoroughly enjoyed living by the book in academia. I have even been able to do research and publish on the pursuit of happiness. Thus, it continues to be an honor and a joy for me to keep up my family's bookish tradition.

AUTHOR NOTE

Joan Aldous is William R. Kenan, Jr. Professor of Sociology.

Address correspondence to: Department of Sociology, 738 Flanner Hall, University of Notre Dame, South Bend, IN 46556.

REFERENCES

Aldous, J. (1956). The relations of Evelyn Duvall's role conceptions to David Riesman's character types. *Journal of Home Economics*, *48*, 2, 761-764.

Aldous, J. (1961). A study of parental role functions. *The Family Life Coordinator*, *10*, 2, 43-44.

Aldous, J. (1962). Urbanization, the extended family, and kinship ties in West Africa. *Social Forces*, *41*, 1, 6-12. Reprinted in Pierre L. van den Berghe (Ed.), *Africa: Problems of change and conflict* (pp. 107-116). San Francisco: Chandler.

Aldous, J. (1965). The consequences of intergenerational continuity. *Journal of Marriage and the Family*, *27*, 4, 462-468.

Aldous, J. (1972). Children's perceptions of adult role assignment: Sex, race and class factors. *Journal of Marriage and the Family*, *34*, 1, 55-56.

Aldous, J. (1974). Observer effects on laboratory behavior: A methodological note. *Récherches sociologiques*, *5*, 1, 84-90 (in French).

Aldous, J. (1975). The search for alternatives: Parental behaviors and children's original problem solutions. *Journal of Marriage and the Family*, *37*, 4, 711-722.

Aldous, J. (1978). *Family careers: Developmental change in families*. New York: John Wiley.

Aldous, J. (1983). Birth control socialization: How to avoid discussing the subject. *Population and Environment: Behavioral and Social Issues*, *6*, 1, 27-38.

Aldous, J. (1985). Parent-adult child relations as affected by the grandparent status. In V. L. Bengtson & J. F. Robertson (Eds.), *Grandparenthood* (pp. 117-132). Beverly Hills, CA: Sage.

Aldous, J. (1996). *Family careers: Rethinking the developmental perspective*. Thousand Oaks, CA: Sage.

Aldous, J. (1998). Public policy and grandparents: Contrasting perspectives. In M. E. Szinovacz (Ed.), *Handbook on grandparenting* (pp. 230-246). Westport, CT: Greenwood.

Aldous, J., & Dumon, W. (1979). European and United States political contexts for family policy research. *Journal of Marriage and the Family*, *41*, 3, 497-505.

Aldous, J., & Ganey, R. F. (1989). Families' definition behavior of problematic situations. *Social Forces*, *67*, 4, 871-897.

Aldous, J., & Ganey, R. F. (1999). Family life and the pursuit of happiness: The influence of gender and race. *Journal of Family Issues*, *20*, 2, 155-180.

Aldous, J., & Hill, R. (1965). Social cohesion, lineage type and intergenerational cohesion. *Social Forces*, *43*, 3, 471-482. Reprinted in Bernard Farber (Ed.), *Readings in family and kinship* (pp. 269-280). New York: John Wiley, 1966.

Aldous, J., & Kamiko, T. (1972). A cross-national study of the effects of father absence: Japan and the United States. In M. B. Sussman & B. E. Cogswell (Eds.), *Cross-national family research* (pp. 86-101). Leiden: E. J. Brill.

Aldous, J., & Kell, L. (1961). A partial test of some theories of identification. *Marriage and Family Living*, *23*, 1, 15-19.

Aldous, J., Klaus, E., & Klein, D. M. (1985). The understanding heart: Aging parents and their favorite children. *Child Development*, *56*, 2, 303-316.

Aldous, J., & Klein, D. M. (1991). Sentiment and services: Models of intergenerational relationships in mid-life. *Journal of Marriage and the Family*, *53*, 3, 595-608.

Aldous, J., Mulligan, G. M., & Bjarnason, T. (1998). Fathering over time: What makes the difference? *Journal of Marriage and the Family*, *60*, 4, 809-820.

Aldous, J., & Tuttle, R. C. (1988). Unemployment and the family. In C. Chilman (Ed.), *Families in trouble: Knowledge and practice perspectives for professionals in the human services*, vol. 1 (pp. 17-41). Beverly Hills, CA: Sage.

Duvall, E. R., & Hill, R. (1945). *When you marry*. Boston: D.C. Heath & Company.

Hill, R., & Aldous, J. (1969). Socialization for marriage and parenthood. In David Goslin (Ed.), *Handbook of socialization, theory, and research* (pp. 885-950). Chicago: Rand McNally.

Kell, L., & Aldous, J. (1960a). The relation between mothers' child-rearing ideologies and their children's perceptions of maternal control. *Child Development*, *31*, 1, 145-156.

Kell, L., & Aldous, J. (1960b). Trends in child care over three generations. *Marriage and Family Living*, *22*, 176-177. Reprinted in Ira J. Gordon (Ed.), *Human development: Readings in research* (pp. 138-139), Chicago: Scott, Foresman & Company, 1965.

Riesman, D. (1953). *The lonely crowd: A study of the changing American character*. Garden City, NY: Doubleday.

Smetanka, M. J. (1999, April 3). Turnover gives the 'U' a chance to rewrite history department. *Minneapolis (MN) Star Tribune*, A1, A12.

Living the Literature: Keeping My Family in Family Sociology

Greer Litton Fox

KEYWORDS. Autobiography, research, family studies, gender, demography

INTRODUCTION

"You Really Do Treat Your Career as a Hobby!"

I wasn't sure whether to laugh or cry when a colleague with whom I was collaborating made that remark. I had been unable to meet with him because it conflicted with my daughter's soccer practice, and I was the assistant coach of her team. Although my professional life and work, including how I came to do it, may look as if I take a casual attitude toward my career, believe me, it has been no hobby! But let me start at the beginning.

Outgrowing My Plans to Be a Stewardess

The first step toward becoming a sociologist was preordained by my genetic inheritance, although I could not have known it at the time. When I was in grade school in a small town in Kentucky in the 1950s, the most glamorous and exciting avenue open to women at the time was to become an airline stewardess. Imagine the travel, the adventure, the makeup, uniforms, and hairstyling! In a time when most women were mothers and housewives only and those who worked were secretaries, nurses, teachers, and check-out clerks, the airline stewardess appeared on the scene as the Wonder Woman of the working world. All my girl friends and I decided we wanted to be one when we grew up. And grow I did. By the time I was in the seventh grade, I was not only the tallest person in my class, but also the fifth-tallest person in the entire junior high school, and that included not only my eighth-grade brother but all the ninth-grade boys as well. By the time it was over, I had outgrown the height restrictions for stewardesses. My glamorous career in the skies was finished before I even got off the ground.

Throughout high school and college, my meager inventory of talents forced me to consider some options and eliminate others. My main talent had always been taking standardized tests. While I was very good at it, it is hardly the thing that wins talent competitions or beauty pageants. Something else had to do. My mother and both grandmothers had been math teachers, so teaching was a well-modeled option, though I hasten to add that according to practice in those days, none of these women continued her teaching career after marriage. Teaching was clearly secondary to their major familial roles, a fallback, not an identity. And until a fateful friendship in college, my own thinking about a professional life was a "doing it," not a "being it" kind of thinking.

Inspirations

I was a junior at Randolph-Macon Woman's College when I met Sally Kenan, a political science major in the class ahead of me. Wholly engaged with current affairs and political action, Sally embodied what became one of the marquee lines of the feminist movement in the sixties, "the personal is political." Sally electrified the campus with her organizing skills, and I was grateful to hang around in her shadows. I was mesmerized by her when she said to me, during a discussion of women's lives and our futures, that, *of course*, I would *be something* and would do more than just graduate into the golf-and-bridge-playing wife-and-mother roles (that we were drifting into). I took her word for it as unquestioningly as any disciple. Even while on campus, she lived day-to-day in a world far beyond the local collegiate community. She was my first real exposure to the tumult that came to characterize the sixties. She was a participant in the world-wide debates about race, about gender, about Vietnam, and she brought the entire campus of women, however reluctantly, into the ferment of ideas along with her. Perhaps such people use up their lives too fully, or too quickly, or perhaps she struggled with other demons of which we were unaware; Sally committed suicide while she was yet a young woman in her thirties.

While Sally gave me the directive, others during that time helped me find direction. Just as during high school at my father's insistence, my schedule of courses at Randolph-Macon was weighted toward math and sciences. But fortunately, Randolph-Macon is a liberal arts college, so I also took several sociology and anthropology courses. These I found intriguing, so much so that I majored in sociology and relegated math to a minor. Because Randolph-Macon was as small as it was excellent, I enjoyed not only superb and dedicated teaching but also a great deal of personal attention. Two of the independent research projects I conducted there continue to be research interests: one was a study of federal correctional institutions, and the second focused on the social contexts of racial prejudice. Since almost all of my own professional career has been spent in state university settings, I can attest to the vast difference in educational experience provided by small independent liberal arts colleges, a national resource that needs to be cherished.

At the urging and nagging of my college professors, I applied for and received a Danforth Foundation graduate fellowship, an enormously important and generous gift of four years of graduate tuition and stipend at any institution of my choosing. In fact, I was one of the first women in years to receive the fellowship. I have to admit that I felt only the responsibility rather than the honor when I received word of the fellowship outcome. After finding the letter from the foundation in my campus mailbox, I retreated to an empty classroom with the letter still unopened so that I could have a few minutes on my own to get used to the results, whatever they were. When I read the letter and learned that I had won, I saw my fate only as more years of hard work stretching indefinitely in front of me, and I sat there and cried and cried. Turning the fellowship down, refusing the opportunity, withdrawing, none of that ever occurred to me as a possibility, although I'm not sure why not. Quitting just because something was hard was not something we did then.

I do know that it was hard for me at that time to give up the ideal of a life pathway that was familiar. The pathway of getting married, having children, and staying home was so compelling (mind you, there was no one in line for the husband position at that point, but that logistical problem didn't dissuade me from thinking about this path as the doable, easy one). The new direction was a foreign and troubling one for which I had no script, no model, no guarantee that it could be done and would turn out all right. I was damn scared. In fact, after graduating from college I spent a couple of weeks in the hospital with ulcers. Nonetheless, when August came, my father drove me to Ann Arbor, Michigan, to begin graduate school in sociology at the University of Michigan. The last words my mother had for me were, "Don't worry. I'm sure you'll meet a nice, tall young man when you get there." Yes, it's true. And this was also a part of the sixties, though not an aspect often written about except by psychologists who were interested in why bright women feared success. As Dad bid me goodbye, the last thing he said was, "Aren't you sure you'd rather be in medicine?"

FINDING OUT HOW TO DO SOCIOLOGY

Graduate School

I loved and hated the University of Michigan with about equal passion and switched feelings just about every week. The course work was simply overwhelming, but the people! Here at last was what I had longed for–people from seemingly everywhere around the world, and the brightest students from coast to coast. I have never felt more challenged or stimulated. The graduate students formed a strong bond, despite large numbers of us originally. Perhaps these close ties were especially urgent because of the Vietnam War, the end of the student deferments, and the subsequent departure of many of the men students.

During the first two years, I studied the gamut of courses, trying to find a home within the department's specializations. The fact that I had a full fellowship excused me from having to work as a graduate assistant, itself a mixed blessing because it also meant that I missed out on working closely with an individual faculty member. But it also meant that I had time to try out several methodological approaches, from survey methods and participation in the Detroit Area Survey, to John Lofland's extraordinary qualitative research seminar, to population studies and demography. Population studies combined everything I liked–the opportunity for cross-cultural work, the discipline of quantitative analysis, and the passion of social relevance (these were the days of ZPG–zero population growth–and the population bomb), and I did well in it. And the faculty in Population Studies had developed a model of professional socialization of their graduate students that is still one of the finest and most effective I've ever seen. I slipped readily into their mold and worked with some of the finest minds in the field.

Meanwhile, the world around us was in flames. I was at Michigan from 1966 to 1970, and during that time we experienced several anti-war marches in Washington and other cities, Detroit's 1968 race riot, the Ann Arbor riot with armed sheriff's deputies marching down the campus streets and billy-clubbing students in their way. The times included the Black Action Movement student strike, antiwar protests, feminist rallies, and general liberations of one sort or another. This general climate of unrest often led to disrupted classes and changed minds–some toward more openness, others toward greater rigidities. My own education as a social scientist occurred as much out of the classroom as in. I brought to that setting a mind-numbing, and perhaps even dangerous, level of naivete about drugs, alcohol, sex, politics and its violent passions, as well as sexual harassment. But I left the University of Michigan in 1970 with a degree, a just-tall-enough husband, and a job where I needed it–within commuting distance of Ann Arbor.

Academic Ropes

Although my Michigan training had provided an excellent conceptual and analytic base for an academic career, it failed to include some of the elementary insider secrets of success in academia: how to develop a research agenda, how to balance course preparations and teaching with pursuit of that research agenda, how to publish, how to get grants, how to be a good colleague and departmental citizen. These I was taught by a host of informal mentors at Bowling Green State University, primarily among the Sociology faculty but including senior faculty from other departments as well. It would be difficult to design a better first job or hand-pick a better set of colleagues. Too bad I didn't realize it at the time.

For two-and-a-half years, I threw myself into teaching, plastered my office walls with posters from the Russian Revolution, and hosted long sessions every afternoon in my office with a cadre of undergraduate students. I brought in guest speakers from Ann Arbor and black activists from Detroit. I also initiated and chaired the Committee on the Status of Women Faculty, which wrote a stunning analysis of gender inequity in salary, rank, tenure, and promotion outcomes at the university (Fox, 1972), resulting in the allocation of a special fund of monies to reverse the salary inequities. I was nominated and won election to the Faculty Senate and Senate Executive Committee. And I received a President's Special Achievement Award. I was incredibly busy and thought I was doing it all, and doing it well.

Then, at my third-year review, my departmental colleagues told me bluntly that continuation on this path would fail to result in tenure! I needed to establish a research-based presence in the field of sociology and do it now. I was stunned. But, rather than leaving me demoralized and floundering, which of course I was, the departmental faculty threw several lifelines my way. One professor showed me how to mine my dissertation for publishable articles, so I published four from that data set (Fox, 1973a; Fox, 1973b; Fox, 1975; Fox, 1978). Several associate professors worked with me to teach more efficiently and to reengineer my heavy engagement with students into a more manageable load. Another faculty member pushed me either to drop or to get publishable mileage out of my concern with sex discrimination among faculty and students; I published two more articles as a result (Fox, 1974; Fox, 1977a). A full professor encouraged me to turn my interest in students' contraceptive attitudes and behaviors into a grant proposal, talking to me about it patiently enough so that I was able to frame my interest into feasible research questions and write the proposal. My application to NIMH was successful (1977b). Within two years, I had several presentations, publications, a federally funded grant, and a research program underway. And I discovered I loved it! I have always enjoyed writing. And what fun it was to put your ideas to the test in the development and analysis of research projects. I loved seeing my words and my name in print. But more even than all that, I discovered I loved the chase, the competition, the pitting yourself and your ideas and your talents against unknown others, and the excitement of not knowing, hoping, waiting for the word that this time you were the winner, the chosen one. Thus I have had to confront the fact that a fair amount of my career motivation has been no nobler or more lofty than that of a riverboat gambler, or a beauty contestant, although I hope the byproducts–the articles and grant reports–have had a modicum of social utility, even if only narrowly.

In the meantime, my husband Bruce continued to work on completing his doctorate in psychology at Michigan. The war in Vietnam altered many lives, including his. While some of our friends were drafted and others contemplated refuge in Canada, Bruce applied for and received conscientious objector status, much as his father had during World War II. Thus, while I had had the luxury of full-time graduate study, Bruce had been forced to interrupt his graduate program to serve out his alternative service obligation. His placement was just north of Detroit at a residential hospital for adults with severe developmental disabilities. When I finished my doctorate in 1970, Bruce still had a portion of his alternative service to complete, and most of his course work and the dissertation ahead of him.

In the spirit of the times, we experimented with different living arrangements. At first we lived full time together in Ann Arbor, and I made the daily commute 90 miles each way to Bowling Green, and Bruce commuted north to the hospital. As soon as the winter weather hit in full force, it became clear that we also would need an apartment in Bowling Green. So for a time one or the other of us commuted on weekends, living alone and apart for most of the work week. This was lonely, wearing, and expensive. Next, we tried "urban communes" at each end of the commute, sharing a home with a female colleague in Bowling Green and with a mixed group of graduate students and young professionals in Ann Arbor. While this took care of the mid-week loneliness, we discovered that our weekends were largely spent doing housework alternately in Ann Arbor or in Bowling Green, with neither set of housemates fully convinced that we were actually doing our share because they only saw us pitching in every other weekend! While all this made great didactic material for the section on alternative lifestyles in my family sociology course, it didn't help either of us as we attempted to handle the pressures of his graduate study and my new job. So we took the plunge, bought a house in Bowling Green, and after almost four years of marriage, starting living together full time. Bruce was able to finish his dissertation while I worked on becoming an academic sociologist.

The Harsh Reality of Dual Careers and Only One Job

By the time Bruce finished his degree in 1975, I was well established at Bowling Green, having been tenured and offered a position as an Associate Dean in the College of Arts and Sciences. I had made some fast friendships on the faculty and could easily have stayed there for the rest of my career. However, there was no position there for Bruce and, understandably, he didn't relish the prospect of a persona on campus as "Mr. Greer." Moreover, I was restless; I wasn't ready myself for a lifelong commitment to one place.

I still wanted to see the world. So we both applied for jobs all over the country. The change in the academic job market between the late 1960s and 1975 was remarkable. Whereas academic jobs had been fairly plentiful when I finished, the job market had largely dried up as Bruce entered it. Moreover, each of us carried some baggage–each other!

It is easy in retrospect to second-guess your decisions and wish you had made different choices. We had two guidelines directing our decision-making: we wanted to be able to live together and avoid commuting again, and we both wanted to work, so we did the best we could with the options we had. I was offered and accepted a tenured Associate Professorship in Sociology at the University of Vermont, and Bruce was promised opportunities for part-time teaching in the Psychology Department there and at a local private college. After a year in Vermont, I knew I did not want to be in a department without a graduate program; moreover, the part-time jobs for Bruce had not materialized. When I left Bowling Green, my department chair had insisted that I take a leave of absence rather than resign outright, and throughout the year in Vermont various colleagues had encouraged us to come back. In retrospect, we should have returned their kindness by being more optimistic and patient about the potential for a job for Bruce there. At the time, however, there seemed to be no point in returning because the situation hadn't changed; and so, like many academic wayfaring couples, we moved on, this time to Detroit. In Detroit I eventually became Associate Director of the Merrill-Palmer Institute and Professor of Sociology at Wayne State University; and Bruce, leaving academia for good, became Director of Information Services at United Way of Metropolitan Detroit.

The statistics on academic women's marital success are not encouraging, and I was well aware of that. At that point in the 1970s, few academic women ever married, and many of those who did had subsequently divorced. Perhaps it will be of solace to some for me to admit that it was not my doing, but Bruce's courage, that kept our marriage together during this period. I myself was demoralized and frantic at his difficulty finding an appropriate job. At one point in Vermont, I recall giving him an ultimatum: get a job within two years or get out. This, despite my having been at the forefront of academic feminist movements, writing, and teaching on sex and gender roles! Intellectually, I was all for change in women's work and family roles and insistent that men needed to shoulder home responsibilities equal to those of women; but I was completely oblivious to my rigid devotion to the traditional male provider-protector role for Bruce and a privileged provided-for/protected status for me. And I was equally blind to the cruelty of my demands for employment when he had so few degrees of freedom to work with. Because of my head start, I was the one who "drove" our employment opportunities and decisions. It never dawned on me that had we switched off, taken turns, or even once given him his first choice, that I would have been equally hard put to find a job I was qualified for.

Two aspects of our life in Detroit worked to pry open my eyes a little. First, during the mini recession of the early 1980s, I began to work with two colleagues at Wayne State on a study of economic distress among Detroit Metro Area residents. Immersion in the research literature on the impact of un- and under-employment on marriages and families was not only an education in itself but a form of self-therapy. And second, I had the opportunity to associate with African American women, some who were colleagues at Merrill-Palmer and others who were neighbors. These women had experienced nontraditional marriages and the lack of social support for the survival strategies that people craft from necessity when normative prescription doesn't fit. In short order I was set straight in unsentimental fashion about living with, supporting, and being supportive of good men who do not fill the provider role as traditionally scripted. Their reframing helped me find a new meaning for the phrase "marriage as a partnership." This form of mutual relationship goes well beyond what is connoted by the traditional Parsonian role-complementary marriage of my parents and, indeed, of my own expectations and youthful aspirations. Perhaps it was this new serenity I felt about the interweave of my personal and professional lives that made our eight years in Detroit such good ones. Whatever the source, I had some of my most rewarding and productive years while at Wayne State/Merrill-Palmer.

Mothers and Daughters and Beyond

My NIMH-funded project on adolescent sexual and contraceptive attitudes and behaviors led to several opportunities, one of which was critical. I was asked to serve as a scientific reviewer for grant proposals to NIMH and, after an apprenticeship of sorts, was appointed to a five-year term on the NIMH Small Grants study section as one of its sociology/social psychology reviewers. This program was quite popular and attracted a high volume of proposal submissions, bringing reviewers five times a year to Washington to deliberate on the reviews we had prepared at home. Although the amount of work involved was considerable, so were the rewards. The experience of writing critiques of more than 100 proposals annually was itself excellent training in grant writing. Then, the process of sharing and comparing one's assessment with that of other reviewers was an unparalleled opportunity to hone and extend one's methodological, analytic, and reasoning skills. More opportunities grew out of the informal interactions during the study section meetings, and that was simply being plugged into an information net of scholars which was national in scope and carefully tuned into the Washington social science research theatre. Conversations over dinner or breaks routinely dealt with such topics as which federal agencies had an especially generous budget or a dearth of proposals, what issues or problems might be addressed in next year's RFPs, which foundations were looking for good ideas, what universities were hiring, and who was doing ground-breaking research on a new area in psychology.

I drew indirectly on these "grantsmanship" experiences in designing my first large research project on mother-daughter communication about sexuality. This project grew out of my fascination with the new area of the sociology of women, as well as my long-standing interest in how fertility, in all of its meanings, affects the sociology and social psychology of women's lives. I wanted to focus on two questions through this project: how do young women learn about sexuality, and what part do their mothers play in this unfolding process? The Detroit city schools offered a readily available pool of young women to sample from, so, with their permission, I applied successfully to NICHD for funds to study my questions of interest among mother-daughter pairs in Detroit. Three weeks after the project began, our first daughter Katherine was born. After that, life became a blur!

Professionally, I was very involved in the mother-daughter research (Fox, 1979; Fox, 1980; Fox & Inazu, 1980a; Fox & Inazu, 1980b; Inazu & Fox, 1980; Fox, 1981b; Fox & Inazu, 1982). It allowed me to keep some distance from the difficult transition of the Merrill-Palmer Institute as it closed its doors as an independent educational institution and began anew as a research institute within the Wayne State University system. I gladly joined the Sociology Department at Wayne State; not only did I know and like the faculty, but it meant we didn't have to move! For the first time, I had the opportunity to teach population courses and to work with students for whom higher education was a difficult and proud achievement, not a taken-for-granted rite of passage.

As I mentioned earlier, I began to work with department colleagues on a study of the impact of the very serious economic downturn of the early 1980s on Detroit's children and families (Kelly, Sheldon, & Fox, 1985). In partnership with a colleague from my department and others from the Law School, we submitted a grant to NSF to study the impact of changes in divorce law on alimony and custody awards. Although the grant wasn't funded, as Associate Director now of Wayne State's new Merrill-Palmer Research Institute, I was able to find a little local money to allow us to collect data from court records in Oakland County so that we could initiate the project (Kelly & Fox, 1993; Fox & Kelly, 1995). And, on my own, I applied for and received a federal grant to extend my research on family constellations as sexual socialization structures to include fathers and sons. This project was special, not only because it was one of the first in the adolescent sexuality program to include fathers and sons, but also because it relied upon long interviews and qualitative analytic techniques (Fox, 1984; Fox & Medlin, 1986; Fox et al., 1988).

Also during this time, I was appointed to a National Academy of Sciences panel on criminal rehabilitation techniques (Fox, 1981a) and also began to be asked fairly regularly to serve on scientific review panels for NICHD, appointments both which involved more travel to Washington.

In the meantime, our family was changing. The longed-for birth of our second daughter Arminta in 1983 not only completed our family, but also meant that we struggled once again with finding decent infant care. As did so many young families then and currently, there were few options that were affordable, accessible, and of high quality (Fox & Allen, 1987). After months of searching and patch-work arrangements, we considered ourselves blessed to be able to hire a young woman who shared our values about child rearing, and who stayed with our children for over a year. Our families had changed in other ways as well. Bruce no longer had his family of orientation living close by in Ann Arbor, and with my mother's death, I was concerned about living so far from Kentucky, where my father, my children's only surviving grandparent, lived. So, when I received a call from an acquaintance from the University of Tennessee asking if I might be interested in their open position as Department Head, I hesitated only moments before agreeing to come take a look.

Big Orange Country

For reasons that are less marked by careful consideration than by the mesmerizing beauty of dogwood blossoms and redbud trees in early March while Detroit was still shivering in the tight grip of winter's frigid air, I decided–against Bruce's advice and my own vague misgivings–to take a department head position in what was then the College of Home Economics at the University of Tennessee. I was 40, Katherine 6, Minta only 15 months old, and Bruce had no job or even the promise of one in Tennessee. I still look back with disbelief at my decision to move. I could not have known then what an intellectual toll would be exacted by the move from a liberal arts orientation to a professional college. I could not have guessed that the kinds of administrative experiences that I brought to the position had in no way prepared me for the conditions I encountered. But, as a family sociologist, I should have realized that dual-career couples with young children need to be very cautious about jettisoning their carefully constructed and precariously balanced lives in one setting for the untested, Circean promises of another. This chapter is not fully written, so I won't dwell upon it except to acknowledge that I made a serious error in judgment for my young family at the time. That we have stayed, that Bruce, now a small business owner, and I have become season-ticket holders who cheer for the Volunteers, and that the girls now call Tennessee home is tribute to human adaptability. When I returned to a faculty position after three years as department head, I was hard put to find courses I was qualified to teach in a curriculum heavy in early childhood education and family development. I turned toward courses in research methods and survey research and gradually developed courses in secondary data analysis and family diversity–all of which allowed me to use some of my research training and sociological perspectives while still fitting into the more applied concerns of child and family studies. For a course on family diversity (taught for more than a decade now), I drew from the sociology of gender, race relations, and group dynamics for theoretical materials. As an organizational framework I used the history of immigration and immigration law. I also was able to draw heavily upon materials from the INS and Census Bureau that used to be mainstays in my population courses at Wayne State.

Additionally, the rich personal experiences I had in Detroit at work were invaluable to draw upon. Moreover, the trauma of my father's homicide propelled me to add a course in Family Violence to the department's curriculum and indirectly has shaped my recent research on fatherhood as well (Fox, Von Bargen, & Jester, 1996; Fox & Bruce, 1999; Bruce & Fox, 1999).

I have always maintained professional association memberships, beginning as a graduate student in PAA, the Population Association of America, and belonging almost as long to the American Sociological Association and NCFR, the National Council on Family Relations. During the years I've been on the faculty at Tennessee, I have become increasingly involved in NCFR, serving as Secretary of the Board, then as Program Vice President, and subsequently as President of the organization. It has been interesting to watch the organization and its membership grapple with a new era, marked by an increasingly public, political interest in family life and family values. But alongside this democratization of interest in families from the lay public has come an increasing interest in families from other professionals–demographers have discovered that human interaction is antecedent to many of the behavioral outcomes (births, deaths, moves) they study; sociologists have discovered children; and psychologists have discovered families. NCFR has a difficult but valuable role to play at the interface of all of these interest groups, and I am hopeful that the major changes in governance that were passed by the Board while I was president will facilitate the organization's work. Some counsel new professionals not to get involved in leadership positions in professional societies; what a mistake! In my experience, professional involvement of this sort is a great way to gain insight and perspective on one's own work and one's institution. Further, not only does it allow for ready access to other scholars, it often provides informal training in a variety of job skills–including turning down committee assignments–that are more difficult to master at home.

In the past few years, my research has drawn together in interesting ways several different threads from earlier parts of my professional work. To give just one example, I am currently a co-investigator with a colleague from the

Sociology Department on a grant sponsored by the National Institutes of Justice, in which we use the National Survey of Families and Households along with Census data to look at the interplay of economic distress and social disorganization on domestic violence. The NSFH is one of the workhorse databases that I have used over the past several years in my secondary data analysis course, familiar to me because I was a consultant on the development of the original interview schedule used in Wave 1. Economic distress continues to be a research interest (Fox & Chancey, 1998), and social disorganization theory is well situated within traditional contextual and ecological explanations of criminal human behavior, material I studied as a young undergraduate interested in people whose lives were marred by crime.

ASSESSMENT

I realize that I have been far more fortunate than most women and men who work for a living to have had the luxury of a career that continues to intrigue me and that has allowed for the healthy growth and sustenance of my ties to my wonderful family. But the flows, of course, are two-way. Without their humor and the reality base, the perspective, that they have provided over the years, I might have continued to treat the academic world as the only world and a career in it as the only worthy grounding of an identity. I know now that Sally Kenan was only partially right about a professional career, not just for women but for anybody. You should "be" it rather than just "do" it; you should take it into your soul as a calling. But it can't be totality of who you are. It shouldn't consume all your passion or be the sole source of how you define yourself. It was a hard lesson for me to learn. As it is, though, as things have turned out, I can hum along now with Johnny Paycheck, that good ol' boy from Tennessee, and think to myself that when I get a little readier, and I admit I'm getting restless, I'll sing his song right out loud with him, "You can take this job and shove it!" And this time I won't look back.

AUTHOR NOTE

Greer Litton Fox, PhD, is affiliated with University of Tennessee.

Address correspondence to: Professor Greer Litton Fox, Department of Child & Family Studies, University of Tennessee, Knoxville, TN 37994-1900 (e-mail: glfox@utk.edu).

REFERENCES

Bruce, C., & Fox, G. L. (1999). Accounting for patterns of father involvement: Age of child, father-child coresidence, and father role salience. *Sociological Inquiry, 69*, 3, 458-476.

Fox, G. L. (1973). Some determinants of modernism among women in Ankara, Turkey. *Journal of Marriage and the Family, 35*, 3, 520-529.

Fox, G. L. (1973). Another look at the comparative resources model: Assessing the balance of power in Turkish marriages. *Journal of Marriage and the Family, 35*, 4, 718-730.

Fox, G. L. (1974). Some observations and data on the availability of same-sex role models as a factor in undergraduate career choice. *Sociological Focus, 7*, 4, 15-30.

Fox, G. L. (1975). Love match and arranged marriage in a modernizing nation: Mate selection in Ankara, Turkey. *Journal of Marriage and the Family, 37*, 1, 180-193.

Fox, G. L. (1977). Nice girl: Social control of women through a value construct. *Signs: Journal of Women in Culture and Society, 2*, 4, 805-817.

Fox, G. L. (1977). Sex role attitudes as predictors of contraceptive use among unmarried university students. *Sex Roles, 3*, 3, 265-283.

Fox, G. L. (1978). Demographic determinants of gender role structure: The case of age at marriage in Turkey. In J. Allman (Ed.), *Women's status and fertility in the Muslim world* (pp. 243-269). New York: Praeger Publishers.

Fox, G. L. (1979). The family's influence on adolescent sexual behavior. *Children Today, 8*, 3, 21-25.

Fox, G. L. (1980). The mother-daughter relationship as a socialization structure: A research review. *Family Relations, 29*, 1, 21-28.

Fox, G. L. (1981). The family and the ex-offender: Potentials for rehabilitation. In S. Martin, L. B. Sechrest, & R. Redner (Eds.), *New Directions in the Rehabilitation of Criminal Offenders* (pp. 406-423). Washington, D.C. National Academy Press.

Fox, G. L. (1981). The family's role in adolescent sexual behavior. In T. Ooms (Ed.), *Teenage pregnancy in a family context* (pp. 73-130). Philadelphia, Pennsylvania: Temple University Press.

Fox, G. L. (1984). Barriers to parent-teen communication about sexuality. *Grosberg Journal, 10*, 15-21.

Fox, G. L., & Allen, J. (1987). Childcare. In J. Figueira-McDonough & R. Saari (Eds.), *The trapped woman: Catch 22 in deviance and control* (pp. 112-142). Beverly Hills, CA: Sage Publications.

Fox, G. L, Blanchard, C. B., Eckman, M., & Merriam, K. (1972). *The status of women faculty at Bowling Green State University*. Pittsburgh: Know Press, Inc. Also reprinted by Educational Resources Information Center, Document No. ER 066 144, 85 pp.

Fox, G. L., & Bruce, C. (1999). The anticipation of single parenthood: A profile of men's concerns. *Journal of Family Issues, 20*, 4, 485-506.

Fox, G. L., & Chancey, D. (1998). Sources of economic distress: Individual and family outcomes. *Journal of Family Issues, 19*, 6, 725-749.

Fox, G. L., Colombo, M., Clevenger, W. F., & Ferguson C. (1988). Parental division of labor in adolescent sexual socialization. *Journal of Contemporary Ethnography, 17*, 3, 349-371.

Fox, G. L., & Inazu, J. K. (1980). Patterns and outcomes of mother-daughter communication about sexuality. *Journal of Social Issues, 36*, 1, 7-29.

Fox, G. L., & Inazu, J. K. (1980). Mother-daughter communication about sex. *Family Relations, 29*, 3, 347-352.

Fox, G. L., & Inazu, J. K. (1982). The influence of mother's marital history on the mother-daughter relationship in black and white households. *Journal of Marriage and the Family, 44*, 1, 143-153.

Fox, G. L., & Kelly, R. F. Determinants of child custody arrangements at divorce. *Journal of Marriage and the Family, 57*, 3, 693-708.

Fox, G. L., & Medlin, C. (1986). Accuracy in mother's perceptions of daughters' level of sexual involvement: Black and white single mothers and their teenage daughters. *Family Perspectives, 20*, 4, 267-287.

Fox, G. L., Von Bargen, J., & Jester, M. (1996). Managing murder: Parents as mediators of children's experience. *Journal of Family Issues, 17*, 6, 732-757.

Inazu, J. K., & Fox, G. L. (1980). Maternal influence on the sexual behavior of teen-age daughters. *Journal of Family Issues, 1*, 1, 81-102.

Kelly, R. F., & Fox, G. L. (1993). Determinants of alimony awards: An empirical test of current theories and a reflection on public policy. *Syracuse Law Review, 44*, 2, 641-722.

Kelly, R. F., Sheldon, A. W., & Fox, G. L. (1985). The impact of economic dislocation on the health of children. In J. Boulet, A. M. DeBritto, & S. A. Ray (Eds.), *Understanding the economic crisis: The impact of poverty and unemployment on children and families* (pp. 94-111). Ann Arbor, MI: University of Michigan.

Aspirations and Possibilities: Coming to Terms with Other People's Reality

Irv Tallman

KEYWORDS. Autobiography, research, simulation games, social psychology, socialization

INTRODUCTION

Recently my two very adult daughters and I have begun talking about the time when we shared our lives together. The most powerful images evoked in these reminiscences centered around their teenage years in the late sixties and early seventies. The memories that surfaced were of peace marches, demonstrations, sit ins, and teach ins–events that energized and ennobled us. Even tedious moments spent stuffing envelopes for the McCarthy for President Campaign or attending rallies in which the rhetoric was often absurd were recalled, in the mellowness of time, with considerable fondness. As these talks continued, however, a more cynical, albeit still light hearted, tone crept into the conversation. My daughters recalled the civil rights rally we attended in 1964 (it was during the ASA meetings in Los Angeles). We were exhorted at that meeting to join a picket line to protest the hiring practices of a bank. My oldest daughter, who was twelve at the time, was so moved that she tearfully demanded that we join the pickets. But we had made plans to go to Marine Land,3 and I determined that we should adhere to our original plans. The unsaid interpretation of that event, or at least the interpretation that I attached to these recollections, was that I was ready to abrogate my commitment to principle in favor of personal pleasure. This interpretation is reinforced as my children gleefully recall how our participation in the Peace March in Washington ended by eating dinner at a good restaurant–not an unusual aftermath of our participation in such activities.

These reflections generally end in my experiencing some discomfort because they bring to light my imperfections as a model for my children. I was not the heroic figure I would have liked them to believe me to be, and perhaps that they would have liked me to be.

I must admit that although my daughters' implicit critiques elicit some guilt, I do not feel either contrition or regret. The effort to balance concern for the collective good with self-satisfaction, if not heroic, is nevertheless a common human response. I mention these reminiscences here because they cast some light on my quandary in writing this autobiographical piece. What is there to say about an intellectual journey that is in its waning years? Did I accomplish all that I wanted to? Clearly not. Could I have done better? Of course. But did I enjoy the ride–you bet. For years I have been paid reasonably well for expounding, pursuing, and testing ideas, many of them my own. There, of course, have been frustrations–colleagues, administrators, peer reviewers, and referees have not always seen and interpreted my ideas and work as I would have liked. But I was allowed to do my work, and it provided me with a degree of autonomy rare in modern life.

My daughters, however, might justifiably argue that the taxpayers have not supported me with salary and grants for over thirty-five years simply for me to "enjoy the ride." I cannot ignore the first part of the collective good-individual benefit balance sheet. Some accounting is due the citizens who supported me, the teachers who trained and launched me, my colleagues who inspired and frustrated me and who shared the intellectual journey with me.

Any attempt to provide such an accounting will have to assess more than my personal contribution. For I am part of a community of teachers, researchers, and scholars, some of whom I have never met but who, nevertheless, influence what I think and what I do. This community is governed by a set of norms that also contribute to the accomplishments and failures of my colleagues and myself. These norms effect the hurdles we must overcome, like tenure, promotion, standards for publication, and the obstacles to obtaining research grants. There were the equally painful processes in which I, along with others, sat in judgment on the future of colleagues, graduate students, and scholars seeking to have their work published or to have research funded–always with the nagging question of whether the standards we applied and the decisions we made were appropriate and valid. Did they contribute to advancing or deterring the continuous development of the discipline of sociology? This, after all, is our raison d'etre.

What constitutes the collective good for the discipline and, more specifically, for the scholarly study of the family? There is no consensus among family scholars as to the answer to that question. So my personal answer represents only a subsection of our profession.

I believe our discipline is best served by focusing on developing a cumulative body of knowledge. We need a system of knowledge building that is generative and can constantly increase in precision and scope. This means we have to go beyond description and be able to generate and test theories. We also have to be able and willing to discard theories that are not useful.

If building a cumulative body of knowledge is the criterion by which we should be measured, my colleagues and I have failed–at least over my professional lifetime. I have seen no systematic development of knowledge statements about the family whether defined as an institution, a social organization, or a small group of interacting personalities. There are, of course, new perspectives, like the life course approach, or the attempt to build a discipline called "familism," or the focus on stress and coping, or the attempts to put new dimensions on what is euphemistically called role "theory." In my view, each of these perspectives is a way of repackaging our limited understanding of the processes through which families develop and change. There have also been valiant attempts to apply systems theory, exchange theory, and behaviorist theories to family functioning, but these have been piecemeal and narrowly focused. In general, our theories are not of sufficient scope, do not have sufficient explanatory power, or do not entail sufficient conceptual precision to provide a basis for building a systematic and cumulative body of knowledge. Our literature is replete with descriptions of aspects of family life as it exists now or in the past. What is lacking are principles that allow us to explain how and why these events occur and the conditions under which the principles are operative. We know the family has changed, but we flounder in our efforts to provide a systematic explanation for the general processes underlying such changes.

We have gained some sophistication in data analysis which has provided us with methods for a more careful and detailed analysis of what goes on within families. Unfortunately, too often these techniques distort rather than contribute to knowledge, as is now evident through the growing misuse of confirmatory factor analysis and structural equation modeling. These statistical analyses rightfully belong in the service of testing theory but are more often used to provide post-datum explanations that last only until the next study.

The literature also abounds in philosophical disagreements about what we should be studying, what is possible to study, and how we should go about studying it. We seem to be chasing our tails. I am unhappy with this state of affairs and, in my way, I have tried to do something about it. What is troubling is that other scholars representing other perspectives can make the same claim. Moreover, they would discredit my contribution as I tend to discredit theirs. Our discipline is, unfortunately, multi-paradigmatic and until one paradigm begins to dominate, we will have difficulty effectively communicating with one another.

So what is to be done? Since this is an autobiographical essay, I can personalize this question. I represent a perspective that is different from many family scholars. Do I pursue that perspective and limit my audience to those few fellow travelers who see the discipline as I do? Or do I try to bridge the differences by debating the merits of the various perspectives? I have opted for continuing to work within my paradigm and letting time be the judge of its value. But the ugly question that my daughters, rapidly becoming a metaphor for conscience in this essay, will not quite let me ignore is, should I do more?

Even more fundamental, given my talents, can I do more? Could I convince anyone to change their perspectives in favor of mine if I tried? Can I be convinced to change? Is my strategy a replica of the decision I made on that July day in 1964: is the choice of letting my work speak for itself the equivalent of going to Marine Land? Am I choosing the pleasure of a comfortable paradigm and colleagues with whom I can easily communicate to the knock-down struggle and frustration of what seems like endless debate?

In a way this essay is an attempt to compromise between these alternatives. By describing my own intellectual development, I will engage the debate, albeit indirectly. Describing how one student of the family developed his perspective and ideas may make some contribution toward understanding why so many of us in this business follow different drummers. Even if this endeavor does not shed light on the paradigmatic disputes that separate us, it may help break down the use of stereotypes and *ad hominem* appeals that inhibit rather than foster effective communication.

There is one more caveat that I must address before I proceed. I was talking with my stepdaughter (my daughters are a source of considerable insight for me) about my misgivings in writing this paper. She understood my concern and noted that in writing this type of essay I could not avoid the fact that I would be choosing what I wrote in order to present myself in a particular light. She said it very bluntly: "You are going to want your readers to like you." This is a shocking statement. For years I have used either data or logic to mediate between the reader and myself, the findings or the theory were to speak for themselves and I, like some medium, was merely the instrument for conveying information to an audience. Indeed, I have never been good at getting people to like me and the idea that I should deliberately set out to do so horrifies me. The best way I can deal with this new and unpleasant insight is to admit that what follows is a subjective and selective depiction of myself as I see my intellectual development and the people and ideas that most influenced me. I leave to the reader (if he or she is so inclined) the task of inferring the motives that underlie my selection of incidents and events.

MY FAMILY BACKGROUND

I grew up in a household in which politics was a central topic of our everyday discussions. My parents were Jewish immigrants from Poland who came to this country by way of Germany. They lived together from the time my mother was 16 until they were married in New York five years later. Although my father was in his teens in Europe, he was active in left-wing socialist revolutionary organizations in both Poland and Germany. As a child I loved to listen to stories of my dad's adventures as a striking coal miner in Germany. Although my parents would define themselves as atheists, my upbringing was more irreligious than atheistic. I had no religious training and grew up without close ties or identification with any religious or ethnic community. I remember going to school on Jewish holidays because no one told me I could stay home until I arrived at school.

The one other childhood experience that I believe must have had an effect on how I view the world is that we moved all the time. I was born in New York City. My parents moved to Seattle before I was two and then moved to Los Angeles when I was five. We moved again to the San Francisco Bay Area when I was seven or eight.

Although I spent my remaining formative years in the Bay Area, my parents constantly moved from community to community. I attended fifteen elementary schools and eight junior high schools before I insisted that I spend three consecutive years in one high school despite the fact that it eventually meant traveling from one end of San Francisco to another. The impetus for these moves was essentially my mother's restlessness; she referred to herself as a gypsy. She simply found what she considered to be better places to live.

These experiences may well have contributed to my sense that the world is in constant flux. I recognize that an adequate explanation of social systems, including the family, involves accounting for both stability and change and that effective systems are those that maintain stability under conditions of change. However, I have always gravitated toward seeking explanations for the change part of the system.

The most obvious outcome of my parents' political radicalism, lack of religious and ethnic identification, and constant mobility, was my sense of isolation and marginality. Lacking traditions and rituals of my own, I look upon the traditions of others with an outsider's curiosity and with an analytical rather than emotional attachment. The same is not true for my perspective on the political and social order. I grew up with a fervent belief that as part of a collective, it is within our power to make the world a better place for everyone. It is this belief and commitment that I share with most, if not all, sociologists. The debate is how to accomplish this end.

WWII

When I graduated from high school, the second World War was well underway, and I was drafted into the Army. Like many who participated in WWII, I consider it the last good war. I went into the army with all the enthusiasm of an eighteen-year-old ready to fight evil and do good. But the fates or my own personal characteristics mitigated any fantasies about or opportunities for heroism. After training in the signal corp, I was sent to the Island of Kauai in Hawaii where I spent the remainder of the war. I served as a radio and radar operator in a radar facility on the northern part of the island. Most of my time was spent playing basketball, swimming, and falling in love with the island, its people, and, in particular, its young women. I have never lost my love for the island and its people. In retrospect I see myself as very fortunate to have spent the war years in that way; at the time I suffered considerable guilt for languishing in safety when many of my friends were in danger and one of my closest friends was killed in combat.

GETTING AN EDUCATION

When the war ended, I enrolled in the University of California at Berkeley. In high school I had anticipated becoming a journalist. This aspiration was spawned by a book Vincent Sheehan wrote describing his adventures as an international correspondent covering foreign wars and revolutions. My experiences in the army, however, awakened an interest in psychology. I'm not sure what all the reasons were, but I remember being aware that, despite our commonalities, my buddies were different from me and from one another. I would go to the library in Kapaa and get books on psychoanalysis, and I took extensive notes on what I was reading. This activity made me the butt of a number of jokes by one or two members of our small unit. The ridicule ended only when I indicated I was ready to fight for my right to read.

So I began my career in higher education in the field of psychology. I remember the years at Berkeley as the happiest of my life. The war was over. Fascism was defeated, and I firmly believed that it was within our power to create a world in which people could be both equal and free. I remember staying up into the early morning talking with friends and roommates about philosophy, economics, politics, and, of course, love and sex. I was active in left-wing youth groups but my choice of romantic partners always seemed to come from more conventional quarters. In fact, I was rapidly becoming disenchanted with what now would be termed extremists and what I saw as adherence to dogma. I never doubted, and still don't, that democratic institutions, whatever their limitations, are the best means for improving the human condition. My disagreements with my fellow radicals also led to those wonderful interminable discussions. Somehow we all thought that we were going to make a real difference in the world and that our talks were an essential part of this process of change.

I remember exciting courses in philosophy, labor economics, and clinical psychology. But most of all I remember the class in motivation that was taught by Edward Tolman. I was intrigued with the way Tolman brought the student into his thought processes. He would put Lewinian topological diagrams on the board, link them to some problem he was working on, take class input into account about the nature of forces operating on the individual and the barriers impeding goal attainment. This involved constantly changing parts of the diagram. The next time he might come into class and say he had changed his mind and introduce still other elements. Despite the indecision and changes, there was a precision and clarity in the way he thought that I greatly admired. I never knew Tolman personally; nor at the time did I know of his contribution to the field of psychology. Nevertheless, he had a profound effect on my image of a scholar both as teacher and writer. He was my first model and he continues to play that role for me. The fact that he led the revolt against signing the loyalty oath at U.C. Berkeley in the fifties did not surprise me.

During the time I was at Berkeley, I worked in a Jewish Community Center Day Camp in San Francisco. The camp provided group activities for children of many races and ethnic groups, some of whom had behavioral problems. The director was a social worker who believed that I had a talent for working with children. She recommended that I go to graduate school in social work and suggested I apply to Wayne State. Social work at Wayne State was noted primarily for Fritz Redl and his work with disturbed and delinquent children. In the absence of any compelling alternatives, and with the approval of a University vocational counselor, I applied to Wayne State and upon graduation went off to Detroit. Being a social worker was consonant with my desire to: (1) be an agent of change and (2) earn a living.

At the time I believed psychological and emotional strength was necessary for people to be actively involved in making society better for themselves and their neighbors. By better I meant primarily more equal. Social work, I believed, could be a vehicle for bringing about such changes. Social work training during those years was predominantly training in psychoanalytic theory and therapeutic techniques. I left Detroit after two years and returned to California a married man with an MSW in psychiatric social work. For three years I worked for the California Department of Mental Hygiene supervising mental patients on leave from state hospitals. I also worked evenings and Saturdays for the San Jose Family Service Agency doing marital counseling. I found the latter job more satisfying but not sufficiently remunerative for me to do on a full-time basis. In fact, I was getting increasingly restless. I was not the agent of change I had envisioned. For the most part what I was doing was trying to keep people from falling apart, and I wasn't doing too good a job of that. I was seriously thinking of going to law school, although I had not worked out how I could afford it since I now had a wife and a child to support. When the opportunity arose to apply for an NIMH fellowship to attend the University of Chicago School of Social Service Administration post-masters program, I seized it, thinking that a PhD in social work might give me the opening I was seeking. I wanted to do more than be a caseworker or supervisor of caseworkers. What part of doing more represented a desire for more money and status, and what part represented a desire to make a difference in the world, remains an open question.

If it were not for the fact that we met fascinating people from all over the world during that year in Chicago, I would consider it a complete disaster. I found myself at odds with the instructors, and I had the feeling that I was wasting my time and learning nothing new. Even more fundamentally, I was beginning to believe that social work, rather than being an instrument for change, served as mechanism for maintaining the status quo. Problem solving, as used in social work, emphasized personal change so that clients could "adjust" to the system rather than change it. It has been over forty years since that terrible year in Chicago, and I am no longer certain that my harsh judgment was fair or accurate. All that I am sure of is that I left Chicago convinced that I must leave social work. It was five years before I could accomplish that end.

San Francisco State

My opportunity came when I was offered a job on a research project at San Francisco State. It was a four-year project designed to study the effects of special education on severely retarded children and their parents. I was responsible for developing the measures and carrying out the analysis for the parent part of the study. Looking back on those days and considering my lack of knowledge about research, I am amazed at my temerity in accepting the job. I knew nothing about scale construction and measurement and was only minimally acquainted with some of the substantive issues involved in doing such a study. Fortunately, I did not know how much I did not know. I was equally fortunate to have colleagues who were able and willing to help me. Their assistance, combined with a great deal of reading in the areas of parental behavior and in scale construction, along with the generous use of consultants hired for the project, enabled me to develop the Parent Adaptability Scale (Kieren & Tallman, 1972; Tallman, 1961, 1965). This is not the appropriate platform for discussing the details of this measure. Suffice it to say that to this day, I am pleased with this accomplishment both for its conceptual dimensions and its predictive utility.

Graduate Study

The job at San Francisco State gave me the opportunity to go to graduate school and still earn enough to support a family now increased by the birth of a second daughter. I decided to study sociology because I thought it was the discipline that would enable me to integrate my current research and past training in psychology and social work. The fact is, I had never taken a course in sociology. I had, however, had lengthy talks with friends who were sociologists, all of whom received their PhD's from Berkeley and recommended that I study at that University. So I began my graduate career in Berkeley in 1957. I took seminars from Erving Goffman, Leo Lowenthal, Seymour Lipset, and Bernard Cohen.

It is both a comment on my naivete and my intellectual preferences that I was thoroughly confused by Goffman's seminar. The seminar was overcrowded, and it seemed as if everyone wanted to speak. Goffman must have been working on *Asylums* at the time because many of his references were drawn from life in mental hospitals. I had worked in and around mental hospitals for a number of years, and I could not relate to these examples. I have since learned to appreciate and admire Goffman's astute insights.

My experiences in the other seminars were quite different. The breadth of the areas of investigation, the explanatory concepts, the subject matter investigated all enthralled me. I had read Marx earlier in my life but the writings of Weber, Durkheim, Simmel, and Mannheim were all new to me. I felt the power that comes with new knowledge and a new perspective on the world. I also felt at home. Although I am sure I experienced the pressure all graduate students feel, my retrospective memory is of pleasurable hours spent in the Berkeley library gathering information for seminar papers. I remember looking for explanations for such questions as to why low-paid office workers resisted unionization and how religion and class combined to stratify Lebanese society. I remember going through old *Colliers* and *Saturday Evening Posts* as far back as World War I to grasp the changing depiction of the family in popular literature. These were all subjects that I believed were not only inherently interesting but also significant in helping to explain why people and collectivities behaved as they do.

Of all of the courses I took at Berkeley, however, the one that turned me on the most was Bernie Cohen's seminar in Small Groups. Here I was introduced to a framework that dominates my thinking to this day. I was learning research methodology both on the job and as a graduate student, but I needed a way of linking the great ideas we had been discussing with research. My professors and fellow graduate students were telling me that sociology was a science–but I wasn't sure how it worked or could work. Certainly data analytic techniques were not sufficient to make us a science. Science required explanation. Ideas, no matter how intuitively insightful, do not constitute explanation–unless we have a way of discriminating which ideas are right or, at the very least, which offer better explanations than others. I began to learn how to make such differentiations in Bernie's class.

He introduced me to the philosophy of science and to elements of the scientific method. I began to understand the importance of deriving hypotheses from theoretical statements, stating the hypothesis *before* making empirical observations, and providing the clear and unambiguous opportunity for falsifying the hypothesis. These are simple premises, ones we have all learned (even if they are rarely applied), but in that seminar Cohen brought them to life. They provided the linkage I needed to understand how sociology can be a science. There was an incisiveness and clarity in Cohen's thinking that I admire to this day. I think his writings on the conditional nature of knowledge and the necessity of stipulating scope conditions in testing sociological theory are major contributions in the ongoing effort to build a methodology for constructing and testing sociological theory.

So I became a positivist. I believed that it was possible to build a science of human behavior. Perhaps, more importantly, there was the embryonic formation of a commitment to building formal deductive theory as the foundation for such a science.

Let me digress for a moment to consider an issue that has troubled me in recent years. There is a growing literature that attacks positivism and even more vehemently the form of positivism to which I adhere (e.g., the emphasis on building deductive abstract theories of behavior) as exemplar of male dominance and capitalist thinking. I have, prior to this essay, avoided debating this issue because I find such debates circular, endless, and, most importantly, unresolvable. It is unresolvable because the opposing positions are based on fundamentally different starting assumptions. Just as one cannot debate or empirically test the premise that "The Bible is the literal word of God," so too the claim that positivism is a manifestation of male dominance is not debatable or testable. In my view such statements are constraining rather than generative or heuristic. I value the scientific method in large part because it helps avoid the interminable and fruitless arguments that stem from such statements. I mention my position here because I think it should be made clear that many of us on the left side of the political spectrum eschew this sociology by fiat.

Having said this, I must add that I consider one of the important new contributions to our discipline to be the literature coming from feminist scholars that has demonstrated the extent to which our theories have been dominated by a male perspective. The most prominent example of this contribution is probably Gilligan's (1982) critique and modification of Kohlberg's theory of moral development, but there are many others that could be cited. At issue are not ideas but the form in which they are put. The two key criteria are whether the ideas are clearly communicable to the community of scholars and whether they can be falsified.

There are those who believe that the very effort to explain human behavior is futile. For them, social life is incoherent and unordered; it is consequently not amenable to systematic investigation. Nor is it possible to build any constitutive meaning about events and their occurrence. For these scholars, sociology can never be science; if anything it is a type of social philosophy. Knowledge, it seems, evolves from a labyrinth of reductionistic (or deconstructionistic) constantly changing interpretations and reinterpretations of meaning. In my view, such orientations not only contribute nothing to building a cumulative body of knowledge, they contribute nothing to efforts to build a better world, however "better" might be defined. They leave us floundering in the tar pits of obsessive discussion without beginning or end.

No matter what kind of a society we desire, no matter what we want to explain, we need to have a way of building knowledge statements that can be accepted or rejected on some shared criteria that extend beyond personal preferences. Logic, in its various forms, is the best mechanism I know for making such judgments.

So when Bernie Cohen went to Stanford as a faculty member, I went there as a graduate student. It wasn't quite that I followed him, although we talked about my going. He was encouraging, and I was enthused. There were other important reasons for my decision. I had talked with Kingsley Davis who was the "Family Sociologist" at Berkeley, and he saw correctly that my work and research interests at San Francisco State were more social psychological than demographic. I had also talked with other faculty at Stanford, and I knew that Paul Wallin was there. Wallin's work clearly was closer to the type of research I was doing. Bud McCord also expressed an interest in my research and asked me to join a study group he was organizing (this was great encouragement for an incoming graduate student).

I learned to appreciate the collegial aspects of graduate school at Stanford. It was much less formal than Berkeley, perhaps because there were many fewer students. We rather quickly called professors and, more importantly, the department secretary, by their first names. Although I had a full-time job that kept me away from campus except for classes, there still was time, before and after class and at parties, for lengthy discussions with fellow students. I remember these discussions fondly; they were a critical factor in my education.

We felt as if we were pioneers. We were part of a new Stanford Sociology. Much of the faculty was new and young, many younger than me. It was a department with a mission and much of what we focused on was the methodology of scientific theory construction. I was introduced to the philosophy of science–to Fiegl, Brodbeck, Cohen, Nagel, Herbert Simon, Carl Hempel, and, most significantly, Carl Popper. I also learned, reluctantly at first, the utility of experiments and observational techniques for studying behavior. If formal theory was the explanatory tool of science, the experiment was the essential mechanism for testing theory. The message took. In my career I have used mail and interview surveys, game simulations, computer simulations, daily diaries, and even videotaped interactions, but I am most comfortable when I am conducting experiments.

For my doctoral dissertation, I recast Merton's theory of adaptation to blocked legitimate means into balance theory as expressed through graph theory. I then designed an experiment in which subjects' chances of successfully attaining their goal were virtually blocked. I also provided an illegitimate, albeit seemingly undetectable, means for attaining the goal. The findings were in keeping with the hypothesis and suggested that subjects who did not take the opportunity to cheat tended to lower their initial evaluation of the success goal. When the findings were published (Tallman, 1966, 1967), I received a complimentary letter from Robert Merton. This was heady stuff for a beginning assistant professor. Since I have not had many such letters in my career, I continue to look back on correspondence with Professor Merton with some pleasure.

THE MINNESOTA YEARS

The research project I was working on at San Francisco State was completed while I was at Stanford, and I took a job at San Jose State teaching sociology and social work. After receiving my doctorate, I was informed by someone at Stanford–I don't remember who–of a position at Minnesota that they felt suited my interests and abilities. Murray Straus had contacted them and wanted someone to do experimental research with families. I remember how helpful Sandy Dornbush, Bernie Cohen, Frank Camilleri, and others were in preparing me for the interview at Minnesota and the negotiations about salary that might take place. I have always wanted, with little success, to replicate the shared sense of mission and solidarity that existed between graduate students and faculty at Stanford in those days.

I was in some awe of Minnesota and its long, illustrious tradition in sociology. This feeling of veneration diminished rapidly, however, as I began attending faculty meetings. Two lasting impressions were initiated in those early faculty meetings and have been consistently reinforced over the years. First, scholarly brilliance and/or eminence is uncorrelated with wisdom; and second, a faculty meeting is the worst possible forum devised by man (here the gender reference is deliberate) to make rational or even useful decisions.

Faculty meetings aside, Minnesota was a stimulating place from the first day I arrived. On that first day, I found on my desk an edited and critically evaluated copy of a draft of a research proposal I had been developing. That was my introduction to that amazing man, Reuben Hill. Reuben had not only carefully read my proposal and criticized it, he provided me with Family Study Center funds to hire a research assistant. This was a remarkable reception for a new assistant professor. From that first day, I became, without ever making a deliberate choice, a member of the Minnesota Family Studies Center.

Even today it is hard for me to sort out Reuben's influence on me and my work. It was important, but I have difficulty in isolating specifics. He was kind, understanding, generous with time and resources. He gave advice easily, and it was usually kindly and thoughtful. He never seemed to push his own agenda, encouraging and supporting my interests in social psychology and political sociology. All of these traits engendered great loyalty toward him within the Family Study Center. He was like a patriarch (albeit an accessible patriarch); he *was* the Family Study Center, and it was difficult to determine where Reuben stopped and the Center began.

Like a patriarch, Reuben was less a colleague and more an instructor. His relationship with the junior faculty and with many "colleagues" was a kind of intellectual *noblesse oblige*. He was generous, accepting, and tutorial. If you disappointed him (as when I got divorced), he was tolerant as if recognizing that even lesser people were deserving of his good will.

In any case, I admired him immensely. I had read his work before I came to Minnesota and was impressed with the ABCX model and his conception of family disorganization at times of crisis and the resultant recovery process. I believe that this still may be his greatest contribution. It is regrettable that those who followed in his footsteps did not do more to explicate and expand on such critical concepts as his notion of the angle of recovery subsequent to family disorganization. Although it became clear that Reuben's epistemology was different from my own, he nevertheless embodied for me the main themes that were important in family sociology. My family writings were, in some ways, a dialogue with Reuben Hill's orientation. When he died, it seemed as if I lost my audience in family sociology. It was the perspective he represented that I was trying to persuade, modify, change, or implement.

Reuben was generally so supportive and his arguments so cogent that it took years for me to understand the basis for our differences. It was not until work began on the *Contemporary Theories of the Family* book (Burr, Hill, Nye, & Reiss, 1979) that I saw clearly the nature of these differences. They are apparent in the methodology adapted for that book and can be best, if superficially, summarized by the gap between inductive and deductive theory building. The difference lies in the emphasis placed on research findings. I will not venture to describe Reuben's position on theory building here. It is available in almost all of his later works, in the methodology chapter of the *Contemporary Theories* book, and in Joan Aldous's writings on theory and family development. I will note only that Reuben and his colleagues had a great respect for empirical findings. He had an encyclopedic mind and tended to incorporate mounds of data into classificatory relationships. From my view, and those who share my perspective, data are ephemeral phenomena; they are tied to a particular time and place–consequently, they are not easily replicated. They are certainly not replicable if they are gathered in natural settings in the midst of multitudes of unmeasured possibly confounding variables.

Thus data cannot provide the basis for building a cumulative body of knowledge. Cumulative knowledge comes from developing, refining, and modifying theory. Theory consists of a set of universal statements about a phenomena that are amenable to empirical testing under specified conditions. Actually, the truth or falsity of a theory is tested at the level of logic. Its power to explain behavioral phenomena is tested at the empirical level but only under specified initial conditions. Data are important for testing the utility of a theory, not for building knowledge. It should be apparent to readers who know the family literature that my approach is discordant with much of family sociology.

By the time the *Contemporary Theories* book was contemplated, these differences were manifest in the decision to write two separate chapters on the theory of problem solving. Reuben and David Klein would write one, and I would write the other in collaboration with Ed Brent. The chapter Ed and I wrote was not acceptable to the editors. It was a wise decision on their part because its format was not appropriate for their approach to theory construction. It incorporated no data, rather it focused on building a stochastic model of the decision processes involved in problem solving. Ed and I never published the paper, but it has served as a take-off point for much of my subsequent writing and research on decision making and problem solving.

Research on Family Problem Solving

Those readers who are aware of the family problem solving research project that was conducted at Minnesota between 1968 and 1973 might wonder how Reuben Hill, Murray Straus, and Joan Aldous, the other members of the research team, tolerated my perspective. In fact, I don't think it was that hard for anyone on the project. Elsewhere, I described the research team as creating a "climate" that was invigorating and challenging. Indeed, our meetings constantly left me charged with renewed enthusiasm and new insights. Although we all had our individual projects, my colleagues were extremely helpful and supportive in my endeavors. We shared the belief that problem solving is a core family activity that can account for how some families function effectively and others collapse. Within the general orientation, I sought, in collaboration with Murray Straus, to incorporate experimental methods and social psychological theory into the research program.

The problem solving grant provided me with the basic support to conduct two research projects. The first used the SIMFAM technique, developed with

Murray Straus, to observe a mother, a father, and a preadolescent child solving puzzle-like problems within their own homes (Straus & Tallman, 1971). The advantage of SIMFAM for this research was that the three-person family could solve the problems conjunctively through motor activities. Thus we were able to design experiments in which the families participated under talking and non-talking conditions. Since our sample was made up of blue- and white-collar families, we could explore whether the reported white-collar advantages in problem solving were due to their greater verbal abilities (Tallman & Miller, 1974). We found that when we counter balanced verbal and non-verbal conditions the white-collar advantage washed out.

This research also provided a beginning effort to test how principles derived from small group research with ad hoc problem solving groups could be modified when applied to families. Our findings indicated that, although family organization was determined by normatively established role expectations, general principles pertaining to the relationship between leadership styles or channels of communication and problem solving applied to families as well as ad hoc groups (Tallman, 1970, 1971, 1988, 1993; Tallman, Leik, Gray, & Stafford, 1993).

These findings led to the development of a second, more ambitious, study. When I returned to Minnesota from U.C. Riverside where we conducted the SIMFAM research, I was asked to participate in a series of seminars at the University's Center for the Comparative Studies of Technological Development and Social Change. These seminars brought together anthropologists, economists, engineers, sociologists, and political scientists to discuss and plan comparative research in developing countries. It was at these seminars that I presented the initial ideas for a comparative study on socialization for social change. It was also under the auspices of this center and its director, Robert Holt, that we opened negotiations for the study on socialization for change comparing Mexican and U.S. families. With Center support, I went to Mexico on two occasions to identify an appropriate research site and to develop a working relationship with the Instituto Mexicano de Estudios Sociales (IMES). IMES provided the staff and supervision necessary for carrying out the research in Mexico. Two Mexican graduate students came to Minnesota to work with us on planning the project. The project was primarily funded by the problem solving grant but was also supported by funds obtained from the Ford Foundation, a midwest consortium for comparative research, and a supplemental grant from NIMH provided needed additional support.

The theory upon which this research was based sought to explain the processes through which children and parents are socialized to function in a changing and uncertain world. The theory's central premise was that family problem solving experiences affected children's abilities to plan for and take necessary risks when confronted with changes in their life circumstances.

In this research we compared peasant, blue-collar, and white-collar families in Michoacan, Mexico, with blue- and white-collar families in the Twin Cities. As much as I would like, I cannot justify, even in this self-indulgent essay, the time and space to discuss in any detail our efforts to solve the methodological problems posed by this kind of research. For the reader who might be interested, I refer him or her to our book *Adolescent Socialization in Cross Cultural Perspective* (Tallman, Marotz-Baden, & Pindas, 1983). I will note, however, that we used a game simulation that enabled us to provide families with behavioral choices that were appropriate for each culture while maintaining their conceptual equivalences. The simulation also enabled us to assess problem solving within constant opportunity structure classes while still enabling us to introduce experimental manipulations. We called the simulation *SIMCAR*, which involved a family of three in planning the career of their twelve-year-old child over a hypothetical ten-year period (Tallman & Wilson, 1974; Tallman, Wilson, & Straus, 1974). Families could invest time and money in 17 choices pertaining to recreation, education, work, religion, and household activities. In the experiment we could create a variety of life changes, such as loss of income, school failures, opportunities in other communities, the introduction of new educational opportunities, and so forth. The research also included face-to-face interviews with a sample of families in the areas studied. It was from this sample that the experimental subjects were selected.

Briefly, some of the key findings from this research pointed to unanticipated gender differences in power relations within the two societies. Despite normative expectations to the contrary, Mexican peasant wives exercised more power than any other class of wives in the study; United States white collar wives displayed the least power. Our hypotheses as to the consequences of experiencing failure within the family of origin held for sons but not for daughters for all groups in the study. Failure within the family led to greater tentativeness in sons and poorer outcomes in sons' planning their own careers. The data also suggested that, when provided with opportunities for success, the Mexicans of all social classes knew how to take advantage of those opportunities. In fact, they were more likely than the U.S. sample to defer gratification for long-term gains (Tallman, 1981; Tallman & Marotz-Baden, 1978; Tallman & Ihinger-Tallman, 1979).

I reached two conclusions from this research that influenced my subsequent work. First, I saw a need to clearly differentiate decision making from problem solving. Not only were the two behaviors distinguishable, but it was also necessary to understand when and how decisions facilitated or impeded the problem solving process. The second conclusion pertained to the assessment of power within families. Our data indicated that self-reports and observations depicted different aspects of the power relations within families. In essence there was a difference between public and private expressions of power.

Even more fundamentally, the data suggested the necessity to go beyond direct measures of power and influence in families to explore structural conditions that affect a family member's power potential. Power potential looms important because the weaker person may often engage in frequent, albeit fruitless, demands; or conversely, he or she may engage in anticipatory compliance. The critical factor in family power potential is the degree of symmetry in power relations. The reader will recognize the correspondence of these notions with Richard Emerson's (1972) theory of power/dependence. Emerson's theory had already had a profound effect on the theory of socialization we developed and would continue to be important in my subsequent work on decision making, commitment, and problem solving.

With the advantage of hindsight, the measures of power used in the SIMCAR study seem remarkably simplistic. They derived from a long line of interaction research in which demands and/or requests of a family member were coded and compared with the coded compliance or noncompliance of the other family members. The next major project provided a much more sophisticated and, I hope, more accurate picture of intra-family power relationships.

Two books were written under the auspices of the problem solving grants. The first, *Passion, Action and Politics* (Tallman, 1976), was an effort to apply problem solving theory to social problems and social problem solving. It was meant to provide a conceptual framework for the study of social problems. The book was generally well reviewed but did not sell as many copies as either my publisher or I had anticipated. It was around this time that I began to wonder if anything I was doing was making any difference. The second book, *Adolescent Socialization in Cross Cultural Perspective* (Tallman et al., 1983), referred to earlier in this essay, was published seven years later. I received favorable reviews in the psychology journals but either indifference or downright anger in the sociological journals. One reviewer simply seemed to doubt the findings, despite the data pertaining to reliability and validity of instruments. Another disliked game simulations, and another accused us of being chauvinistic because our theory predicted that the American adolescents would perform better than the Mexicans.

The pain I experienced at the criticisms of my book was somewhat ameliorated when I considered the spate of reviews of James Coleman's much more important book, *Foundations of Social Theory* (1995). If my personal pain was alleviated, my frustration at the inability to effectively communicate within the discipline was enhanced. Admittedly, Coleman's intent was monumental. He sought not only to provide a theory that bridges the micro-macro gap, but also to establish the foundations for a unified theory of social action. Such a cosmic endeavor in this day and age of diversified perspectives can be expected to elicit a rash of criticism. It is hard to understand, however, why so many of the attacks seemed to take on hysterical dimensions. In general, the critics did not address Coleman's work in terms of whether or not it succeeded in accomplishing the goals he had set for it; rather, they focused on what the reviewers would have liked the book to accomplish.

Interestingly, the critics seldom agreed with one another. The critiques covered the gamut from attacks on his ahistoricism, to his use of individual behavior as a point of departure, to his use of aspects of rational choice theory. The assessments were so disparate that they suggest a discipline without a central core. Coleman, reflecting on the range of criticisms, used the word "anarchy" to describe the discipline's inability to identify its essential problems.

And so we seem to keep talking past each other, protected by our values and reinforced by the small cadres of people who think as we do. In my experience we cannot even agree on basic definitions of key concepts. In fact, I think we thrive on ambiguities. Consider, for example, whether we can effectively communicate with one another using terms like "family," "alienation," "social capital," or even "problem solving." Part of the difficulty is the reliance on English rather than some more precise symbolic language. The meanings of words tend to decay as they are folded into common usage. A more profound part of the problem in my mind is that the ambiguity of the terms gives us freedom to apply them broadly, while giving the illusion that we are dealing with profound issues. Never mind that we are not effectively communicating either the range or boundaries of the concepts we are employing.

THE WASHINGTON STATE YEARS

Despite the support I received from the faculty at Minnesota, and the Family Study Center, it was only in my last year there that I had a colleague who shared my vision of what sociology should be and how to get there. Bob Leik came to head the Family Study Center in 1975. The next year I followed my future wife to Washington State.

It is a testament to the power of love that I am at Washington State. With the arrival of Leik, I came to realize the advantages of co-workers who share one's perspective. Free of philosophical debates, sharing the same priorities and the same universe of disclosure, Bob and I were able to let our imaginations soar. We have remained colleagues and continue to work on joint projects over the years.

I was ambivalent about leaving Minnesota, and I still keep close ties with many of the faculty whom I count among my best friends. I have returned often as a visiting professor and consultant. I continue to be interested in the research of my Minnesota colleagues and still care about how the department fares.

It is ironic and perhaps a kind of perverse justice that while I have never been comfortable with the rural life afforded at WSU (it is a standing joke that I have to leave Pullman for an urban fix every six weeks), I have found here a highly productive and stimulating group of scholars. There are among them several whose visions of sociology as a discipline are compatible with my own. Chief among these is Louis Gray, who, incidentally, was a student of Bob Leik's at the University of Washington. Not only do Louis and I share the same perspective about theory in sociology, but we also have in common similar substantive interests. Louis's mathematical sophistication was of tremendous help to me in clarifying my thinking and in developing theories of decision making, group commitment, and problem solving, all of which we have published together. Louis also made me more sensitive to the contributions of behavioral psychology in building our theories of decision making. My interest in exchange theory and my early training in psychology made me aware of the explanatory power of behaviorist principles for explaining aspects of human learning. Gray showed me how these principles could be expanded and modified to explain human choice and decisions. The principles were critical in the decision model we built and in our theory of problem solving. They are also at the core of my theory of socialization, our explanation for the inter-generational transmission of marital conflict and the conditions under which changes can be produced in previously learned destructive patterns of marital interaction. Neither Gray nor I were constrained by some of the limiting assumptions of the behaviorists. For example, we incorporated elements of cognitive psychology, particularly the work of Kahneman and Tversky, symbolic interaction, and exchange theory in our developing framework.

My work with Gray, and less frequently with Bob Leik, has returned me to the laboratory, although with some embellishments. The ability to use computers in interactive modes has enabled us to develop rather interesting experiments and simulations. For example, we are now working on an experiment that can test our theory of commitment to long-term relationships and the conditions leading to exploitation in those relationships (Gray & Tallman, 1984; Tallman & Gray, 1990; Tallman, Gray, & Leik, 1991).

At the same time, I am continuing to apply our theoretical framework to conduct research with natural families. I have just completed a five-year longitudinal study of newlyweds with the intent of testing a model that explores the impact of the family of origin on couple behaviors and the conditions under which such influences are enhanced or mitigated. The research, which included Peter Burke and Viktor Gecas as co-investigators, was funded by NIMH. It was designed to investigate the processes through which couples are socialized into marital roles, and the influence of these processes on the quality of the marital relationship. Couples were studied by means of face-to-face interviews, daily diaries, and videotaped couple interactions. We have written several papers on this research, and I plan to write two or three more before writing what I expect to be my last book (Tallman, Burke, & Gecas, 1998; Tallman, Gray, Kullberg, & Henderson, 1999).

ASSESSMENT

And so it goes. Every new project offers new hope that I can convey what I have learned to my colleagues and that this will make some difference in our understanding of human behavior. Except for a student here and there, I cannot see that my efforts or the efforts of my colleagues have had any appreciable influence on the state of sociological knowledge. Or, for that matter, on our knowledge about the family, either as a small group or as a social institution. This, of course, may be the result of my own limited abilities. I am drawn to simple explanations which I justify by arguing that parsimony is not a bad thing and that we should exhaust simple explanations before we add complications. Nevertheless, my reliance on linear logical models is probably too limiting as we look to explain developmental processes in human behavior.

Regardless of my personal limitations, it is reasonable to ask why, for over a hundred years, we have not been able to effectively move beyond the contributions of Durkheim, Mead, Simmel, Weber, and Marx? Why has it been so difficult to build a systematic, cumulative body of knowledge? One possible explanation is that we have become so fragmented that we have lost interest in a collective effort beginning, as it must, with effective communication.

What is the solution? Given the reaction to James Coleman's heroic effort, or Parsons before him, attempts to unify the discipline under some general theory appear at best to be premature. Perhaps the best course of action may be to accept our fundamental differences and for each scholar to work within his or her paradigm in the hope that in the future one paradigm will demonstrate its utility and predictive power so effectively that it will dominate the field.

All of this may be a rationalization for keeping on doing what I do. I continue to apply social psychological theories and methods to the study of the family. I have also tried to build some theories pertaining to general behavioral processes such as commitment and problem solving and to explore their relevance in explaining family behavior. I have done so not because I believe families are necessarily wonderful types of social organizations that need saving, nor am I prescient enough to claim that it is an institution that will exist forever. I have focused on the family because right now and for the foreseeable future it is the arena within which people's essential behaviors and orientations are forged. It is within the family that we learn to live with each other, learn to fear, tolerate, love and hate one another. It is within the family that we develop the skills and abilities to shape the world of the future.

I have just recently retired. I don't think this will change my life appreciably. I still love to do and plan research, to analyze data, to talk with colleagues, to influence young minds, and to be part of the University environment. I know I should feel that my best work is behind me, but I don't. I am looking forward to the next book. As I said at the beginning of this essay, I have enjoyed the trip. Is this enough to justify my continuing to draw on resources and get grants? My daughters would say no–and so would I. I owe something more to the community that has allowed me to have this rich and fulfilling life and to the discipline that has trained and sponsored me. I hope I can do better in the future.

AUTHOR NOTE

Irv Tallman is Professor Emeritus, Washington State University.
Address correspondence to: 22 Smith Ranch Court, San Rafael, CA 94903.

REFERENCES

Burr, W. R., Hill, R., Nye, F. I., & Reiss, I. L (Eds.). (1979). *Contemporary theories about the family.* Vol 1. New York: The Free Press.

Cohen, B. P. (1989). *Developing sociological knowledge: Theory and method (2nd edition).* Chicago: Nelson-Hall.

Coleman, J. S. (1990). *Foundations of social theory.* Cambridge, MA: Belknap Press of Harvard University Press.

Emerson, R. M. (1972). Exchange theory part II: Exchange relations in networks. In J. Berger, M. Zelditch, & B. Anderson (Eds.). *Sociological theories in progress, vol 2.* Boston: Houghton-Mifflin.

Gilligan, C. (1982). *In a different voice.* Cambridge, MA: Harvard University Press.

Gray, L. & Tallman, I. (1984). A satisfaction balance model of decision making and choice behavior. *Social Psychology Quarterly, 47*, 2, 146-159.

Kieren, D. & Tallman, I. (1972). Spousal adaptability: An assessment of marital competence. *Journal of Marriage and the Family, 34*, 2, 247-256.

Straus, M. A. & Tallman, I. (1971). SIMFAM: A technique for observational measurements and experimental studies of families. In J. Aldous, T. Condon, R. Hill, M. A. Straus & I. Tallman. (Eds.). *Family problem solving: A symposium on theoreti-*

cal, methodological and substantive concerns (pp. 381-438). Hinsdale, IL: Dryden Press.
Tallman, I. (1961). Adaptability: A problem solving approach to assessing childrearing practices. *Child Development, 32*, 4, 651-668.
Tallman, I. (1965). Spousal role differentiation and the socialization of severely retarded children. *Journal of Marriage and the Family, 27*, 1, 37-42.
Tallman, I. (1966). Adaptation to blocked opportunity: An experimental study. *Sociometry*, 29, 2, 121-134.
Tallman, I. (1967). The balance principle and normative discrepency. *Human Relations, 20*, 4, 341-355.
Tallman, I. (1970). The family as a small problem solving group. *Journal of Marriage and the Family, 32*, 1, 94-104.
Tallman, I. (1971). Family problem solving and social problems. In J. Aldous, T. Condon, R. Hill, M. A. Straus & I. Tallman. (Eds.). *Family problem solving: A symposium on theoretical, methodological and substantive concerns* (pp. 324-350). Hinsdale, IL: Dryden Press.
Tallman, I. (1976). *Passion, action and politics*. San Francisco: W. H. Freeman and Co.
Tallman, I. (1981). Social structure, family socialization and children's achievement goals: A comparative analysis. In J. Trost (Ed.). *The family in change* (pp. 75-87). Varteras, Sweden: International Library.
Tallman, I. (1988). Problem-solving in families: A revisionist view. In J. Aldous & D. Klein (Eds). *Social stress and family development* (pp. 102-128). New York: Guilford Press.
Tallman, I. (1993). Theoretical issues in researching problem-solving in families. *Marriage & Family Review, 18*, 3-4, 155-178.
Tallman, I., Burke, P. J., & Gecas, V. (1998). Socialization into marital roles testing a contextual, developmental model of marital functioning. In T. N. Bradbury (Ed.). *The developmental course of marital dysfunctioning* (pp. 88-105). Cambridge, England: Cambridge University Press .
Tallman, I. & Gray, L. (1990). Choices, decisions and problem solving. In W. R. Scott & J. Blake (Eds.). *Annual Review of Sociology, 16*, 405-433.
Tallman, I., Gray, L., & Leik, R. K. (1991). Decisions, dependency and commitment: An exchanged based theory of group formation. I. Tallman, L. Gray, & R. K. Leik (Eds.). *Advances in Group Processes, 8*: 227-250.
Tallman, I., Gray, L., Kullberg, V., & Henderson, D. (1999). The inter-generational transmission of marital conflict: Testing a process model. *Social Psychology Quarterly, 62*, 3, 219-239.
Tallman, I. & Ihinger-Tallman, M. (1979). Values, distributive justice and social change. *American Sociological Review, 44*, 4, 216-235.
Tallman, I., Leik, R. K., Gray, L., & Mark Stafford, M. (1993). A theory of problem solving behavior. *Social Psychology Quarterly, 56*, 3, 157-177.
Tallman, I. & Marotz-Baden, R. (1978). A comparison of U.S. and Mexican parental aspirations for sons and daughters. *Adolescence, 13*, 3, 251-268.
Tallman, I., Marotz-Baden, R., & Pindas, P. (1983). *Adolescent socialization in cross-cultural perspective*. New York: Academic Press.

Tallman, I. & Miller, G. (1974). Class differences in aspects of family problem-solving. *Sociometry, 37*, 1, 13-37.
Tallman, I. & Wilson, L. (1974). Simulating social structures: The use of simulation games in cross-national research. *Simulation and Games, 5*, 2, 147-167.
Tallman, I., Wilson, L., & Straus, M. A. (1974). SIMCAR: The use of a simulation game in cross-national research. *International Journal of Social Science Information, 13*, 2, 121-144.

Constructing a Life Course

Phyllis Moen

KEYWORDS. Autobiography, research, life course, gender, aging

INTRODUCTION

I consider myself a *life course* scholar, because I am interested in patterns and pathways at all ages and stages, as well as the strategies individuals, couples, and families adopt in the face of expected and unexpected change (Moen & Wethington, 1992). My research spans the adult life course–from the early parenting years through retirement and life after retirement (Moen & Yu, 1999; Moen, Dempster-McClain, & Williams, 1989, 1992; Moen, 1997). A central focus of my research and writing is *gender*: the ways that gender shapes the choices and life chances of men and women as they move through roles and relationships (Han & Moen, 1999a; Han & Moen, 1999b; Moen, 1995, 1996, 2000; Moen & Han, 1999; Quick & Moen, 1998). This points to the importance of a *role context* approach, placing lives in the context of gender, cohort, and other markers of location in the social structure (see a discussion of the role context approach in Moen, Dempster-McClain, & Williams, 1989).

In thinking about my own biography, I can see the value of taking a life course approach in the study of lives. Who I am today, and what I do, reflects the interaction of various life course processes: *context, linked lives, transitions, and trajectories.*

CONTEXT

Historical Location

I was born in 1942, the year after America entered World War II, which meant that I have moved through life just ahead of the large Baby Boom cohort born in the years following the war. I imagine my parents might not have even married had it not been for the war, but they did so hastily right before my father, an officer in the army, was shipped out to fight in Europe.

The war affected my life directly in two ways. First, my father, who I assume experienced stresses related to his combat experience, wrote my mother to ask for a divorce. (His father had always opposed the marriage.) Second, since my mother became a single parent and had to support us both, she worked full time as a hairdresser and put me into one of the excellent day care facilities created to encourage women to join the workforce during the war.

Historical circumstances have continued to shape my life course. As a teenager in the '50s, I was spared the drugs and disillusionments common to the Baby Boomers coming of age in the 1960s. I loved sports but wasn't given the opportunity to play, although I was permitted to be a cheerleader for the Little League. In high school we could play basketball but were restricted to half the court since the full court was "too strenuous" for girls. (Also we could only dribble three times before passing the ball so as not to tax our "female organs.") And even then, we could play only when the boys' teams weren't using the court. Upon graduating from high school, I began college but then married at the age of 18! Marriage was common to young women in Georgia in 1961, and 18 did not seem "early" to me.

I became a full-time housewife and soon the mother of two girls. I did not feel I could go back to school to continue college until my preschoolers were also in school. So I took correspondence courses and an occasional class at night. When I did return to school, graduating with undergraduate and graduate degrees in the 1970s, I benefited from the spirit of the women's movement as well as student loans that opened new opportunities for me. At the same time, I felt I was going against the grain of the times; most mothers of school-aged children that I knew (by then I was living in northern Minnesota) remained homemakers.

Other Contexts

I was born in the South (Hazelhurst, Georgia), which has shaped my identity, my food preferences, and my life-long love of iced tea. But much more consequential to me was the fact that I left Georgia at age six. My mother had remarried and, with my stepfather, a professional in the Army, we frequently moved and lived all over the world. This was key to my developing an understanding of the importance of *cultural context*. When I was six, we moved to Frankfurt, Germany, where I marveled that "their" Santa Claus and "their" Easter came on different days than ours. I then made what was one of my first independent decisions: I decided to celebrate "theirs" and "ours" to get more goodies!

Moving back to the United States (to the Presidio in San Francisco) at age 10 was a culture shock. There were things I hadn't experienced before: popsicles and paper dolls. There were people who ate differently than we did and talked differently (I still had my Southern drawl). I also learned even more about cultural relativity and the importance of *situational context*. In the fifth grade I was seen as nothing less than brilliant in that I already had learned fractions (as no one else in my class had). But then my status plummeted. I didn't know how to speak even as well as kindergartners in San Francisco: I pronounced "Yosemite" phonetically as Joesmight, "San Jose" as San Joe's. Unfortunately I did this in a presentation before the whole school. What I learned from this important incident is that identity doesn't simply lie within the individual, but changes as the context changes.

Notions of *cultural relativity* and the *flexible self* were reinforced when we moved to Japan, where I attended three different military high schools, as well as when we moved back to Georgia for my senior year. The topic in the public eye that year was *Brown v. the Board of Education* and whether our school was going to have to be integrated. I had attended "integrated" schools all my life and had had friends from all racial and ethnic backgrounds, so this was a difficult time for me. The South was in turmoil, with sit-ins, bus boycotts, and the thundering rhetoric of Martin Luther King. I remember taking the only seat left on a bus, in the back, and being berated by a young black woman for trying to "save" her people. Actually I wasn't reading a Bible (as she accused me), but another book and was too embarrassed to tell her. I had never before been on a bus that had a color line drawn in the middle. I could not believe there were "white" and "colored" drinking fountains. All in all, it was the United States, specifically "my" South, not Germany or Japan, that provided the most culture shock.

Linked Lives

Urie Bronfenbrenner (my colleague and dear friend at Cornell) always says, "You are the people in your life," and I believe this is true. Yet I also think that the people *not* in your life matter as well. My biological father (who never saw me when he returned from the war) was always in the recesses of my mind. I've always wondered why he divorced *me* as well as my mother.

But the ones who were in my life remain with me in who I am today. My grandfather's unstinting love, no matter what. My mother's style of helping out and caring for others. (Though her emphasis on personal looks and stylish clothes made me feel that I could never manage to meet her expectations [she was a strikingly beautiful woman].) My stepfather opened up a new world of books and learning. Before he came into my life, I had had only one book, an alphabet picture dictionary. He got me a library card! Read to me! Actually discussed things with me. Without a doubt, he raised my awareness of the intellectual dimension of the world around me. But he too was a product of his *historical location*, having come of age during the Great Depression and losing all his savings for college when the banks closed. He never did go to college, but instead instilled the desire and expectation for higher education in me.

My brother Dennis came along when I was almost ten. I had so wanted a baby brother and saw him as much "my" baby as my mother's. I babysat with him from the time he was born (even though I now realize I was far too young then to do so). Over the years, my sense of responsibility for Dennis has not faded, and events since (his leukemia, brain damage, loss of memory) mean that I continue to care for him.

My first husband, Arnie, and I both grew up together, since he was not yet 21 at the time of our marriage. The real reason we got married was that my mother felt it would be improper for a young girl and a boy to travel by bus from Georgia to Minnesota, where he wanted me to meet his family. Rather impetuously, we decided to marry so she would not object to our traveling together. We not only visited northern Minnesota, but eventually moved to a small farm there, raising Arabian horses while he supported us (barely) by working as a medical technologist at a local hospital. To me this was just another in a series of moves, since I had spent my life moving. But I found myself isolated on the farm with only my two girls for company, and started taking night classes and continuing with my correspondence courses. Soon after I had received my bachelor's and then master's degrees at the University of North Dakota, 20 miles distant from our farm, we learned that my husband had cancer.

A key person in this time of trial was the pathologist who was also our friend. Everyone said, "You can beat this thing," recalling all the people they knew who had been cured of cancer. But the doctors' sober expressions belied their words of encouragement. Our pathologist friend volunteered to examine the tissue slides and give a second opinion. After doing so, he bluntly told me, "You are married to a dead man. He will be dead in three months. What are you going to do after he is dead?" This brusque way of talking took my breath away, but it also made me angry. I glared at him and said, "I am going back to school to get my PhD." He quickly said, "Then show me your application next week." My anger with him encouraged me to do it, and I soon sent the application in. Had that not been the case, I doubt that I ever would have had the strength to apply then or even consider it three months later when, in fact, Arnie was dead.

Arnie taught me much about love and life. But his greatest legacy was seeing how thoughtfully he handled dying. We talked about everything, and he underscored his confidence in me to "carry on," raise our children, and build a life without him. His confidence gave me the strength I needed to get through the grief and depression that made me want to end my own life as well. In April I received a letter from the University of Minnesota, saying that not only had I been accepted but that I would receive a trainee scholarship, working with a professor I had never heard of, Reuben Hill.

The notion of *linked lives* underscores not only the ways individuals influence one another but the ways that lives are lived in tandem. My two girls, Deborah and Melanie, experienced all these changes with me, but from a different vantage point. Only 12 and 10 when their father died, they lost not only Arnie but also the social network and lifestyle they had known, as we moved from the farm to student housing in Saint Paul. They blamed this wrenching change on me, not on the death of their father. And then, in another three years I uprooted them once again, this time to move to Ithaca, New York, where I had accepted an offer from Cornell. My two daughters provided me with a sense of purpose in life when I thought all was lost. I had to be cheerful for their benefit, taking them to the zoo instead of crying in my bed. And I had to get a job and support us all so they too could go to college.

My ongoing source of emotional support during graduate school was Carla Howery, my office mate at the University of Minnesota, and Janet Kelly (now Janet Kelly Moen after she married my former brother-in-law), who helped me go on when I thought it was impossible to do so. The first day I met Carla, I placed a heavy burden on her. I told her that my husband had just died, that I had two kids who were unhappy that we had moved to the Twin Cities, and that I knew no one there. I needed a friend and asked her to be my friend. Even though she was in her early 20s (I was only 32 but felt *much* older), she rose to the challenge and has been my close friend ever since. Jan also has always been there for me, from our first days in the master's program at the University of North Dakota. She was like a sister to me and an aunt to my girls long before she married my brother-in-law. She received a PhD from Cornell and now teaches sociology at the University of North Dakota.

Another aspect of *linked lives* is, as Robert Merton reminds us, the fact that our intellectual development occurs because we stand on the shoulders of giants. The "giants" in my life have been Reuben Hill, Jeylan Mortimer, Glen H. Elder, Jr., Robin M. Williams, Jr., and Urie Bronfenbrenner. Reuben Hill challenged all of his students to be all they could be. His emphasis on the *life cycle* sparked my life-long interest in locating people and families by where they are as well as where they have been in their life course. I found his (then) recent book on three generations fascinating. Jeylan Mortimer, who was a junior faculty member at Minnesota while I was there, became something of a role model. She impressed upon me the importance of persistence. She also taught one of the first courses, I am sure, on women's labor force participation, sparking my interest in gender, work, and family. Glen Elder came to the University of Minnesota to give a talk. When I picked him up at the airport, I was surprised that someone so young could have written such an important book (*Children of the Great Depression* had just been published in 1974). He has been a mentor and a model of the way one engages in life course research. When I came to Cornell, Urie Bronfenbrenner offered what Vgotsky said was the key to optimal development: maximum demand and maximum support. And Robin Williams became a mentor, a collaborator, and a good friend.

Others have offered encouragement and assistance along the way. At Minnesota, Robert Leik served as my dissertation advisor while Reuben Hill was on sabbatical. Joe Galaskiewicz raised my sights from seeking jobs at only junior colleges in Minnesota and marked up the employment bulletin to indicate the schools to which I should apply. When I accepted the Cornell job, my department chair, Phil Schoggen, helped me to locate a house, let me put his name down on school records ("in case of an emergency . . ."), and encouraged me to follow my own interests in research. Phil and his wife Dikkie, along with Urie and Liese Bronfenbrenner and Robin and Marguerite Williams, became close friends as well as colleagues. In fact, my second marriage took place at Phil and Dikkie's house.

Graduate students, faculty, and staff over the years have made work fun, taught me much, and have become lasting friends. I've been blessed with a wonderful network in Ithaca: Donna Dempster-McClain and John McClain, Joan Jacobs Brumberg and David Brumberg, Mon and Eva Cochran, John and Cathy Eckenrode, Jenny Gerner, Steve and Mary Agnes Hamilton, Ritch Savin-Williams, Joyce and Henry Walker, Jerry and Pat Ziegler, Ron Breiger, Xueguang Zhou, Irene Pitcher, Kim Rosenstein, and Sarah Jaenike Demo.

I have had the pleasure of co-authoring articles, books, and chapters with many scholars, including Penny Becker, Urie Bronfenbrenner, Marin Clarkberg, Glen H. Elder, Jr., Vivian Fields, Francille Firebaugh, Leonard Goodwin, Shin-Kap Han, Carla B. Howery, Jungmeen Kim, John Krout, Kurt Lüscher, Karl Pillemer, Pat Roehling, Alvin L. Schorr, Steve Sweet, Pamela Tolbert, Nancy Tuma, Henry Walker, Elaine Wethington, Robin M. Williams, Jr., and Yan Yu.

I have also had the pleasure of writing and publishing with former students Ellen Bradburn, Donna Dempster-McClain, Mary Ann Erickson, Kay B. Forest, Heather Hofmeister, Stacey Merola, Melody L. Miller, Heather E. Quick, Julie Robison, Deborah B. Smith, Ken Smith, and Loreen Wolfer.

The last chapter in the *linked lives* process brings me to meeting (through Donna Dempster-McClain) and marrying my husband, Dick Shore. Even though we had a commuting marriage for years (he was at the Department of Labor in Washington, DC), we have been together in Ithaca since 1990. Dick is my confidant, critic, companion, colleague, and closest friend. Both the professional and personal aspects of my life have benefited from his wise counsel, common sense, and wry sense of humor.

TRANSITIONS AND TRAJECTORIES

Transitions

The key transitions that have shaped my life course thus far include my two marriages, becoming a mother, becoming a stepmother (of Linda Shore and Roberta Maguire), becoming a grandmother (of James, Kiri, Tara, and Matthew), going back to school, getting a PhD, securing a job at Cornell, becoming a program director at the National Science Foundation (while on leave from Cornell), and institution-building at Cornell (the *Bronfenbrenner Life Course Center*, the *Cornell Gerontology Research Institute* [with Karl Pillemer], and the *Cornell Employment and Families Career Institute*). I focus here on the academic transitions, but want to stress how even academic transitions are embedded in relational contexts.

I took the job at Cornell because Ithaca seemed like a good community in which to raise children, and, of all my three offers, it was the closest to Georgia, the home of my mother and brother. I didn't realize at the time that I had unwittingly made another choice: to go into a department of Human Development rather than Sociology. Though I became a member of the Sociology Department at Cornell as well, my Human Development colleagues have really impressed upon me the importance of cross-disciplinary research.

I went to work as Assistant Director and then Director of the Sociology Program at the National Science Foundation in 1987, frankly to be able to live with my husband Dick in Washington, DC. It turned out to be a transformative experience. Robin M. Williams, Jr., gave me this advice about going to work for a federal agency: "Keep your back to the wall and keep looking in both directions." He was right! The mostly male, mostly natural science environment at the Foundation challenged me in ways I can't begin to describe here. The result was that I became an advocate for the social sciences and for women scientists. Working with various "bosses" as well as collegial program directors in sociology, law, psychology, political science, and economics–Stanley Presser, Murray Webster, Bob Althauser, Felice Levine, Roberta Miller, Dan Newlan, and Mary Clutter–broadened my understanding not only of sociology but also of social research more generally and of science policy "writ large." It became clear to me that if sociology is to make a contribution, it must be seen (and see itself) as a legitimate science, one that may use a range of methods (from qualitative to quantitative to simulation), but that is as rigorous and as cumulative as the natural sciences. I also was reassured as to the importance of fundamental (basic) science in addressing issues of societal concern.

I returned to Cornell from NSF in 1990 and experienced a bit of culture shock. While I had been dealing with the "big picture" at NSF, I was suddenly focusing only on my own research. Donna Dempster-McClain, Robin M. Williams, Jr., and I continued our work on the *Women's Roles and Well-Being Project*, funded by the National Institute on Aging. Following up women that Robin had interviewed in Elmira, New York, in the 1950s, we reinterviewed them 30 years later in 1986, as well as their (by then adult) daughters. The analysis of this exciting panel data produced fascinating findings regarding women's lives: the importance of multiple role occupancy for longevity, health, and well-being; the complex links between caregiving, employment, and psychological well-being; the ways that daughters and mothers changed and influenced one another along with the concomitant changes in women's roles in the larger society.

I believe, because of my experience at NSF, that I followed up on Dean Francille Firebaugh's interest in establishing a center on aging. After a series of breakfast meetings with faculty from a variety of disciplines (food always helps to bring people together!) and a stimulating visit by Vern Bengtson, it became clear to me that we lacked the numbers to establish a center on aging, and so I convinced Dean Firebaugh that what we *could* do was create a center on the life course. Thus, the Bronfenbrenner Life Course Center came into being, a university-wide center named in honor of a psychologist who has always emphasized the importance of person, process, context, and time. Its mission is to engage in fundamental life course research addressing issues of national concern.

When Karl Pillemer came to Cornell, he and I became codirectors of CGRI (*Cornell Gerontology Research Institute*), an institute under the umbrella of the Bronfenbrenner Center supporting applied research on social integration and aging. From the funds provided by the National Institute on Aging in support of this institute came the *Cornell Retirement and Well-Being Study*, a three-wave, six-year study of older workers and retirees from six employers in upstate New York. Findings from this study of a pre-baby boomer cohort include: (1) a mapping of their various pathways to retirement (and how women traverse many paths, while men are located in two), (2) how caregiving affects the timing of retirement (encouraging women to retire, delaying men's retirement), (3) the correlates of retirement satisfaction, (4) how community participation promotes well-being among retirees but not among the not yet retired still in their career jobs, (5) how marital quality changes with the retirement transition (the transition itself produces more conflicts and less marital satisfaction), (6) the ways couples perceive each spouse's influence regarding the other's retirement transition (he sees her as having more influence than she felt she had), and (7) the way life after retirement affects psychological well-being. We found that men in post-retirement jobs married to women who are not employed report the lowest depressive symptoms (Moen, 1998; Moen, Fields, Meador, & Rosenblatt, 2000; Moen, Fields, Quick, & Hofmeister, 2000; Quick & Moen, 1998; Smith & Moen, 1998).

I am now engaged in a study, also funded by NIA, of the Baby Boom Cohort and their plans and expectations regarding retirement (the *Midcareer Paths and Passages Study).* The retirement transition of this group will be a unique experience for the large Baby Boomer Cohort; we are interested in comparing them with the pre-Baby Boomers in the *Cornell Retirement and Well Being Study.* (Other research by Karl Pillemer, Elaine Wethington, and Nina Glasgow has also been conducted for this Institute, but I am reporting here on *my* life course!)

The most recent "transition" for me was the establishment in 1997 of another institute under the umbrella of the Bronfenbrenner Center, the Cornell Employment and Family Careers Institute, a center for the study of working families funded by the Alfred P. Sloan Foundation. The Cornell Careers Institute has solidified my interest in the intersection of work and family roles at all stages of the life course. It has supported work with Shin-Kap Han to chart men's and women's career pathways, and with Penny Becker to show how working couples with children scale back their obligations. Other foci are defined by Marin Clarkberg on variations in work time and work-time preferences among couples as well as by Yan Yu on who feels successful at work *and* at home. Finally, a related area is specified by Jungmeen Kim and Heather Hofmeister on changes in marital quality in late midlife (Becker & Moen, 1999; Clarkberg & Moen, 1999; Han & Moen, 2000; Moen, Kim, & Hofmeister, 1999; Moen & Yu, 1998). A signal contribution of the Cornell Careers Institute has been its focus not only on work/family issues over the life course, but also on how *couples* strategize about their three jobs–his, hers, and their families.

Trajectories

Becoming a professor at Cornell was my first full-time job, though the nature of it has evolved as my experiences and research/teaching interests have developed over the past 21 years. But I can see threads of continuity in my intellectual agenda. First, I have had an ongoing interest in policy, writing two chapters on family policy in the editions of *Handbook of Marriage and the Family* (Moen & Schorr, 1987; Moen & Forest, 1999. See also Moen & Firebaugh, 1994; Moen & Jull, 1995). I want to do work that addresses contemporary concerns, and that helps to define and frame key issues. One of my favorite courses has been *Families and Social Policy,* in which we look at the deliberate and unintended impacts of social policies on families, couples, and children. A second thread throughout my intellectual biography is a focus on continuity and change, the *transitions* and *trajectories* so fundamental to life course research (Robison & Moen, 2000; Erickson et al., 2000; Krout et al., 1998).

These threads became clear to me in my first study on women and work. Using data from the 1977 *Quality of Employment Survey,* I looked at women who worked part time versus full time, noting all the significant differences between them. Then I turned to the *Panel Study of Income Dynamics,* finding that women who worked part time one year were often either working full time or else had moved out of the labor force the next year, and that women who worked full time one year typically moved to part-time work or full-time homemaking the next year. This impressed upon me the need to get data both on where people are now and where they have been. Data of this kind could be acquired either through prospective studies following people over time or by collecting life history data in cross-sectional studies. This research made me question cross-sectional research on the impacts of mothers' paid work on their children–they may be working or not working at the time of the interview, but in the previous year they could well have been in the opposite circumstance. Capturing past trajectories of roles and relationships has characterized all my own data collection: the *Women's Roles and Well-Being Study,* the *Cornell Retirement and Well-Being Study,* the *Cornell Couples and Careers Study,* and now the *Cornell Midcareer Paths and Passages Study.* In 1992, in recognition of my life course scholarship, I was awarded an endowed chair; I am now "The Ferris Family Professor of Life Course Studies."

A third thread of continuity concerns what Reuben Hill emphasized as the importance of *comparative analysis*. He said we should always think as comparativists. True to his training, I always look for differences, primarily by gender, but also by class and race. I wrote a book on working parents in Sweden (see Moen, 1989; Moen & Forest, 1990) comparing and contrasting, where possible, the Swedish cultural and policy climate with that in the U.S. And my work with Nancy Tuma and Xueguang Zhou has examined the labor force experiences of men and women in China (Zhou, Moen, & Tuma, 1998; Zhou, Tuma, & Moen, 1995, 1997).

Reflections

This life-course approach to my own biography illustrates the ways choice and chance–along with constraining and changing opportunity structures–have opened some doors and closed others. I am a product of my times (the pre-baby boomers), my childhood experiences, and the people in my life and my work as a sociologist. I look forward to the next life course stage!

AUTHOR NOTE

Phyllis Moen is affiliated with Cornell University.

Address correspondence to: Phyllis Moen, Ferris Family Professor of Life Course Studies, Department of Human Development, G58 MVR Hall, Cornell University, Ithaca, NY 14853.

REFERENCES

Becker, P. E. & Moen, P. (1999). Scaling back: Dual-career couples' work-family strategies. *Journal of Marriage and the Family, 61*, 4, 995-1007.

Clarkberg, M., & Moen, P. (1999). The time squeeze: Married couples' work-hour patterns and preferences. In P. Voos (Ed.), *Proceedings of the 51st annual meeting, Vol. 1* (pp. 15-23). Madison, WI: Industrial Relations Research Association Series.

Erickson, M. A., Dempster-McClain, D., Whitlow, C., & Moen, P. (in press). Social integration across the transition to a continuing care retirement community. In K. Pillemer, P. Moen, E. Wethington, & N. Glasgow (Eds.), *Social integration in the second half of life*, Baltimore: The Johns Hopkins Press.

Han, S. K., & Moen, P. (1999a). Work and family over time: A life course approach. *The Annals of the American Academy of Political and Social Sciences, 56*, 2, 98-110.

Han, S. K., & Moen, P. (1999b). Clocking out: Temporal patterning of retirement. *American Journal of Sociology, 105*, 1, 191-236.

Han, S. K., & Moen, P. (2001). Coupled careers: Men's and women's pathways through work and marriage in the United States. In H. P. Blossfeld & S. Drobnic (Eds.), *Couples' careers in a dynamic perspective.*

Krout, J. A., Moen, P., Oggins, J., & Bowen, N. (1998). Reasons for relocation to a continuing care retirement community. Pathways Working Paper #2. Ithaca, NY: Bronfenbrenner Life Course Center.

Moen, P. (1989). *Working parents: Transformations in gender roles and public policies in Sweden.* Madison: University of Wisconsin Press.

Moen, P. (1995). Gender, age and the life course. In R. H. Binstock & L. George (Eds.), *Handbook of aging and the social sciences*, 4th Edition (pp. 171-187). San Diego, CA: Academic Press, Inc.

Moen, P. (1996). A life course perspective on retirement, gender, and well-being. *Journal of Occupational Health Psychology, 1*, 2, 131-144.

Moen, P. (1997). Women's roles and resilience: Trajectories of advantage or turning points? In I. H. Gotlib & B. Wheaton (Eds.), *Stress and adversity over the life course: Trajectories and turning points* (pp. 133-156). New York: Cambridge University Press.

Moen, P. (1998). Recasting careers: Changing reference groups, risks, and realities. *Generations, 22*, 1, 40-45.

Moen, P. (2001). Gender, age and the life course. Forthcoming in R. H. Binstock & L. George (Eds.), *Handbook of aging and the social sciences*, 5th Edition. San Diego: Academic Press, Inc.

Moen, P., Dempster-McClain, D., & Williams, R., Jr. (1989). Social integration and longevity: An event history analysis of women's roles and resilience. *American Sociological Review, 54*, 4, 635-47.

Moen, P., Dempster-McClain, D., & Williams, R., Jr. (1992). Successful aging: A life course perspective on women's roles and health. *American Journal of Sociology, 97*, 6, 1612-1638.

Moen, P., Fields, V., Meador, R., & Rosenblatt, H. (in press). Fostering Integration: A Case Study of the Cornell Retirees Volunteering In Service (CRVIS). In K. Pillemer, P. Moen, E. Wethington, & N. Glasgow (Eds.), *Social integration in the second half of life*. Baltimore: The Johns Hopkins Press.

Moen, P., Fields, V., Quick, H., & Hofmeister, H. (in press). A life course approach to retirement and social integration. In K. Pillemer, P. Moen, E. Wethington, & N. Glasgow (Eds.), *Social integration in the second half of life*. Baltimore: The Johns Hopkins Press.

Moen, P., & Firebaugh, F. (1994). Family policies and effective families: A life course perspective. *International Journal of Sociology and Social Policy*, (Special Issue), *14*, 1-2, 30-53.

Moen, P., & Forest, K. B. (1990). Working parents, workplace supports, and well-being: The Swedish experience. *Social Psychology Quarterly, 53*, 2, 117-131.

Moen, P., & Forest, K. B. (1999). Strengthening families: Policy issues for the twenty-first century. In M. B. Sussman, S. K. Steinmetz, & G. W. Peterson (Eds.), *Handbook of marriage and the family* (pp. 633-663). New York: Plenum Press.

Moen, P., & Han, S. K. (2000). Gendered careers: A life course perspective. In R. Hertz (Ed.), *Work and family: Today's realities and tomorrow's possibilities*. Berkeley: University of California Press.

Moen, P., & Jull, P. M. (1995). Informing family policy: The uses of social research. *Journal of Family and Economic Issues, 16*, 1, 79-107.

Moen, P., Kim, J., & Hofmeister, H. (1999). Couples' work status transitions and marriage quality in late midlife. (Unpublished manuscript).

Moen, P., & Schorr, A. L. (1987). Families and social policy. In M. B. Sussman & S. K. Steinmetz (Eds.), *Handbook of Marriage and the Family* (pp. 795-813). New York: Plenum Press.

Moen, P., & Wethington, E. (1992). The concept of family adaptive strategies. *Annual Review of Sociology, 18*, 233-51.

Moen, P., & Yu, Y. (1998). Does success at work compete with success at home? In *Conference proceedings, women's progress: Perspectives on the past, blueprint for the future* (pp. 171-174). Washington, DC: Institute for Women's Policy Research.

Moen, P., & Yu, Y. (1999). Having it all: Overall work/life success in two-earner families. In T. Parcel (Ed.), *Research in the sociology of work, Volume 7* (pp. 107-137). Greenwich, CT: JAI Press.

Quick, H., & Moen, P. (1998). Gender, employment, and retirement quality: A life-course approach to the differential experiences of men and women. *Journal of Occupational Health Psychology, 3*, 1, 44-64.

Robison, J., & Moen, P. (in press). Future housing expectations in late midlife: The role of retirement, gender, and social integration. Forthcoming in K. Pillemer, P. Moen, E. Wethington, & N. Glasgow (Eds.), *Social integration in the second half of life*. Baltimore: The Johns Hopkins Press.

Smith, D. B., & Moen, P. (1998). Spouse's influence on the retirement decision: His, her, and their perceptions. *Journal of Marriage and the Family, 60*, 3, 734-744.

Zhou, X., Moen, P., & Tuma, N. (1998). Educational Stratification in Urban China: 1949-1994. *Sociology of Education, 71*, 3, 199-222.
Zhou, X., Tuma, N., & Moen, P. (1995). Social stratification dynamics under state socialism: The case of urban China, 1949-1993. *Social Forces, 74*, 3, 759-796.
Zhou, X., Tuma, N., & Moen, P. (1997). Institutional change and job-shift patterns in urban China, 1949 to 1994. *American Sociological Review, 62*, 3, 339-365.

Following a Non-Linear Career Path: Dietetics + Child Development + Special Education = Family Studies

Marilyn Coleman

KEYWORDS. Autobiography, researcher, child development, professor

INTRODUCTION

Two years ago a former college roommate and sorority sister of mine sent letters to me and several others asking us to tell her what we had been doing the last 30+ years. She would compile the results and share them with us. As an example, she summarized her life with a sort of listing: taught school, married and became a stepmother, gained a lot of weight, and retired. I was appalled by some of her life markers (why do women define their lives by pounds gained and lost?), but I also was so intimidated by the task that I managed to "lose" the letter before I got around to responding. If I could not cough up a reasonably short response about my life to an old college friend, how on earth could I respond with an essay for this project? I was even more intimidated when I read the two remarkable essays that were provided by Gary Peterson and Sue Steinmetz as examples. Unlike the careers of many in our field, my early career was primarily based on avoidance rather than a drive to achieve. I spent far more effort eluding things (e.g., boredom, learning to sew) than I did pursuing lofty goals, or goals of any kind.

WHY I AM NOT YVES ST. LAURENT

I grew up in a small town (less than 2,000 population) in northeast Kansas. It was the kind of place where your classmates had nicknames like Shorty, Bucky, and Goose, and where your every move was closely watched and duly reported. If you ever got in trouble, your parents would have been informed by the time you got home. Intellectual stimulation was not a community goal, and, as I recall, the only community-wide entertainment, other than summer band concerts and the county fair, was an annual minstrel show that was incredibly racist. I was pretty oblivious to the racist jokes that our blackened-faced, white-gloved town leaders conveyed to an appreciative audience, and I am sure that sexist jokes abounded as well. I was even less aware of sexism than racism. I was at least conscious that, except after sporting events, the three or four African American students in my high school were not allowed to eat at Jim's Waffle Shop where the rest of us hung out. Those who suffered the most from discrimination, however, were the Native Americans. My hometown bordered the Sac and Fox/Kickapoo reservation, now the location of a very lucrative casino. I can barely imagine how the casino might be changing the community dynamics–and I haven't been back to see. It was not until I got to college, however, that I really gave thought to the destructiveness of discrimination and stigma, and I have worked hard to alleviate it my entire career. One major theme running through my record of publication is related to this topic. Since 1983, I have published two dozen articles dealing with stereotyping and stigma. The bulk of the research has been in relationship to family structure stereotyping (Bryan, Coleman, Ganong, & Bryan, 1986; Bryan, Ganong, Coleman, & Bryan, 1985; Coleman & Ganong, 1984; Coleman & Ganong, 1987a; Coleman & Ganong, 1995; Ganong, Coleman, & Mapes, 1990), but I have also looked at racial stereotypes (Bryant, Coleman, & Ganong, 1988b). For example, my late colleague and friend, Lois Bryant, and I investigated race and family structure stereotyping in introductory family textbooks (Bryant & Coleman, 1988a), a study that caught the eye of publishers and resulted in changes in the way that nonnuclear and nonwhite families are now presented in family textbooks.

My favorite location in my town when I was growing up was the public library, and my favorite activity was reading. It still is. In retrospect it was a very small library, but it seemed adequate at the time. If you wanted to read something "racy" (any book that mentioned sex, and I am not talking about pornography), you had to ask the librarian, who would then retrieve the book from under the counter if she thought you were old enough to read it. I was too embarrassed to ask, but my mother was a part-time assistant librarian, and I would sometimes sneak the books when she wasn't looking. I would read them while waiting for her to get off work and shelve them in a place where only I could find them. I could then continue my reading the next time I was in the library. The remainder of my sex education came from a column in the *Ladies Home Journal* called, "Can this marriage be saved?" The case study presented each month always fascinated me, and perhaps that was the beginning of my interest in family studies. But I doubt it.

My father was a highway patrolman, and there was always the possibility of transfers, so we always lived in rented houses. Evidently our leases ran out rather quickly, because I had lived in 14 different houses by the time I finished junior high. Part of the reason for leasing rather than buying was the strong "depression mentality" my parents shared. They never bought anything unless they could pay cash for it–including houses. My father did get transferred to different communities a couple of times, so I spent 4th and 6th grade in other school systems, but the remaining years of school were all spent in the same building. We didn't have kindergarten, but all the rest of the grades (1-12) were under one roof. We also didn't have school lunches, Latin, foreign language, art, or much other variety in the curriculum. I think this was due to a limited budget rather than conservatism, but I'm not sure. We did have some excellent teachers, however, and those of us who went on to college did well.

On to College

In spite of always knowing that I would go to college, my only goal was to marry and have children. That is what successful women did in the late '50s. My parents had no particular ambition for me either, and I was never pressured by them to succeed at anything. I had a fairly contentious relationship with my mother, and it always seemed to me that her major concern was that I not embarrass her in any way. She was extremely judgmental and controlling and provided little positive feedback. On the other hand, my father seemed pretty happy with anything that I did or didn't do, and it is to him that I am indebted for escaping childhood with a reasonably intact sense of self. It was my Dad who read and praised the truly terrible short stories that I wrote throughout my childhood and even into high school.

English was always my favorite subject, and writing themes was my favorite part of English class. I had some vague notion of becoming a writer, but I had no clue how to do that, so I began college at Kansas State University as a Home Economics Journalism major. Why home economics? I have no idea. Home economics was a required subject for girls at my high school, and I blundered through project after project, showing a fair amount of ineptitude in the subject, especially anything to do with sewing. My sophomore year in high school, I rebelled and refused to take any more home economics classes, a decision which infuriated the school superintendent. Why he cared, I don't know, but I remember his apoplexy as he threatened me with NEVER being able to take a home economics course again. Of course, that was my goal–to never take a home economics course again. The only course I was allowed to substitute was world history; a subject that triggered an interest in art and travel that has heightened through the years.

Refusing to continue taking home economics classes was my first memory of "kicking against the traces" and feeling personally rewarded for having taken the risk. It is a pattern that has served me well throughout my career.

Unlike high school, my college English classes were both disappointing and frustrating. The disappointment stemmed from their focus on literary criticism rather than writing. The frustration was due to my lack of success. I had trouble adjusting to the fact that I would have to spend time studying for my classes if I were going to do well. Although I assumed that college would be more difficult than high school had been, I did little to rise to the challenge my freshman year. I was also naïve about my strengths and weaknesses and made some incredibly stupid decisions in choosing a major. After the shock of getting a B in English, I decided that journalism was probably not for me, and I changed majors before even taking a journalism class.

I switched to Dietetics and Institutional Management for three reasons, none of which was good. First of all, I had enjoyed a first-semester foods laboratory class that was required of Home Economics Journalism majors. I think much of the appeal was that you could get up and move around during class. Secondly, when I was in college, graduating in 4 years was the norm. I could not afford an additional semester or year of school, so I needed to switch to a major that would still allow me to graduate within 4 years. This meant finding a major that could incorporate the previously mentioned 5-credit foods laboratory. Finally, I needed a major within Home Economics that did not require any aspect of clothing construction. From my high school experiences I knew that sewing was my nemesis, so majors that required it were out. That left few choices. I was only vaguely aware when I chose it that the dual major of Dietetics and Institutional Management basically combined a science major with the skills needed to run a large food service business. Science is not my forte, especially chemistry, yet I ended up with 21 hours of it and even incompetently taught it one year at the high school level.

My memorable chemistry class experiences included burning a hole through my shoe and part of my foot via carelessness with a pipette full of sulfuric acid. Another memory is ruining a lab partner's blouse by my inattention to sodium that I was heating over a flame–it shot out of the test tube and ate holes in her blouse and possibly her back. Prominent among my memories was when my non-English speaking biochemistry lab partner accidentally set himself on fire (this one was *not* my fault)–so I learned very little.

My other science classes were more interesting and less catastrophic, but disaster followed me into the dietetics lab. My ignorance of gas ovens (I didn't realize they had to be lit, and thought you just turned them on like electric ovens) caused an explosion in the kitchen where I was conducting a time-management experiment. The blast blew a cook across the room, burned off her eyebrows, and sent her to the emergency room. Fortunately, she wasn't seriously hurt. I never admitted to being the culprit because I was afraid I would be kicked out of the program. That event was only slightly more memorable than being chased around this same kitchen by various football players, the sole occupants of the dorm serviced by the kitchen. The level of testosterone coursing through these guys must have been monumental if they were attracted to young women wearing hairnets, baggy white uniforms, and "sensible" shoes. These players were much more aggressive and effective at hassling dietetics majors than they were opposing team members. I don't think they won a single game when I was in school, but they ate well.

Even though I never worked in the field of dietetics, I appreciate the scientific rigor of my undergraduate coursework. I think the training I received provided excellent research preparation. I still feel badly, however, at my ecstasy when my rat died early in my vitamin deprivation study in experimental dietetics. Its early demise greatly shortened the number of twice-daily trips I had to make to the dark, spooky attic of the home economics building to feed and weigh it. I have yet to wish the early demise of anyone in my studies of humans, but some have pushed it a bit.

When I originally decided to go to college, there were only two things that I wanted to avoid–teaching (my mother had strongly promoted this because you could always "fall back" on teaching if something happened to your husband) and sewing. Although I managed to evade anything related to those two topics in college, I couldn't sidestep them forever. I married during spring break my senior year of college, and, after graduation, I followed my husband to his job in a community that had no positions for dietitians. Before giving up on dietetics or a career in food service, I even faced the humiliation of being turned down as the lunch counter manager at the local Woolworth's because I was overeducated. Out of desperation I took a post-graduate year of classes in education and began a career in teaching that has spanned most of my life.

Teaching High School

My first two years of teaching were at a small rural high school in a poverty-stricken town in western Kansas. This was a foreign culture to me. My students' sports heroes were rodeo stars, and one's father was arrested for cattle rustling while I was there. The school was so small that basketball was the only competitive sport offered until 6-man football was added my first year of teaching. I taught all of the science courses, all of the home economics courses, and directed the junior play. I was also sponsor for the pep club, in charge of the junior/senior prom, and sponsored the yearbook as well as the senior class. The average university teaching load has seemed like a breeze in comparison.

The school board made it clear that I would have to offer sewing classes my third year. So I reluctantly prepared by taking a clothing construction class at the same small Catholic college where I had previously taken education courses. When a nun cried in frustration after I ruined some expensive material by ineptly following her quite detailed instructions, I decided to give up sewing forever. I not only hated it and was bad at it, but I was endangering the mental health of others with my incompetence! So, my third year of teaching was at a junior high school in Salina, Kansas, where I had completed my student teaching.

My teaching career was soon to be ended, however, because I was pregnant, and schools had rules against letting pregnant women teach. The purpose of this rule was to protect impressionable young children from being exposed to the end result of SEX. I was not pleased with the rule, but I didn't consider challenging it any more than I considered challenging the fact that male faculty were paid more than the women, theoretically because men had families to support. Not surprisingly, women who were heads of households did not receive the extra compensation. Although the principal waived the pregnancy rule (because he couldn't find a suitable replacement for me), I moved to Columbia, Missouri, that summer, and my opportunity to warp the students by flaunting my pregnant body became a moot point.

SEW-ON TO GRADUATE SCHOOL

When my oldest son was 18 months old, I decided to return to school. I was very nervous about this decision and unsure about whether or not I had the ability to succeed. I didn't know anyone who was going to graduate school, especially anyone who was married and had a child. Although I was now interested in teaching, my sewing phobia remained, which meant that my career as a home economics teacher was over. I had to choose another field, a task that was not easy.

I had hated my child development class as an undergraduate. We were required to sit in the child development lab and observe the children, but we could not talk to the children or interact with them in any way. As a result, the children treated us as if we were inanimate objects, a situation that gave me the creeps. I also found my family living classes extremely boring, and if the elderly, unmarried family health instructor who taught me that the pain of childbirth is all psychological had been in the delivery room when I was having my first child, I would have strangled her.

Even more boring were classes in interior design and clothing selection. I didn't have to sew, but I was required to have a frightening nude silhouette taken and to design clothes to fit my lumpy silhouetted "body type." Most of us worked on our projects surreptitiously, praying that no one would look over our shoulders and ask us to identify that black, oddly shaped thing (the silhouette).

The interior design class had different sorts of challenges. I spent the first 6 weeks of the class completing a color wheel. That may sound like a simple task, but I met my Waterloo trying to make neutral gray by mixing red, yellow, and blue. At least I think those were the colors. God knows I should remember after spending at least 2 hours/week for 6 weeks trying to mix them. I tried to cheat by mixing black and white, but the teacher always caught me. I assume there was a point to this exercise, but it was not clear to me then, and it continues to escape me. I wasn't interested in pursuing graduate studies in dietetics or nutrition because it would require more chemistry, and I had clearly risen to my level of incompetence in that area long ago. By the process of elimination, I decided that, because I was now a mother, maybe child development was worth revisiting.

The graduate program in child and family development at the University of Missouri was very small, and I got to work with two phenomenal women. Dr. Ruth Cook, a University of Chicago graduate in Human Development, was the department chair, and Dr. Virginia Fisher was the Director of the Child Development Laboratory. Ruth had a very dry and somewhat wacky wit that was lost on most of the students. She was diagnosed with multiple sclerosis after I started my master's degree, and she coped with this horrible disease in amazing and courageous ways. She was a rather shy and very proud woman who was afraid that students who saw her staggering gait brought on by the disease would think that she was an alcoholic. Her mind remained active even as her body totally betrayed her, and she continued to keep up with the field and the department until her death.

Ginny Fisher had a very different personality from Ruth Cook's. She had flown planes during World War II (delivered them from the U.S. to England) and was pretty nonconformist in most of what she did. She was working full-time and completing her PhD in social psychology at Mizzou when I was working on my master's degree. Because she had so many irons in the fire, she assigned tasks to me that were probably inappropriate to delegate to a master's student. However, she provided me with incredible opportunities to do things like develop upper-level classes and even graduate courses. When Ruth Cook was forced to resign because of her illness, Ginny took over as department chair. She established an air of openness to people of all races, colors, and creeds that pervades our department to this day.

When I began my graduate work, and for many years afterwards, the department budget was minuscule. Ginny basically held the department together with purchases from Army surplus and hard work. At one point the children in the child development lab were using old Army ammunition canisters as soup bowls! Eating hot soup out of a metal bowl is not for the fainthearted! Ginny never threw anything away because even the worst junk had potential for children's art projects. An advocate of the A.S. Neill school of childrearing, she believed that warm loving behavior (plus singing) could turn the most recalcitrant child around. This technique worked well until the late '60s when Ginny decided to incorporate Head Start training into the department offerings. The switch from predominantly children of faculty members to children from the broad spectrum of the community required a much more structured approach to teaching, although I think at heart, Ginny never gave up on warmth and singing.

I loved graduate school and found working with the children much more interesting than merely observing them as I had as an undergraduate. In fact, my biggest obstacle in graduate school had nothing to do with motivation or academics; it was finding adequate childcare. I probably spent as much time lining up childcare as I did studying. Making 15 phone calls to find childcare for each class period I attended was not unusual. Because of my frustrating experiences, I was later active in developing the Student Parent Center on our campus, although it opened much too late for my use. The overt philosophy of the central campus administration at the time, all males, of course, was that the University would be encouraging women to shirk their duties as mothers if childcare were provided for students. Overcoming that philosophy was neither easy nor rapid.

I finished my master's degree a few weeks before I gave birth to my second child. I had intended to take some time off but an opportunity to write television scripts for a University Extension project occurred, and I was soon involved in half-time work. Within a few months, I added off-campus instruction of Head Start teachers to my agenda. I flew to two locations in Missouri each week to teach these incredibly motivated women. These teaching experiences were surreal. The first class period I discovered that *all* of the students had already read *all* of the books. I am pretty satisfied if traditional campus students have *bought* the book by the first class period. The small single engine plane that delivered me to the class locations also provided some unique experiences. Particularly memorable was a day that we flew low enough that I could read the names on tombstones in the cemetery we were circling waiting for cows to move off the small rural landing field.

Child Development Specialist

As my flying/teaching opportunities wound down, I began job-sharing an Extension Child Development Specialist position with another woman. We worked closely with the state day care licensing staff, prepared training materials, and provided quite a bit of day care training throughout the state. When the "other half of the job" left the community, I heard that the full-time Extension Child Development Specialist job was going to be offered to someone who was already working full-time with Extension. I was upset about not being considered for the job, and I finally mustered enough courage to ask why. I found out, not for the last time, that assumptions had been made that I would not be interested in the position because I had two small children. The underlying message always seemed to be that I *shouldn't* be interested in working because of my children. I spent a lot of my early career feeling guilty for wanting to work, in spite of the fact that my children were thriving (and have turned into great young men). When I made it clear that I wanted the job, it was immediately offered to me, and I continued in the position for the next seven years.

I loved being a Child Development Specialist. It was the perfect job for me at the time. There was a great deal of autonomy, and much of my time was spent developing and writing materials. My favorite project was creating the *Preschool Quarterly*, a publication for day care providers that I edited for 10 years and that reached 3,000 subscribers. I worked with an exceptional journalist on the project and learned a great deal about the process of editing lay publications.

I don't remember when I started working on my doctorate, but it was probably shortly after I began the full-time job with Extension. University employees had to pay only 25% of course fees, and my entire degree was accomplished through this employee assistance plan. I felt badly enough about what was perceived as the self-indulgence of pursuing additional education; if I had had to pay full fees, my guilt would have only escalated.

Although I had completed my master's degree with a 4.0 and had far exceeded the admittance criteria for the doctorate, when I met with my program committee, questions were raised. More specifically, one of the committee members asked me why I wanted to pursue a graduate degree when I had two preschoolers and was working full-time. Such behavior obviously seemed quite deviant to him. I don't remember how I answered the question; my decision to pursue a doctorate was probably not something that I understood all that well myself. I just knew that it was something that I had to do.

I had taken all the graduate courses in Child and Family Development and had even developed and taught some of them, so, I once again had to find a new field of study. This was not an era when husbands followed wives who wanted to pursue degrees or careers, and it was certainly not a time when wives left husbands in charge of the children while they left the state to pursue degrees. My choices, therefore, were limited. The closest thing to child development on campus was Learning Disabilities, so my doctorate is in Special Education/Curriculum and Instruction. I now have two degrees that I have never used professionally. Even more ironic, I do not have a degree in family studies–the area where I have built my career–and I had very limited formal coursework in the field.

I must have subconsciously felt that to pursue an advanced degree I also had to do everything else as well as stay-at-home mothers. Therefore, for several years, I not only worked full-time and took at least 6 hours of graduate credit each semester, including summers, but I was also a Cub Scout leader and a room mother at my children's school. I even made elaborate cakes for my children's birthday parties, cakes shaped like trains and animals or decorated to replicate football fields. My cake-decorating phase came to a bitter end when my ingrate oldest son wistfully told me that he wished I would buy one of those "pretty" birthday cakes from the store with big frosting roses on them. I was clearly a victim of the Superwoman phenomenon, and I think an unfortunate result of pulling that off is my lack of patience with graduate students who don't appear to me to have much drive.

THE PATTERN OF MY CAREER

By the time I had finished my degree, I was bored with my Extension position. In fact, I was so bored that when there was a last-minute faculty defection, I volunteered, as overload, to teach the only large lecture class offered by the department. I enjoyed this experience so much that I decided that what I really wanted was a regular faculty position. That same year, Ginny Fisher decided to resign as department chair, so my first opportunity for a regular faculty position was one combining the department chair responsibilities with teaching the department's largest lecture class. Because I was desperate to make a change, when a couple of faculty members encouraged me to apply for the position, I screwed up all my courage and did it. Keep in mind that when I applied, I had never had a regular department position, had absolutely no administrative experience, and had just completed my doctorate the previous year. This was in 1976, a different era to say the least!

Not surprisingly, I was not the first choice for the department chair position. However, choice number one managed to shoot himself in the foot several times during the negotiation process, and I ended up with the job more or less by default. I was so happy to have a regular faculty appointment that I didn't even ask for a salary increase. Luckily, Dr. Fisher continued to serve as Director of the Child Development Laboratory, so I had an outstanding consultant the first few years to guide me through the hazards of administration.

I had two major goals as chair. One was to broaden the curriculum, and the other was to increase the research productivity of the department. To help make this happen, in addition to administrative responsibilities, I taught three courses a semester for years and even taught four courses one semester. I also reasoned that the best way to increase departmental research efforts was to lead by example. I had a nice data set from my dissertation research, a classic experimental design testing a parent education model that I called the Parent-Child Interaction (PCI) program. It was based on The Far West Laboratory Toy Lending Library concept, which had never been evaluated. In five areas of the state, parents of preschoolers signed up to attend six sessions of instruction in how to use six different toys with their children. The parents (all mothers) were randomly assigned to either a control group (who attended a later PCI program) or the experimental group. I developed videotapes to instruct the parents, accompanying guidesheets, and a pre/post measure (the *Cognitive and Perceptional Skills Test* or *CAPS*) of the children's ability to master the concepts being taught. That was the easy part!

Because I had very limited funding, I had to figure out a way to get the lending toys made. I put a graduate student in charge, and he marshaled the forces of the child development laboratory children to sand and paint the many different colored blocks that were used in the program. We were operating a little preschool sweatshop, but the children seemed to enjoy it and I was desperate. I later got a federal grant from Extension Service to expand the program nationwide. We required people in other states to make their own toys, but my graduate students and I had to assemble a number of CAPS test kits for other Child Development Specialists to use. So, it was back to the sweatshop for a few weeks.

Research and Publications

The first article I published from this study was pure serendipity. I had continued to collect data on the PCI expansion, and was doing a follow-up on the IQ scores of the children who had been enrolled in the original program (my dissertation study). One of the graduate assistants who was collecting the data forgot to take a copy of the PPVT, the IQ test I had used in the first study, but had taken a copy of the SIT, a shorter IQ test that I also had planned to use. His memory lapse resulted in the *Psychology in the Schools* publication, "A Comparison of PPVT and SIT Scores of Young Children" (Coleman, Brown, & Ganong, 1980). I am not sure what sort of omen it is to have your first publication be the result of a mistake, but it was certainly more motivating than a rejection!

The PCI project resulted in five publications with the guts of the research published in the *Journal of Social Psychology* (Coleman, Ganong, & Brown, 1980). Parenting has been a bridge between my early work in child development and my later work in family. The PCI project was followed by a North Central Region Agriculture Experiment Station Project using the *Q-sort Inventory of Parenting Behaviors*. In spite of being developed by a committee, the instrument worked well and resulted in three committee publications and one based only on Missouri data (Coleman, Ganong, Clark, & Madsen, 1989).

I ended my first marriage about the same time that I finished my doctorate and assumed the department chair position, although I don't think there was a relationship between these events. In 1979, I remarried and my husband and research colleague, Larry Ganong, and I embarked on a challenging, stimulating, and extremely satisfying dual-career marriage.

I met Larry when he was a graduate assistant at the Student Parent Center I had helped organize. I was so impressed with him that I hired him to manage two funded projects that I no longer had the time to manage on my own, the national PCI expansion and a rural preschool screening project. Thus began a 24-year research partnership and a 21-year marriage partnership, both of which have exceeded any expectations that either of us ever had. We have co-authored over 100 articles and book chapters and three books in the 21 years we have been married.

Larry and I have long felt that our work together is synergistic, that neither of us would have accomplished as much working alone. A down side of being married to your research colleague, however, is that potentially you could be always working–we can't go home to get away from each other! Nonetheless, we think we have found a satisfactory solution. When we travel or are on vacation, we don't even mention work-related issues, which allows us to come back fresh and ready to take on new challenges.

Although people probably assume that our research interests in remarriage and stepfamilies, the area of scholarship most closely identified with us, came about because of our own remarriage, that was not the case. Larry had grown up as the child of a remarried couple. He became interested in the topic partially for those reasons, but his thesis advisor was also remarried and living in a blended family household. Larry used to babysit with her children and stepchildren. I think those experiences probably piqued his interest in the topic, and he hooked me. One of our first publications related to remarriage was a reworking of his thesis data on the attitudes towards marriage and divorce of adolescents from differing family structures. Being published at all was pretty thrilling to me in 1980, and having four articles accepted in that first year was just phenomenal and incredibly motivating (Bryan, Coleman, & Ganong, 1981; Coleman, Brown, & Ganong, 1980; Coleman, Ganong, & Brown, 1981; Ganong, Coleman, & Brown, 1981). This was the first step in changing the department culture towards more emphasis on research. Considering the current climate, it is hard to imagine a time, only two decades ago, when faculty members who had not published at all were tenured and promoted, including those who had only a master's degree.

I remember a conversation between Larry and me early in our publishing careers when we shared that we would feel our careers had been successful if we could just get one article published in the *Journal of Marriage and the Family*. It was years before we were courageous enough to even submit a paper to *JMF*, but with trepidation, we finally submitted two articles in 1985. Jetse Sprey, the editor at that time, responded that he thought both articles "could be salvaged," but because he was at the end of his term, he was passing them on to Alan Booth, the new editor, for his consideration. We didn't know whether to be encouraged or have our feelings hurt by Jetse's comments, but we were delighted when both articles were published in the 1986 volume of *JMF* (Bryan, Coleman, Ganong, & Bryan, 1986; Ganong & Coleman, 1986a).

Editor of JMF

Considering my early awe of publishing in *JMF*, not in my wildest dreams could I have imagined being selected as editor in 1992. I have no idea who nominated me for that position, but I would never have considered applying for it on my own. I was so nervous during the interview with the publications committee that I thought I was going to throw up.

A goal I had for my term as editor was to include more women in every facet of the journal operation, from Board membership to publication. This goal was not unique; I think previous editors had focused on accomplishing this as well. My sense of obligation was a little different, however. With the exception of a one-year term held by Gladys Groves in the 1950s (and I have no idea why her term was so short), I was the first female editor of *JMF* in the history of the journal, a travesty that should shame NCFR. The journal averaged nearly a submission per day during those 4 years, so the workload was heavy, but I enjoyed having the opportunity to shape family scholarship for a brief time. I especially liked the opportunity to encourage new scholars, many of whom were women.

Midway through my term as *JMF* editor I decided to resign as department chair. This decision was partly because I was spending nearly all my time working. Mostly, however, it was because the department had improved to the extent that I thought we would be able to attract a strong chair who would continue to augment the quality of the faculty and the national status of the department. It was a good time to bow out, in other words. Additionally, of the three "hats" I was wearing, teaching, research, and administration, the administration hat was the one I thought I would miss the least.

This decision was met with great relief by my husband, who was eager for me to be able to devote more time to our joint research projects as well as to have time for more extended travel. And I was right about not missing administration. It was another one of those experiences that I am glad that I had, but enough is enough. Perhaps if I had become department chair because I was seeking an administrative position, it would have been different, but it had never been my intention to be an administrator. As a result, I continued to teach and engage in research throughout my 17-year term as chair, which made it easy to slip over into a regular faculty position.

Now that I have more time to devote to research, I think Larry and I have been able to take on more interesting and creative projects. In the last 5 years, we have published two books (*Remarried Family Relationships* [Ganong & Coleman, 1994] and *Changing Families, Changing Responsibilities: Family Obligations Following Divorce and Remarriage* [Ganong & Coleman, 1999]), completed 13 different studies related to various aspects of family obligations and responsibilities after divorce and remarriage (see reference list), and have collaborated with Mark Fine on a stepfamily study with a heavy qualitative component, a methodology that was relatively new to the three of us (e.g., Coleman, Fine, Ganong, Downs, & Pauk, in press; Ganong, Coleman, Fine, & Martin, 1999; Ganong, Coleman, Fine, & McDaniel, 1998). I am now engaged in grounded theory studies of women in stepfamilies (stepdaughters, residential and nonresidential stepmothers, and biological mothers), an almost ignored area, and Larry and I have several other grounded theory studies of remarriage planned. We also would like to return to some themes of earlier research. For example, we have done several studies of partner expectations and have also conducted a series of studies on sex roles (e.g., Coleman & Ganong, 1985a; Ganong & Coleman, 1992; Ganong, Coleman, Thompson, & Goodwin-Watkins, 1996). We have more than enough studies planned to keep us busy for a couple more lifetimes.

When looking back, I cannot identify a seminal study that I could point to as a highlight of my career. I think the impact of my work would have to be taken as the total effort. In fact, in looking through the 1999 edition of the *Handbook of Marriage and Family*, Larry noted that we were cited in nearly every chapter, but almost every citation was different from those in the other chapters. One thing that Larry and I have consistently tried to do in our stepfamily work is move away from pathologizing stepfamilies (Coleman & Ganong, 1985b; Coleman, Ganong, & Gingrich, 1985). This is not to say that stepfamilies are problem free. However, the vast number of studies conceptualized from what we term a "deficit comparison" model tells us little about *why* stepfamilies have problems, nor are they enlightening about how successful stepfamilies got that way. The goals that Larry and I typically share for our research are to find ways to help stepfamilies be more functional and to better understand the reasons why some families are not successful (Coleman, Ganong, & Weaver, in press; Coleman & Ganong, 1990; Coleman & Ganong, 1987b; Coleman & Ganong, 1995). Our approach no doubt stems from our training in the applied field of family studies, but it also stems from our research experiences.

One of the most influential research experiences came from what we have facetiously referred to as our "concrete baby" study. The idea for the investigation resulted from a survey of self-help books for an article we were planning for *Family Relations* (Coleman & Ganong, 1987c). In seven different books we came across the advice that remarried couples should have a baby together in order to *cement* their union. Whether or not having a baby would *cement* a remarried union seemed like a researchable question to us, so, in 1984, we interviewed 105 stepfamilies to find the answer to that and other questions. There was no evidence that these concrete babies made much difference, at least to things that we could measure, but we did find out a lot about stepfamily dynamics (e.g., Coleman, & Ganong, 1987d; Ganong & Coleman, 1988). I should note that a *JMF* reviewer was appalled by the image of a concrete baby and nixed the use of the term in the title of the article. So much for humor in academe.

We reinterviewed 79 of the families in 1989 (Ganong & Coleman, 1994), and we are planning another follow-up soon. We also collected survey data from the families, but it was the interviews that influenced me the most. I think that listening to all those family stories gave me insight that has led to impatience with yet more studies indicating that stepchildren have lower GPAs, get married earlier, have babies sooner, etc. I don't question the findings of those studies, but I am much more interested in family process. What is it about living in a stepfamily that is related to lower GPA, underachievement in school, early marriage, etc.? I think the answer to the "why" is probably to be found using qualitative methods, and, for that reason, I think that my best work is still ahead of me.

James Matthew Barrie, novelist and dramatist, was quoted as saying, "Nothing is really work unless you would rather be doing something else." By that definition, I am a real slacker. I cannot imagine that doing anything else would be half as satisfying as the life of a college professor. There is nothing that I would rather be doing.

AUTHOR NOTE

Marilyn Coleman is Professor, Department of Human Development and Family Studies, 411 Gentry, University of Missouri, Columbia, MO 65211.

REFERENCES

Bryan, L., Coleman, M., & Ganong, L. (1981). Geometric mean as a continuous measure of androgyny. *Psychological Reports*, *48*, 3, 691-694.

Bryan, L., & Coleman, M. (1988a). The Black family as portrayed in introductory marriage and family textbooks. *Family Relations*, *37*, 3, 255-259.

Bryan, H., Ganong, L., Coleman, M., & Bryan, L. (1985). Counselor's perceptions of stepparents and stepchildren. *Journal of Counseling Psychology*, *32*, 2, 279-282.

Bryan, L., Coleman, M., & Ganong, L. (1988b). Race and family structure stereotyping: Perceptions of black and white nuclear families and stepfamilies. *Journal of Black Psychology, 15*, 2, l-16.

Bryan, L., Coleman, M., Ganong, L., & Bryan, H. (1986). Person perception: Family structure as a cue for stereotyping. *Journal of Marriage and the Family, 48*, 1, 169-174.

Coleman, M., Brown, G., & Ganong, L. (1980). A comparison of PPVT and SIT scores of young children. *Psychology in the Schools, 17*, 2, 178-180.

Coleman, M., Fine, M., Ganong, L., Downs, K., & Pauk, N. (in press). When you're not the Brady Bunch: Identifying perceived conflicts and resolution strategies in stepfamilies. *Personal Relations.*

Coleman, M., & Ganong, L. (1984). Effect of family structure on family attitudes and expectations. *Family Relations, 33*, 3, 425-432.

Coleman, M., & Ganong, L. (1985a). Remarriage myths: Implications for the helping professions. *Journal of Counseling and Development, 64*, 2, 116-120.

Coleman, M., & Ganong, L. (1985b). Love and sex-role stereotypes: Do "macho" men and "feminine" women make better lovers? *Journal of Personality and Social Psychology, 49*, 1, 170-176.

Coleman, M., & Ganong, L. (1987a). The cultural stereotyping of stepfamilies. In K. Pasley & M. Ihinger-Tallman (Eds.). *Remarriage and stepparenting: Current research and theory* (pp. 94-140). New York: Guilford.

Coleman, M., & Ganong, L. (1987b). Marital conflict in stepfamilies: Effects on children. *Youth and Society, 19*, 2, 151-172.

Coleman, M., & Ganong, L. (1987c). An evaluation of the stepfamily self-help literature for children and adolescents. *Family Relations, 36*, 1, 61-65.

Coleman, M., & Ganong, L. (1987d). Sex, sex roles and irrational beliefs. *Psychological Reports, 61*, 2, 631-638.

Coleman, M., & Ganong, L. (1990). The use of juvenile fiction and self-help books with stepfamilies. *Journal of Counseling and Development, 68*, 3, 327-331.

Coleman, M., & Ganong, L. (1995). Insiders' and outsiders' beliefs about stepfamilies: Assessments and implications for practice. In D. Huntley (Ed.), *Understanding stepfamilies: Implications for assessment* (pp. 101-112). American Counseling Association Press.

Coleman, M., & Ganong, L. (1998). Attitudes toward men's intergenerational financial obligations to older and younger male family members following divorce. *Personal Relationships, 5*, 3, 293-309.

Coleman, M., Ganong, L., & Brown, G. (1980). Effects of multi-media instruction on mothers' ability to teach cognitive skills to preschool children. *Journal of Social Psychology, 115*, 89-94.

Coleman, M., Ganong, L., & Cable, S. (1997). Beliefs about women's intergenerational family obligations to provide support prior to and following divorce and remarriage. *Journal of Marriage and the Family, 59*, 1, 165-176.

Coleman, M., Ganong, L., Clark, J., & Madsen, R. (1989). Parenting perceptions in rural and urban families: Is there a difference? *Journal of Marriage and the Family, 51*, 2, 329-335.

Coleman, M., Ganong, L., & Gingrich, R. (1985). Stepfamily strengths: A review of the popular literature. *Family Relations*, *34*, 4, 583-589.

Coleman, M., Ganong, L., Killian, T., & Kusgen-McDaniel, A. (1998). Child support obligations: Attitudes and rationale. *Journal of Family Issues*, *20*, 1, 46-68.

Coleman, M., Ganong, L., Killian, T., & McDaniel, A. (1998). Mom's house? Dad's house? Attitudes toward physical custody changes. *Families in Society*, *79*, 2, 112-122.

Coleman, M., Ganong, L., & Weaver, S. (in press). Maintenance and enhancement in remarried families. In J. Harvey & Wenzel (Eds.). *Close romantic relationships I: Maintenance and enhancement* Hillsdale, NJ: Erlbaum.

Ganong, L., & Coleman, M. (1986a). A comparison of clinical and empirical literature on children in stepfamilies. *Journal of Marriage and the Family*, *48*, 2, 309-318.

Ganong, L., & Coleman, M. (1986b). Sex, sex roles, and emotional expressiveness. *Journal of Genetic Psychology*, *146*, 3, 405-411.

Ganong, L., & Coleman, M. (1988). Do mutual children cement bonds in stepfamilies? *Journal of Marriage and the Family*, *50*, 3, 687-698.

Ganong, L., & Coleman, M. (1992). Gender differences in self- and future partners expectations. *Journal of Family Issues*, *13*, 1, 55-64.

Ganong, L., & Coleman, M. (1994). *Remarried family relationships*. Newbury Park, CA: Sage Publications.

Ganong, L., & Coleman, M. (1994). Adolescent stepchild-stepparent relationships: Changes over time. In K. Pasley & M. Ihinger-Tallman (Eds.), *Stepparenting: Issues in theory, research, and practice* (pp. 87-104). Westport, CT: Greenwood Press.

Ganong, L., & Coleman, M. (1999). *Changing families, changing responsibilities: Family obligations following divorce and remarriage*. Hillsdale, NJ: Lawrence Erlbaum Associates.

Ganong, L., Coleman, M., & Brown, G. (1981). Effect of family structure on marital attitudes of adolescents. *Adolescence*, *16*, 62, 281-288.

Ganong, L., Coleman, M., & Mapes, D. (1990). A meta-analytic review of family structure stereotypes. *Journal of Marriage and the Family*, *52*, 2, 287-297.

Ganong, L., Coleman, M., Fine, M., & Martin, P. (1999). Stepparents' affinity-seeking and affinity-maintaining strategies with stepchildren. *Journal of Family Issues*, *20*, 3, 299-327.

Ganong, L., Coleman, M., Fine, M., & McDaniel, A. (1998). Issues considered in contemplating stepchild adoptions. *Family Relations*, *47*, 1, 63-71.

Ganong, L., Coleman, M., Thompson, A., & Goodwin-Watkins, C. (1996). African American and European American college students' expectations for self and future partners. *Journal of Family Issues*, *17*, 6, 758-775.

PART III: ENVIRONMENTAL AND FAMILY INFLUENCES SHAPING FAMILY SCHOLARS

In Memoriam
Carlfred B. Broderick
(1932-1999)

The future belongs to the new breed of well-tooled, eclectic, hardheaded, family research scholars. I see a generation of them just emerging from graduate school, and, like all commencement speakers everywhere, I am encouraged that the future of the field is in good hands.

Environmental and Family Influences Shaping Family Scholars

Suzanne K. Steinmetz
Gary W. Peterson

Whenever you have a large number of contributors involved in a project, you can expect a number of life-course changes. Scholars marry, divorce, have children, send their young to college (or off to live with a spouse) as well as face the illnesses and/or deaths of parents, siblings, and partners. When a project such as this involves senior scholars, death becomes a reality–and, unfortunately, we have had to face this circumstance during the progress of this project.

This section is dedicated to Carl Broderick, who died over a year ago after a long battle with cancer. Broderick's autobiography is the lead article in this section. Each of us has our memories of Carl–bright, energetic, loveably devilish in humor, gracious, and caring. One of the Editors, for example, fondly remembers Carl not only for his excellent scholarship, but also for his talent as an illustrator of complex family concepts through the creative application of physical comedy–in particular, Carl's seemingly natural gift to dramatically represent basic principles of a family system "metaphorically" with his body. Carl would commence to rotate and swing his arms and legs in contrary directions (demonstrating remarkable coordination), combined with other body movements and contortions. Meanwhile, and quite remarkably, he would carefully describe how family systems are composed of interconnected components, each with some independence, but also forming part of the pattern and redundancy that defines the whole. He was indeed a sight to see!–and everyone in the audience immediately got the point as they laughed uproariously at his performance. He indeed is dearly missed by all of us today. His wit, scholarly achievement, and humility are clearly evident in the pages of his essay.

This section, "Environmental and Family Influences Shaping Family Scholars," might be interpreted as presenting a point of view somewhat akin to the "Nature versus Nurture" controversy as it applies to the shaping of family scholars. For some scholars, individual and family characteristics influence their choices, while, for others, the social-historical environment of the time clearly shapes their lives and the themes explored. A particular common theme of note in these essays is the extent to which the historical, political, and economic circumstances become intertwined with individual and family circumstances to shape the personal and scholarly lives of these distinguished contributors.

In Carlfred B. Broderick's essay, "An Autobiographical Sketch," he demonstrates that growing up in a blended, somewhat unstable family does not always have negative consequences. What might be described today as a difficult childhood–one characterized by several stepfathers and a confusing, though colorful, set of relatives–gave him strength to leave a legacy as an innovative, brilliant academic, father of nine children, with an enduring marriage. He also reveals his perceptive understanding of the politics of academe. Specifically, Dr. Broderick describes that, although he was offered a full professorship at an extremely young age, he astutely read how the realities of this circumstance might not bode well for his future in the department. Moreover, although he became known as a guest on the Johnny Carson show, as an expert "Sexologist" because of his research in this area, Dr. Broderick eventually declined invitations to appear because it did not appear to be in the best interest of more staid academic scholarship. He details the various stages of his life with humor and helps us understand how relatively new the field of family studies was during the early years of his career.

In her essay, "How I Got This Way: Memoirs of a Liberal," Margaret Feldman gives us some insights into the early workings of the family field. Although the word "sexism" has been a part of our language for several decades, Margaret Feldman appears to be the person who first coined this word in 1969. Feldman demonstrates how being raised in a family environment embedded in charity work was an important component throughout her own professional career. Characteristic of many women of her generation, she obtained her PhD later in life, yet continued to exert her academic influence for years after formal retirement, and continues to do so today. Her life also illustrates how family professionals can devote themselves in very constructive ways to political action and to advocacy of social policy that supports families and the field of family studies.

"The Autobiography of a Sex Researcher: Short Version," by Ira L. Reiss's illustrates how one's family environment as well as one's neighborhood can have a lasting impression on one's personal and academic life. Early in childhood, Reiss tells us that he made extra money by telling men where they could find the local "cat" houses in his community. This peaked his interest in obtaining accurate information about this most intriguing aspect of life–sexuality. While serving in the army, Reiss's knowledge about sex propelled him to provide fellow service men with information about sexuality, a practice that furthered his interest and made him aware of just how sexually illiterate his peers were. Not only will his research have a lasting effect, but he was also instrumental in developing, in conjunction with Indiana University and Kinsey Institute, a PhD program in sexuality.

Catherine Street Chilman's essay, "My Family and Me: A 20th Century Saga," provides insights into the struggle that women face when obtaining graduate education in the middle years. Chilman's family was represented by several generations of well-educated men and women who were extensively involved in humanitarian and charitable activities. Chilman did not return to obtain her PhD, however, until she was faced with the facts that her husband had a terminal illness and that she would need to find a way to adequately provide for her children and herself. Beginning her career as a researcher for the federal government, she worked in the area of family policy, especially as it applies to the issue of unplanned pregnancy among teens. Chilman's scholarship provided a foundation in these areas that many have since used to build upon. Her extensive training and experience as a social worker in such areas as Appalachia, a region with pervasive poverty, provided powerful influences on her scholarly interests. Chilman also suggests that her work was influenced, to a considerable extent, by major historical-political developments of the 1960s, the most prominent of which were the ambitious social programs promoted by President Lyndon Johnson.

In "A Personal and Intellectual Journey," John Scanzoni provides a connection between his early family experience in a fundamentalist church and the academic climate of the 1960s. Discussing a connection that is similar to that noted by Weber in the *Protestant Ethic and the Spirit of Capitalism*, Scanzoni notes the importance of his church both in terms of providing him with a middle class, well-educated model to emulate, and of instilling the values of hard work. His essay demonstrates the push and pull of early values in a changing society on both his academic and personal life. Scanzoni carefully describes how his own conceptions of families have evolved into a very malleable construct that is not constrained by structural specificity. He clearly places himself at odds with those in our society who seek to define and make value judgements about families in terms of specific structural definitions.

Harold T. Christensen, clearly one of the fathers of family sociology, documents how his religious background, Mormonism, provided him with both a curiosity about families and a stable set of guidelines that emphasized the importance of this focus. His essay, "My Life Story: Reflections of an Early Family Scholar," clearly demonstrates his intense curiosity about what makes families work, combined with strong values about the importance of family. These dual themes are evident in his first book, a family text, written both for empirical accuracy, but also suitable for his church. During the 1960s, Christensen was committed to conceptions of the family nurtured by his religious community and, at the same time, became editor of the *Handbook of Marriage and the Family*, the definitive compilation of scientifically and theoretically- based reviews on family scholarship of its time. His long and productive career resulted in both a body of prominent academic publications as well as numerous thoughtful works for his church.

Glen H. Elder, Jr.'s essay entitled "Families, Social Change, and Individual Lives" demonstrates how life in the tumultuous 20th Century drew his attention to longitudinal analyses of "changing lives in changing times." Elder increasingly became interested, not only in individual life changes, aging concepts, and transitions, but also in how major historical forces, cohort membership, and the timing of major social events shaped the meaning and life experiences of individuals and families. As a consequence of these interests, his extensive scholarly program has made him the foremost proponent of what has now become known as the "life course" perspective. His work stands as a truly classic example of how systematic, cumulative social science can carefully sketch out the meaning of family life and the lives of family members during a particular historical time period and within the context of specific kinds of social change. Elder's empirical work demonstrates both the discovery of lawful patterns in family life as well as how larger historical-social forces set normative parameters for the choices available to individuals and families across the life course.

Katherine R. Allen, in her essay "Making the World Safe for Difference," describes her early experiences of observing and experiencing marginalization based on race, class, gender, and heterosexuality. Both her life and work illustrate how these obstacles can be identified, deconstructed, and challenged. She notes that her intellectual goal, to deconstruct marginalization and reconstruct social arrangements that gain respect for diversity, are features of both her academic work and personal life. She offers that these two aspects of her experience are inextricably intertwined, a stance she believes is essential to becoming a reflective scholar, teacher, and person. For Allen, her professional and personal lives are experiences in which feeling and being are as important as thinking and doing. She also describes an interesting dilemma rooted in her current positions of academic prominence in family studies, gender issues, feminist thought, and aging. Specifically, she describes the dilemma of being in simultaneous positions of status and influence as a family scholar, while, at the same time, being a member of other marginalized social statuses in our society.

Thus the intertwining of environmental and family influence on one's academic life is a common theme in essays authored by men and women who faced very different family influences in very different environmental settings over nearly a century.

An Autobiographical Sketch

Carlfred B. Broderick

KEYWORDS. Autobiography, family therapy, marriage, religion

FAMILY BACKGROUND

My Birth and Naming

My parents married on a dare. Fred Broderick, an Irish Catholic Brooklynite, had arrived in Salt Lake City by "Poorman's Pullman" (i.e., by hopping a freight car) only a few months before. My mother, Napina Bartholomew, had grown up a Mormon in the city of Mormons, but was at a vulnerable place in her life. She was living at home and unhappy to be there, and she had a job working in a "Mom and Pop" neighborhood grocery store where "Pop" was, in modern parlance, sexually harassing her. To her, Fred Broderick, 10 years her senior, a world traveler, and a veteran of the World War, seemed like a sophisticate. They had been dating off and on for some months when a couple of friends decided on the spur of the moment to run off to Sin City (alias Ogden, the Las Vegas of its day) to get married and invited them to be the witnesses at their wedding. On the way to Ogden, the eloping couple rode in the front seat of the open coupe, my parents-to-be in the rumble seat. About two-thirds of the way there the bride-to-be leaned over the back seat and yelled, "I dare you guys to get married too." And so they did. My mother says of that marriage that I was the only good thing that came of it.

My entrance into the world a year and a half later was an extended family event. I was born April 7, 1932, in my maternal grandparents' home on Roosevelt Avenue in Salt Lake City. In attendance were a large number of relatives, including, of course, my grandparents, Elizabeth and Carl Bartholomew. She had been head nurse at the Latter-day

Saint Hospital and was an experienced obstetric assistant, but, on the occasion of my birth, she exercised her Victorian prerogative and fainted. Grandfather, on the other hand, a hale-fellow-well-met traveling salesman noted for his practical jokes and inexhaustible store of off-color stories, was calling the color shots. "I can't tell if its a boy or a girl yet," he yelled over his shoulder to those who couldn't get a close view, "but it's a blond."

In this crowd my father was the outlander. All of my newborn features were immediately parcelled out among the maternal kin; the nose was my grandfather's, the chin was my Aunt Adah's, my ears were a direct legacy from Uncle Jasper. His genetic contributions ignored in the general consensus, Fred Broderick was heard to mumble, "Well, thank God he's got my brains." And, perhaps I did.

There was a certain amount of contention over what to name me. The local clan felt that, since I was the first grandchild, I should be named Carl Bartholomew Broderick, after my grandfather. My father was firm in the opinion that I should be named Fred Broderick, Jr. A conciliatory aunt finally hit on the compromise, Carlfred [no middle name] Broderick to which everyone agreed. Ultimately, however, my grandfather performed the naming ceremony in front of the congregation in the Mormon fashion, and he pronounced me Carlfred Bartholomew Broderick, "by which name he shall be known throughout his life and on the records of the Church." My parents and a number of others gasped at the perfidy, but the deed was done. My grandmother (whom I suspect of being confederate) commented only, "Well, thank heavens he's not a small child."

Paternal Ancestors

My paternal ancestors came to America from County Waterford, Ireland during the Potato Famine era. My father's grandfather, Richard Broderick, was listed as a 20-year-old with an occupation of carpenter. The 1851 passenger manifest of the overcrowded *Universe* out of Liverpool listed him as traveling alone, but he was probably ready to take on the new world. He managed to find work with a contractor in Yonkers–and love. According to family tradition, Ellen Ryan had also recently arrived on these shores in the company of her sister, the last of seven Ryan children sacrificially sent to America by their parents, before they themselves perished from the famine. Richard and Ellen married in 1857. By the time of his death twenty-two years later (of dysentery), he had become proprietor of his own contracting business and was an officer in the local Democratic Party organization. He left his widow with 7 surviving children (out of 11 births), all minors. Ellen was a feisty woman and, although illiterate, had a good head for business. For a few months, she tried to operate his contracting business by herself, but, even after it became clear that this was not going to work, she was successful in selling it to a former competitor. She invested the money in tenements and died many years later with an estate substantial enough to cause her surviving children several years of litigation over its distribution.

My father's father, John R. Broderick, was Richard and Ellen's fourth child. He was 16 at his father's death. At 25 he married Susan Murphy, the daughter of another contractor in the area. After trying his hand at several enterprises, he eventually bought and operated the Broderick Bar and Grill on Third Avenue and 39th Street in Brooklyn. My father, the youngest of their eight children, was born in the family apartment over the bar in 1899. Apparently, it was not a happy marriage because when Fred was only 18 months old, his mother abandoned her husband and children for reasons that can only be surmised. The five younger children, including my father, were placed in the Orphanage of the Diocese of Brooklyn. A few months later, their father, John R. Broderick, died of cirrhosis of the liver at age 39. Two years later his widow, Susan, also died, leaving the children orphans, indeed.

One by one the Broderick children ran away from the orphanage. The last to leave was my father, the youngest, who finally made his escape when he turned 14, as he believed. My own research into the baptismal records of the family prove that he was, in fact, a year older than he thought (and that his "twin" brothers were actually born a year apart). It is poignant evidence of the emotional poverty of the orphanage environment that these children did not even know their own ages. In any case, he joined the Army in 1914, lying about his age (but by one year less than he thought). He served in France, driving a munitions truck back and forth to the front. After the War, he bounced from job to job and town to town, ending up, as we have noted, at the somewhat unlikely destination of Salt Lake City, Utah.

Maternal Ancestors

My Bartholomew ancestors came to Pennsylvania from Germany in the early 1700s, working their way west, generation by generation, through Ohio and Illinois. It is a curious fact that somehow Carl Bartholomew, my mother's father, managed to find his way to the copper mining community of Bingham Canyon, Utah, and there became the proprietor of a bar and grill. Clearly, if a family coat of arms were ever designed, it ought to feature a bar and grill in the foreground.

It seems to me that my maternal grandparents were an exceedingly unlikely pair. He was a thoroughly worldly man with no religious interests or pretensions, a hard gambling, hard drinking, fun loving man. She was a starchy Mormon nurse working at the local hospital. He was four years younger than she and four inches shorter and roughly the dimensions of Santa Claus. It is reported that she married him to reform him and "because he was the cutest man I ever met," and he is said to have married her because she was the only woman he ever met that he couldn't get into bed without marrying her first. Their first child was born in a little apartment over the bar, but by the time my mother was born, Grandma had "prayed him into bankruptcy" to get him out of the tainted business. He went straight and became a traveling salesman. By the time I was born, he had also became a Mormon, of sorts, but the kind that drank coffee (and more than once offered to let me taste it, to my grandmother's horror). It was a continuing family embarrassment that he never really gave up having a couple of drinks with his friends from time to time.

Family of Orientation

Nearly everybody liked my grandfather, but my mother did not, and I think that getting away from home was a part of her motivation to elope with my father. If so, it didn't work. He couldn't keep a job, and they lived with her family for the entire duration of their marriage. She divorced him when I was 18 months old and, leaving me with my grandparents, went to California to find a job. On my third birthday, we were reunited in Los Angeles where we came perilously close to starving while trying to live on what she made working in the Sears-Roebuck employee cafeteria. She confesses to having stolen food to feed me, although she would not eat purloined provender herself. When we were finally rescued, she weighed, at 5′4″, only 89 pounds.

Our benefactor was an older second cousin of hers, Allen Howard, whom her mother had sent to check up on her welfare. Within a few months, she had married him. I give my mother credit: she learned from her marital mistakes (one at a time). Allen Howard was no itinerant ne'er-do-well, but a financially well established divorced man who, having taken an early retirement as president of a steel company, had invested in Southern California real estate. To that extent, he was a clear improvement over Fred Broderick (who, incidentally, soon after this, disappeared over the horizon, never to be heard from again). From my point of view, however, the new marriage was, at best, a mixed blessing. We did manage to ride out the rest of the Great Depression in comfort and security. But from the beginning, Allen Howard did not like me, and I returned the sentiment. I was never physically abused (thanks to my mother's commitment to the sound principle that "If you don't love him, you can't hit him"), but I yet remember him, without fondness, as my "wicked step-father." To the best of my recollection, he never permitted a kind word toward me to cross his lips. It was his often expressed view that I was lazy and stupid and worthless and badly *needed* the thrashing my mother wouldn't let him administer. (He used to tell the apocryphal story that when my mother took me to kindergarten on the first day, she told the teacher, "Carlfred is a very sensitive child; if he does anything wrong, hit the child next to him.") Fortunately, my mother's alternative view was that I was an extraordinary child, whose destiny was, like cream, to rise to the top in any situation. I dare say that the determination to prove her right and him wrong has been a governing dynamic throughout my life.

He died when I was twelve. I did not mourn his passing; in fact, my unseemly attitude toward his demise so offended one of my school teachers that I felt compelled to explain that I had not personally done him in, I just was happy that he was gone. Mother married a third time when I was 14, this time to Victor Astley, the mail carrier who had walked our route as long as we had lived there. In my view, he was by far the best of the bunch. For one thing, he had enough sense not to try to parent me, and we managed to work out what began as a pretty good relationship and evolved over the years into a very warm and meaningful one. Vic Astley is the grandfather of my children, and when I use the word "Dad," I refer to him.

I suppose it must be admitted that I was raised in a "dysfunctional" family, but in truth, I do not think I had any sense of that as I was growing up. Probably part of the reason was that all of my extended kin had families at least as dysfunctional as mine. Just to give a little of the flavor of it, my "Aunt Fern," who lived just across the street and was one of the most present and puissant female relatives in my life, was, to be genealogically precise, my mother's brother's, first wife's, second husband's, father's, 3rd, 4th, and 5th wife (She married "Uncle Lew" three times in the course of her seven matrimonial ventures). But beyond the lack of a more functional comparison group, I think I was not a particularly introspective or socially insightful child. My interests were in the hard sciences. In the summer between elementary school and Jr. High, I managed to smuggle myself into a high school physics course and got the highest grade in the class. In high school I was always on the math, physics, and chemistry teams that competed for state-wide recognition. In several such competitions I placed among the top ten in the state. On the application form for admittance to Harvard, it seemed natural to declare myself a math major. My early conversion to the social sciences was partly a function of the intellectual energy in the Social Relations Department at Harvard in that era. But I wonder if the ground was softened a little by having had an Aunt Fern.

Before moving on into my academic history, one other aspect of my growing up deserves mention. I grew up Mormon. None of my mother's husbands were believing members of the Church, although long after I left home, Vic Astley eventually joined the Church and even became a Mormon Bishop, serving the local congregation I had grown up in. But growing up, one of the axial tensions in the household (I was the other) was the unresolvable conflict between my mother's unwavering, unsophisticated commitment to her faith and Allen Howard's very well documented and highly sophisticated attacks on all religion. I remember a very early, very conscious decision to aspire to her faith and his scholarship. From an early age, I became a student of the scriptures, of comparative religion, and of church history. And I have never wavered from the faith.

Family of Procreation

I met Kathleen, the woman I eventually married, at church when we were both three years old. Our family picture album begins with a picture of our kindergarten class: I was the tallest one in the back row, and she was the shortest one in the front. In third grade we were in a play together. I was William Tell, and she was my son. The dramatic scene where William Tell was forced by the wicked Austrians to prove his fabled marksmanship by shooting the apple off his own beloved son's head was rigged. I was supposed to aim high, and she was supposed to pull on the string attached to the apple. In any event, I knocked the apple cleanly off her head with my first shot. Not too shabby, considering I had never pulled a bow before (nor since). For reasons that escaped both of us, her mother got very upset over the incident, and, I think, held it against me all her life.

I had a perpetual crush on Kathleen from kindergarten forward. At 14, she was my first date, but in high school we both dated other people, and the first clue I had that she really liked me as more than just her oldest friend was when I got admitted to Harvard and she cried and cried. Between our junior and senior years in college, we married. By graduation, the first of our eight children was already on the way. Since then, over 40 satisfying years of marriage have come and gone; the children, too have come and gone, and we are enjoying those much touted (and doubted) pleasures of the empty nest that have evaded so many of our contemporaries.

ACADEMIC TRAINING

Undergraduate Years

I count it a great good fortune that the years I spent at Harvard (1949-1953) were also part of the golden age of the Social Relations Department there. In a somewhat unusual configuration, it combined Sociology, Social Anthropology, Social Psychology, and Clinical Psychology into a single major. George Homans taught the introductory course in sociology, Talcott Parsons taught social structure, Gordon Allport taught social psychology, Clyde Kluckholm, social anthropology, Robert Sears, child development, and Samuel Stouffer and Fred Mosteller taught the two semesters of social statistics. By any measure, this was a star-studded cast.

Of particular importance to me was Carle Zimmerman, who taught the family course. He and his good friend Pitrim Sorokin were out of favor in those years. Their offices were on a different floor from the main-line group, and they were never assigned teaching assistants. Zimmerman remained an associate professor until his retirement, his style of sociology considered passe (partaking neither of the rigorous empiricism of Stouffer nor the grand theorizing of Parsons). It was definitely not politically correct to study with him, but he was the only one teaching about families, so I took his courses anyway (thus establishing a pattern of nonconformity that has served me well ever since).

Carle had let a colleague at the medical school persuade him that a lobotomy would effectively relieve his hypermania with few intellectual side effects. It resulted in slurred speech and a peculiar scrambling of his order of presentation. To compound his problems, I believe he kept a bottle in his desk, and it was easy for colleagues to explain and dismiss him as an alcoholic, but I learned a great deal of good sociology from him. There was an order underlying his presentations, and, once I figured out how to decode him, I found his scholarship to be impressive and his ideas exceptionally logical, creative, and thought provoking.

He sponsored my first empirical study. He had developed a theory about the functions of the informal networks of families, and he realized that the temper of the times was such that no one would take his idea seriously without empirical support. Together we developed a questionnaire, and I took it back to Long Beach and, as my undergraduate honors thesis, collected information on almost 2000 families and their closest friend-families. In 1954, we published a report on it in *Marriage and Family Living*, the forerunner of the *Journal of Marriage and the Family* (Zimmerman & Broderick, 1954). It was my first publication. This study together with those by Marvin Sussman and Elizabeth Bott (published about the same period) were the first on the nature and function of family networks. In our case, we were interested in network size and homogeneity of the network and how these variables impacted various family issues. We found strong correlations between both variables and the ability of the family to avoid divorce, delinquency, and school dropouts. Somehow in the printing of the article the tables got scrambled so that they could not be readily understood. I have never seen the article cited (except by the authors, of course). Later, another of Zimmerman's students, Lucius Cervantes, a Jesuit Priest, oversaw the replication of the study in eight additional cities, substantiating my findings.

Unfortunately, Zimmerman's chief conclusion from this massive empirical effort was that one should protect one's children from having anything to do with families who were blemished by divorce, delinquency, and school dropouts. There was probably never a good time for such an idea; certainly it was not in the year John F. Kennedy was elected President of the United States on a platform of social conscience, involvement, and outreach. The book was stillborn, an instant antique. The only reason to mourn its demise was the fact that it reported one of the most substantial investigations of family networks, then or since.

Harvard was not all classes and theses, of course. It was a good deal of fun, especially after I was able to bring Kathleen back as my wife. She sang in the Radcliffe Choral Society and I in the Harvard Glee Club. Together we performed some marvelous music with the Boston Symphony under the baton of Charles Muensch: Bach's B-minor Mass, St. Matthew's and St. John's Passions, Berlioz' Requiem, and Hindemith's Oedipus Rex. Also, having an apartment of our own, we became something of the social center of the little community of Mormon undergraduates. We all became very close and have maintained contact over the years. Nearly all of them have gone on to become professionals of substantial reputation, university presidents, and the like.

Graduate School

I applied to three graduate schools. Harvard admitted me, but offered no financial support. I had heard of Reuben Hill at North Carolina and of Robin Williams at Cornell, so I applied to both schools and got accepted at both. Cornell offered me $100.00 more, so I went there. In later years, after I got to know Reuben, I have sometimes wondered idly what it might have been like to have worked with him, and whether my professional interests might have been shaped differently by such an experience.

Cornell was an exciting place. It turned out that, since my application was to work in the family, I was admitted into the Department of Child Development and Family Relations in the School of Home Economics. Although I was not in the Sociology Department where Robin Williams had his appointment, I did succeed in getting him as a member of my Committee. Urie Bronfennbrenner was there and so was Harold Feldman, a clinical psychologist of the Rogerian persuasion who had an influence on my later clinical work. Coming to Cornell from Harvard turned out to be a happy circumstance because everyone at Cornell was in awe of the things happening at Harvard. I had just come from the feet of the gods and was viewed as retaining just a bit of the Olympian aura. For example, several faculty refused to let me sign up for their seminars because they were certain the material would be "old hat" and "derivative." One seminar on Parsons and Bales' new book on the family was canceled after only two or three sessions when it became clear that the instructor didn't understand the somewhat opaque material as well as one of the class members. I confess that this sort of thing did not distress me as much as it might have had I been of a less arrogant disposition. In any case, I plowed right on through the degree in three years, passing the French and German exams on schedule and, if it may be believed, actually enjoying the five-day written and oral qualifying exams. My dissertation followed a class of 100 entering freshman Home-Ec majors and predicted the friend-formation process over the first several months, utilizing a similarity/opportunity matrix. It worked out well, although for years I dreamed about that 100 by 100 matrix laid out on the apartment floor. At 24 I had my PhD, three children (the third, born the Summer after I got the degree), and an exciting new job at the University of Georgia.

CAREER AS A PROFESSOR AND RESEARCHER

Carle Zimmerman had always said that no one ought to be allowed to practice Sociology in the United States unless they had lived at least four years in the South. I had job offers from Brigham Young University and Merrill Palmer; in fact, the job market for PhDs was so favorable in those far-off, balmy days that I actually received telephone calls from the presidents of these institutions. But I chose Georgia because, in addition to my finding Zimmerman's reasoning persuasive, they offered an absolutely top salary and–as a measure of how competitive the bidding for new faculty could get in that era–the rank of Associate Professor.

Georgia

In many ways, 1956 was an exciting time to be in that place and situation. The *Brown v. the Board of Education* decision had been handed down by the Supreme Court, and the gears had been set in motion that led to the civil rights movement and eventually reshaped American society. But none of that change had been effected yet. When we got off the plane in Atlanta, we walked into a Quonset hut air terminal with separate drinking fountains and bathrooms, a cafe open only to whites (no place at all for blacks to get food), and segregated cabs. As a matter of principle, we went to the Black and White cab stand. The name sounded progressive. The cabby was very patient with us: "You folk from the North, ain't you? Well, you see the thing is this, I can take you where you want to go, but if I do, won't be no cab for any colored folk. Why don't you folk just take one o' them nice Yellow cabs down there."

At that time segregation was the fundamental principle upon which all race relations were founded throughout the South. I remember in 1957 the Southeastern Council of the NCFR had its annual meeting in Tallahassee, Florida. We had a handful of black members. There was literally no public facility in Tallahassee that would accommodate us: not a hotel or motel or restaurant, not a civic center, and most shocking to me, not the University. We finally met in an Episcopal church whose pastor came from New Jersey. It feels as though centuries, rather than decades, have intervened in the social history of the United States since those days.

Everything at Georgia seemed tailor-made for me. I had this remarkable salary and rank, the established faculty were welcoming (and somewhat in awe of my Ivy League education), I had a third of my workload freed to develop research projects. But as a matter of fact it was one of the hardest periods of my life. The problems were not in the setting, but in my own expectations for myself. This was my big chance, at last, to do some significant work–under my own name. So I would sit down at my desk, hour after hour, with a set of sharpened pencils and a blank yellow pad trying to think of something really significant to study. I would covenant with myself that I would know neither food nor water nor woman until I had put something *important* on that pad. But in the end I would get nauseous and headachy and come crawling home–where, incidentally, my wife was already fully occupied with three rambunctious, demanding, preschool kids and didn't much need a fourth.

This was the period when I got into therapy as a client. My choice of therapist was fortunate. She had been one of Carl Rogers' early trainees at Chicago, and, in a relatively short time (I think I went for six sessions), I managed to work through my block and get some research going. The first project (on pre-school friendship formation) was a useful learning experience for me, but eventually fizzled. It led me, however, to a second project with a colleague, Stan Fowler, which established the foundations for the following twelve years of my scholarly life. We got a grant to study the normal sociosexual development of children.

At that time the Freudian theory of psychosexual development reigned supreme. But it did not square either with my personal experience or with my observation of how actual children developed in their relationship to the opposite sex. In particular, in the aborted study of preschool children's friendship patterns, I had observed informally that there was an unmistakable difference in the emotional tone children used in describing same-sex and cross-sex friends. This was not consistent with Freudian doctrine. Moreover, I never experienced Freud's famous Latency period. I *always* liked girls and suffered unrequited crushes during that post-Oedipal period when I was supposedly oblivious to the whole heterosexual issue. On checking it out with my students, I discovered that my own experience was replicated in most of their memories.

So Stan and I decided to challenge the paradigm and study children in the supposed latency period directly, using a mix of direct questions and projective techniques. The results were dramatic. Among the fifth and sixth graders we surveyed in that first study, romantic fantasy and heterosexually structured social interaction reigned supreme. Not a whiff of latency anywhere, among about 80% of the kids. There was, of course, the often observed segregation of the sexes at the lunch table and elsewhere, but far from being the result of lack of interest in the opposite sex, it grew out of the lack of social skills that made them self-conscious and awkward, effectively preventing their acting on their all too present awareness of the heterosexual potentials of these social situations. But in their fantasies and dreams and even in their conversations with same-sex peers, they exhibited a pervasive attraction to the opposite sex, and the majority explicitly looked forward to dating, courtship, and eventual marriage (Broderick & Fowler, 1961).

Meanwhile, having found no established congregation of Mormons nearer than Atlanta, 70 miles away, we invited the scattered members of the Church we were able to locate in that area to meet in our home every Sunday. Only a few months after we arrived in Athens, a formal Branch of the Church was formed, and I was called to be the first Branch President. We soon outgrew our living room, and, by the time we left in 1960, we were meeting in a rented hall and had purchased property for our own building. During those same four years, we had two additional children, girls, whom we always referred to as our Georgia Belles.

Penn State University

In 1960 when I was 28 years old, I was invited to join the faculty of the College of Home Economics at The Pennsylvania State University as a full professor. Fortunately, I had enough sense to insist on coming at the associate level. Although I had never developed a good nose for departmental politics, it did occur to me that a number of associate professors on that faculty had a good deal more seniority than I and that some of them just might feel some resentment over such an appointment. It took them nine years to get around to offering me the rank again, but I have never doubted that my decision at that time was the right one (and I can still take private pleasure in knowing that I *could* have been the youngest full professor in the profession if I had been foolish enough to accept the offer).

Based on the work that Stan Fowler and I had done at Georgia, I was able to get a grant from the U.S. Department of Mental Health to expand the research on children's normal sociosexual development. In the end we obtained data from 6,000 children from rural, urban, and suburban areas in three states, ages 3-18, plus interview data from a sub-sample of parents. It was a very comprehensive data set with direct questions, projective material, sociometric data, and cross-validation from both parents of some of the children. I feel that it is safe to claim that no one else before or since collected as much information on that aspect of children's development (Broderick, 1965, 1966a, 1966b, 1967, 1968a, 1968b, 1969; Heltsley & Broderick, 1969; Hicks & Broderick, 1970; Mahan & Broderick, 1969).

Since the topic was a "sexy" one, I suddenly found myself getting a lot of media attention. For the most part, this was a positive experience. I enjoyed finding my work the subject of articles in all of the news magazines not to mention *Life, Playboy,* and the *PTA Magazine.* I enjoyed the talk-show interviews. There are certain risks in this kind of exposure, of course, and early on I stubbed my toe on some of them. For example, in my very first encounter with a major news magazine, at the end of an extensive discussion of my findings, their social implications, and so forth, the reporter thanked me for a good interview, closed his notebook, and asked conversationally how Kathleen and I handled the issue of pre-teen romantic crushes among our own children. I guilelessly regaled him with a really funny incident that had occurred just that week when my 4th grade daughter had been "dumped" by the boy she loved. It didn't seem such a funny story when it turned up as the final two paragraphs of *Newsweek's* story on my research. For some time thereafter my name was Mud at home.

In that same interview, on the other hand, I learned about the power of the press in a more positive sense. At one point, the reporter had asked me if I considered myself an expert on this subject. Half in jest, since all the topic we were discussing was my own research, I said, "Well, I suppose on this subject I'd have to be considered the world's foremost authority." But even I was taken back at the sheer *hubris* of the headline in the *Newsweek* article "WORLD'S FOREMOST AUTHORITY ON CHILDREN'S ROMANCES SAYS. . . ." Even more surprising was my colleagues' reaction to this claim. Far from being offended, most of them saw that headline and said to themselves (and each other), "By golly, I hadn't realized that Broderick was such an authority." Before that, it had not occurred to me that professionals tend to believe what they read in *Newsweek* just as others do. That headline did more for my professional reputation than an article in *ASR* would have.

I did, of course, publish articles on my findings in professional journals, but I made a mistake in agreeing to publish the comprehensive monograph on the study in a foreign press. Rovalt Verlag of Hamburg, a respected scholarly press, invited me to have the book brought out as one volume in a truly impressive series on human sexuality to which virtually every European and American scholar in the field had committed a volume. Through arrangements with other publishers, the series was to come out not only in German, but also in French, Italian, Dutch, and, of course, English. The German, French, Italian, and Dutch versions came out as promised (Broderick, 1970, 1972a, 1972b). Negotiations on the English version broke down, however, and, alas, my first scholarly monograph never came out in the language of the great majority of my professional colleagues

Clinical Training: Marriage and Family Therapist

About that time, I came due for a sabbatical. I applied for a Fulbright to go to Ghana and teach for a year at the University of Accra. The application was accepted and both my family and I were looking forward to a truly enlarging experience in a new cultural setting. (Also, the family was not unmoved by the fact that visiting faculty were treated royally with housemaids and cooks and private swimming pools.) But then we began to see disturbing reports from West Africa. There were anti-colonial uprisings in the interior. One white missionary couple was massacred less than a hundred miles from the University. There were reports of student unrest. Although we were assured that we would be perfectly safe, I simply could not bring myself to put my family at potential risk. So instead I applied for a post-doctoral clinical fellowship to be trained as a Marriage and Family Therapist at the University of Minnesota. As it happened, my old friend and mentor, Harold Feldman of Cornell, replaced us in the Fulbright spot. The Feldmans had a life-enhancing, pampered year of tropical stimulation and delight. We got the coldest, longest, dreariest winter in memory in Minnesota. For the family, it was a miserable experience, and I think they never quite forgave me for the switch. A few years later I was recruited as a candidate for Reuben Hill's spot at The University of Minnesota, probably the most prestigious position in the field at that time, if only because of the stature of the predecessor. When I shared the exciting news of the invitation with my always fully supportive wife, she smiled encouragingly and said, "I think that would be a wonderful opportunity for you, Dear, and I want you to know the children and I will write to you every week."

As for me, weather aside, the year in Minnesota had been a stimulating one. I had been doing marriage counseling for a number of years without the benefit of much training or supervision. This was the norm in those days. There was no licensure anywhere and little formal training available. People just worked out their own approaches without anyone telling them what they could or couldn't, should or shouldn't do. But when I became aware of the formal training program at Minnesota with Jerry Neubeck and Dick Hay, I figured I might as well take advantage of it. The hardest part of that year was the return to the lowly status of student. One forgets that the respect freely offered professors in a university community is strictly a function of rank. Students, by contrast, are treated condescendingly by gum-chewing departmental secretaries and are ranked as unemployed bad risks by bank personnel.

The academic part of the program was old stuff for me, but I learned a lot from my clinical internship at the University Hospital and the VA hospital outpatient clinics, and I became facile at interpreting MMPI's. Most encouraging was the discovery that the clinical style I had already developed survived the scrutiny of my more experienced supervisors.

Publishing

Coincidentally, that year I was invited to a workshop sponsored by the recently formed Sex Education and Information Council of the United States, better know by its acronym, SEICUS. Mary Calderone had assembled a board of experts to help coordinate and shape the national resurgence of interest in getting better programs of sex education in the public schools. At that time, most schools had a menstrual education film for the 6th grade girls, and that was about all. The purpose of this workshop was to put together a resource handbook for the new breed of sex educators, because there was really nothing out there for them to draw upon. I was appalled at the stuff they had assembled for us to review for inclusion in this new source book. It was scientifically inaccurate, badly out-of-date, and heavily burdened with sermonizing. I'm afraid I was characteristically tactless in my outspoken negative opinion of the material and managed to alienate nearly everyone there, including the usually patient chairman, David Mace. I remember leaving the conference feeling that all I had accomplished was making an ass of myself. "Broderick," I said to myself, "when are you ever going to learn to keep your mouth shut! These people did not really want to hear your opinion. All you managed to do was spit in their soup." No one could have been more surprised than I when a few months later Jessie Bernard, who was head of the SEICUS publication committee, called me and asked if I would be willing to be the editor of this source book. I said, " Can I throw out all of the articles you have already collected and start fresh?" She said "yes." The result was the first book in English with my name on it, *The Individual, Sex and Society,* co-edited with Jessie Bernard (Broderick & Bernard, 1969). Putting that book together was a good experience, and the advance they gave me for taking the job saved the family from an otherwise enveloping poverty that had resulted from trying to maintain two residences and live on a Sabbatical income.

Editor

We returned to Penn State for three more years that turned out to be productive ones for me. In addition to continuing to publish research papers, I was invited to succeed Marvin Sussman as the editor of the *Journal of Marriage and the Family*. That was an exciting time to be editor of the most prestigious journal in the family field. Family scholarship was exploding in every direction during the late '60s. After a year of trying to keep up with all of the new developments, it occurred to me that it would probably be helpful to publish a review of the decade's achievements. The result was the first *Decade Review* (Broderick, 1971a), which, it pleases me to note, was imitated by later editors and so became only the first in a series of decade reviews in the *Journal*. Another innovation that I believe was a step forward was the establishment of an international section and editor. U.S. family scholars tended to be altogether too insular, and this was intended as a partial corrective.

Issue on Feminism. By all odds, the most hair-raising (actually hair-graying) experience as editor of the *Journal* grew out of a decision to sponsor an issue featuring the new, and at that time somewhat militant and raw, feminist family scholarship. It was a well-intended effort to expose our readers to a challenging new approach to the analysis of matters familial; I suppose it constituted a watershed event in the history of the field, but as a personal experience it was simply horrific.

I commissioned a distinguished feminist scholar to edit the special edition, gave her the page constraints, a number of copies of the *JMF* author's style guidelines, and a firm deadline for the edited manuscripts to be in my hands for final copy-editing. She didn't come within a month of meeting any of the deadlines, and she commissioned twice as many papers as I had authorized. The bibliographic references at the end of each article were unfinished or absent, the manuscripts were single-spaced, frequently written on both sides of the paper, and coffee-stained. They were peppered with four lettered words and, even worse from an editor's perspective, poor grammar and sentence structure. About 3/4 of the pieces had no scholarship to them; they were just hate pieces against men and the patriarchal establishment. The remaining 1/4 I thought had some merit, though even these needed an extraordinary amount of editorial work to put them in shape for publication. I told her which ones I would agree to publish; she told me that I would damn well publish them all or she would pull them all. Mind you, we were already running two months late on getting out this quarterly issue and in jeopardy of losing our Second Class status with the post office if we delayed much longer. It was an editor's worst nightmare–these women were not into compromise for the good of all. As far as they were concerned, the *Journal* (as surrogate for patriarchal society) owed women for thousands of years of injustice. From my point of view, it was blackmail, pure and simple.

In the end, I absolutely refused to publish a few of the articles and insisted on strongly editing some of the others to try to bring them into some approximation of acceptable journal style. We finally had to give up two entire issues of the *Journal* to accommodate all of the pages of manuscript that were left. When the issues finally reached *Journal* readers, they were not charmed with this, which seemed to them as unaccountable dedication of many pages to material of uneven quality. Reuben Hill, for one, charged me with "selling out" to the feminists.

In retrospect, I still think it was a good idea to expose our traditional readership to the winds of feminist critique that were beginning to make themselves felt in the early '70s and that have since truly reshaped the field of family scholarship. But the actual experience literally turned my hair white. I try to think of my snowy crown as a marker on the path of gender liberation.

Student Revolts

At Penn State I maintained my active participation in Mormon affairs and eventually ended up presiding over the Central Pennsylvania District of the Church. I was also more active than I have ever been before or since in campus politics. At various points I chaired the Graduate Faculty of the University and the Academic Standards Committee of the University Senate. This was the late '60s and early '70s, and, like other campuses, we had to face a student revolt. Students occupied buildings and tried to burn down the ROTC Building. I remember sitting up all night in one of the entrances to our college office building to try to discourage students from setting it to the torch. Other faculty sat in other doorways. We were not armed; we didn't even have any way of communicating with each other, but we believed that the students would not want to hurt anyone just to make a statement about the establishment. It was a scary night, but nobody came to torch our building (although there were fires set elsewhere). The University President fared less well. A mob of students took an ax to his front door, and, while he, his wife, and his eighty-year-old mother fled out the back door, they entered and ransacked the house. The next day we had a full complement of state militia, armed, in white helmets and spats, guarding the campus. It was just after the Kent State tragedy, and, given that we were in very similar circumstances, it was probably luck that no one got hurt.

Those were interesting days on many campuses. I remember the day the students shouted down the Faculty Senate and grabbed the microphone from the President. Some of the younger faculty were very sympathetic to their cause and style of pursuing such goals. It became necessary to disband the Senate for a period of months.

The spirit of the times also pervaded the classroom. I remember one graduate seminar when I asked the students to assume that the student revolt had fully triumphed, the establishment was overthrown, and local student soviets ruled supreme. What, if any, of the old society's norms would be worthy of preservation? After some heated debate, they agreed that there would be no laws against murder or rape because in order to support such laws you would have to reinstitute the whole hated apparatus of society: police, jails, judges, governments–better to suffer a few murders and rapes. It is a tribute to the depth of commitment to ecological values and the Zero-Population dogma that they would have defined only one act as a capital offense: having more than two children. The revolutionary passions and certitudes of those days are difficult to credit in these more laid back times, but they were fiercely real then.

University of Southern California

In 1970 I got an offer to come to the University of Southern California to head up their PhD program in Marriage and Family Therapy. It was housed in the department of sociology, a real anomaly then and now, but that's where James Peterson had his academic appointment when he started the pioneering program in the early 1950s. When Jim moved over to help establish a new School of Gerontology in 1969, the department had to decide if they wanted to keep this clinical option as part of their offering. There were arguments on both sides, but persuasive on the plus side was the fact that, then and now, some of the best students who applied to the department were attracted by the opportunity to be trained as a marriage and family therapist while earning a respectable PhD in Sociology. So they decided that if they could find a bona fide sociologist who also was qualified to train clinicians, they would retain the program. In the interview, it appears that I was able to persuade them that my somewhat marginal credentials as a sociologist, or, for that matter, as a clinical trainer, were sufficient for the purpose. Perhaps it helped that I brought the *Journal of Marriage and the Family* with me. In any case, in the fall of 1971 I returned to the area where I had grown up, where all of my relatives still lived, as Professor of Sociology and Executive Director of the PhD Program in Marriage and Family Therapy at the University of Southern California.

It had not been an easy decision to leave Penn State. It would not be overstating the case to say I had it made there. I had tenure, quality colleagues, and an ongoing PhD program in Family Relationships that attracted excellent students and was regarded as one of the strongest in the field. Moreover, at that point in my career I was heavily involved in campus politics (for example, being a member of the President's "Kitchen Cabinet," a circle of informal advisors that had a great deal of influence on what went on at the University). State College, Penmnsylvania, was a beautiful place to live and raise a family. Taking it all together, I asked myself: why would I want to move? Then it hit me. At 39 years I was already feeling seduced by the siren song of a serene and certain future. That settled the question; I had better move on to new challenges before hardening of the arteries set in. And besides, the children could get to know their grandparents and cousins.

The new position was a challenge. I don't suppose I had ever before in my life felt a greater need to master an unfamiliar literature in a shorter time, so as to bring myself "up to speed" as both a sociologist and a clinical trainer. Because, to be perfectly honest, although I knew a great deal about the family and human sexuality, there were oceans of pertinent information that a competent, all-purpose sociologist might be expected to know that were not within my scope of expertise. Moreover, I had a great deal of clinical material to cover before I could feel comfortable as a graduate mentor to these students. It would only be a slight exaggeration to say that the move forced me to take a second, informal, graduate degree in the areas of my deficits. I liked that.

Organizational Roles. At USC I managed to keep out of local campus politics, but got involved, instead, in the politics of the profession. Once my term as editor of *JMF* was finished, I managed to find myself elected, first, President of the Southern California Association of Marriage and Family Counselors (1974), then, President of the National Council on Family Relations (1976), and, finally, President of the Association of Mormon Counselors and Psychotherapists (1982).

I took particular pleasure in serving as President of NCFR because that organization had always been, and remains, my professional home base. Most of the people who have been important in my professional life are regularly attending members. I think I have only missed one annual meeting (1975–I had the flu) since 1960. There is not much that one can do of lasting significance in a one-year term of office, but I think fondly of three accomplishments that year. First, I was able to persuade the organization to sponsor the first few years of operation of the *Journal of Family History* under the editorship of Tamara Hareven. To a small extent, I was a sponsor of the then new and now thriving sub-discipline of family history. Second, I represented NCFR and American family scholars in helping the Australian Family Life Movement, under John Robison's leadership, celebrate their fiftieth anniversary. And third, I held the very first nonalcoholic President's reception. The event turned out to be a big success, but up to the last hour there were rumblings that the traditionalists and heavy drinkers would either blackball it, or usurp it, bringing their own liquor to spike the punch. With the money we saved on drinks, we were able to afford a very nice buffet indeed.

The seventies marked something of an intellectual watershed for me. Prior to that period most of my scholarly work had centered on children's sociosexual development. I had always been interested in family theory, but until I assigned myself the task of reviewing the family theory literature of the 1960s for the decade review (Broderick, 1971a), I had never done any serious writing in this area. I believe I am correct in stating that my 1971 article, "Beyond the Five Conceptual Frameworks: A Decade of Development in Family Theory" (Broderick, 1971b) was the first to bring the new family systems approach to the attention of mainline family scholars. Prior to that, it had pretty much been confined to family therapists. Later that year Reuben Hill came out with a paper on family systems theory, comparing it to his own developmental approach. However, it was published in a Belgian Journal and not many American scholars saw it. Towards the end of the decade, I was one of the participants in the major theory construction project headed by Wesley Burr, Reuben Hill, Ivan Nye, and Ira Reiss that eventuated in the two-volume handbook, *Contemporary Theories About the Family* (1979a; 1979b). I had a chapter, coauthored with a graduate student, in the first volume that attempted to summarize the family process theory of socialization (Broderick & Pulliam-Krager, 1979c). For Volume II, Jim Smith and I tried the more challenging job of attempting to present a digest of the general systems approach to family processes (Broderick & Smith, 1979d). Subsequently, I have attempted to follow up on those initial efforts with an article on family process theory (Broderick, 1990a) in Jetsey Sprey's theory book, and finally with a book-length treatment of the subject, *Understanding Family Process: The Basics of Family Systems Theory* (Broderick, 1993).

Besides theory, my interests included the clinical branch of family scholarship *The Therapeutic Triangle,* (Broderick, 1983), historical aspects of family therapy (Broderick & Schrader, 1980), and a historical study of the field of family studies in the 1930s (Broderick, 1988a). I also wrote a reasonably successful trade book entitled *Couples* (Broderick, 1979a) and a college text that had four editions, *Marriage and the Family,* (Broderick, 1979, 1984, 1988, 1992), and a text, *Understanding Families* (Broderick, 1993).

I've continued as an active Mormon, serving as a Bishop and as a Stake President (the next higher administrative level over bishops), and I even wrote a book on marriage for the Mormon audience, *One Flesh, One Heart* (Broderick, 1986).

As one of the more senior statesmen in the field, I get invited to do a fair number of workshops, keynote addresses, perspective pieces, and chapters in other people's books. I even get invited to do commencement addresses from time to time, surely one of the stiffest challenges for any speaker. I continue to head up the Marriage and Family Therapy program in the Department of Sociology at USC.

As one with deep roots in the field, I am easily seduced into projecting my own view of its future (although, as a social historian I am painfully aware of how mis-aimed most future-telling turns out to be). Perhaps the most prevalent contemporary view is that the future belongs to the feminist and conflict theorists and to the postmodern constructivists. As my publications document, I am betting that the most profitable direction for future research and theory lies in the investigation of what Hess and Handel, years ago, called the psychosocial interior of the family. The immediate challenge is to discover the metarules governing the patterning of family processes through the careful observation of families in real time (that is, over the course of seconds, minutes, and hours, rather than merely in developmental time or in cross-sectional stop-time). In my view, that is the frontier that beckons. The effort to understand how families operate in real time started with the observations of family therapists, and I trust that this group of professional family observers and manipulators will continue to make important discoveries. But the future belongs to the new breed of well-tooled, eclectic, hardheaded, family research scholars. They will discover still better ways to probe the interior of families and to take advantage of the enormous laboratory provided by the variety of family forms and the high rate of family formation, dissolution, and reformation that is prevalent in this historic period. I see a generation of them just emerging from graduate school, and, like all commencement speakers everywhere, I am encouraged that the future of the field is in good hands.

REFERENCES

Broderick, C.B. (1965). Social heterosexual development among urban negroes and whites. *Journal of Marriage and the Family, 27*, 2, 200-203.

Broderick, C.B. (1966a). Sexual behavior among preadolescents. *Journal of Social Issues, 22*, 2, 6-21.

Broderick, C.B. (1966b). Socio-sexual development in a suburban community. *Journal of Sex Research, 2*, 1, 1-24.

Broderick, C.B. (1967). Going steady: The beginning of the end. In S.M. Forbes & R.H.L. Wilson (Eds.), *Teenage marriage and divorce* (pp. 21-24). Berkeley, CA: Diable Press.

Broderick, C.B. (1968a). Preadolescent sexual behavior. *Medical Aspects of Human Sexuality, 2*, 20-29.

Broderick, C.B. (1968b). Dating and mating among teenagers. *Medical Aspects of Human Sexuality, 2*, 16-19.

Broderick, C.B. (1969). Normal sociosexual development. In C.B. Broderick & J. Bernard, *The individual, sex and society* (pp. 23-40). Baltimore: John Hopkins Press.

Broderick, C.B. (1970). *Sexuelle entwicklang in kindheit und jungend.* Hamburg: Rowohlt.

Broderick, C.B. (Ed.) (1971a). *A decade of research and action on the family.* Minneapolis: National Council on Family Relations.

Broderick, C.B. (1971b). Beyond the five conceptual frameworks: A decade of development in family theory. *Journal of Marriage and the Family, 33*, 1, 139-160.

Broderick, C.B. (1972a). *Kind, jeugd en seksualiteit. Utrecht AulaBoeken.* (Dutch Translation)

Broderick, C.B. (1972b). *La Sessualita nell'jnfanzia e nell'adolescenza.* Milano: Informazione Sessuale Bompiani (Italian Translation).

Broderick, C.B. (1979a). *Couples: How to confront problems and maintain loving relationships.* New York: Simon & Schuster. (Paperback, Touchstone Press).

Broderick, C.B. (1979b). *Marriage and the family.* Englewood Cliffs, NJ: Prentice-Hall.

Broderick, C.B. (1983). *The therapeutic triangle: A source book on marital therapy.* Beverly Hills, CA: Sage Publications.

Broderick, C.B. (1984). *Marriage and the family.* 2nd Edition. Englewood Cliffs, NJ: Prentice-Hall.

Broderick, C.B. (1986). *One flesh, one heart.* Salt Lake City, UT: Deseret Books.

Broderick, C.B. (1988a). To arrive where we started: The field of family studies in the 1930's. *Journal of Marriage and the Family, 50*, 3, 569-584.

Broderick, C.B. (1988b). *Marriage and the family.* 3rd Edition. Englewood Cliffs, NJ: PrenticeHall.
Broderick, C.B. (1990). Family process theory. In J. Sprey (Ed.), *Theorizing about the family* (pp. 171-206). Newbury Park, CA: Sage.
Broderick, C.B. (1992). *Marriage and the family.* 4th Edition. Englewood Cliffs, NJ: PrenticeHall.
Broderick, C.B. (1993). *Understanding families.* Newbury Park, CA: Sage.
Broderick, C.B. & Bernard, J. (Eds.) (1969). *The individual, sex and society.* Baltimore: John Hopkins Press.
Broderick, C.B. & Fowler, S.F. (1961). New patterns of relationships between the sexes among preadolescents. *Marriage and Family Living, 23,* 1, 27-39.
Broderick, C.B. & Pulliam-Krager, H. (1979). Family process and child outcomes. In W.R. Burr, R. Hill, F. I. Nye, & I. L. Reiss (Eds.), *Contemporary theories about the family.* Vol. 1 (pp. 604-614). New York: Free Press.
Broderick, C.B. & Rowe, G.A. (1968). Scale of Preadolescent Heterosexual Development. *Journal of Marriage and the Family, 30,* 1, 97-101.
Broderick, C.B. & Schrader, S. (1980). The History of Professional Marriage and Family Therapy. In A.S. Gurman & D.P. Kniskern (Eds.), *Handbook on family therapy,* Vol. 2. (pp. 3-40). New York: Brunner/Mazel.
Broderick, C.B. & Smith, J. (1979). Systems theory and the family. In W.R. Burr, R. Hill, F.I. Nye., & I.L. Reiss (Eds.), *Contemporary theories about the family,* Vol. 2. (pp.112-129). New York: Free Press.
Burr, W.R., Hill, R., Nye, F. I., & Reiss, I.L. (Eds.) (1979a). *Contemporary theories about the family.* Vol. 1. New York: Free Press.
Burr, W.R., Hill, R., Nye, F. I., & Reiss, I. L. (Eds.) (1979b). *Contemporary theories about the family,* Vol. 2. New York: Free Press.
Heltsley, M.E. & Broderick, C.B. (1969). Religiosity and premarital sexual permissiveness: Reexamination of Reiss's traditionalism proposition. *Journal of Marriage and the Family, 31,* 3, 441-443.
Hicks, M.W. & Broderick, C.B. (1970). The functions of sex in courtship. In J.M. Henslin (Ed.), *The sociology of sex.* Edwardsville, IL: Southern Illinois University Press.
Mahan, C.S. & Broderick, C.B. (1969). Human reproduction. In C.B. Broderick & J. Bernard, *The individual, sex and society* (pp. 175-220). Baltimore: John Hopkins Press.
Shope, D.F. & Broderick, C.B. (1967). Level of sexual experience and predicted adjustment in marriage. *Journal of Marriage and the Family. 29,* 3, 424-427.
Zimmerman, C.C. & Broderick, C.B. (1954). Nature and role of informal family groups. *Marriage and Family Living, 16,* 2, 107-111.
Zimmerman, C.C. & Broderick, C.B. (1956). The family self protective system. In Zimmerman, C.C. & L. Cervantes, *Marriage and the family* (pp. 91-100). Chicago: H. Regnery.

How I Got This Way: Memoirs of a Liberal

Margaret Feldman

KEYWORDS. Autobiography, sexism, family policy, women's movement

INTRODUCTION

Any story of my development in the field of the family has to be thought of as inextricably entwined with that of my husband, Harold Feldman. When we met in 1943, we were attracted to each other because of our similar interests and social work degrees. Right at the beginning we started collaborating on a talk he had contracted to give, and we continued to collaborate until his final passing at the Groves conference in New Orleans in 1988.

Early Years

Of course, our early years and our early family experiences also play a part in how we turn out. My father and mother, Frederick Eichbauer and Lillian Fowler, both trained physical education teachers, met on a playground in Pittsburgh when he was the director and she was the girls' worker. My younger sister, Betty, and I were both born in Pennsylvania, but we moved around to several cities as my father was called during WWI to provide recreational activities for the troops.

In 1920 we finally ended up in the Los Angeles area of California where my father had a variety of teaching and playground jobs. My mother did not work out of the home, but both parents were concerned that their two girls have a good start in life. Thus, our education began at home. When I would have been ready for the 2nd grade, we moved to a new area. My mother judged the local school to be inadequate and decided to run a private school in our garage. Schooling at home without schoolmates would not provide the interaction with children we needed, so a private school was the obvious solution. I did go to a new school, which opened up in our area, for 5th and 6th grade.

Only about 10 to 15 children were in the school, but we experienced an educated and innovative mother-teacher who worked–but worked at home with us. One of the innovative activities of the school was a school club. Since I was the oldest in the school, I was the President and, at the early age of about 8, learned about *Robert's Rules of Order* (1915) and how to conduct a meeting. We also did folk dancing, which was a specialty my mother had learned on a trip to Europe. That trip, which came after her graduation as a physical education major from Oberlin, was a highlight in her life. For her, and us, folk dancing was a way to develop an interest in people from other countries. I was always proud that my mother had a college education, and I found her knowledge and interest in helping others an inspiration.

When it came time for me to go to junior high school, I commuted to Los Angeles with my father to the school where he was teaching. I spent three happy years there, participating in the homeroom intramural sports for girls and boys that my father promoted, and becoming a cheerleader. My sister spent two years there.

In 1929 my father was appointed Superintendent of the Pacific Lodge Boys Home in Girard, now Woodland Hills, California. Mother became Assistant Superintendent in charge of all health, diet, and housekeeping activities. Although my sister and I attended the local high school, we lived far from the town and really did not participate in high school activities. Instead, we participated in activities around the Lodge, learning how to keep score for boy's games, and accompanied the band. Of course, we spent a lot of time on our studies and got good grades, but we were also learning a great deal about the field of social work.

The boys at the Lodge had families who were unable to care for them. My father often talked to us about the "broken families" that the boys came from and told us how difficult it was for their families to come to see them. My mother was able to get health care for the boys, many of whom had come to the Lodge in poor physical shape. The probation officers who had placed the boys at the Lodge used to talk about the wonders that had been accomplished with the health care provided and the activities scheduled. My father's philosophy of changing behavior was based on structured group activities with feedback and instruction, which made it possible for a child to succeed and develop self-esteem.

The sixty boys at the Lodge were divided into four teams, selected to be as equal as possible, with A and B squads. The teams played an intensive intramural schedule for the four seasons: basketball, football, baseball, and track. Boys from A squad coached the B squad and encouraged the younger boys, and each squad cheered for the other since points from both squads contributed equally to the final score for the team. Each season ended with a banquet at which the winning team members were the guests of honor and all the rest were the waiters, planners, and entertainers. Every boy attended and had a part. This philosophy of involvement and sharing created a wonderful spirit among the boys and did bring behavior change because the workers as well as the boys reinforced it.

I was always close to my father, and he taught me many things about the world of business, social work, and life itself. Since Mother and Dad were supposed to cover for each other on days off, we often had happy weekends and times with each parent alone.

EARLY ADULT YEARS

College

Because of my involvement with the Lodge and my parents' profession, it was clear that social work was what I should also do. In 1933 I entered California Christian College, which had been recommended to my father by Mr. George Pepperdine, the President of the Lodge Board of Directors (and later the organizer of Pepperdine College). This was depression time and the College was in very bad financial straits–students were being given scholarships to assist professors and the professors were to use the student help instead of having a salary. Mr. Charles Chapman, a benefactor of the College for whom the College was later renamed, had a ranch but was unable to sell his produce, so he would bring crates of avocados and artichokes to school for our meals. I became active in student government and in my senior year was elected student body president, the first woman to hold that office. In spite of my closeness to my father, he did not seem to approve of my running for student body president. When I was elected, I asked him why he had not been more supportive. He said, "I didn't want to see you hurt." That was one of the first times I really realized how women were supposed to stay out of leadership roles.

Even though my parents were employed and were able to pay my tuition, room, and board, the experiences of the depression made a strong mark on me. When I went away to graduate school at Western Reserve in Cleveland, my parents did not want me to accept a position with the Youth Corp because they said other students needed it more. I was studying social work with a major in group work. As graduate students doing fieldwork, we learned about multiracial and multiethnic communities and the many varieties of families. I worked in the Polish area and learned about the labor movement since the Steel Workers Organizing Committee was meeting each Sunday in our local parish church. During the two years at WRU, I was exposed to Freudian thinking but in general rejected it. I was much more comfortable with a cognitive approach and felt that the problems so many of our clients were experiencing were the results of their family and external factors in their environments. I fully rejected the idea that women were passive.

After completing my master's degree, I went to San Francisco to work in the Italian neighborhood in an old fashioned settlement house. After one year, I went to Fairbanks, Alaska, and found that with a degree in group work I could not get a job because they were looking for child welfare workers. This was an early contact with credentialing, which seemed too rigid to me. I got a job as a waitress but never told anyone I had a master's degree; a college degree was already enough to make people think I was strange. In frontier Alaska in 1940 they were building an airfield to protect us from the Japanese. Experiencing the life of a shift worker gave me empathy for low-income workers, which has been invaluable in shaping my thinking.

But I did have a professional degree and wanted to use it. After a year in Alaska, I got a job in Amarillo, Texas, as Director of the Social Settlement for Girls. There were very poor families in Amarillo at that time, and I especially remember one family living in a cellar dug out of the plains. Many girls were getting pregnant.

Marriage

During the first winter in Amarillo, Pearl Harbor changed our lives forever. A new army force moved in to town and with it came Harold Feldman. In 1943, we were married in Washington, D.C., where Harold had been sent for three months in the Officer's Training School. After a preliminary three-month tour in Omaha, he was sent back to D.C. for special training as Personnel Officer. In 1944 he was sent to Indianapolis to work in a unit training men to read.

I was able to get a job as a school social worker in the Indianapolis city schools. To the children, my job was truant officer. I worked closely with the school nurse, and we saw the families whose mothers had to go to work leaving younger children in charge of older ones who had to stay home from school. Housing in those days in my area of Indianapolis was very poor with outside privies.

Our daughter, Dorothy, was born in 1945, shortly before the war was over. When Harold got out of the army, we moved to Michigan where he attended graduate school in psychology. His major was clinical psychology, and, during one summer, he worked on the "Assessment of Men" project at Michigan as Urie Bronfenbrenner's graduate assistant. In 1948, as an ABD, Harold went to Cornell in Ithaca, New York, to work with Urie on a large multidisciplinary project on social creativity. Harold finished his PhD in 1952.

Our son Dick was born in 1947, and Larry arrived in 1951. During these years of being at home with children, I was more and more restless and depressed. It became clear that I would have to spend my life in therapy or else get a job. I started as a paid Play Lady at the local hospital's children's ward.

Beginning in 1953 and until 1962, I ran a summer camp for children based on the group work principles from my social work days. More than a hundred children experienced this camp, some several summers, and many consider it one of the best experiences in their childhood. My children, like my sister and myself in our childhood, had an activity run by their mother, but with playmates. Dorothy grew up and became a junior counselor at the camp, which provided her with valuable leadership training. Dick also became old enough to be involved in camp leadership during the last year we had it, but for him, the greatest benefit was an abiding interest and knowledge about birds and the out-of-doors.

Larry also finally became a junior counselor but his greatest claim to fame, in my mind, was that he became my computer assistant during the analysis of the data for my thesis in the summer of 1963. He grew up to be a teacher of math and computers.

In 1954, I was able to get a teaching job at a semi-rural school with 31 first and second grade children. Trying to provide experiences for each child at his/her level was very difficult, and I enlisted parents to help. I only lasted until after Thanksgiving because I came down with hepatitis. On the basis of that semester teaching, and my prior years with the Indianapolis schools, in 1955-56 I was able to get a one-year position at Cortland State Teacher's College, while a faculty member was on sabbatical. College teaching seemed much more compatible than elementary school.

In 1956, Harold received a Fulbright Teaching Award, and we went to Ceylon for a year. During the long vacations offered by universities following the English system, we had marvelous opportunities to travel within India and by sea to Japan. Returning from Japan, we had to drop our expected visit to Saigon because the Suez Canal was closed and our connecting ship had to go around Africa.

Cornell

During the year in Ceylon, I turned 40 and made the decision to enter Cornell in the fall of 1957 to work toward a PhD with the goal of college teaching. Only one other wife we knew of had gone back to school for such a degree. I loved being in school again. Harold and the children were very supportive of my work, even though it did require more cooperation on their part. Although my interests were very similar to Harold's, it seemed I should not be in his department. I majored in educational psychology but worked as a graduate assistant in the general psychology department with a number of different professors. My thesis was on programmed learning, and I became an advocate of behavior modification as useful in the armamentarium of the classroom teacher and the therapist, but not to be used exclusively (Feldman, 1964; Feldman & Feldman, 1965). I finally received my PhD in 1964 with Harold in the procession and the rest of the family watching. It was a family achievement.

During my three years as an active student at Cornell, Harold and I learned from each other, he about behaviorism and I about therapy and personality theory. It was an excellent mix, which benefited us both. During this time, I attended all the colloquia offered by psychology, sociology, and family studies. One I recall very clearly. It was a two or three day seminar on Talcott Parsons and his theory of the four-fold table of family functioning in which women were clearly in their separate realm. It was widely applauded, but not by me. I continued to believe that men also had to participate in the socio-emotional aspects of interpersonal relationships and that women could be, and were, instrumental. How else did the work of the family get done?

Ithaca College

In 1960, as an ABD, I got a position teaching educational and child psychology at Ithaca College. It was a wonderful job teaching at the college. Working with and knowing the students and the faculty was a joy. After a few years, when the college wanted to have a social work course and later a minor in social work, I became the coordinator. My experiences in supervising field placements for students gave me an opportunity to learn about the social services of the community and to know people in all areas of Ithaca.

The college went through its amazing growth streak while I was part of it. I served on many committees, including the long-term planning committee. While on that committee, I stood firmly for a college of strong professional training at the bachelor or master's level, with a strong liberal arts background. When compared to the alternatives of a mini-university for professions only, or a medium sized liberal arts college, this middle ground seemed best. This was the final choice that the college has followed. I have always been proud of my association with a college which has done so well with its mix of professional and liberal arts.

THE MIDDLE YEARS

Harold was an excellent therapist and psychologist but wanted to broaden his knowledge. He spent one year reading and preparing himself to become a family sociologist. At that time at Cornell, and most other land grant colleges, the Home Economics Departments divided their departments into child development to be taught by psychologists, and family relations to be taught by sociologists. Harold and I agreed that this division was unfortunate and not like real life. We became early advocates of life-span psychology and of the importance of parental and family influences, as well as community, on children as they grew. Harold's interests were always with "people who made it," those who would be expected to fail because of their family or living situation but who became successful in their lives. His whole research career was directed toward aspects of this idea. The summary of his life work, which he prepared after his retirement in 1981, was entitled, "People Who Made It."

Harold's interests were always an influence on my thinking, and several of his studies were planned as we took long trips together, sharing insights, experiences, and theoretical ideas. In 1957, when we returned from Ceylon, Harold began a series of studies on marriage. The first was a cross sectional study sponsored by NIMH on the development of marriage over the life cycle.

The Influence of Ghana

In 1964 Harold had a second sabbatical, and I took leave from Ithaca College to go to Ghana for a year to experience another culture. I taught psychology classes there and did some research on eidetic imagery. It was a useful year in experiencing life in a socialist country with a very anti-American administration. We made friends with Eastern European communist teaching staff from the Kwame Nkruma Ideological Institute which shared our town, and had most interesting peaceful co-existence in afternoons on the beach. We greatly enjoyed the people we lived among and worked with as well as learning the pitfalls of cross-cultural research.

When we returned, Harold turned to the topic of poverty. He had always been interested in the experiential aspects of learning and in his classes on poverty used some unusual techniques to get students involved. He had his college students go to spend a weekend with a welfare family in Ithaca and had welfare mothers come to class to instruct the students. During the winter session of 1966, Harold arranged trips for students to New York City and Morgan Town, West Virginia, to observe the situation of people who were accepting welfare and to learn from those people. It was an eye-opening experience for all of us who went.

Pursuing this interest in welfare and especially welfare women, Harold designed a very large study to determine what characteristics of welfare women's lives, personalities, and communities were related to their getting off welfare. The proposal to carry out this work was not accepted the first time he submitted it to HEW so he divided it into two parts: one for HHS and the other for the Department of Labor. Much to his surprise, both were funded, and, in 1968, he had two very large studies going in three different communities: urban, rural, and rurban (his term for small towns like Ithaca). The experimental questions, in addition to the welfare question, were to determine the effect of father absence on teenagers and the effect of low-income mothers' working on their teenage children. These studies came to a conclusion in 1971. That summer we worked on the statistics with a large crew of assistants, and that fall we both had sabbaticals which we spent writing up the results of the studies (Feldman & Feldman, 1971, 1972, 1974; Feldman, 1975a; 1975b; Feldman, 1973).

In December of 1971 Harold was invited to Washington, D.C. to talk with grants managers and other welfare researchers and to share the results of studies. I went along, and it was very interesting to see that the grants people all wanted to be doing research while the researchers all were interested in the policies their research might influence. This visit to Washington was influential in our decision to come to Washington in 1978 on our next sabbatical and whetted our interest in federal policies that could improve the lives of families.

Until the late 1960s, I had not participated in Harold's professional meetings, but, as the children grew up, it was possible for us to be away at the same time. I started to attend meetings of the Groves Conference and the National Council on Family Relations. At these meetings I was a "spouse," joining in discussions and participating in workshops, but I did not feel I was a real member. In 1972, Harold became the president of Groves Conference, and I joined him in making plans for the three meetings of his presidency. It was during those years that I felt I became a member of the "family field." The Groves Conference in Dubrovnik in 1975 was a high point in our lives, and in the lives of many others. We had an opportunity to meet people from both east and west.

Studying Family Life Cycle and Family Careers

Our interest in the international study of families was always present, but our stays in Ceylon and Ghana and our other travels heightened that interest. In 1973, we attended the International Sociological Association's Committee on Family Research in Paris, France, and found ourselves very stimulated by the papers that added new dimensions to the ordinary conceptualizations of the family life cycle. As a result of our reactions to those papers, we wrote our paper, "The Family Life Cycle: Some Suggestions for Recycling," which appeared in *Journal of Marriage and the Family* (Feldman & Feldman, 1975). We thought this paper was our most important contribution to the field.

In the paper, we distinguished between the family life cycle and the family career. The family life cycle is the lineage of families, with different roles being filled by different people as families are formed; babies are born who in their turn become parents and grandparents, etc. The family career is the lifetime career of a person who starts as a baby, becomes a parent, and ultimately a grandparent through his/her life.

Because of the wide differences in timing of family changes, which had been documented at the Paris conference, we thought it was essential to distinguish between various sub-careers of the family career. We recognized that the active sexual career, marriage, parenthood, and, finally, what we called the filial career could all be separated out and looked at independently. This breakdown makes it possible to more nearly describe the varieties of families of today. Many individuals begin an active sexual career before marriage, perhaps become a parent before marriage, perhaps never enter marriage at all or never become a parent. Perhaps a couple has to take back a child who had left the home and reassume the parental career. Some people are never called upon to be responsible for their parents' care.

Our inclusion of the filial career in the list may be surprising. It is a different dimension than the others, but, when defined as "responsibility," it has the characteristics of the others, which involve care and commitment. In the usual paradigm, the children leave home and the parents are left with the empty nest. The couple, during their child-rearing years, have been expected to be on their own and the parents on their own. Cordial and loving relationships often exist. But with old age, especially after one parent dies, the need for filial responsibility and care emerge. The need for this has increased in recent years because of the tremendous increase in longevity. My memory is that there are estimates that as many as 40% of families will be caring for a parent for some period of time. Some estimates are that the years spent in caring for an elderly parent may be more than the child-rearing years. This phenomenon has given rise to concern for the "sandwich generation," another way to describe the filial stage.

The different sub-careers have different durations. A person can be in an active sexual career but later decide to be celibate. Marriages can break up. The fact of parenthood can hardly be reversed, unless we count giving a child up for adoption, but the stage of active parenting can end. Filial responsibility is time-bound by the longevity of the parent. Gone are the days of an expected passage from one stage to the next in the family life cycle, as usually described in the standard textbooks. The combinations of these sub-careers make up the family career. Typologies of families can be defined and the frequency of each determined.

Each of the sub-careers exists without the others and can be studied independently. We proposed that the intersections where the careers join or dissolve are points of special interest for study: a couple marry, become parents or step-parents, lose children because they grow up and marry, divorce, or take on the responsibility for a parent and become grandparents and even step-grandparents. The intersections become the points at which natural experiments take place as some members of a cohort experience the new status and others do not. The census has been wrestling with the problem of how to define families. Perhaps some of these typologies would be useful.

Washington, D.C.

We took our 1978 sabbatical in Washington, D.C. Harold worked at the Center for the Family at the Home Economics Association, and I worked for two months in a Health Education and Welfare agency that was disseminating materials about sex education primarily to diminish the teenage pregnancy problem. This had been my research interest at Ithaca College. The last two months of our time I worked in the office of the Assistant Secretary for Evaluation and Planning in the section, which was writing a bill to define and set up a new office of Adolescent Pregnancy Prevention. I attended hearings on the bill and learned about the tremendous barriers that continue to exist to keep information from young people. For example, I was told by an important lay person that, "Yes, girls should have access to contraceptives before marriage, but only after they had a child!" This was called "secondary prevention." I found that the Hubert Humphrey Health Education and Welfare building was "littered with burned out adolescent pregnancy workers," as one man told me. It was then that I learned the meaning of "intractable problem" when values clash.

Back in Ithaca, I continued my interest in the adolescent pregnancy problem by working with a group of Ithaca College students as a research team. We tried some innovative projects, such as training high school students to go into drug stores to ask for condoms and, if they were made to feel uneasy, to say to the druggist, "Well, would you rather I got the girl pregnant?" No druggist said that and soon the New York law against open display of condoms and other contraceptives was overturned and our students were emboldened. We also developed a game to be played by adolescents based on real probabilities and on chance.

RETIREMENT

In 1981, Harold and I retired. Our retirement plan was to spend the summer and fall of each year back in Ithaca but three months of the spring of each year in Washington to put our expertise to work in the policy arena.

During the fall semesters at Cornell, Harold continued teaching a very large class on human sexuality. After a few semesters of this, he and his assistant, Andrea Parrot, decided to edit a book making use of new essays, which would give two or more sides to arguments regarding sexuality. The book, *Human Sexuality: Contemporary Controversies* (1984) was published by Sage. At the end of each paper and section were questions and suggested activities to encourage active learning, which grew out of Harold's preoccupation with teaching. That book became the model for *Current Controversies in Marriage and Family* (1985), which Harold and I co-edited.

During our previous encounters in Washington, we had both been impressed with the openness of the bureaucracy. Following our pattern of researching and working in areas of concern to our own life stage, we thought it would be appropriate for us to work in the field of aging. Over several springs, we each found opportunities to work with the Senate and House Committees on the Aging or a variety of non-profit and semi-governmental agencies. We attended meetings and worked to promote programs and policies to improve conditions for the elderly.

In meetings we noted that discussion of health of the aged was always addressed as a problem for the elderly person. We became outspoken advocates for the caregivers, who were most likely to be the women in families. My mother had been the responsibility of my sister and myself so we recognized the filial stage. We were gratified after a few years to see that caregiving was recognized as a problem and that opportunities were expanded for respite care. Long term care of the aged is still a major problem.

Back in Ithaca during five summers and falls we organized the local Gray Panthers. A small group of us produced a number of meetings and rallies for national health and a celebration for the 40th anniversary of Medicare. We got a group together to do a survey of doctors' plans to take Medicare as full pay and assessed doctor's attitudes about payment and about patient questions. Results were published in the local paper.

Each time we were in Washington we joined the NCFR policy committee and added our strength to the ongoing activities. We became more and more concerned with policies of the government which affected families. When we moved more or less full time to Washington in 1987 we were both on the NCFR policy committee. Harold became the NCFR representative to the Coalition of Family Organizations (COFO) while I continued work in the field of aging. After Harold's passing in 1988, I became the volunteer NCFR Washington Representative, a position that the policy committee had outlined. I also represented NCFR on COFO and in 1991 assumed the rotating job of chair. From a focus on aging, I turned to full time on families.

In 1992, I chaired the Program Committee for the very successful Groves Conference held here in Washington. Catherine Chilman, who moved into my neighborhood two years earlier, was co-chair, and arranged the workshops. It was good to be able to call on previous contacts to develop the resources needed to have the Conference be a success.

ADDITIONAL CONCERNS

Religion

Religion was never a big concern for me, as it was not for my father. He used to take us to church and sit outside in the car to read the paper. My mother was constantly seeking a more responsive religion and turned to Christian Science and to other deist, as opposed to Christian, religions. I was interested in her search but found none of them really appealed to me. The college I attended was a Christian college, and I am glad I had the courses on religion that we were required to take. However, I was very disappointed by the unethical behavior of some of the strongest churchgoers at the college, so I realized that exhortation does not always result in the expected behavior.

On a train trip during my years at Western Reserve I met a woman who told me about the Ethical Culture Society. The idea that there could be an organized group with an ethical basis for action that did not depend on religion was a wonderful insight. In later years I somehow found out about the *Humanist* magazine and subscribed. I sent for the Humanist Manifesto and realized that I was a humanist and became a card-carrying member of the American Humanist Association. I attended several national conventions but was disappointed at first to see how sexist the Humanists were, and was later cheered by the vigorous efforts of the Humanist Women's Caucus. I feel that we can act according to ethical principles, which turn out to be remarkably like those of social work: to treat everyone with dignity, to foster cooperation, to appreciate the value of each person, and to base our plans on reason. I have tried to follow these principles.

During our years in Ithaca we were members of the Unitarian church, and our children attended the Sunday school there. Humanists and Unitarians are very close in philosophy.

The Women's Movement

A major job for a girl growing up is to try to find out what she can do in society. I have mentioned several incidents which were important in my life in this regard: my relationship with my father who had no son, his reaction to my becoming student body president, my mother's example of an educated involved woman, and the ways in which my parents could work together. I was interested in being a professional person in my own right, so one of Harold's characteristics that was especially endearing was the fact that he said he wanted a strong woman who could be a partner. We tried to run our marriage on that basis.

On our trip to Ceylon I read Simone de Beauvoir's *The Second Sex* and found it tremendously consciousness raising. Betty Friedan's *The Feminine Mystique* came along in 1963 and, after a personal appearance by Betty Friedan at Cornell in 1965, our interest in the women's movement was very high.

During 1968, Harold sponsored a student-led course on racism. In the fall, the same students wanted him to sponsor a course on women. He encouraged the women to find a woman professor to be the sponsor but, when no one would take on the job, he agreed. The women did a number of projects in the Cornell and Ithaca communities and started collecting data about the ways in which women were controlled and discriminated against. Harold became identified with the women's movement as a result of this class and became the token male in the women's studies program board that eventually resulted. At one point he agreed to be the secretary, but not the president.

Coining "Sexism." In the fall of 1968, Andrew Hacker, a professor in the Government Department at Cornell, was invited to address the Ithaca College community about racism. In the course of his remarks he said, "Just as there is racism, there is discrimination against women." He went on, "I am a womanizer myself." I was astonished at his use of that term and said to myself, "What he means is that there is sexism." That fall I went around to all the parties asking people if they had ever heard the term sexism, and no one had. Some got the idea right away but some had to have it explained. No dictionary contained the term.

In January 1969, the first women's conference on a university campus was held at Cornell, organized by Sheila Tobias. On a panel, I used the term "sexism." In her book, *Women at Cornell*, Charlotte Conable gives me credit for inventing the word which now is universally used (Conable, 1977). Of course, it was just a matter of time for the word to be invented since it was such a natural, but I have enjoyed the credit for it. Dictionaries now list the term and give it the date of around 1970.

In 1970 another woman and I organized a large celebration in a park in the center of Ithaca to commemorate the 40th anniversary of the 19th Amendment giving women the right to vote. In 1972, I organized a local meeting similar to a women's political caucus. The speakers were women office holders, and the attendees were encouraged to participate in the political process by being candidates and campaign managers rather than just envelope-stuffers and phoners.

At Ithaca College I participated in all the women's activities, including an effort to get a women's studies program. I found that a few people with very rigid ideas and an inability to compromise could sabotage the efforts of a group. In my contacts at Ithaca College I worked to raise people's consciousness about the use of male pronouns and collective nouns. The high point of this effort came one morning as I was walking down the hall and the chair of the English Department greeted me with, "Good morning, Margaret Feldperson."

In 1977, I chaired a core group of women who organized a second Seneca Falls Women's Conference. This event, preliminary to the 1977 National Women's Houston Conference, was very well attended and provided a boost to Seneca Falls, which was the site of the events of the first wave of feminism. Harold and I both attended the Houston Conference. We were very annoyed to find that the TV commentators felt they had to give equal time to Phyllis Schlafly's counter group.

Out of the 1977 conference came a Continuation Committee with which I worked for several years. In 1987 there was a "Decade After" Conference in Washington. One of the main speakers was Riane Eisler who had just come out with her book, *The Chalice and the Blade* (1987), which stimulated us all. Her book is based on "revisionist" archaeology, mainly by women, and takes as the thesis the idea that the original religion was worship of the female earth goddess. The coming of the Bronze Age brought with it the conquest of earth worshipping Neolithic peoples by the nomads from Asia and the patriarchal Hebrews from the deserts. Patriarchy was forced on the goddess worshippers, and the Old Testament is in large part the story of the difficulties of this forced change from the goddess. Others have told this same story but the grounding in archaeology and myth seemed better done in this book.

The idea within the book that was most meaningful to me was also not a new idea, but seemed newly relevant. Riane Eisler said that there are two forms of organization for society, the vertical and the horizontal, the hierarchical and the partnership. She said that if you were brought up in one of these, it was very difficult to take the mind-set of the other. It was clear that what the women's movement had been looking for and working toward was partnership, and what patriarchy and the men in charge had in their heads was hierarchy. The men were having a very difficult time understanding the other concept. Men's idea was that, according to the hierarchical form of organization, someone had to be on top. If men were not in charge, then women would be, and men did not want a matriarchy. Women, on the other hand, did not want to be on top–they wanted to be partners and share in authority and planning. Women had a hard time understanding why men were so afraid of letting women share as partners. There were some men, of course, who had the partnership idea and these are the "new men." We need a new name for these men because many find it hard to think of themselves as "feminists."

With this framework, and others that we had been considering for a long time, it became clear that the major part of the problem was with men–the hierarchical-thinking men (and women). How could we raise, or retrain, men in a new form of thinking? To my mind, this is now perhaps the most serious question we have for society. When we look at the behavior of many of our elected officials, and certainly the minds of our military planners, we see that winning dominance is their major value. When we look at male administrators in business, many are the same. In the family, men who feel they must be dominant and that anything is appropriate to maintain that dominance, including violence, are the ones who are battering their wives and children. In many cases, dominating and violent men also are those who did not experience true nurturing and respect as children.

Put more broadly, the question is how to organize society in a way which will contain the violence of men and make them feel important as partners–not dominators. Can family life education and parental training provide this training?

As I was writing this essay in the middle of April 1992, the *Washington Post* had just reviewed a book by, of all people, Andrew Hacker, the same professor who spoke at Ithaca College in 1968 and who made me think of the word "sexism." His book, published in 1992, was entitled

Two Nations, Black and White, Separate, Hostile, Unequal. As I read the review, every time the white race was mentioned I could substitute "male" and it all fitted very well.

In his book, Hacker has described the racial equivalent of Riane Eisler's thesis of built in hierarchy and partnership as two forms of societal organization. The reviewer, Lynne Duke of the *Washington Post*, says, "when Hacker is talking about whiteness, he thinks of it as a 'condition' like a 'virus' of the psyche. It makes whites react to blackness as a 'stain,' like a drop of ink in water. Whiteness is a delusional state of mind that was used to justify slavery and that persists to this day to justify white privilege."

Ms. Duke goes on to say, "Hacker's words, and Hacker's book, are almost a dare. Dare to consider that the basic racial problem in America might not be about blacks and their troubles, as so many social critics contend, but about whites and their delusions."

Since gender, like race, is a characteristic one is born with and cannot hide, it is clear that it would be easy to identify those who are not male as having a "condition" like a "virus" which precludes their positioning at the top of the hierarchy. The problems women face may truly be the problems of male delusions.

Community Participation

In 1979 I ran for mayor of Ithaca. I was encouraged to do this to provide a liberal option and to provide a candidate who opposed a large environmentally damaging road project. Young people in the liberal and environmental movements were my staffers. Although I was fourth in a field of 5, 1 got 20.9% of the votes; The winner only got 29% of the votes, which showed how close the first 4 candidates were. Number 5 was a Right to Life Candidate who got 45 votes. The old time politicians were amazed at my votes and became aware of how many supported the environmentalist position.

Running for this office, with Harold as a devoted telephoner and associate, was a major event in my life. It was exhilarating because of the need to be on top of so many issues, to learn so much in a very short time, and to be able to speak to a crowd. Even in a small town, the candidates made a total of 68 appearances, debates, interviews, etc. On the street when I was campaigning, I would get comments from some of the older women and men: "Why aren't you home with your children?" I was pleased that at the same time my little granddaughters were going around town with t-shirts saying "Grandma for Mayor."

In the summer of 1980 I organized a group of clergy, therapists, educators, and parents around the issue of family violence. We held several open meetings, held some workshops, and, finally, came out with a set of four TV shows on ways to deal with anger and prevent aggression in the home. We did not assess the effect but felt it was worthwhile to do something about this problem, which was being experienced in more and more families.

In Washington, when we decided to become more or less residents in 1987, we bought into an old time cooperative with many professional federal workers and retirees. Our co-op, River Park, is located close to the museums, congressional buildings, and the river, in a racially integrated and diverse community. We thought it was like the "real world" and wanted to be in "the city," not a suburb. River Park was going to have its 25th anniversary in 1988, and a small group of us, with me as chair, decided to prepare a celebration. I began work on this in the fall of 1987. When I had to return from the Groves Conference in 1988 without Harold, it was a great help for me to be able to return to a very supportive co-op and to have something which needed to be done. The 25th Anniversary Celebration was a huge success. It enlisted the work and enthusiasm of a great number of residents and other community people.

The next spring, I was asked to become the president of the local civic group. Although I had not been a previous member, I agreed to run and was elected. I served in this position for three years, until March, 1992, then passed the leadership on to a young man from the neighborhood. His mother was a welfare mother who got all her eight children through college and into responsible positions in teaching, social work, and the government. Working in this organization was very rewarding because of the opportunity to get to know and work with all kinds of people in our mixed community. As president, I received many invitations to meet politicians in other parts of the city, which was fun. I am still continuing my interest and involvement in the community as president of a less active group affiliated with the old organization.

Our concern in the civic organization has been with neighborhood improvement, which often means crime and welfare. I have become very concerned about the prospects for the black women who cannot find a good husband or get a good job, and with the black men who cannot find meaningful work with dignity and respect. We are spending too much time finding the money for jails and courts and "changing behavior" of those who are in difficulty, and not enough money and effort spent in training and in changing the behavior of those in charge so they in turn could change the environment.

Even though I am living in a racially integrated neighborhood, whites in general live in the better housing, and we have several housing projects which are almost all black. The questions of race are always here–at least dormant. I truly believe that I am not racist and do relate to people as individuals of value. Still, in America, and in our communities, the questions of race must be addressed. Our community is filled with wonderful people of all colors and religions who are interested in working toward the betterment of the community.

CONTINUITY AND UPDATE ON FAMILY

Reading back over this account has given me an opportunity to try to draw out the common threads and consistent concerns. It is clear that there has been great continuity throughout my life. The influence of my parents as models and the upbringing they afforded was powerful in my continuing interest in the welfare of society and its members. Following their lead, I have tried to live an ethical life not based on any religious dogma, have been willing to take on leadership roles and, in being a leader, have tried to include people so that they can have a sense of participation. I see my father's ideas in this. My mother's strengths and interest in healthy living and the health of society have also influenced me.

Family, but now my children and grandchildren, all seven of them, are important in my life and provide strong support. I find that each is different but each shows an aspect of Harold's and my interests, which has been emphasized in that child's life.

Dorothy has become very artistic, which I thought I had abilities to do when I was young. She and her family returned to Ithaca when Kira was 4 and Sarahjane was 2. She continues to do excellent work as a community leader and organizer in Ithaca. She has been the mainstay for the schools her children have attended, always willing to be the homeroom mother, the chaperone, the band mother and the PTA worker. She has taken on a craft profession, which allows her to plan her own time to accommodate the needs of the family. Her family is buying a new house with a room for me. Her husband John has been a wonderful addition to the family and a resource for us all with his tax preparation skills.

Dick has continued an interest in words, which I learned from my father and also enjoy. Dick teaches English to foreigners at Cornell and is the coordinator of the teaching assistants. He feels respect for his women colleagues, which shows the continuation of Harold's attitudes.

He is also an excellent computer person and a very creative teacher. While in the Peace Corps in Africa after college, he learned gardening, so he has continued this interest by participating in the farm he and Beth have near Ithaca. At the moment, their four children, Heather, Ann, Ethan, and Ben, and a neighbor child are enjoying a home school which Beth is teaching during the day, making use of the farm and country environment. Dick brings computer skills and its learning possibilities to the children when he is home evenings and weekends.

Larry for a while took on the radical attitudes his parents sublimated but eventually joined the academic world. He and his wife Margaret, both PhDs, are tenured full professors at Indiana University of Pennsylvania in the math department with a focus on preparing teachers in the new math. In 1991, they welcomed Keith, their only child. They each took a semester of quarter time so they could take turns being the home parent. They work together and encourage each other, true partners.

Policy and the Family Field

We are all informed by our own experiences, and we all believe this is especially important in the family field. In Harold's case, and by association my own, and I think many family researchers, interest often follows the stage in the family career in which one finds oneself.

Perhaps because it was so remote to young family scholars, the area of aging was a latecomer to the field, long after marriage and parenting. However, the area of the middle-aged family was later still, which does not follow the age-stage hypothesis. I recall thinking about this middle stage when we were thinking of lifetime individual development and wondering why people had not paid more attention to it. One explanation was that it was much easier to study "them" than to probe too deeply into oneself. Perhaps it is not our stage in life that determines the area of interest but other factors, possibly including a particularly emotional event or situation, or even the research interest of our major professor! Perhaps this is an interesting area for further study.

Harold and I were both interested in the potential effect our research could have. Even though the paradigm of a proper research paper includes in the conclusions the "implications for further study and for policy," many research interests do not lend themselves to policy at all. It is interesting that there has been an increasing trend in NCFR for members to indicate an interest in policy. Perhaps this has come as a response to the deteriorating condition of the family, our subject of study.

It is likely a response to the decreasing support for families and our increasing bewilderment when it comes to figuring out what to do.

Although I have had a very deep interest in women and their full functioning, I find that my affection for my father, my love and respect for Harold, and the empathy I have for both men and women has made me very sympathetic to the plight of men and boys in the present climate. I can understand how beleaguered many of them feel when their self-esteem has come from being strong and in charge to then find that women want to be partners in their work–or worse still, to find that they have been laid off with no work at all. The recent conditions in the farms, the factories, and in all the construction trades have been devastating to the self-concept of men. And boys have lacked role models to whom they could realistically aspire to model themselves. Being a male of any age has its hazards–but, of course, so does being a female. Society is not well organized at present to lead to the best development of its citizens. There is despair in our country, but even more despair when we look at what is happening to large groups of people in other parts of the world.

"Doing policy" at this time (1992), is extremely frustrating. I find I am not willing to go out in the streets for revolution, but, on the other hand, I feel impotent to help change what is going on. I do feel the United States is not living up to its ideals. I love the interactions I have with the people who are still trying, and I am still trying, but I feel the possibility for real structural change is very remote. In my analysis of what is needed to bring more equity and more opportunity to our people, I feel a national health program is the bottom line. Without it there can be no real movement of many people off of the welfare rolls. We need housing and more income for people. Yes, people do need to take responsibility for themselves, but there have to be real opportunities for them.

During times like these, when it is so difficult to see where progress can be made, it is easy to slip into personal involvement with the everyday and forget the outside problems. So long as every thing is going well for us, why should we worry? We can slip into "complacency," which some writers are bemoaning. However, it is important to continue the struggle. For those of us who grew up in social work-oriented homes, it seems to be part of our nature to be concerned and to feel that without working toward the betterment of something, we really are failing in our job of being a good citizen. My mother had this feeling very strongly, and I share it.

I am more invested in the family field than ever. Working with the National Council on Family Relations as their Washington Representative and with the Consortium of Family Organizations provides a needed legitimacy for my activities and allows me to focus on the policy needs of families. We are trying to help bring family needs to the attention of the policy makers.

The NCFR Policy Committee, based here in Washington, has started the Family Fax system which we designed to make it possible for NCFR members back in all states to become active in policy by writing or phoning Representatives, Senators, or other key people when family-relevant issues are being decided. This is a new program, which we hope will increase the sense of involvement of NCFR members.

Finally . . .

In many ways, the present years have been some of the most rewarding, even though I miss having Harold with me. Without Harold as a companion and colleague, it was a great support for me to be in Washington where I had made so many friends and had activities that enlisted my interests. Among the best groups are several connected with women's interests.

Over the years, working for and with NCFR has given me the stimulation and focus I need and an opportunity to contribute. Working with the civic association in my neighborhood continues to be very rewarding, even if we find we cannot accomplish all we would like to. Washington is a wonderful city, full of exciting activities and people. With sufficient income, it is possible to pursue my own interests and to travel when I wish. I am going to Brazil this summer with Elderhostel. So long as I have my present good health, I am happy to do what I can here and to enjoy my loving and supportive family where they are.

Another spring has come. The flowers are out and each wave of new blooms brings its joy to us all. We can hope that with another spring will come a new breakthrough in national commitment to the needs of citizens and to an awareness of the need for human capital as well as financial capital. We are still trying. And we have not given up the liberal belief that government has a part to play in maintaining the "general welfare."

UPDATE: 1999

It is now 1999, and I see that much of what I wrote in 1992 is still relevant–as it should be since our lives are continuous. I am still the Washington Representative for NCFR, but COFO is no longer operating. I continue to write on families and policy (see Quarterly Policy Reports 1990-present). I am still taking a leadership role in many activities within my neighborhood to try to improve conditions for the people in public housing. My social work ideals are still active, and I am still interested in the women's movement.

I was able to attend two of the Vienna planning meetings for the Fourth World Conference on Women and then attend the Beijing Conference in 1995. Being there and seeing women from all over the world, hearing them talk about their problems that were similar worldwide, was a fascinating experience. Here in Washington, I have attended Beijing follow-up meetings held by the President's Interagency Council. The U.S. government has been opened up and is much more woman friendly, human and family-friendly, than it was before this work got underway. It was gratifying to hear officials from the State Department, for instance, talk about what a positive difference had been created for both women and men by having a woman Secretary. The Armed Services are more concerned with families and run the largest day care operation in the country. Each agency has had to provide a plan for their agency to forward the twelve issues in the platform of action.

I have continued traveling. A return trip to Ghana with an African-American woman we had met while there in 1965 brought back fond memories. Another memorable African trip was to Benin at Christmas of 1995 to visit Dick and his family. Dick had a Fulbright at the University to teach teachers of English. Larry joined us, and we had a fascinating drive north into the country of Niger where, among other things, we visited with some Nomads camped on the desert.

Two trips back to Alaska have been exciting. One, with Elderhostel in 1994, provided a week in Fairbanks and 10 days in Siberia to see the different ways two cultures have dealt with permafrost living. The other, in 1995, was with Larry, Margaret, and Keith in which we retraced the trip I took in 1940. This was a wonderful chance to relive my earlier trip with family members. A trip to Norway is planned for this June for another international women's meeting.

Family

Dorothy has degrees in counseling and sports medicine but given the job market in Ithaca, now is an aid for special children, especially teens. John is a rural mail carrier, which allows him to be his most efficient self. Both their girls are now graduated from college and have married classmates from their colleges. Kira, my granddaughter, is an excellent mother to her two little boys, thus I am now a great-grandmother. Sarahjane is teaching music on Long Island, which includes teaching all the elementary grades and leading the band.

Dick is still teaching English to foreigners at Cornell, but Beth is now teaching languages at the local middle-high school. They essentially gave up the farm the year they went to Africa. All the children are doing well in public school in academics, music, and athletics.

Larry and Margaret are still teaching at IUP, working together on some projects. Larry has been part of a team working to encourage teachers to use real math statistics with academic subjects. Keith is now going to be 8 years old and is enjoying music lessons, ice-skating, and swimming. Indiana, PA, is a comfortable town to live in and raise a child.

I do not see all the children as much as I would like, but we keep in very good contact through phone and e-mail–a wonderful help. We have family gatherings but also individual visits as they get down here. I do not relish the drive up to Ithaca by myself, but have been going at least twice a year for family gatherings, often to celebrate family milestones.

Finally. So life continues to be interesting and hopefully productive. At this age, one becomes concerned with what is to come, but we enjoy family and old and new friends and take advantage of all the opportunities we have.

REFERENCES

Conable, C. (1977). *Women at Cornell: The myth of equal education*. Ithaca, NY: Cornell University Press.

Eisler, Riane (1987). *The chalice and the blade: Our history, our future*. New York: Harper and Row.

Feldman, M. (1964). Learning by programmed text and format at three levels of difficulty. *Journal of Educational Psychology*, *56*, 3, 133-139.

Feldman, M. (1973). Low-income liberated woman. *Human Ecology Forum*.

Feldman, M. (1990-present). Quarterly Policy Reports printed in NCFR Report. Minneapolis, MN: National Council on Family Relations.

Feldman, M. & Anderson, E. (1993). Family-centered health policy. In S. Price (Ed.), *Vision 2010: Families and Health Care*. Minneapolis: National Council of Family Relations.

Feldman, H & Feldman, M. (1965). *Mental hygiene and the project method of teaching hygiene*. Bombay: Oxford University Press.

Feldman, H & Feldman, M. (1971). Differential academic coping behavior of siblings in three geographic areas. Research Report for the National Center for Educational Research and Development, U.S. Office of Education.

Feldman, H. & Feldman, M. (1972). Impact of the welfare woman's working on her family. Research Report for the Office of Manpower Research, Department of Labor.

Feldman, H. & Feldman, M. (1974). The relationship between the family and occupational functioning in a sample of urban welfare women. *Cornell Journal of Social Relations, 9*, 1, 35-52.

Feldman, H. & Feldman, M. (1975a). Helping families leave welfare: Four strategies. *Forum, 5*, Spring, 16-19.

Feldman, H. & Feldman, M. (1975b). Effect of father absence on adolescence. *Family Perspectives*, Fall, 3,

Feldman, H. & Feldman, M. (1975c). The family life cycle: Some suggestions for recycling, *Journal of Marriage and the Family, 37*, 2, 277-284.

Feldman, H. & Feldman, M. (1984). *Human sexuality: Contemporary controversies.* Beverly Hills, CA: Sage Publications.

Feldman, H. & Feldman, M. (Eds.) (1985). *Current controversies in marriage and family.* Beverly Hills: Sage Publications.

Hacker, A. (1992). *Two nations, black and white, separate, hostile, unequal.* New York: Charles Scribner.

Robert, H. M. (1915). *Robert's rules of order: Revised for deliberative assemblies.* Chicago, Scott, Foresman & Co.

The Autobiography of a Sex Researcher: Short Version

Ira L. Reiss

KEYWORDS. Autobiography, research, premarital sex, sexuality

ENVIRONMENTAL INFLUENCES

Learning to Tell a House from a Home

Besides the love they showed for me, the most significant gift given to me by my parents was their acceptance of my personal choices. My mother, in particular, supported everyone's right to challenge the choices society imposed. My mother was an iconoclast who felt betrayed by a world that permitted so much injustice and unhappiness in our lives. My father was more of a pragmatist, and less confrontational, but he had high regard for intellectual questioning and the search for new knowledge. He was more willing than my mother to adapt to the world as it was, and then quietly and privately make what adjustments were needed. My mother was more like Don Quixote, compelled to battle, even though deep down she knew she could never really win. But, her efforts were not without value, for as George Bernard Shaw has noted, reasonable people conform, and so all progress depends on the unreasonable person.

The city I grew up in afforded me an ideal laboratory to develop my own ideas about sexuality. Scranton was an anthracite coal mining town in northeastern Pennsylvania. My father moved there from New York City in the early 1930s, just after my sister and I started school. He was trying to rebuild the clothing factory he lost in the early years of the depression. Scranton, like most cities at that time, was in deep economic trouble, and we lived close to poverty for a few years until finally my father's persistent struggles paid off and he was able to establish a new clothing factory.

At the same time, other entrepreneurial souls in Scranton were founding a different sort of business as their way of surviving the depression years. Houses of prostitution opened–scores of them, in the alleys behind twelve of the downtown streets. The impact on Scranton economically and culturally was dramatic. Prostitution brought in a large amount of wealth to many parts of the city and, as a result, the sex industry gained considerable political support, and it thrived throughout the depression years. On a Saturday night the population of Scranton increased tremendously. Scores of cars came in from New York City and Philadelphia and many other smaller cities, loaded with men eager to "try out the Scranton girls." The "cat" houses were painted gaudy colors like orange, purple, and yellow to make it easy to distinguish them from private residences.

Some houses were known by their color–one of the most famous being called the "Orange Front." It became well known in part because it was centrally located, less than a block from the YMHA, the Jesuit College of St. Thomas, and from Central High School. Its status was marked by having its own small parking lot. It was called the "Orange *Front*" because it was located at the start, or "front," of the colorful collage of twelve blocks of houses in the alleys of downtown Scranton. A gas station at the end of one of the alleys displayed a large sign that read "Always One Dollar." Supposedly that meant a car wash and shine, but it also happened to be the price in the houses for sex with a white prostitute. Societal views on race, class, and gender were indelibly written during the 1930s and early 1940s in the social and economic structure of Scranton's houses of prostitution. Sexual services from black and mulatto prostitutes were less expensive than the same services from a white prostitute. The houses were a very early first course for me in the social context of race, gender, and sexual relationships.

The houses brought money into the eager cash registers of the hotels, restaurants, gas stations, and bars. Prosperity also was evident for those who were connected directly to the running of the cat houses. As a young boy, even I benefited economically from their existence. No, I did not become a child-pimp or a child-performer. My part-time role was more indirect than that. It was impossible to grow up in Scranton and not know where these brightly painted "pleasure houses" were located. I recall that when I was about 9 or 10, cars would stop by me when I was walking with friends near the downtown area. The male passengers would lean out the car window and say: "Hey kid, where's the cat houses?" When I gave them directions, the men in the car would usually toss me a nickel or a dime. I was fascinated by the power of sex to so easily bring so many men, so far from their homes, into an economically depressed coal mining town. It reinforced the idea to me that there must be something very special about sexuality–something mysterious, powerful, and extraordinarily rewarding.

Prostitution was illegal but the police patrolled the alleys and let customers know that they were supposed to be over 16 to get into the houses, although they didn't always enforce that very carefully. The felt need for prostitution was in part an inevitable outcome of the fact that our society then labored so hard to restrict female sexuality. The ancient double standard demands "bad girls" as sexual partners for men, in order to keep men from bothering the "good girls" that they would later marry. Even as a teenager, the double standard seemed to me to be contradictory, unfair, and very poor preparation for both men and women for any sort of enjoyable marital sex life.

At times I would stay in the parlor after having sex to talk to and get to know the "working girls" better. Many of them were high school ages, about 16 to 18. They would make it clear in their conversations with each other and with me that they were not going to be like the friends or sisters they knew who worked for years in some factory sweat shop for low pay, with no future. They hoped to earn good money, save it, open up a beauty shop or dress shop and eventually get married. I saw some of these same women years later, and a few had achieved that goal. But many of them found it wasn't such an easy path and left or headed downhill.

Bear in mind that a good deal of the condemnation of prostitution was not from people who supported equality in society for women. A negative view of sex without affection and particularly a negative view of female casual sexuality, underlay much of the conservative criticism of prostitution. Some of today's feminist opponents of prostitution have similar views and would not accept prostitution even in a fully gender equal society. Much of this anti-prostitution view is based more on a narrow view of what is acceptable sexuality, than on a striving for gender equality. In my mind, the harm in prostitution is not in the recreational approach to sexuality, but in the gender inequality and the illegality that still permeates that profession.

FAMILY INFLUENCES

Partaking of the Religious Script

Although my parents did not live strictly according to orthodox Jewish rules, they wanted me to be exposed to that way of thinking. Both my mother and father had parents who were very strict in their religious observances. In the early decades of this century, my father's mother, Rachel Goldworm Reiss, helped found a female rights movement within orthodoxy. She was an educated woman who, in addition to speaking English and Yiddish, could speak Hebrew, the language of the Torah. This ability was a rarity even among religiously educated Jewish men, and it gave my grandmother more influence in her efforts to equalize women's rights in Judaism. She was a very strong woman, just like my mother was, but, unlike my mother, she had the good fortune of having found a cause to which she could commit her energies.

Every day after public school, for almost ten years, I was sent for two hours to attend an orthodox Jewish religious school. Every Saturday morning I would attend a four hour religious service. I wasn't too enthusiastic about this extra schooling but, like it or not, that religious training did have a profound impact on my views concerning sexuality. The orthodox religious school focused mostly on learning to read Hebrew and very little on learning to speak it. Reading Hebrew was all one needed to pray and that was their focus. But, as we got older, we also spent a lot of time interpreting the meaning of the Bible, which in Judaism is the Old Testament. We studied the Torah, the five books of Moses, line by line, word by word. We started with the assumption that the Torah was true, but we were all obligated to examine it very carefully and argue the case for different interpretations. I did not know it then, but I was learning a respect for logic and reasoning and careful examination of the deeper significance of human belief and behavior. Later in life that was to serve me well in my professional scientific work.

When I was about ten years old I had a memorable experience in Hebrew School which illustrates the respect for learning that I was being given. I usually did not volunteer answers to the questions the Rabbi or other teachers would raise with us. I often was more interested in being outside and playing with friends. One day a particularly difficult biblical passage was thrown out to us for interpretation. No one offered an answer and Rabbi Schachter kept pushing for us to think it through and find the answer. I was caught up in the challenge, and I raised my hand and gave what I thought was the answer. The Rabbi walked over to me, stopped, stared at me, and then backhanded me hard across the face. Slaps and whacks with a ruler were not uncommon when we acted up, but I wasn't acting up this time. I was hurt and confused and I asked: "What's wrong? Was I that far off?" The Rabbi said: "No, you were correct." "So why did you hit me?" I asked. The Rabbi looked straight at me and said: "Because your answer showed me that you could do far better work than you have been doing all year. To fail to use the talent God gave you is a sin. I wanted you to know that." I felt, despite the pain of the slap, that I had been praised. I learned from that experience and from my years in Hebrew School a respect for the value of thoughtful inquiry that I still carry with me.

But along with the logic and reasoning of my religious education came the value assumption that we ought to avoid sexuality outside of marriage. This was at the same time that I was giving directions to out-of-towners as to where the cat houses were located! The religious restrictions included masturbation as well as petting and intercourse and so there was not much room left for acceptable sexuality. This religious perspective inserted a third element in my thinking: I had a pleasure emphasis from my mother; a pragmatic emphasis from my father; and now, from my religion, an ethical emphasis that promoted guilt and shame. I was receiving, in spades, a typical conflicted American sexual socialization. I was to spend many years trying to personally sort out these powerful but conflicting messages.

When I was about 14, I decided orthodoxy was too restrictive, and I became far less observant of its rules. I wanted to go to movies on Saturdays and play football and I was tired of the four hour Saturday morning religious services. I have never lost my belief in God even though my God became more generic and less Jewish. I continued to celebrate most of the Jewish holidays, but I felt I could not accept the narrow lifestyle restrictions demanded by orthodox Judaism. Years later, when I married, I returned to organized religion, but not to orthodoxy. My wife, Harriet, and I joined a Reform Jewish Temple that permitted us to bring our minds as well as our feelings into our religion. But all those changes did not automatically exorcise all the qualms I had about the rightness of the sexuality I had experienced. That part of my background was much more difficult to set aside.

My Sexuality Troika: Pleasure, Pragmatism, and Purity

My father always strongly advised me to use condoms so as to avoid pregnancy and disease. As a result, I was using condoms and practicing "safer sex" in the early 1940s, several decades before it became popular in America. But I wanted more than just knowledge of how to avoid the negative outcomes of sex. I wanted to get insight into how to achieve the positive outcomes that sexuality could involve and how to better understand why there was so much societal opposition to enjoying sexuality. To do this I felt I had to gain a broader overview of what were the full range of choices in heterosexual relationships. I began to work out a sort of analysis of sexual ethics and the rewards and costs of different life-styles. That sort of exploration has occupied me, on and off, throughout my academic and personal life. The freedom my parents gave me to work things out coupled with the restraints of my religious upbringing, encouraged me to search for a way to put these opposing pieces of my sexual puzzle into a meaningful guide for living.

The earliest part of my search involved me in questioning the double standard that gave men more sexual rights than women. The restraints on women's sexuality inevitably led to restraints on the range of partner choices that men had, and so self interest alone spoke against the double standard. Another reason for my gender equality attitudes came from the fact that my mother was a very assertive woman who did not take a back seat to anyone. She also was a woman who let me know that she felt that part of the reason the world had shortchanged her was simply because she was a woman. Furthermore, my sister, Carol, who was just 16 months older than me, was one of the two best students in her high school class and a very talented person. Also, as I've mentioned, my paternal grandmother had been an active Jewish feminist and had fought against special male privileges in religion in the early 1900s. With all that in my background, how could I accept any theory of inherent female inferiority and male dominance? I was lucky to be able to endorse male equality!

It interested me that many of the men I knew were unaware of any inequity or hardship imposed by the double standard on women. The argument they often used was: "Women like it that way," or, as Marilyn Quayle put it at the 1992 Republican Convention, "Most women do not want to be liberated from their essential natures as women." That kind of explanation did not cut much ice with me. Some women accepting male dominance didn't make it right anymore than some slaves accepting slavery made that right. Furthermore, as I've said, I knew many women who, even in the 1940s, outright rejected such inequality and the reasoning underlying it.

A SEX EDUCATOR IN THE ARMY

Another important influence on my thoughts and feelings regarding sexuality came from my hitch in the U.S. Army (1944-1946). I was drafted just weeks after turning 18 in December of 1943. After testing, I was placed into a unit that was supposed to be sent to college for special training. Many of the men in this outfit were already a few years into college when they were drafted and many came from upper middle class homes. Very few came from a coal mining, open prostitution town like Scranton. What most surprised me about these men was that, although they were about 18 to 22 years old, many of them were still virginal or had very limited sexual experiences. I had thought the world was like Scranton where very few boys passed age 18 without sexual experience–but I soon learned otherwise. The Army changed its plans to send us to college for special training and instead sent most of us for basic training as part of a combat engineer battalion at Camp Chafee, Arkansas. The Army taught us how to build roads and bridges and then how to blow them up when we were done. They then sent us overseas to try out our skills.

Many of my army buddies saw in me someone who could help them get involved with women. I saw in these better educated men a chance to learn about things they knew, such as good books, a wider range of music, how to play chess, and much more. As things worked out we made a fair exchange; I shared with them what I knew about sexual relationships, and they shared with me what they knew about "high" culture in America. I think we all benefited from the exchange. I sharpened my awareness of the world and became more eager to go to college, and I believe they broadened their skills in relating to women. My army experience convinced me more than anything that biology is not the major determinant of one's sexual attitudes and behaviors. These army friends were no different than my Scranton friends in their biological inheritance, but they were a world apart in sexual attitudes and behavior–at least they were when we first met.

CLIMBING UP THE ACADEMIC TREE

Undergraduate Years

Neither of my parents ever went beyond the eighth grade, but they both believed passionately in the value of education, and they encouraged me to go to college. I knew that my father expected me to work in his clothing factory after I finished college and so when I went to Syracuse University I majored in Business Administration (now, euphemistically called the School of Management). However, most of the courses I enjoyed were not in Business Administration but were in psychology, economics, and philosophy. I found the business courses to be largely a waste of time for me. I had serious doubts about whether I would enjoy working in my father's clothing factory, and I began to think of other professions.

A philosophy course I took in my senior year was particularly important in moving me in the right career direction. Our professor was critical of all premarital sex because he had witnessed how it could lead to pregnancy and disease. I rejected that negative view because safe sex had worked very well for me in avoiding disease and pregnancy outcomes. I argued my ideas with him in class and included them in what I wrote for that course. I continued discussing this issue in depth with the six college roommates with whom I shared the second floor of a home near campus. In the fall semester of 1948, in order to try to convince my roommates about the worth of my ideas, I wrote a paper on choices among premarital sexual standards. This was my first written attempt at integrating the conflicting elements regarding sexuality that existed in my own socialization. In this paper, I presented marriage as the ideal place for a sexual relationship, but I suggested that it was also acceptable to have sex if you liked or loved your partner. Recreational sex I saw as borderline in rewards and risky in costs, and I argued that the comparative consequences of different types of premarital relationships strongly favored affection-based sexuality. One could experience recreational sex, but it was not worth your primary emphasis.

But, although I was somewhat conservative in my sexual rankings, I still rejected abstinence as *the* answer. I stressed the importance of the spirit or intention in a relationship rather than following the strict letter of some demanding orthodoxy. I saw virginity as a mental state and not a physical state. Each new sexual relationship actualized something very new in the world and so the fact of having had prior sexual relationships was not very important. To me, in a new caring relationship, both partners were, in a psychic sense, virginal. I put forth these idealistic views equally for both men and women and thereby rejected the double standard.

I was taking a position in accord with the standard I would call "Permissiveness With Affection" and that I would herald as the wave of the future in my first book in 1960. The satisfaction I gained in writing this 1948 paper and talking about it with my roommates encouraged me to plan to someday write a book on premarital sexual standards. I had, unknowingly, begun a lifelong search for an understanding of sexual choices in American society. Clearly, I was working out my own personal problems, but equally so, I saw that my problems reflected the cultural and social confusion regarding sexuality that has disturbed so many of our people for so long a time.

The Choice of a Career

When I finished college, I worked for a year at my father's clothing factory. During that time, I wrote a 150 page essay on religion and science that made the case for science being a better guide to moral action than organized religion. I maintained my belief in God, but I heralded careful scientifically based thinking as a better measure of truth than that offered by organized religion. This was another step in freeing myself from the constraints of orthodox religion while still maintaining a comforting belief in a Deistic type of God who planned the entire universe, although not in accord with the Biblical script. The sort of analysis and synthesis of ideas in this manuscript was what excited my interest the most. The business world contained very little of that sort of intellectual nourishment, and it did not challenge me sufficiently to hold my interest.

By the end of my first year in my father's factory, I was convinced that I would not be satisfied in the business world despite the possibility of good financial reward. My father worked very hard, and I respected his dedication and achievements, but I wanted a type of occupation that would allow me to follow my interests. I felt that to be able to choose a profession that is tailor made for oneself is a rare opportunity. I was fortunate enough to have that opportunity, and I worked to find a path to follow. As my unhappiness at work increased, I discussed my feelings with my old high school friend and one of my Syracuse roommates, Mort Friedman. We were both back in Scranton after college and neither of us was too happy about it. I always liked to argue and debate controversial issues, and, one night after work, we were having our usual debate about some social issue, and Mort sighed, paused, and turned to me and said: "You know Ira, you really enjoy battling over these controversial issues. Maybe you ought to be a college professor and get paid for doing that." This was a landmark experience–like the slap in Hebrew School when I was 10 years old. Now at age 24 I had the chance to do what Rabbi Schachter told me to do; not to waste what talent I had but to nurture and develop it. Mort's suggestion was so much in harmony with my gut feelings that I knew my life was about to take a dramatic turn.

I began to think intensely about going back to graduate school and getting a PhD and becoming a college professor but I wasn't sure what field to choose. My first thought was philosophy, for I loved the open questioning of that field, but I still had my old feeling that philosophy left too much up in the air because it lacked an established tradition of empirical verification. I wanted a field that dealt with philosophical issues but that used scientific methods to help resolve differences. Psychology, I felt was too morbid. Another college friend of mine came to my rescue. Ralph Forest in our college conversations had encouraged me to think about sex with affection as preferable to casual sex and thereby influenced my thinking in my 1948 sex standards paper. Now, Ralph was again giving me good insights. He told me that he believed sociology was just right for my type of interests and advised me to get my PhD in that field. I still wasn't fully certain, so I decided to start my graduate work in sociology but take courses in philosophy too and decide which one to major in during my first year in graduate school.

I had to tell my Dad about my plans. I dreaded doing that. I knew he was expecting me to eventually take over his business. But somehow I had to tell him of my hopes to become a college professor. I remember the day I broke the news. It was the late afternoon of July 15, 1950, and I was sitting in the living room with him. I just said it right out: "I'm thinking of leaving work and going to graduate school to become a college professor." Now it was finally out. My Dad saw my anxiety and said to me that only now, after telling him outright, could I really get in touch with my true feelings. We talked and I told him that even if I was a fantastic success in business it would not make me feel satisfied, whereas if I was an average professor, I would be very happy. Our priorities were not exactly the same. He questioned whether I would earn enough and I stressed how I would respect myself so much more as a teacher. After we discussed the issue for some time, he and my mother spent about two hours alone talking about it. I knew my mother was willing to accept anything I wanted. She was always supportive, and I was sure she only wondered why I hadn't yet been elected President of the U.S. They both came back after their discussion and informed me that they had decided that the best thing would be for me to try graduate school and see what happened. I was much relieved and exhilarated. Their acceptance of my desires made my plans much easier to pursue.

Academic Hurdles and the Race to the Finish Line

Two months later I was in graduate school at Penn State. There was a small but very tight knit group of graduate students in sociology, and I was soon integrated with them. The sociology department at Penn State was relatively new and had given its first Ph.D. just four years earlier, in 1946. The recipient was William J. Goode who was to make his mark in sociology soon afterwards with his classic study of divorce in Detroit, and eventually would become president of the American Sociological Association.

My first sociology course in Sociology of Religion decided my career choice for me. Luther Lee Bernard, a former president of the American Sociological Society, was my first professor. He was 69 years old and this was to be the last year of his life, but he exuded excitement about sociology and it was contagious. A few weeks into the semester, I gave my first graduate report (on Egyptian religion) to L. L. Bernard's class. I can still see L. L. staring at me with his blue eyes gleaming approval during my talk. My fellow grad students also responded with enthusiasm. Afterwards they followed me out of the class, asking me how I knew so much about Egyptian religion and how was I able to conceptualize it so clearly. I was thrilled. I had only read one book. I thought to myself: Imagine what I could do if I really knew the area I was reporting on!

This very positive reaction gave me the confidence that I could organize ideas into coherent patterns and make them interesting and understandable. I now knew that I could be a teacher and perhaps a writer and that I could contribute something to sociology. Sociology was now my chosen major area. Philosophy, with a specialization in ethics, would become my minor area for my PhD. The fire to learn was fully lit, and I was eager to earn my degree and start my career. I had found a pathway into the academy, and I was anxious to fully explore what lay ahead.

I never took a family class at Penn State, and there were no sexuality or gender classes in the 1950s. So my interest in studying sexuality was not reinforced, but I held onto it. I did have Jessie Bernard, L. L. Bernard's widow, as the advisor of my MA Committee, and I did read some of her family and gender publications. But by far the most influential professor for me was a young, imaginative, free thinking sociologist named Edward J. Abramson. I took his course in social change and liked the breadth of his qualitative view of sociology, the paradoxes he saw in society, and the personal respect he gave to even my sometimes far out ideas about society. As a newcomer to the field, I needed that sort of support, even though I covered that need up with my brash presentation of self.

Another very influential person in my first year was a fellow graduate student, William Bensch. He had just returned from a year's trip around the world, and he was always willing to argue and discuss new ideas. We often disagreed, but we clearly showed the mutual respect that gave the lie to the ridicule we hurled at each others' views. Bill and I ended up doing a joint master's thesis with Eddy Abramson as our advisor. We asked Jessie Bernard to be our official advisor because another professor, Arnold Green, objected to Eddy chairing our committee since he had not finished his PhD. Bensch, like Eddy, had the depth of cultural background and tolerance of difference to which I was attracted. I knew I had a lot to learn, but I also was not about to give up my right to decide what I accepted. I always questioned things before I would accept them, even such widely accepted things as the poetic value of Shakespeare or the power of Wagnerian music. Bensch, like Eddy Abramson, accepted that feistiness in me and so enabled me to continue my cultural education that had been nurtured during my stint in the Army.

My first and most lasting love in Sociology was the development of theories that make sense out of some part of our social lives. And so theory construction became my major area for my PhD. I was fascinated to find out how things worked in society and why things worked the way they did, especially in areas of controversy, like sexuality. I minored in Cultural Anthropology for my MA and in Philosophy of Ethics for my PhD. Both of these minors opened up windows into the universe of ideas that I eagerly wanted to explore. The years in graduate school were an intellectual feast for me, and I gorged myself as much as I could. But I wanted to be a professor and be free of other people's rules and regulations. I rushed through and earned my MA and PhD degrees and made up the undergraduate sociology courses, all in just three years.

One of those three years was spent at Columbia University. In between my MA and PhD I went to Columbia to take my PhD course work and to gain a different perspective. Once there I was very impressed by the theoretical abilities and interests of Robert K. Merton. He was only 41 then and four years later he was to be president of the American Sociological Association, but most importantly he was a very stimulating and exciting scholar. Unlike Eddy Abramson and Bill Bensch, Robert Merton was not that approachable and was far more systematic and scientific in his thinking. Nevertheless, his vast knowledge and ability to explain social events was exciting. He influenced me to accept many of the ideas of the structural/functional approach and to put more emphasis on the scientific aspects of sociology.

In my third and final year I went back to Penn State to take my language and prelim exams and write my dissertation. I will tell you the interesting story of my final PhD oral that took place on August 21, 1953.

This event will give you insight into my "chutzpah." My dissertation was an ambitious project aimed at comparing viewpoints concerning how sociologists can obtain the subjective thoughts and feelings of people in society. I compared the qualitative vs. quantitative methodological positions on this issue and developed my own perspective. This issue held great interest for me and was part of the widespread debate about just how scientific sociology could be used in studying our subjective beliefs. It combined my interest in theoretical explanation with my interest in controversy.

A heavy dose of departmental politics interjected itself into my dissertation project. One of the faculty members on my committee, Walter Coutu, thought he had written the answer to my dissertation inquiry in his recent book (Coutu, 1949). I did mention this professors' ideas in my first dissertation draft, but I had not given them prominence, nor had I endorsed them. He and I had previous disagreements on other issues in a course of his and that may have exacerbated our dissertation clash. I strongly believed in my right to academic freedom but I was soon to find out how academic politics can compromise academic freedom, particularly if you are a graduate student.

My PhD advisor, Arnold Green, was an associate professor. Walter Coutu was a full professor, who would vote on my advisor when he came up for promotion. This worried Arnold Green, and he told me that he hesitated to set up my final oral while my conflict with Coutu was unresolved. I had made some compromises in my dissertation on the advice of another committee member, the chair of our department, Seth Russell. The heart of my dissertation dealt with whether you gave priority to the meaning and significance of what you were studying or whether you gave priority to the reliability of evidence concerning what you were studying. I felt that the significance of what was being studied about people's subjective viewpoints was of prime importance even if it could not easily be replicated. I did not disregard the value of reliability but I thought of it as secondary in importance. This position was part, but by no means all, of the debate I was having with Coutu. I followed Seth Russell's advice to take a more middle-of-the-road position in my final dissertation draft, and I gave both significance and reliability a more equal position of importance.

But that was not enough to end the conflict. Coutu felt that his social psychological approach had resolved the conflict of significance and reliability. He favored the importance of reliability over significance, but he tried to include them both in his theorizing. He had taken the "stimulus/response" approach and added to it the element of "meaning." So instead of S-R, he presented S-M-R. I did not think this resolved the conflict between significance and reliability. One still had to decide how to get at the meaning of an act, even if you put the word "meaning" into a formula. Accordingly, I mentioned his view in my final draft but did not describe it as having resolved the controversy. I had compromised as far as I was willing to go. But I had only a few weeks left in which to schedule my final oral before leaving for my first job, and Green was still unwilling to schedule it.

If rank was the issue between Green and Coutu, I decided I would play that trump suit. Seth Russell was the chair of the department and was, therefore, the highest ranking person on my committee. I could not talk directly to Russell about Green's hesitancy to set up my final oral without aggravating the interdepartmental conflict further and so I took another path. I called Russell and told him that Green and I had talked about having my oral on the 21st of August. I asked him, as chair of the department, for his approval to finalize this date. Russell thought my statement meant Green had agreed to set up my oral and so he endorsed the date. My statement was a half truth: I had talked about that date with Green, but he had not agreed to schedule it–he wanted Coutu to feel more comfortable with my dissertation before he would move on it. But, I was about to finesse that opposition.

After I spoke to Russell, I proceeded to call Green and told him that Russell wanted my final oral to be scheduled on the 21st. I knew that Green would not deny what he thought were the chair's wishes–he respected rank. Also, by Russell making the decision, Green knew he could not be criticized by Coutu. Green agreed with setting up the oral. I then called Coutu and told him that Russell and Green had agreed to set up the oral on the 21st. He did not object. The rest of my committee all accepted the date. I had played the cards in the power game and won that opening round. But what would happen at the oral was still up for grabs.

My oral was scheduled at 3:30 on Friday the 21st of August. It was the last of three orals on that day and that day was the last day possible for holding an oral before the Fall semester. The oral began with the usual formalities. The differences of opinion between Coutu and myself came out during the oral but in muted form. Coutu was not as critical as I had feared. Also, Green sought to shift the oral discussion to areas that would not arouse Coutu's disagreement. Russell, of course, knew of the conflict, and he tried to reduce the tension by suggesting minor changes that should be made in the dissertation. Russell had shown support for me throughout my stay at Penn State, and he provided the needed leadership to keep the oral on track towards a successful completion. During the oral, the other four members of the committee expressed support for my dissertation. Then the discussion ran its course, and Green asked me to leave the room so they could decide if I passed.

When I went out in the hall to wait the final decision of the committee, I knew the start of my career was in jeopardy, and I was very unsure of the outcome. The committee could have decided to ask me to radically rewrite and thereby delay my degree a full year. I very much wanted to start my first job without this burden. Finally, Green called me back into the room and informed me that although I had to make a number of minor changes in the dissertation, I had passed. He did not express much in the way of congratulations but informed me in a matter of fact fashion. But, being passed was the only outcome that mattered to me. I don't know how Coutu voted, but I could not have received more than one negative vote or else I would have failed. Also, I do believe he voted to pass me because he came to the party that my friends had that night and personally congratulated me. He told me that I better write a book on my thinking soon, because he was about to write one on his views. So perhaps the problem on my dissertation was more with Green's anxiety about promotion than with Coutu's disagreement with my dissertation. That night I called to thank Seth Russell, and he told me that he too was leaving Penn State. He was very kind and said: "I was not about to go, Ira, without first getting you through that political minefield." His support for my final oral was the key that opened the door to my successful finishing of my degree.

My friends and I had one wild celebration that night. It was like breaking the bank at Monte Carlo. I had played the academic system at its own game and I had won. It was an early lesson in the role of power in the realm of ideas. There surely was an adversarial dimension to academic freedom. Jefferson was right: the price of liberty was eternal vigilance. And that certainly is still true in regard to academic freedom at our universities today.

The Professional World: The Early Years

A few weeks later, in September 1953, I started in my first job at Bowdoin College in Maine. Kinsey had received his bachelor's degree there thirty some years earlier. I learned that the College was thinking of giving Kinsey an honorary degree, but they changed their mind for fear of criticism from Senator Joe McCarthy who was then spewing his bigotry even into the colleges and universities of our country.

The chair of my department at Bowdoin, Burton Taylor, asked me to teach a family course. I did not know it then but that course was to afford me my first legitimate platform for expressing my ideas about gender and sexuality. Having never taken a family course, I wrote away for all the texts in that area and proceeded to try to select one. I felt I knew something about sexuality–after all I was the unofficial sex educator of the 1273rd Combat Engineer Battalion and the author of a 1948 college position paper. I decided I would read the chapter on sexuality in each textbook and choose on that basis. What I found was shocking.

Almost without exception, every textbook in the family area condemned premarital sexual intercourse. Sex before marriage was painted as inevitably involving negative outcomes like pregnancy, disease, guilt, social condemnation, and the weakening of your future marriage. Your relationship might escape one or two of these; however, you could never escape all of them. The positive consequences of premarital sex, such as physical pleasure, psychological satisfaction, or preparation for marital sexuality, were ignored or distorted. In general, pleasure outside of marital sex was conceptualized as evil and lustful. In the perspective of these textbooks, affection was removed from premarital sexual relationships and selfishness and irresponsibility took its place.

Some premarital sex, of course, fits the portrait being sketched in these textbooks, but there was so much more that was left out or misrepresented. The acceptance of what was said in these texts would be equivalent to accepting as accurate a politician's description of his opponent. These textbook treatments of sexuality were not scientific, nor were they even carefully reasoned. Data from such authorities as Kinsey were either ignored or distorted. The texts were simply boldface traditional sexual propaganda.

I was taken aback by the presentation of such dogma as social science. One of my major career goals was set by this experience. I vowed that I would present a more empirically based and logically reasoned view of sexuality in my family class and in my writings. Also, I would work hard not to allow my values to bias my presentation. I would be conscious of alternative values and alternative evaluations. In the years that followed, much of my writing on sexuality and on the family was aimed to achieve these things. Some of my hesitancy to take a strong policy stance as part of my sociological analysis was tied to the destructive mix of value positions and sociology that I had found in those family textbooks. As I will note later, my views on the integrating of value stances into science have liberalized somewhat for I now promote being explicit about our value assumptions and with conscious care, and caution, still not allowing that position to compromise our scientific integrity as it had in those early 1950s family textbooks.

Just as I was writing my first two articles (Reiss, 1956, 1957) criticizing the family textbooks I had examined, I met the woman who has been my life companion ever since: Harriet Marilyn Eisman. Harriet has been my intellectual sparring partner as well as my editor and my emotional support. This has been true since I met her in late January 1955, fell in love with her, and married her in September 1955. She discussed all my writings with me and gave me much to think about. But it was only in my 1990 book that she allowed me to even list her name on the cover of the book. So as I explain my academic career, I want to here give major credit to the wonderful collaboration that Harriet and I have had on all my work since our marriage in 1955. She combined the finest traits of both my parents: the complete devotion of my mother and the pragmatism of my father. Having Harriet in my life has made everything else in my life much more enjoyable.

Just weeks after we married I began a position at the College of William and Mary in Williamsburg, Virginia. I wrote the early drafts of my 1960 book on premarital sexual standards in the summers of 1956, 1957, and 1958. It was in that book, in the last chapter, that I predicted the sexual revolution that I believed was to fully appear in the late 1960s (Reiss, 1960a, pp. 239-241). William Kephart at the University of Pennsylvania reviewed that book in sociology's top journal, *The American Sociological Review* in April of 1961. He commented on my prediction of college students leading a new sexual revolution by saying that in ". . . the last chapter . . . Reiss apparently lost control of the typewriter" (Kephart, 1961, p. 294). But that's exactly the way our country went, and so don't put too much of your faith in book reviewers.

I interpreted the textbook bias against premarital sexuality as a defense by conservatives against admitting that there are new sexual standards that are replacing abstinence and the double standard and thereby promoting a new sexual revolution. This change was threatening to those with traditional views and so they fought back with their one-sided condemnation of all premarital coitus. I saw the major cultural trend among young people in our country as a rejection of abstinence as "the one and only" sexual standard. The trend, as I saw it, was an endorsement of permissiveness with affection as an acceptable choice in its place. In connection with writing about this new affection based standard, I developed my ideas about how love develops in dyadic relationships and presented them in the form of my "wheel theory of love," which has over the years been one of my most popular articles (Reiss, 1960a, pp. 136-144; 1960b).

By 1960, my views on permissiveness without affection had liberalized from those in my 1948 college paper on sexuality. My book conceptualized permissiveness without affection as having two subtypes: (a) sophisticated–pragmatic pleasure lovers who take precautions against disease and pregnancy, and (b) orgiastic–pleasure lovers who de-emphasize taking precautions against disease and pregnancy. I had problems personally accepting only the orgiastic sub-type. Even though I had, since my college days, become more pluralistic, I still emphasized the acceptance of affectionate coitus as the trend in America, and it was the one that I personally preferred. I analyzed what data we had and cultural trends in as fair and unbiased a way as I could. I think I succeeded in this. The fact that permissiveness with affection did indeed become the most popular new sexual standard supported the fairness and accuracy of my empirical analysis and my theoretical interpretation.

As I was writing my first book, I began to correspond with Albert Ellis–a therapist who was writing some very innovative books about sexuality. It was my questioning of sex without affection that led me to correspond with Albert Ellis and eventually establish a friendship. It was in 1956 that I first contacted Ellis, the founder of today's very popular Rational Emotive Therapy. I wrote to Ellis about my qualms concerning the strong support for casual sex that he expressed in some of his writings. We corresponded and discovered that we were not quite as far apart as we thought. A year later we met for the first time in a rather interesting way.

We had set up a time for meeting at the Eastern Sociological Society meetings in New York in April of 1957. I was presenting a paper stressing trends in premarital sexual standards towards acceptance of permissiveness with affection. After my talk, a man in the audience stood up and asserted that I was stressing affection not fully acknowledging the increase in permissiveness without affection. In 1957 that sort of "liberal" viewpoint was so rare that I wondered to myself if the questioner could be Ellis. I half jokingly asked the speaker if he were Albert Ellis. My hunch was right–it was indeed Albert Ellis, and that was the beginning of a long personal relationship. I have always admired Ellis's openness in expressing unconventional views and his dedication to developing and applying his ideas to the field of therapy. As the years have passed, I have come to share more and more of his rational/emotive psychological perspectives. He is the person who first thought of founding the Society for the Scientific Study of Sexuality. He convinced me to become a charter member of that organization when it began in 1957. Ellis is still a leader in confronting the dogmatism of the radical right. All of us who value choice in sexuality owe him a debt of gratitude for the many battles he has fought–and won.

The years at William and Mary rounded out my basic background in sociology and also in anthropology. There were only four of us in the department and so we each had to teach many different courses. We required a senior research paper for sociology majors. In 1958, with the encouragement of my chair, Wayne Kernodle, I started a major study of premarital sexual standards. It was my way of testing the idea that many young people do indeed believe in newer sexual standards such as the one I called "permissiveness with affection." It was the popularity of this new standard that I felt heralded a new sexual revolution in our country. Four of our senior majors chose to work with me on my project: Ron Dusek, Martha Fisher, Richard Shirey, and John Stephenson. John was the leader of the group and the one who would go on to get a PhD in sociology and become president of Berea College in Kentucky. All four students worked very hard during their senior year on this project. They had been caught up in the passion of this project and were excited about the possible findings.

I discussed with this group of four students the development of my Guttman scales to measure premarital sexual permissiveness and informed them that their senior research would be its first testing ground. The 12 item scales measured premarital sexual permissiveness attitudes in terms of the place of affection as related to the acceptance of kissing, petting, and coital behavior. This scale in both its original and in its shortened form has been used in scores of other research projects (Reiss, 1964a, 1967, 1989a, 1998a, Reiss & Miller, 1979; Schwartz & Reiss, 1995). But to test these scales and our hypotheses about causes of changes in the permissiveness levels they measure, we needed to get permission from local high schools and colleges to administer our questionnaire to their students. In Virginia, or anywhere in 1958, this was not an easy thing to do. Once more social and political reality set up a barrier to a project of mine. But I was to find a way to overcome that.

When my four senior students approached the principal of the white and the black high schools in Williamsburg, they were turned down. I knew that these principals feared public reaction, but I also hoped that they would see the usefulness of knowing more about their students. Now I had to figure out how to change their minds. I went to see the white principal first, and, when he repeated his opposition to administering my questionnaire, I asked him how many of his high school girls had become pregnant last year. I then asked him whether he felt any responsibility to lessen the risk of pregnancy for these and for future girls. I said to him: "Do you want to be seen as someone who chose to pass up the opportunity for increasing awareness of sexual standards that might help reduce unwanted pregnancy?" I let him know that this research was important to gaining knowledge of how to control outcomes like pregnancy. I also made it clear that I might well make a public issue of it if he continued to deny us permission. He finally came around and said he would not let us give our questionnaire to the 9th graders but the 10th, 11th, and 12th graders could participate. I was reminded of my PhD final oral conflict some five years earlier. I saw clearly how the social context of our life space had to be thoughtfully navigated if we were to carry out our so called "pure science" research.

The response from the black high school principal was more of an enigma. My chair, Wayne Kernodle, was friends with this man, and he took me to his office and introduced me. The three of us sat down to talk, and I explained the importance of this research for gaining better control over unwanted sexual outcomes like pregnancy. But instead of responding, he kept changing the topic to the anti school-integration politics in Virginia. I kept trying to turn the conversation back to my study and he ignored my efforts. Finally, I realized that he wanted to see where I stood on the still hot issues of racial integration which the powerful Byrd political machine, represented by Governor Almond of Virginia, was resisting. I turned to him and shared a political joke I had heard: "The Byrd machine has inbred so much that it finally had produced an idiot–the Governor." He gave a loud laugh and said to me: "When do you want to give out the questionnaires?" Once more the importance of the social context of social research was vividly impressed upon me.

We gave out our questionnaires to the two Williamsburg high schools and also to two colleges (William and Mary and Hampton Institute). The four students on the project worked with our primitive McBee card system. It was a pre-computer method of analysis used to test whether our premarital questions produced a usable Guttman type scale. The answer came in the Spring of 1959. I remember the night very well because we lived right across the street from the campus, and there was a "panty raid" that night. Harriet and I were observing the event with interest from our window. The phone rang, and I thought it must be about the panty raid on campus. But it was John Stephenson and with great emotion he said to me: "They work! They work! The scales work! They meet all Guttman scale criteria, they are valid!"

The students and I celebrated that event with much gusto. It was like the discovery of some new chemical element, for there was no existing scientific scale to measure premarital sexual permissiveness. This was an important step towards systematizing the analysis of premarital sexuality and getting away from the very unscientific presentations that abounded in the textbooks and in the media. As I mentioned, these scales have since come to be very widely used, and, in 1989, I published a 4-item version that can be used instead of the two 12 item male and female scales (Reiss, 1989a, 1998a). This new very short version has been tested in the U.S. and Sweden and found to meet Guttman scale requirements (Schwartz & Reiss, 1995). The four-item scale is more convenient, and one could even use a single item (#3) if a dichotomous response was adequate. That item asked about acceptance of premarital coitus if one was in a relationship that had "moderate" affection. As of the 1980s and 1990s, responses to that question tended to divide college students into two equal groups and thus it was a convenient measure.

After we gathered data from our four schools, Wayne Kernodle, a very supportive and very helpful chair, encouraged me to apply for a government grant to further analyze the data I had gathered. Wayne was an important supporter of my work in those days. I recall talking to him about some traditional students in my family course telling me that I was spending too much time on sexuality. Wayne's response was that *they* had a problem and that I should cover whatever I felt needed to be covered. In my early work on sexuality, I very much appreciated that sort of intellectual support.

In 1959 I left William and Mary and went to Bard College. I followed Wayne's advice and applied for a National Institutes of Mental Health (NIMH) government grant to support analysis of my research data. In 1960 I received approval of the first of three NIMH grants that for four years were to support my analyses of these data and my gathering of a new nationally representative sample of adults to further test the scales and the predictors of scale values. When I was awarded the grant, NIMH told me to change the title of my grant so that it did not contain the word sexual, or else, the grant might not get through all the official government checks. Even in the 1990s, this same higher risk applies to grants researching sexuality–it is sad to see how powerful the uninformed and narrow minded still are in our government.

My new research grants would test out many of the ideas in my 1960 book. That book sought to explain sexual standards in America and predicted dramatic sexual changes by the end of the 1960s (Reiss, 1960, pp. 239-241). The notion that someone could fairly analyze our society and accurately predict such changes was not widespread at that time. I hoped that my research grants would yield knowledge that would dissuade many such pessimistic beliefs. A job offer from the University of Iowa followed very soon after the book appeared, and I decided that it was time to leave the liberal arts college world and explore the Big Ten Universities. I've always valued my three liberal arts college positions–particularly William and Mary. But I thought it was time to move on and explore an environment that would provide me with better scientific support for analyzing the data and other work connected to my NIMH grants.

The University of Iowa afforded me good technical support in the way of staff and equipment. The first day I was on campus I came in contact with Don McTavish, a PhD student in sociology. I told him I was looking for a research assistant. He took me on a tour of the computer center and in the process demonstrated the research skills he possessed. I hired him as my research assistant that same day. For the next three years, he was a major collaborator in the analysis of my data. In 1962, I applied for and received a supplement to my NIMH grant that allowed me to try out my scales on a nationally representative sample of the country. The National Opinion Research Center (NORC) at the University of Chicago was doing "amalgam" surveys where you could buy a segment of time and have your questions asked of a nationally representative sample. My questions were added to the NORC June 1963 national sample. It was the first scale analysis of sexual attitudes done on a representative national sample, and today it affords us a benchmark measure of the premarital sexual attitudes in this country just shortly before the sexual revolution exploded forth in the late 1960s. These data are now archived at the Kinsey Institute at Indiana University and are available for use by other researchers. I have recently used this national data on premarital sexual permissiveness levels for analyzing trends in premarital sexuality from the early 1960s to the early 1990s (Reiss, 1996).

The academic priorities at the University of Iowa and my intense involvement in the analysis of my national and student data moved me further in a hard science direction. The scientific script that I was then following allowed sociologists to explain the trends but mostly left to politicians the making of recommendations for resolving any social problems. I surely did do some social commentary on sexual problems during the 1960s but that was not my main thrust. What I eventually came to realize was that often those who would use my research had values that were very different than mine and might well distort my findings. I also increasingly felt the responsibility to present what I thought was the most effective solution to a particular sexual problem.

During the 1960s and 1970s the trends in the country were towards increased acceptance of a supportive view of sexuality. This societal trend made it easier to not take positions on how to reduce sexual problems in our society–the society at large often seemed to be making the same moves that I would have suggested. So I could focus more on just explaining what the trends were and why they were happening. When those trends stopped and sex negative resistance surfaced in the 1980s, I felt the need to speak out and suggest directions that we as a society should be taking in order to resolve our sexual problems. I believed that if I was aware of my own values and made a conscious effort to avoid bias, I could make my value assumptions explicit and still do a good job of analyzing the sexual situation in a scientific manner. The increased resistance to sexual changes had made me more conscious of the inevitable mix of science and values when we study human behavior of any kind.

In 1967, my book, *The Social Context of Premarital Sexual Permissiveness,* which analyzed the national sample and the regional school samples, was published. It received a very favorable reception, and the "autonomy theory," which I put forth to explain change in sexual permissiveness, has inspired scores of research studies in the years since (Reiss & Miller, 1979; Schwartz & Reiss, 1995). In this second book, I tested my Guttman scales measuring premarital sexual permissiveness and also tested a number of explanatory variables derived from my 1960 book and elsewhere. I used a 1963 national adult sample and 6 student samples that consisted of two high schools and four colleges in three different states (I had added Bard College and the University of Iowa to my Virginia college sample). The autonomy theory that I developed explained changes in premarital sexual permissiveness as due to increased freedom for youth from adult institutions and increased acceptance of sexuality in the culture at large.

This autonomy theory was a broad theoretical integration of the seven theoretical propositions that I developed in this book to explain more specifically the social forces that alter premarital sexual permissiveness levels (Reiss, 1967, Chapter 10). The events that happened in America in the late 1960s and 1970s fit very well with the predictions that the autonomy theory made about causes of changes in sexual customs in our country. For example, the theory predicted that the group whose autonomy (ability to run their own life) increased the most would be the group whose premarital acceptance of sexuality would increase the most. Of the four race/sex groups, white females were showing the greatest increase in autonomy and so I predicted their increase in acceptance of sexuality would be the greatest. That was precisely what happened in the decade from the late 1960s to the late 1970s.

The Move to Minnesota

In 1967, I was at a crossroads–what to do next? My two books had attracted a great deal of favorable attention and job offers and other opportunities were coming my way. I received a call from Jack Weiner at the National Institutes of Mental Health inviting me to undertake a national study on homosexuality and heterosexuality. I was exhausted from having just finished my 1967 book and so I regretfully declined. Albert Klassen and his colleagues at Indiana University took on that project. At that same time, activist sociologists were asking me to help lead a movement to advocate politically for more liberal changes in sexual standards. This was the late 1960s and the sexual revolution was beginning to become more obvious to everyone. I was tempted by this suggestion but to do so would have likely required that I make my scientific research and theory work secondary to advocacy efforts. Then and now, I give my scientific work top priority and so I felt I had to decline even though I publicly made it clear that I personally supported more pluralistic changes in sexual standards.

I chose to write a sociology of the family textbook. Ever since 1953 when I had reviewed family textbooks in preparation to teach a course on the family, I had wanted to write my own textbook in order to present a sociological analysis of the family in what I believed was a more reasonable and accurate fashion. I had been teaching family courses regularly since I received my degree. In 1965 I published an article arguing that nurturance of the newborn was the only family function that was present in every society (Reiss, 1965a). I tied that conception into a deeper understanding of the place of the family in society. I should note here that it was Marvin Sussman as editor of the *Journal of Marriage and the Family* who liked this article enough to publish it in record time–just three months after it was submitted. I wanted to follow up on my ideas concerning the family. I also wanted to write a text that integrated human sexuality into the understanding of the family more than current textbooks did.

This family textbook eventually went into four editions (Reiss, 1971, 1976, 1980, 1988). That textbook took up a good deal of my energy from the late 1960s to the late 1970s (the 4th edition had Gary R. Lee as a co-author). I sometimes wonder just how different things might have been had I followed through on my work directly in the sexuality field and not ventured so strongly into the sociology of the family area. But, I did use my sexuality research and theory perspective in my family textbook. Also, during the 1970s I was increasingly moving back to research and theory directly in sexuality, because that was still clearly my number one substantive interest (Reiss, 1970, 1972, 1973; Reiss, Banwart, & Foreman, 1975; Reiss & Miller, 1979; Reiss, Walsh, Zey-Ferrell, Tolone, & Pocs, 1980a; Reiss, Anderson, & Sponaugle, 1980b).

In January 1969, as I was working on my family textbook, the University of Minnesota offered me a position in the Department of Sociology as the Director of the Family Study Center. Reuben Hill wanted to step down from that position in the Family Study Center he had helped found. Interestingly, he selected me despite the fact that he knew I had long been critical of some of his views about sexuality (Reiss, 1957). I accepted the offer and joined what probably was then the strongest program in family sociology in the country. Oddly enough, Reuben Hill, the conservative Mormon, and Ira Reiss, the liberal Jew, got along very well with each other. Reuben's and my acceptance of diverse viewpoints and our strong sense of loyalty to good research and theory were the things that bound us together during the 16 years we were colleagues at Minnesota. Reuben was the most helpful colleague I had during those years. He and his wife Marion had also become our friends. I was very grieved by his death in 1985.

At the 1971 National Council on Family Relations meeting, Reuben Hill and I, together with Ivan Nye and Wesley Burr, organized a major project to present all the existing theories in the family field in a formal, scientific fashion in a two-volume work. In 1979, after eight years of effort to gather some of the best people in the family field and have them present their formal theories on specific substantive areas of the family, we published this two-volume work (Burr, Hill, Nye, & Reiss, 1979). Wesley Burr was the junior member of the team, and he did the bulk of the work organizing the contributions to these volumes. I now feel that this work stressed too much the presentation of formal theory and contributed too little to the qualitative understanding of the family or to the possible use of this work for social problem resolution. But in the 1970s, I was more of a believer in the need to formalize theory and to encourage others to do so. In that way, we could best develop our theoretical understanding of the family. Many family scholars found that work useful and told us that our work helped shape the field. But today I would want to add a broader methodological and theoretical sweep and move the focus of the field more to containment of socially rooted problem areas of the family.

The role of Director of the Family Study Center at the University of Minnesota stressed administration work and the obtaining of research grants and Fellowship Grants for graduate students. It left too little time for me to nourish my interests in building theoretical explanations and too little time for researching sexuality and gender issues. I have never liked administering other people's problems, for I have always enjoyed doing my own chosen work. I stayed as director for five years, but in 1974 I eagerly stepped down. I once again was free to focus more fully upon my own research and theory work. I wanted to move back more into sexual science and gender issues. I was once again searching for a new challenge.

I had a sabbatical in 1975-76. In order to gain a broader view of how gender and sexuality are tied into different societies I spent that year teaching and doing research at Uppsala University in Sweden. By being a foreigner for that year, I learned how important it is to understand the cultural and social context of sexuality and gender. It was obvious that the Swedes had a deeper acceptance than we do of premarital intercourse as a legitimate option for young people. The public display of condom advertisements on billboards and their availability in street machines was one indicator of this. The lower disease and pregnancy rates in Sweden made me aware that this greater acceptance and better preparation for sexuality was indeed working very well. I wrote some papers on this experience and have found my experience in Sweden very helpful in developing my cross-cultural perspective on sexuality, gender, and the family (Reiss, 1980).

Part of what I learned about Sweden concerned extramarital sex, and I decided I wanted to focus more on American extramarital sexual attitudes. Together with one of my doctoral students, G.C. Sponaugle, and my colleague, Ron Anderson, I undertook to analyze U.S. national data and develop a theory explaining attitudes towards extramarital sexual permissiveness. We used four different years of the General Social Surveys data on extramarital sex. That sample was gathered annually by NORC and was representative of the nation. They used only one rather general question to measure extramarital attitudes. But this was the best data available, and we carefully analyzed some hypotheses about possible predictors of changes in extramarital sexual attitudes. It turned out that there were three major factors influencing extramarital attitudes. I would sum them up as: (1) how happy one's current marriage was,

(2) how highly one valued sexuality, and (3) how intellectually flexible one's attitudes were (Reiss, Anderson, & Sponaugle, 1980b). The findings contradicted the popular, simplistic view that the first factor, unhappiness of marriage, was the key answer to why extramarital sex was accepted. It was not even the strongest predictor. Several replicative studies of our work followed (Glass & Wright, 1992; Sponaugle, 1993; Reiss, 1998b) and the 1980 article won an award from the National Council on Family Relations. I had thought about doing a book on extramarital sexuality, but I felt I had done enough in this major project and I resumed my search for another area to explore.

COMING FULL CIRCLE

By 1980 I had finished the third edition of my family textbook and increasingly wanted to find a major project in the sexuality and gender area. But this time I wanted to reach a broader audience than just sociologists. One dissertation project that had interested me even back in graduate school was to examine the writings and data on sexuality cross culturally with the aim of arriving at a sociological explanation that would be useful in understanding sexuality in any society. This sort of cross-cultural explanation I thought would be useful to any social scientist and also to some clinicians and social workers who dealt with the area of sexuality. I had always had a strong cross-cultural interest and had taught Anthropology for four years at William and Mary. My goal in this new book project was to find those parts of human societies that are most strongly linked to our sexual customs and to build an explanation of how and why those linkages differed in various societies around the world. This was a very demanding project but that was what I was seeking–I wanted a new challenge. To be sure, this project was a major challenge; it was to occupy me for almost the next five years. Good thing I did not take it up as a dissertation topic!

I read all the anthropological literature I could find on sexuality in various societies. In addition, I used the Standard Cross Cultural Sample (SCCS) of 186 non-industrial societies to check out a number of my ideas (Murdock & White, 1969). I arranged to get permission to add to the SCCS several new sexual codes from other researchers working with this sample. My project was very broad, and there were times I wondered if I would ever be able to finish this work. But eventually I developed my "PIK" theory which stated that the crucial linkages of sexuality in any society were in the areas of Power, Ideology, and Kinship (PIK). I tried to explain why and how the specific nature of this triple linkage differed as it did in various societies as well as why sexuality was always linked to PIK (Reiss, 1986, Chapter 8). I felt I had made a breakthrough in producing a sociological theory that explained similarities and differences in human societies ways of handling sexuality. I had developed a broad macro theoretical perspective within which others could reexamine and could develop additional specific theoretical ideas.

The comparative approach I used was contrary to the fads and fashions, that is, the politically correct view of the day. The popular view then and still now is that each society is unique and thus we cannot really compare different societies in any meaningful way. I accepted the distinctiveness of each society, but I rejected the view that comparisons were not possible. I felt the same way about comparing different people in a group. People are surely different from each other but surely we can compare them without denying that they differ in some respects. Science is not possible if such comparisons cannot be made. I published this book in 1986 and it met with surprisingly strong support from Ron Moglia at the graduate program in human sexuality in New York University, and elsewhere. But my ideas did not reach the broader professional audience as much as I had hoped. Nevertheless, I have noticed in recent years that this book is being cited by other writers who share my desire to understand the similarities as well as the differences in sexuality around the world (Suggs & Miracle, 1993; Devin & Meridith, 1997). Perhaps the politically correct academic stranglehold on cross-cultural comparisons is beginning to weaken. Science thrives best in an open atmosphere rather than in one where certain types of projects are blocked by prejudgments of their worth.

In this book, I had taken a significant step away from writing only for sociologists and I wrote for a broader range of social scientists. The change was refreshing to me but now I wanted to reach an even broader segment of the public as well as reach other professionals. I once more anguished over how to do this and what sexuality topic to explore. The answer came to me loud and clear one day in the fall of 1986 when I heard Letty Cottin Pogrebin talk about the American family at a National Council on Family Relations meeting in Detroit. Her comments emphasized what the family "could be" much more than what the family is or what the trends might be. The phrase "could be" hit me with great impact. I was tired of writing about what is and why it is and what the trends are. I wanted to put a more personal and ethical touch on my work and talk about what I thought was the way to build a better society.

I was picking up the writing task I had begun back in 1948 when I wrote my philosophy course paper on premarital sexual ethics. I wanted to present, with reason and evidence, a personal position on resolving our major sexual problems. Letty Pogrebin's approach gave me the encouragement I needed for such an approach. I thank her for that.

A second major motivation for my new project in 1986 was the increasingly strong radical right emphasis on returning to an abstinence only solution for our sexual problems such as HIV/AIDS. I knew that approach was doomed to failure, but I also knew that the American public was very poorly informed and still harbored the Victorian virus that supported a return to past sexual standards. I wanted to do what I could to show the public that the resolution to our sexual crises was not present in the past but in a changed future.

Projects that have a broad societal applicability have always been most interesting to me. I see as my strength the ability to interpret and explain very diverse phenomena. But I had not applied that ability to finding solutions for our society's sexual problems quite as directly as I was to do now. I chose four American sexual problem areas that begged for problem resolutions: HIV/AIDS, rape, teenage pregnancy, and child sexual abuse. I explored what in our society had produced our high rate of these problems and what changes in society would best bring these four unwanted problems under better control.

As my analyses of these four problem areas proceeded and I examined the major studies in these areas, I found myself confirming that the traditional sexual ethic of our society had seriously exacerbated, rather than helped, in all these problems. It was also increasingly clear that a new pluralistic sexual philosophy was evolving that would help us to manage these sexual problems. That new philosophy was what I called HER sexual pluralism. My wife Harriet suggested the HER acronym to me. This sexual ethic asserted that if a sexual relationship was Honest, Equal, and Responsible (HER), then it was morally acceptable whether it was between two men, two women, a man and a women, two sixteen year olds or whatever. Also, the amount of affection was not the number one value. The honesty, equality, and responsibility in a relationship were the key moral criteria of sexual choices in that relationship. Love by itself was not the answer to a moral choice. Surely there are many love relationships with severe gaps in HER and non-love relationships with greater HER. This change toward a HER sexual standard in America in the late 1980s was as significant to me as the change to permissiveness with affection was in the late 1950s. It heralded a new way of conceptualizing sexuality by the American public. This was, I believe, the final phase of the sexual revolution that had become visible a generation earlier.

Writing this book afforded me such an exhilarating feeling. I was finally openly involving so much more of myself in my professional work. Now, I was speaking as a whole person and not just from a scientific position. Now my work was more of a human endeavor and less of an antiseptic, "pure" science project. Now I could develop a more humane model of science. I was clearly prescribing as well as theorizing. It was about time!

But I want to be clear about this new sexual standard. HER sexual pluralism does not say anything goes. It demands an ethical approach that shows concern for one's partner. That concern is the minimal price of admission to the arena of ethical sexual choices. What choices one makes within a HER negotiation will vary by where one is in their life and what other values one holds. This minimalist HER philosophy would encourage people to take responsibility for working out such ethical choices and to change their specific preferences when their life situations and their values changed. But it was not a carte blanche. It did not require a commitment to deep affection, but it did require a concern for treating the other person in an honest, equal, and responsible fashion. To me, HER sexual pluralism surely qualifies as a revolutionary perspective compared to our Victorian and Puritan ethics. It is also a significant change from the much more narrow permissiveness with affection standard.

In this 1990 book I was directly confronting the absolutism of those traditionalists who said we should reject teenage sex, reject homosexuality, reject sex outside of marriage. I examined the evidence of trends all over the Western world towards HER sexual pluralism and argued that we are now in the midst of a new Western sexual revolution. This one will complete the sexual revolution that began in the late 1960s. Today's revolution concerns sexual attitudes and not so much sexual behavior. It is a more silent revolution. And it is only partially recognized as such, but it is rapidly spreading in the Western world, and we will increasingly become aware of it.

I made a number of predictions in this 1990 book that could be checked in my revision of that book in 1997. Among other things I had predicted lower teenage pregnancy rates, increased condom use, decreased HIV/AIDS rates, decreased rape rates, and greater tolerance for gays and lesbians (Reiss, 1990, pp. 234-236). By 1997 almost all these changes were happening (Reiss, 1997, pp. 13-14). I also had predicted that by the end of this decade our country will have explicitly endorsed the HER sexual pluralism ethic and our rates of all sexual problems will be declining (Reiss, 1990, Chapter 10). The evidence from national surveys indicated that I was right on the money (Reiss, 1997, Chapter 10). The American public's reaction to President Clinton's affair with Monica Lewinsky perhaps most clearly indicates that we as a nation have moved toward a more pluralistic approach to sexuality. Two-thirds of the public consistently said that no matter what they thought of his affair, they felt that it was not the business of the public and that he should remain in office. Few of us would have predicted such a supportive view for the privacy of sexual behavior that most Americans personally reject.

My 1990 book exemplified a much more direct legitimate role for sociological work in coping with social problems. My approach today surely does not deny the value of "pure" science and mainstream research work. Rather, I am validating the need to add a prescriptive dimension to our work and to develop a portrait of what we "could" be like, rather than focusing only on what we are like. This stance also incorporates elements of my views as a graduate student emphasizing the importance of what is significant and keeping as essential, but lowering the priority on, what is precisely measurable. It is a reemphasis of my admiration for the work of people like Gunnar Myrdal (1944), who were bold enough to suggest how we might resolve our "American Dilemma" about race and equality.

After my 1990 book appeared, I applied my more problem solving view of social science here in Minnesota. The Minnesota State Legislature authorized a committee to plan an Institute for Child and Adolescent Sexual Health that would aid in the reduction of sexual violence against children and youths. In 1992, The Governor, Arne Carlson, asked me to chair that committee. From September of 1992 to February of 1993 this 14-person committee met a number of times. I focused our committee on defining what we meant by "sexual well-being" so that we would have a clearer vision of what tasks the new Institute should undertake. I felt that if we believe that promoting sexual well-being was the primary prevention method for sexual violence, then we must clarify our thinking about the concept of sexual well-being.

I was amazed at the remarkable amount of agreement on a very positive view of sexual well-being that emerged from our committee. This is further evidence that our society is indeed ready to do the type of prevention that is needed to produce less sexual violence and more sexual rewards. I learned a great deal about bureaucracies and about state politics, but, more than anything else, I developed a deep respect for the very diverse group of members of our planning committee. We submitted our proposal to the legislature, and, for three successive years, we were able to get financial support for this new institute of child and adolescent sexual health. By promoting the making of our own policy proposals, I sought to take back some of the powers that so many social scientists abdicated to the politicians. I am convinced that we in science need to work together with those in power to develop a common vision of how to change society, and not give the "vision thing" completely over to the politicians. I fully believe that we can do this and at the same time we can maintain fairness and balance in our scientific work.

Quo Vadis?

I see now more clearly than ever the place of science in the making of ethical decisions. The connection to my own ethical decisions was surely part of the role that sociology has played in my life. But I want to be very clear that I still firmly believe that our personal moral views should not be allowed to overwhelm our scientific integrity. I do not want to reproduce the biased stances taken in the 1953 family textbooks. The rigor, logic, empiricism, and openness to new ideas, of science must be preserved. But instead of seeking the impossible goal of being value free, we need to work harder to be value aware (Reiss, 1993, 1997b). In that way we become more conscious of how our values may shape not only the projects we undertake but also the evaluation of the evidence we examine in our explanations. Instead of allowing our values and assumptions to unknowingly creep into our work, or pretending that values have no impact on our work, we need to stress value awareness so as to prevent our values from overwhelming our science.

I finally have reached a much broader audience, not a mass audience, but a broad audience of educated Americans. Groups like Planned Parenthood responded enthusiastically to my 1990 book. I wrote the book without jargon and with no tables or graphs. I worked for 18 months with my nephew, Spence Porter, a New York playwright, who helped me learn how to add dramatic quality, use anecdotes, and make my ideas relevant to current events. My wife, Harriet, increased my awareness of the reader's needs and gave me insights into a woman's perspective on gender equality issues. By the end I had improved my ability to write in clear, plain, and interesting English, and I hope I have retained some of that in this chapter. In 1997, I responded to a request from my publisher to revise and update this book and publish it in paperback

(Reiss, 1997a). This updated version is now reaching an even broader audience. I encourage others to write for this broader audience.

Finally, let me mention that I felt for years the need for a separate discipline of sexual science in order to advance the credibility and quality of the work in that field. In 1998 a committee was formed to work to encourage such a PhD in sexual science by one of our major universities. The committee was founded by both the Society for the Scientific Study of Sexuality (SSSS) and the American Association of Sex Educators, Counselors and Therapists (AASECT). Since I retired from the University of Minnesota in 1996, I had time to chair this committee. In May of 1999 we met at the Kinsey Institute at Indiana University and were successful in persuading the Kinsey Institute to share our goal and work towards the establishment of a Ph.D. program in sexual science at Indiana University. The first major step in this direction is to produce a summer institute that will bring in a number of top faculty from around the country to teach in sexual science. John Bancroft, the director of the Kinsey Institute, is currently applying for government and private grants that would allow this first summer institute to take place in the summer of 2001. This PhD program is the first at a major American University, and it will do much to establish the legitimacy and creditability of sexual science (Reiss, 1999).

There is much that needs to be done to promote the scientific treatment of human sexuality. I just recently wrote up my thinking about this (Reiss, 1999). We can make a very important breakthrough in the legitimation of our field as we enter the next millennium. There is more government funding for supporting sex research now than ever before. The public is more accepting of such research. Assuming success with the PhD program in sexual science that the Kinsey Institute is working to found, we will make the 21st century a time during which we may as a people finally achieve significant progress on containing more of our sexual problems than ever before, while at the same time achieving more of the rewards of sexuality. I intend to continue to work to contribute to this trajectory as much as I can. I believe that we are on the threshold of major achievements in sexuality both in science and in our society.

REFERENCES

Burr, W., Hill, R., Nye, I., & Reiss, I. L. (Eds.) (1979). *Contemporary theories about the family, volumes I & II*. New York: The Free Press.

Coutu, W. (1949). *Emergent human nature*. New York: Alfred A. Knopf.

Deven, F. & Meredith, P. (1997). The relevance of a macrosociological perspective on sexuality for an understanding of the risks of HIV infection. In L. Van Campenhoudt,

M. Cohen, G. Guizzardi, & D. Hausser (Eds.), *Sexual interactions and HIV risk: New conceptual perspectives in European research* (pp. 142-158). London: Taylor and Francis.

Glass, S. P. & Wright, T. L. (1992). Justifications for extramarital relationships: The association between attitudes, behaviors and gender. *Journal of Sex Research, 29*, 3, 361-387.

Hopkins, K. W. (1997). *An explanation for the trends in American teenagers' premarital coital behavior and attitudes between 1960-1990*. Unpublished Doctoral Dissertation, University of Minnesota.

Kephart, W. M. (1961). Book review of: *Premarital sexual standards in America. American Sociological Review, 26*, 2, 294-5.

Murdock, G. P., & White, D. R. (1969). Standard cross cultural sample. *Ethnology, 8*, 3, 329-369.

Myrdal, G. (1944). *An American dilemma*. New York: Harper & Brothers, 1944.

Reiss, I. L. (1956). The double standard in premarital sexual intercourse: A neglected concept. *Social Forces, 34*, 2, 224-230.

Reiss, I. L. (1957). The treatment of pre-marital coitus in marriage and the family texts. *Social Problems, 4*, 2, 334-338.

Reiss, I. L. (1960a). *Premarital sexual standards in America*. New York: The Free Press.

Reiss, I. L. (1960b). Toward a sociology of the heterosexual love relationship. *Marriage and Family Living* 22, 2, 139-145.

Reiss, I. L. (1964a). The scaling of premarital sexual permissiveness. *Journal of Marriage and the Family, 26*, 2, 188-198.

Reiss, I. L. (1964b). Premarital sexual permissiveness among negroes and whites. *American Sociological Review, 29*, 3, 688-698.

Reiss, I. L. (1965a). The universality of the family: A conceptual analysis. *Journal of Marriage and the Family, 27*, 4, 443-453.

Reiss, I. L. (1965b). Social class and premarital sexual permissiveness: A re-examination. *American Sociological Review, 30*, 3, 747-756.

Reiss, I. L. (1967). *The social context of premarital sexual permissiveness*. Holt, Rinehart & Winston.

Reiss, I. L. (1970). Premarital sex as deviant behavior: An application of current approaches to deviance. *American Sociological Review, 35*, 1, 78-87.

Reiss, I. L. (1971). *Family systems in America*. Holt, Rinehart & Winston, Inc. (1976 2nd ed., 1980 3rd ed.; 1988 4th ed. with Lee, G.L.).

Reiss, I. L. (1972). Premarital sexuality: Past, present and future. In I. L. Reiss (Ed.), *Readings on the family system* (pp. 167-189). New York: Holt, Rinehart, & Winston.

Reiss, I. L. (1973). Heterosexual relationships: Inside and outside of marriage. In H. L. Wilensky & L. Mayhew (Eds.), *University programs modular studies series* (pp. 1-29). Morristown, NJ: General Learning Press.

Reiss, I. L. (1980). Sexual customs and gender roles in Sweden and America: An analysis and interpretation. In H. Lopata (Ed.), *Research on the interweave of social roles: Women and men* (pp. 191-220). JAI Press.

Reiss, I. L. (1986). *Journey into sexuality: An exploratory voyage*. New York: Prentice-Hall Inc.

Reiss, I. L. (1989a). Is this my scale? *Journal of Marriage and the Family, 51*, 4, 1079-1080.

Reiss, I. L. (1989b). Society and sexuality: A sociological explanation. In K. McKinney & S. Sprecher (Eds.), *Human sexuality: The societal and interpersonal context.* (pp. 3-29). Norwood, NJ: Ablex Pub. Corporation.
Reiss, I. L. (1990). *An end to shame: Shaping our next sexual revolution.* Amherst, NY: Prometheus Books.
Reiss, I. L. (1993). The future of sex research and the meaning of science. *Journal of Sex Research, 30*, 1, 3-11.
Reiss, I. L. (1996). Sexual behavior. In G. T. Kurian & G. T. T. Molitor (Eds.), *Encyclopedia of the future. Volume 2* (pp. 828-830). New York: Macmillan Publishing Co.
Reiss, I. L. (1997a). *Solving America's sexual crises.* Amherst, NY: Prometheus Books.
Reiss, Ira L. (1997b). An introduction to the many meanings of sexological knowledge. In R. T. Francoeur (Ed.), *International encyclopedia of sexuality, volume 1* (pp. 21-30). New York: Continuum Publishing Group.
Reiss, I. L. (1998a). Reiss male and female premarital sexual permissiveness scales. In C. M. Davis, W. L. Yarber, R. Bauserman, G. Schreer, & S. L. Davis (Eds.), *Handbook of sexuality-related measures, 2nd edition*, (pp. 496-498). Thousand Oaks, CA: Sage Publications.
Reiss, Ira L. (1998b) Reiss extramarital sexual permissiveness scales. In C. M. Davis, W. L. Yarber, R. Bauserman, G. Schreer, & S. L. Davis (Eds.) *Handbook of sexuality-related measures. second edition.* (pp. 226-228). Thousand Oaks, CA: Sage Publications.
Reiss, I. L. (1999). Evaluating sexual science: Problems and prospects. In Raymond Rosen (Ed.), *Annual review of sex research, Volume* 10. Mount Vernon, Iowa: Society for the Scientific Study of Sexuality.
Reiss, I. L., Anderson, R., & Sponaugle, G. C. (1980b). A multivariate model of the determinants of extramarital sexual permissiveness. *Journal of Marriage and the Family, 42*, 2, 395-411.
Reiss, I. L., Banwart, A., & Foreman, H. (1975). Premarital contraceptive usage: A study and some theoretical explanations. *Journal of Marriage and the Family, 37*, 3, 619-630.
Reiss, I. L., & Leik, R. K. (1989a). Evaluating strategies to avoid AIDS: Number of partners vs. use of condoms. *Journal of Sex Research, 26*, 4, 411-433.
Reiss, I. L., & Miller, B.C. (1979). Heterosexual permissiveness: A theoretical analysis. In W. R. Burr, R. Hill, I. Nye, & I. L. Reiss (Eds.), *Contemporary theories about the family, volume I* (pp. 57-100). The Free Press.
Reiss, I. L., Walsh, R., Zey-Ferrell, M., Tolone, W., & Pocs, O. (1980a). Research on heterosexual relationships. In R. Green & J. Wiener (Eds.), *Methodology in sex research: Proceedings of the conference held in Chevy Chase, Maryland November 18-19, 1977* (pp. 1-57). Washington, D.C.: U.S. Department of Health and Human Services.
Schwartz, I., & I. L. Reiss (1995). The scaling of premarital sexual permissiveness revisited: Test results of Reiss's new short form version. *Journal of Sex and Marital Therapy, 21*, 3, 76-86.
Sponaugle, G. C. (1993). *A study of attitudes toward extramarital relations.* Unpublished Doctoral Dissertation, University of Minnesota.
Suggs, D. N., & Miracle, A. W. (Eds.) (1993). *Culture and human sexuality; A reader.* Pacific Grove, CA: Brooks/Cole Publishing Company.

My Family and Me: A 20th Century Saga

Catherine Street Chilman

KEYWORDS. Autobiography, policy, adolescence, pregnancy, social work

INTRODUCTION

This is a story about my family and me during most of the 20th century. It is also about my career as a social scientist specializing in family services, research, and public policy. Since I was born in 1914 and it is now 1999, it is also about my social history as I traveled through much of the turbulent 20th century, a century that saw enormous changes, including fantastic shifts in the roles of women and the patterns of family life.

Family Origins

My parents both descended from the first settlers of Ohio–then the Western Reserve. Most of them emigrated from England to New Engand during the 17th and late 18th centuries. Later, they moved west for free land available through the Revolutionary War land grants. They became farmers, teachers, ministers, lawyers, physicians and–in a few cases–businessmen.

As a child, I thrived on romantic fantasies of myself as an intrepid adventurer on the new frontiers only somewhat hampered by being female. This problem was solved by reading books for girls telling about the intrepid adventures of women as partners of their men in forging new homes in the wilderness, battling starvation, disease, savages, and exhaustion. This heroic, pioneering tradition throbs within me to this very day, even though I sadly realize that the dream has drastically faded and that it lacked many elements of reality from the first.

I was my parents' firstborn and came close to arriving in the middle of Lake Erie, near Cleveland, Ohio, where my athletic parents had been canoeing with Mother paddling stern "of course." My physician grandfather delivered me with the help of my grandmother, so it was very much a family affair. Three years later in 1917, I was joined by my brother, Tom, to my mother's intense joy, but to my own decidedly ambivalent feelings. What's so *special* about having a "son and heir" in the family?

His preeminence, as a male, was further established three years later by the arrival of *twin daughters*, Sarah and Sibyl. Now this was my domain as big sister and model for twin baby girls. I paraded down the street beside the twin baby carriage, proud in my role as protector of this exciting and adorable package. My father said that his family seemed to be proceeding by geometric, rather than arithmetic progression, so it was time to come to a baby halt–a proclamation applauded by Mother, who was perpetually in conflict about parenthood. It got in the way of ambitions of her own to have a "real career," unthinkable for a married woman with children in that period (1914 to 1940).

Early Days

My parents were devoted to ideals of higher and higher education together with better and better community service. This included their intense personal involvement in politics and liberal causes. My first memory of their political passions revolves around the tragedies of World War I and their commitment to Woodrow Wilson's plea for a League of Nations. While I was much too young to understand international policies, I dimly recall their joy at the Armistice of 1918, their aid to wounded friends returning from the war, stereopticon slides shown in our home of the war's devastation, and descriptions of war trials by friends who had been Red Cross nurses in Europe. The Red Cross nurses seemed incredibly exciting to me. I devised my own nursing uniform from old pillow cases and imagined myself as an angel of mercy saving suffering victims of the War–a heroic woman at the front, as brave and necessary as any man.

My next memory of parental social concerns goes back to 1920. My mother sobbed violently over the morning newspaper with its news that Democrat Cox had been defeated for the Nation's presidency and Republican Harding had won. It was an intense personal tragedy for my mother, who had taken me at age six to march with her in parades for women's sufferage and the Democratic Party. The 1920 election marked the first year that women had been allowed to vote in federal elections. My mother was devastated because she thought that women's suffrage had failed to produce the vastly improved government she had hoped and believed it would. The election tragedy, which was definitely a family affair, and my mother's passionate devotion to good government and social welfare still vibrates for my siblings and me.

My father was less openly emotional about the social good, but devoted to it, nonetheless. At the time I was six, he was founder and director of the Louisville Community Fund (a far more idealistic version of today's United Fund or United Way). He was also Director of the Council of Social Agencies, a planning organization for all the community's private health and welfare organizations. His conscientious devotion to his job involved the whole family in many social welfare activities. Much was said about understanding and appreciating people of all kinds; about feeling sympathy for "the poor"; about my own obligations as a child of privileged parents. My father often intoned his family motto: Non Nobis Solum Nati–Not born for ourselves alone.

MID-CHILDHOOD

These lessons became part of my own identity before I was seven when I drove with my family one hot summer evening through the dismal slums of St. Louis–a city to which we had recently moved. I was overcome by my own sorrows for others when I saw many children and adults trying to sleep on the steps and sidewalks of their darkly looming tenements. I wept at my parents' explanation that this was the way these families had to spend the night in the heavy summer heat when their crowded flats became intolerable.

This became not just a problem for my parents but a deeply felt experience for me. It was part of a marked movement in my life from early childhood into the middle childhood years. This shift to my own involvement in the social well-being of others still forms a core part of my identity along with my fervent hopes for effective government in the name of social justice, even though these hopes have taken many batterings over the years.

There were special friends, including highly competent professional women whom my parents, particularly my mother, especially enjoyed. At home, in my growing up years, I rarely met the supposedly normative woman of the 1920s. Almost all the women I remember were strong, independent, vital people. They included Sophie Nelson, public health director of the John Hancock Life Insurance Company; Blanche Renard, who became an executive of the National Jewish Welfare Federation; Doctor Martha Elliot, Chief of the U.S. Children's Bureau; Belle Sherwin, President of the National League of Women Voters and her successor in that position, Anna Lord Strauss. There were others, less prominent, but brilliant women. My mother described these people in hushed, worshipful terms as "fine professional women with a *wonderful* education."

Education was of first importance to her, as it was for her grandmother, mother, and her maternal aunts, all of whom had been trained as teachers and had taught school until they were married. Her older sister, Beth, trained at Ohio State University in the Montessori method of education (1907) and eventually went to Burma to establish nursery schools there. She went as the wife of a lawyer, Joseph Pawtun, a citizen of Burma who later became Prime Minister of that then-British colony. The King of England knighted him for his service, and my aunt became Lady Elizabeth Pawtun. Now there's a role model for you and a bit of British colonial history!

My mother, Augusta, was an Oberlin graduate in physical education. She had taught this subject at Case Western Reserve University for a short year before both her marriage and my subsequent arrival blighted her aspirations to become a doctor like her father, a well-known Cleveland physician and professor of obstetrics. In time, her own career, mostly as a volunteer, became impressive.

My mother did not really approve of my father's mother, Josephine, who was devoted to feminine frills and laces, not the severe tweeds my mother fancied. Nonetheless, Josephine was an outstanding pianist and gave music lessons for most of her life to help support the family. I was particularly devoted to my music teacher grandmother, who seemed to greatly enjoy having me visit since all her four children had been sons. Much to my delight, she curled my hair, sewed frilly clothes for me, and advised me to sleep with my cheek on a shoe button so that I could develop a dimple. She laid the foundations for my interest in later research on grandparenting and my much later attempts to be a "perfect" grandmother–indeed, one who still tried to play the piano.

Josephine's sister, my great-aunt Catherine, was a school principal and helped develop a settlement house in her native Cleveland to help recent poverty-stricken immigrants. Both of these relatives were loved and well known to me.

My other grandmother, Cora Jewitt, seemed to be full of complaints and petty concerns. She was something of an intellectual, having been trained as a teacher and continuing as a constant student in adult education courses. Her husband, a physician (my grandfather), had a strong sense of who was boss. It appears that my Grandma Jewitt was more typical of women of her period than my more ebullient, creative, and congenial Grandma Street.

What of the men I knew in my early years? First and foremost there was my adored father, who also adored me–what a delicious feeling! He made me feel special and loved, just because I was his daughter, and also because he thought that girls, just as much as boys, could grow into strong, intelligent, creative adults. He thought women were attractive if they had both brains and beauty. You didn't have to choose between one or the other. Obviously, he was far ahead of his time; and what a difference that has been to me! He further empowered me by frequently saying: "Don't be bound by other's ideas. Be yourself, kid."

Dad was not only an eminent social work executive, he was also an ardent photographer, inadequate violinist, brutally competitive tennis player, hiker, student, writer, professor, and enthusiastic father. He read to all of us nearly every evening. He read poetry instead of grace before every meal and brought us floods of books from the library. He encouraged our hobbies when he considered them worthy (wild flower study as opposed to cigar band collecting in my case), took us to museums, on arduous hikes, and talked to us (especially to me, I think) about his interests in literature, philosophy, and history. If there was ever a cognitive developer, it was my father, and my mother was close behind. Far before the writings of Piaget, my parents were devotees of cognitive enrichment, then called intellectual development.

In later life, when I met leaders in social work, they often referred to my father in almost worshipful tones. Many referred to him as a legendary person, remarkable for his unfaltering honesty, kindness, courtesy, and bright humor. Then, too, Dad was an incredibly well organized person. He had a plan for every hour of every day–for every week, month, and year but also included "be nice to Augusta and the children" and get plenty of recreation. To put it mildly, Dad's planfulness was heavily complementary to Mother's impulsivity.

Other men were also important in my early years. My mother's father, Grandpa Jewitt, the obstetrician and professor, was devoted to me as his first granddaughter and delighted in singing to me, telling stories, and taking me on house calls in his Model T Ford. My father's father, Grandpa Street, was a dreamy Quaker. He was an impractical, gentle person, who had a vague junior manager job in a large Cleveland factory. His chief pleasure was in learning new languages, listening to my grandmother read, telling his rather weak jokes, driving the family car on back country roads where he usually got lost, buying me ice cream cones, and going dancing with Grandma. These grandparents were close to poverty, lived in a tiny cottage, but seemed to intensely enjoy life.

Emulating her father, my mother's volunteer work often centered on such topics as maternal and child health, rights of women, free access to birth control services, and family life education. Throughout her adult life, she was an ardent devotee of the League of Women Voters. Among other things, she served on its national board as finance chairman during the 1930s. In this same period, she helped found the national Groves Conference on marriage and the family. In the 1940s and 1950s, her activities included being President of the Tri-State (New York, Connecticut, and New Jersey) Council on Family Relations. When my father was Director of the Community Fund in Houston, she was a traveling lecturer (a veritable mental health evangelist) for the Texas-based Hogg Foundation for Mental Health (her first paid job).

In the late 1950s, when she was sixty-five, she taught Marriage and the Family at Hartford (Connecticut) Theological Seminary. She preempted my father's appointment as lecturer for this course, since she was sure she could do a far better job in this field than he could. She was probably right! She also obtained the first National Institute for Mental Health (NIMH) grant for an interfaith training program for pastoral counseling. She said that a meeting of priests, rabbis, and ministers went well once she could get them down from their pulpits.

In thinking about the historical context of my parents' lives as I was growing up, I see them as avant garde people, pioneers like many of their ancestors. My parents not only talked about their liberal beliefs, but also acted on them vigorously. In a time of widespread anti-Semitism, they were particularly devoted to their Jewish friends. In a time when racial segregation was absolute and severe, they included black people in their social activities. My father accepted the job as originator and Director of the Community Fund and Council in Washington, D.C., only on condition that all social agency meetings would be integrated–a first in Washington in 1928.

All during childhood I loved school. I felt supremely competent as a student most of the time (with a few deflations in math and later in Latin). I missed most of first grade because of a severe case of scarlet fever and a double mastoid infection. However, I soon more than made up for this deficit by skipping virtually every other semester through the eighth grade. This unfortunate practice of double promotions left me seriously lacking in some basic math skills (woe to fractions and algebra). It also plunked me into the freshman year of high school at the awkward age of 12. My misery was compounded by being distressingly tubby, and by my family's frequent moves from Louisville, to St. Louis, to Washington, D.C. in pursuit of my father's expanding professional career.

LEAVING HOME

High school miseries were eventually lightened, mostly by academic shining and growing up. I was also over-involved in extracurricular social and school activities. Finally bursting the bars of adolescent life with family, I was off to Oberlin in Ohio in 1931 at the age of 16. Of course, this still closely involved my mother, an enthusiastic, active alumna of Oberlin (1911).

Overlooking a number of stresses, such as grueling hard work, heartbreaking romances, incredibly restrictive college rules, Oberlin's horrid gray-cold climate, and my rather dimly perceived threats of the Depression and looming world war, I was generally in an excited state of academic rapture during most of my college years. At that time, Oberlin was famous for its remarkably talented and committed teachers. I was bowled over by such personal discoveries as the fundamental universality of knowledge and creative endeavors over time, place, and subject matter. I saw within this universality a simultaneous relativity of values and goals by different peoples in differing times and life situations. Gone, alas, was my assurance that certain behaviors were inherently right or wrong. I also came to the reluctant recognition that some students were actually brighter than I, no matter how hard I worked, but there was also a deeply felt joy mixed with tears of rapture in response to poignantly discovered glories of literature, art, and music.

My wonderful education at Oberlin enriched my whole life. I acquired a solid foundation for later graduate work through rigorous courses in the social and biological sciences. Life, itself, was forever celebrated through my deepened acquaintance with literature, art, music, history, and all the rest–even including folk dancing and field hockey. At Oberlin I gave my intellectual potential a really big test and found both my abilities and my limitations–all useful, though at times depressing, information.

I was torn in my choice of majors. I was far more deeply moved by literature and art than by the social sciences. I soared to the aesthetic splendor of literature, especially poetry. Time raced unnoticed when I plunged, with total absorption, into my own compositions. The mechanistic emotionless approach of psychology and sociology was essentially a dreary betrayal of my spirit, I thought. However, I majored in sociology because of my social reformist ideals, my empathy for people in trouble, and the practicalities of this major as a background for graduate education in social work. A career in this field had many attractions, including the fact that the worse the Depression became, the more the demand for trained social workers grew.

I have always felt, unhappily, that I "sold out" through my choice of the social sciences and my relative desertion of the arts. On the other hand, I know if I had chosen the latter I would have been in a perpetual state of guilt. Better to starve my aesthetic sensibilities than to starve others who might be in far more desperate need. The bipolar pull of the arts vs. the sciences goes on to this day, though in my later years I have managed a somewhat shaky bigamous marriage with my differing loves.

Throughout college, I and my women friends were torn over the issue of the central need "to get your man and hang on to him through marriage," and our own intellectual and career interests. Our own hard academic work was to be put on hold, more or less indefinitely. All the effort at learning–for what? To help a husband in his career and to raise his children? Dismal! We were further trapped, not only by the social norms, but by our own frail tendencies to fall in love (or something that seemed like love) which was often a mixed mask of biology and social pressure. I barely managed to escape the Oberlin marriage mania.

First Jobs and Graduate School

I graduated in 1935, and, after much difficulty and taking a number of Civil Service examinations, I found a job as a file clerk in the Washington, D.C., government. This was supposedly a good job at $18 a week. My visions of being a national leader for social reform, or even a noted poetess, faded rapidly before the dark realities of a file drawer. I who had trained for higher things was in the dismal depths of one of the most routine junior jobs in the whole imponderable bureaucracy. Frazzled by filing and by engagement to a handsome but limited youth, I approached a total breakdown. I was pulled from the brink of collapse partly by my no-nonsense mother, who frequently urged "Get up and get going; there's no such thing as being tired, or scared, or confused or depressed." I was also saved by my decision to accept a scholarship offer from the School of Social Service Administration of the University of Chicago! What an experience in the depths of both the Depression and the coldest winter in decades (1936). Chicago–a brutal, frightening, desperate city. This is where I worked for my room and board with ultraliberal family friends who lived a long, frozen mile from the school to which I trudged day after day.

The School of Social Service Administration was presided over by an impressive over-worked, brilliant trio of maiden (the then-used term) women: Edith Abbott, Grace Abbott, and Sophinisba Breckenridge–all in their 60s and beyond. These famous women, trained in law and social sciences, were fiercely committed to causes of social justice, reduction of poverty, establishment of social insurances, ending of child labor, expansion of public welfare, improvement of low income housing, fair labor standards, and equal rights for women.

The trio was basically impatient with "Band-Aid approaches to social problems." They barely tolerated social service methods in the curriculum such as casework and group work, especially when these techniques involved such basically "indecent" concepts as those emanating from psychoanalytic theories. However, in the name of practicality and employment opportunities, we did have a few courses in social work practice and psychiatry, along with heavy doses of law, public welfare, medical issues, research, and community organization.

Besides all my walking to and from school, working in the library for my scholarship, studying, and weak attempts to help my clients, I was ecstatically busy falling in love; and this time it was one hundred percent for real. Bill Chilman, a fellow social work student, had escaped from a frigid climate and family severity in Maine to the relatively gentle permissiveness of Chicago. We dated within the first month of meeting in a Child Welfare class and strengthened our attachment in coffee breaks during Social Insurance and Legal Aid. After one date, I was totally in love with this strong, tall, handsome, hearty advocate for music, art, poverty solution, wholesome food, and a woman just like me. Our partnership flourished through shared homework, union meetings, and writing and acting in skits that lampooned our school. We also marched for social justice, welfare reform, improved curriculum, and world peace–to name a few causes. Clearly, Bill was a perfect companion and husband-to-be. With a mixture of guilt and relief, I broke my engagement to the outraged boy at home. My mother steamed out to Chicago to assess the damage, but stayed to celebrate the implausible–her daughter was finally attracted to a magically perfect man who, also incredibly, was attracted to her.

Bill was a super-achiever in his profession and a super work partner on the home front. Unlike most men, he did at least half of all domestic tasks. He was a gifted cartoonist and pianist, as well as an enthusiastic interior decorator. Perhaps most fundamentally, he seemed to be exceptionally calm, never losing his temper and almost always a patient but bewildered standby helpmate for my–alas–occasional dramatic tears and tempers. Bill's mother had become an invalid with rheumatoid arthritis when he was five years old and died when he was fifteen after ten long tragic years of suffering and helplessness. Chronic illness was Bill's bug-a-boo. Early in our dating he told me about his poor mother and swore that he would ask for a divorce if he ever became seriously ill so that I would not have to go through the horrors he had experienced living with an invalid. I was touched by tales of his troubled childhood and wanted to somehow make it up to him in our life together.

Getting Married, Getting Jobs

Let the wedding bells ring, even though this threatened the end of my scholarship and even my affiliation with the school. Edith, Grace, and Sophinisba were joined in their conviction that married women were disasters as professional social workers and it was impossible to be both a wife and competent graduate student, not to mention a career woman. Giddy with the importunity of love, I gave little heed to the triumvirate and, by early fall, was a thoroughly married woman. Bill, ever a champion of women's rights, especially mine, pledged his small savings to help me finish my Master's degree. Incredibly, the three academic furies capitulated and even gave us wedding presents. The news of the great surrender flashed through the school, setting off an epidemic of marriages by women students, some of who had actually been married for quite a time.

After we finished our courses, both of us got what were considered plushy social work jobs in Chicago. Bill was employed by an ultra-progressive agency for the treatment of disturbed children. I was a caseworker with the elitist Family Service Bureau of the United Charities of Chicago, an agency dedicated to the treatment of families primarily suffering from psychological problems rather than families with economic difficulties. The latter were to be referred to the professionally lower-status public welfare agencies.

Ever planful and persistent, Bill made excellent progress on his Masters thesis, but I struggled more haphazardly and emotionally with mine. He seemed to be even more determined than I that we should both finish our theses and get our degrees; we had to prove the positives of career cum marriage to the Trio. With much help from Bill, I did complete my thesis on time, though his had been finished some weeks before, and we passed our written and oral Comprehensive Exams under the basically benevolent but collectively beady eyes of the Three. We received our Master's degrees in 1938–the only married couple from the whole University of Chicago to manage this feat. Much newspaper publicity and considerable crow-eating by our pleased but puzzled mentors: Grace, Edith, and Sophinisba.

Off to Appalachia

As to our jobs, after a year or so, we became restless with our lowly status as practitioners in Chicago. We moved south where Bill became state Child Welfare Services representative for the appallingly poor isolated 13 counties of southwestern Virginia. I became a caseworker for the tiny Family Service Agency in Roanoke.

By 1940, we were immersed in the overwhelming problems of Appalachia where deep poverty had been a way of life for probably a third of the families for generations, but had become even more serious and widespread because of the Depression. These problems included severe child abuse or neglect, widespread venereal disease, alcoholism, homicide, malnutrition, tuberculosis, pandemic school truancy, mental retardation, and mental illness. Many adults, both black and white, suffered from extreme poverty and endemic unemployment. Modern casework, with its emphasis on counseling, made hardly a dent on these issues.

I was asked by the State to participate in a survey of the welfare recipients in Roanoke City. I was overwhelmed by the primitive conditions I found. I visited families of seven or more living in one tiny shack with no windows, light only from a kerosene lamp, and water only from a city well. These families had a cash grant of only $10 a month, which bought a diet of fatback and dry beans. They had no money for rent or clothing, and there was virtually no health care for anyone. When I asked people how they got along on their meager welfare grants, the usual answer was "by the hardest." Among other things, the "hardest" often meant picking up coal off the tracks, bootlegging, odd jobs, and petty thievery. Chicago's poor families at their most desperate were far better off than these people of Appalachia.

Bill and I did accomplish one professional goal. In our own living room, as volunteers, we put on a series of night classes for all the 20 area social workers who needed to pass upcoming Civil Service exams. As a team, we gave them a remarkably tight survey of our entire University of Chicago curriculum. They did pass the exam, but it remains unclear as to whether their new knowledge had any appreciable impact on the extremely complex problems they encountered.

Those were the days when we thought that professionally trained social workers could manage to change the behavior of the people they were supposed to help and that this, in turn, would cure poverty. As we learned later from research reports, it is exceptionally difficult to change human behavior, especially if underlying social and economic problems are not solved or, at least, reduced. No amount of education, training, or counseling will help people obtain poverty-escaping jobs if such jobs at adequate wages are not available. We learned this in the 1930s and again in the 1960s. This learning needs to be reacquired in the 1990s as calls arise on all sides to "make welfare recipients quit lolling around on welfare and go to work."

Motherhood and Migration to Syracuse, New York

I more or less escaped my professional dilemma in 1940 by having a glorious baby girl, Peggy. Bill and I were both ecstatic. I had thought childcare would be boring and I would want to go back to work soon after Peggy was born. Much to my astonishment, I couldn't stand the idea of leaving my incredibly precious infant for more than a few hours. The allure of a job faded before the marvels of motherhood. Bill's reaction to parenthood intensified his already sturdy efforts to become a successful and well-paid professional. Within a few months, he managed a miracle, and we were off to Syracuse, New York, where he was to administer the casework services component of the Council of Social Agencies.

Now that Peggy was six months old I was getting rather restless as a full-time mother/homemaker. My first part-time job in Syracuse was to develop exhibits on the theme of strong community social agencies, as a crucial part of an overall Civil Defense program, for the New York State Fair. I was shocked to find that we could not include the Planned Parenthood Agency in this exhibit. To do so would incur a wrathful boycott by all Catholic agencies. This was a brutal reminder of earlier barriers I had encountered in both Chicago and Roanoke when I had tried to give birth control information to families who very much needed this help.

Aside from the family planning "No-No," other social services, renamed Civil Defense Programs, were high on the community agenda. They were particularly promoted by people who thought that the U.S. should go to war, especially since England was being so severely battered by Nazi Germany. Bill and I, like many of our friends, were highly ambivalent about such a move since we had been so deeply indoctrinated as children and adolescents by peace movements. Later, we were impressed by the communist arguments that World War II was simply a battle between imperialist nations. However, our own reluctance faded when the Soviet Union briefly made a pact with Hitler and later when the Japanese bombed the U.S. ships in Pearl Harbor.

Our own partial personal response to the U.S. involvement in World War II was to have another baby. After baby Jeanne was born, we moved to the suburbs. Our isolation plus two little children, plus a carless existence (gasoline had gone to war) cut me off from volunteer activities. I was stranded in a neighborhood bursting with other young mothers and their demanding little ones. It meant separation from the larger world and almost total immersion in neighborly domesticity.

This may be why I accepted a part-time job as senior social worker with the Home Services Division of the American Red Cross. I also wanted to make my own heroic contribution to the war effort. I also wanted to escape the twenty-four-hour grind of a homebound mother. It was a vast relief to dress up and go to an office where I was treated as a person with a brain, not just a body, and as important in my own right, not just as Bill's wife or Peggy and Jeanne's mother.

My job was to develop social and family histories for overseas counselors of psychologically disturbed soldiers who were having problems. The histories were needed to build treatment plans for these men. I visited and interviewed the men's families to get the needed information. Obviously, this was sensitive work since the families were usually extremely upset by my visit and to find that their son, brother, or husband was having problems. This called for using all of my professional training and skills, including attempts on my part to avoid my own heartbreak for these unhappy people who often had many other serious problems.

I was soon forced to give up my job–it became increasingly clear that our children were suffering from my absence five half-days a week. The only baby sitters I could find were elderly women who were simply unequal to the task. With regret, I returned to being a full-time homemaker and was even featured in a Syracuse newspaper as the ideal mother who stayed at home with her little ones. This experience, plus later struggles in trying to combine child care with employment, has given me special empathy and concern for working mothers with little children. This has led to study, research, and writing on this topic, plus involvement in social action for better childcare and parental aid.

Having quit my job at the Red Cross, I became restless again with the urge to be useful in the larger world. Thus, I was soon involved with other young women to start a League of Women Voters in our suburb. This ushered me into local politics where I did the impolitic thing of joining the American Labor Party–not a good move as Bill's wife in conservative Syracuse. The President of Bill's board called me saying that they would like to promote Bill, but couldn't do it if I remained active in the "New Dealish" League of Women Voters and the "communist" American Labor party. I said I would think it over but I couldn't promise to become a different person without talking it over with Bill.

Then followed one of the glorious moments in our marriage. Bill said he couldn't ask me to betray my convictions, that he didn't want a job that depended on my obedience to his Board, and that our mutual integrity was of first importance. My hero! Bill explained this to the Board and they backed down; I continued as a social activist, although one of a rather mild sort. Bill's action on this point, plus his full partner behavior throughout much of our life together is one of the main reasons that I am only a semi-feminist. Of course, this "semi-feminist" stance was nourished by my early family and school life and many of my job experiences over a lifetime.

We became expectant parents again, and our son was born in the spring of 1942. Tragically, he was exceedingly frail and lived only a few months. This was a desperate loss. During his short life, Bill and I lost our ability to really communicate with each other. I was in poor physical shape and devastated with grief. I felt Bill did not share this–that he was distant and that I could no longer depend on him. I found out much later that Bill received his draft notice just as our baby was born. He was horrified at the prospect of leaving me with my multiple problems, at leaving his little daughters and dying son and didn't want to worry me with the draft notice. The Big Secret built a Big Barrier between us, confirming what much of marriage research shows about the prime importance of open communication.

Of prime importance, too, is the strength that children bring to a family crisis, an under-researched topic. I will always remember Peggy's contribution to my decision that I must surmount my grief, worries, and hurts of that time. As I lay on the living room couch, trying to pull myself together, she brought bouquet after bouquet of drooping dandelions and clover, knowing how intensely I loved wild flowers. She then stood sturdily before me, dark eyes shining, round cheeks aflame, golden curls bobbing up and down as she shook her head and proclaimed: "You don't have to worry about me. I'm right here and little girls who are four years old don't die." Brave assurance for both of us. Eventually, we had three daughters, for Cathy, a special consolation prize, was born in 1948, a precious part of the postwar baby boom.

Over the years, my daughters have been a source of joy, of deep emotional involvement, of fun, wonderment, and companionship. While mothering has relatively little intellectual content (that is for sure), it did stimulate me to learn as much as I could about child development and parenting. Of course, this induced wracking waves of guilt in me as I was not the ever-giving, perpetually competent mother described in books. Probably no mother can be that good. This is a perception that I used a lot in my later parent education leadership and writing activities. I also found that mothering vastly broadened and deepened my personal growth, though it often didn't feel like it.

My urgent sense of kinship with my children has been essential to my development as a mature woman. It seems that these feelings go beyond socialization but are also connected to deep biological evolutionary roots that intertwine with cultural prescriptions. Especially when my children were young, I, along with my friends, often felt almost destroyed by the demands of mothering plus homemaking. However, most of us also felt that the enormous love and joy our children brought balanced the agonies of submersion. Life with kids was lacerating; life without them threatened death itself.

My development as a mother, and eventually a grandmother, has spilled over to my lifelong career. Over the years, I have written extensively for and about parenting; I have done research about parenting and grandparenting; I have become involved in numerous advocacy efforts on behalf of parents and children; I have taught and counseled about parenting. Partly because of my own experience, I am particularly moved by the sufferings of children and parents in trouble–physical, economic, psychological, or social trouble. I want to help them all. Naturally, I can't do this, but my efforts to help my own, and other, children have been essential to my own personal growth. Much has been said in the past thirty years or so about the supreme importance of personal and professional growth, especially about growth of women as individuals, but somehow the individual has to be balanced with the familial.

In 1947, Bill was offered a splendid job opportunity as an outstanding expert in child welfare and research director for all the public child welfare programs in New York State. This meant he would have to travel for months and would only be home on weekends. I was pregnant again and was terrified at the thought of being left alone during each week with my young children. Surprise! I found I could manage very well on my own and even liked it. It was easier, in many ways, not to have to fix large dinners every night, not to keep the house in shining order, not to dress up myself and the children every evening in honor of Dad's return. I continued happily in my presidency of the local PTA, shocking many citizens by presiding over large programs when I was eight months pregnant–very daring at that time.

I also continued activity with the village League of Women Voters where I had a number of close and supportive friends. The League, with its excellent national and state program materials, importantly increased my education in government affairs. It also eased my "bomb anxiety" as we worked hard for the United Nations and global control of the atomic bomb.

Cathy was born in the spring–a perfect baby on a perfect day in May. She was a baby who brought a profound renewal of an ongoing sense of springtime to both Bill and me. Bill was a marvelous father, sharing equally with me in childcare. At least he did this insofar as his new job would permit. He had finished, with distinction, his child welfare study and was now promoted to the directorship of the city's Council of Social Agencies.

Academic Teaching

Responding to a part-time job offer from the College of Home Economics of Syracuse University, I began to teach a senior course in social work one night a week. Another surprise! I loved teaching even more than social work practice. It was easier and more hopeful to deal with college students than with deeply troubled social work clients. It was far less harassing to teach about social work than to practice it.

Who took care of the kids while I did all this teaching, writing, and community work? Why, Bill, of course. People often asked me in those days why I always looked so happy and alive. I usually answered, "Why, it's love, naturally!" And that was true, especially when I considered our joy in our children (less arduous now with two in school), Bill's support of both my home and budding career activities, and his own blossoming career. We considered ourselves exceptionally fortunate, especially when we contemplated the problems some of our friends were encountering.

Bill was widely loved and admired in the community. I swelled with pride and a touch of jealousy when he was given an award for outstanding achievement at the 1950 annual meeting of all the community's social agencies. By this time, he was also teaching a course at Syracuse University and was president of the local chapter of the National Association of Social Workers. The latter led to TROUBLE. As President, he gave support to a group of social workers who joined in bringing liberal Henry Wallace to a Syracuse meeting in support of his candidacy on the Socialist ticket for President of the country. We learned soon that a local ultraconservative radio station was accusing Bill of being a communist member of the "Red Network." To put it mildly, Syracuse was not a liberal town, especially during the McCarthy era. It is probable that Bill would have been fired had it not been for the intervention of several prominent, wealthy members of the Establishment who particularly admired and respected Bill as a person.

This job threat increased our reluctant recognition that social work occupies an unhappy place in the social and economic structure of society. It is supposedly oriented to serving the poor, but, in my reluctant view, this service is equally aimed at keeping the poor quietly submissive. Non-public social agencies for poor people depend for their support on the gifts from more fortunate citizens, especially those who are fortunate in both terms of wealth and power. I felt that a basic (but often rationalized) aim of most money givers is to retain their own good fortunes, at least partly, through the "cooperation" of the poor who, as recipients of a generally stingy largesse, are not to agitate for good jobs, inexpensive quality housing, adequate wages, and all the rest.

Bill's Illness

Now comes the hardest emotional part of my story. At this time, my beloved Bill, age thirty-four, was stricken with amyotrophic lateral sclerosis. He had noticed increasing weakness in his hands and feet. This was first diagnosed as exhaustion because of his tendency toward huge amounts of overwork. However, within a year of his first symptoms, an examining neurologist told us Bill had ALS (Lou Gehrig's disease), that it would progress steadily with increasing involvement of the entire neuromuscular system, that nothing could be done to help the victims of this rare and poorly understood disease, that no one knew its cause, and that Bill would die shortly.

A major reaction to my family's predicament and my own grief was to delve deeper into further career advancement so that I could somehow manage to earn enough money to support all of us. I wanted to hold a job that was consonant with my own values and that also carried enough social status to maintain a sense of prestige and self-respect, particularly for our children. If Bill could no longer provide the social and economic base for our sense of pride and security, I would do it in his stead. I would do it for myself, for Bill, for our children, and for my parents, too. And I would do it as a kind of highly principled, respected, contributing community member that Bill had been–and was still struggling, tragically, to be. I would do it in such a way as to be a "complete mother" for my children, a loving and "non-threatening wife to my husband.

This was in the retrogressive traditional 1950s–a time in which women were socialized to take central responsibility for building their mate's sense of superior strength and wisdom, to never threaten his sense of masculine adequacy, to never be–Oh horrors!–a "castrating female bitch." I should manage to be strong, calm, competent, and endlessly dependable for my family. I should serve brilliantly and with apparent happy ease in both female and male roles. However, since no one knew the cause of ALS, I feared that my charade of super-competence was defeating him–was leading him to seek an escape through illness.

I had to take my career seriously. Upon reading the U.S. Department of Labor reports, I found that women with ill husbands and young children were at the very bottom of the economic heap unless they had either outstanding abilities as an aggressive business executive or possessed exceptional advanced training in a field of high demand. In no way, either by personality, values, or family tradition, could I be a successful businessperson. I had already found that I was a supremely happy, highly approved university teacher in my very part-time university teaching job. My teaching had been eagerly sought by Syracuse University. There was a huge demand for faculty members for the returning GIs who were flocking back to universities for free higher education under the GI Bill of Rights. My university hours and vacations fit wonderfully with the children's needs. Furthermore, I enjoyed dressing up, sitting down at work, being treated as a human being that should be listened to with respect, and finishing my job at a specific time. All this was in sharp contrast to the experience of homemaking and mothering. University teaching was perfect for me. I also loved the students and sharing with them as potential social workers my knowledge, ideals, and skills for what I saw as the finest, most arduous, most beleaguered of professions.

Becoming a Professor and PhD

However, my situation was seriously flawed. Relegated to the tail end of the academic procession at graduation time, I could quickly see that success in academic life required a PhD. Little did I know then how much more it required. At any rate, after consulting with my Dean in the College of Home Economics, I found that the University definitely wanted me as a full-time lecturer, and that this full-time status would entitle me to free tuition and nursery school for our youngest daughter.

After submitting to a huge battery of intelligence and personality tests and consultations with university Pooh-Bahs, I was eventually launched on a PhD program in counseling psychology plus a full-time teaching load (social problems, social work, and marriage and the family). I thought I would hate the required research and statistics in the PhD program, but, after many fantastic struggles, I eventually conquered and became fascinated by statistics. Virtually all of the professors in my PhD program were men, as were virtually all of the university administrators. Though my feminist friends will be horrified and unbelieving, I have to admit that nearly all of these academic males were wonderfully kind and helpful to me. They had almost never before encountered a youngish wife, mother, and full-time university teacher who was simultaneously a PhD student. Most frankly thought it couldn't be done and that I should be gently treated (at least part of the time) as one of the walking wounded. I was that all right, but a wounded person who was determined not only to recover, but also to move on to a far more glorious state of well-being. I was glad for the male help. I admit that I often behaved with a mixture of seductive flirtation and a massaging of the male ego, combined (I hope) with a necessary overdose of professional dignity. Part of my student role was that of a game player, but part was an earnest, eager scholar–the tough mind and tender heart that has been a central part of my life.

Some of my professors made mockery of what they called my bleeding heart emotionalism and paraded their own "rigorous scientism" (I couldn't help thinking they were really bragging about their erectile potencies). I was outraged by their rejection of compassion, empathy, and emotionality. My entire PhD program took seven years, including my dissertation. Much to my amazement, I heartily enjoyed the latter endeavor even though it was extremely fatiguing and consuming work. I liked the intellectual challenge, the creativity and the independence involved in this venture even though many hours were spent in achieving perfectionistic detail.

While I was teaching a 15-credit hour load and working for my PhD, I also became involved in other career-related activities. As a volunteer, I led many parent education groups in Syracuse. I also worked part-time as a research associate for the New York State Community Mental Health Department and wrote articles for *Parents* magazine. Then, too, I led Camp Fire Girl groups, worked for the League of Women Voters and the Syracuse Association of Social Workers, and chaired programs for the Parent Teacher Association of my daughters' school. The extra jobs were undertaken chiefly to make more money for the family; the volunteer activities were mainly to try to meet my model of the perfect citizen and mother.

I taught in a dilapidated but somehow homey prefabricated building, which housed the Department of Family and Child Development. My three department colleagues were all older married women with grown children. They all had a keen empathy with my plight and stood ready to help when emergencies like measles and Bill's broken hip struck. We all taught the department's course in Marriage and the Family. It was tremendously popular throughout the university; so much so that we could teach endless numbers of sections and still not meet the student demand. All four of us worked hard and cooperatively to build this course, replete with excellent readings, films, psychodramas, outside lecturers, and group and individual counseling with students. Many of our students, including the returning GIs, were burning with the desire to become marvelous marital partners and parents and to manage graceful separations from their own mothers and fathers.

Six male professors attended the defense of my dissertation. They probably thought it a bit strange that I brought a bouquet of my favorite lilies of the valley from my garden to buoy me up. After a barrage of questions and an unseemly recessed waiting period, they finally called me into their august presence. The Chair said, "Congratulations, Doctor Chilman. Now you know what hard work really is." With trepidation, I asked: "*Doctor* Chilman? Are you sure?" In response to their chorused "Yes," I said, "Gentlemen, I have news for you. The hard work for my PhD was mainly a pleasure, a mere trifle compared to the grueling, endless work of bearing and raising three children, nursing an ill husband, and caring for a large house." A bit baffled, the "gang" tried to pass off my remarks as a joke. I gave them each a lily in appreciation and rushed home to spread the glad word–at age forty-four I was finally a PhD.

In 1959, I was probably the first wife and mother to obtain a PhD in psychology at Syracuse University. How times have changed since then! Perhaps a third or more of PhD degrees today are won by mothers who have returned to school in later life. This is a gorgeous part of the feminist revolution. My own mother, who had given up her aspirations to become an MD to become a MAMA, as she often said, was thrilled to have a doctor daughter, and I was thrilled to become one, partly for her sake.

Soon after the doctoral excitement passed, I engendered more excitement by getting a large research grant from the Education Division of the Department of Health, Education and Welfare (HEW). I had applied for a grant to study the educational and familial outcomes for married college undergraduates compared to their unmarried counterparts. At this time, combining marriage with being a college student was thought to be a near impossible undertaking–a road to academic and marital disaster and a threat of corruption to academia, itself! Again, how times have changed.

My grant provided for a staff of research assistants, which gave me crucial help for an overly ambitious research plan. It also gave me lots of good experience in supervision and administration. Moreover I won a raise in rank and a badly needed increase in what had been a minuscule salary. I was into the academic game for real. Some major findings of the study were that women who continued their education after marriage were usually high in perseverance, strong in motivation, and high in self-confidence. In general, married students did better work, on average, than single ones.

A NATIONAL JOB

My academic game was soon ended by an irresistible call from Washington. The federal government wanted *me!* Incredible, exciting, fantastic! I was sought for the position of parent education specialist in the research division of the Children's Bureau of HEW. At that time, the Children's Bureau shone with a brilliant luster, at least to all of those with a background in social work. It symbolized the acme of professional excellence, the beacon of leadership in the cause of social reform for the well-being of mothers and children, the arbiter of impeccable parenting guidance through its publications such as *Infant Care* and

Your Child from Six to Twelve. Among other things, I was to rewrite the latter, bringing it up-to-date on the basis of recent research (Chilman, 1966a).

The Children's Bureau also had deep personal meaning to me. My main and heartily admired professor at the University of Chicago had been Grace Abbott, the former Chief of the Children's Bureau during the early 1930s. Then, too, my mother had been on the Citizen Advisory Committee for the maternal and child health programs of the Children's Bureau. I had also brought up my own children, especially my first baby, by slavishly following detailed directions of Infant Care. To top it off, this call came in 1961 at the dawn of the Kennedy Administration.

I am confident that the revolutionary changes in our society made a huge contribution to my own career advancement in this job. I benefited enormously from being in the right place at the right time, a beneficiary of both "cohort and period" effects. For example, when I finished my graduate work in psychology I was one of the few people in the whole country who had both an MA in social work and a PhD in psychology. As an entrant into the federal government in 1961, I was there near the beginning of the fabulous 1960s–an opportune time for social scientists and social reformers in the federal government. I was there when "the best and the brightest" joined the government or served on its advisory committees. I benefited tremendously from the heady intellectual climate and from knowing so many talented people. Many factors combined to make the 1960s a time of jet-propelled career growth for me both in terms of academic publishing in family studies (Chilman, 1964a, 1964b, 1966d, 1966e, 1968a, 1968b, 1969a, 1969b) and policy (1965, 1966f, 1966g, 1967) and writing a number of government publications regarding child and family development, families in poverty, family planning and population problems, and family measurement (Chilman, 1966a, 1966b, 1966c).

For me, the move to Washington had formidable, positive career effects. My delight in the move included not only the job, but also my love of the city and the fact that my parents and siblings all currently lived in the Washington area. Then, too, Bill, now very severely handicapped, had no job and two of our three daughters were away at their colleges. It was essential that I earn more money.

Eventually I became so exhausted, depressed, and anxious about mounting work demands, Bill's increasing illness as well as psychological problems in my daughters and myself that I sought the help of a psychiatrist. His assistance was immensely important. Among other things, he helped me recognize that Bill's illness was not of my doing and that I was not centrally responsible for everyone in my extended family (especially my mother). I also learned that I could tend to my own needs at least some of the time. I was encouraged to take a firm stand about such realities as putting limits on household expenditures and extreme overwork in house and yard. This exceptionally skilled psychiatrist even made me like myself again. My self-image had been badly damaged by Bill's growing hostility and depression. It sounds simple that I could change some of my feelings and behaviors, but it certainly wasn't. These experiences not only helped me in my own living, but deepened my recognition that psychotherapy can be subtly helpful in many complex ways over a long period of time–ways that frequently resist short term quantitative measurement.

This experience contributed to my skepticism that the costs and benefits of all human service programs could be totally assessed in terms of objectively measurable, quantitative goals. Important as such evaluation may be, it is not enough by itself. My conflicting concerns on this subject continued to disturb me in my government work that eventually involved administration of research and development programs and analyses of their implications for public policies. My work covered an astounding range of topics: educational and counseling services for families in poverty, family planning programs (new and controversial for the federal government), child care, job training for welfare mothers, and mental health services for children and youths. I served on numerous government task forces. Along with many other idealistic civil servants, I worked endless hours of overtime. Part of me really believed that if I learned enough, thought hard enough, and worked hard enough, I really could contribute to the solution of poverty problems.

Wilbur Cohen, Secretary of HEW part of the time I was there, was a heady inspiration to many of us. He was one of the Nation's leading architects of progressive programs in health, welfare, and education. How thrilled we were when he took leadership in the development and passage of Medicaid and Medicare! Little did we suspect that both these programs would grow to be so enormously expensive and so heavy a budget burden today. Even so, I believe that their benefits have far exceeded their costs, and I, along with others, will always honor Wilbur Cohen (now deceased) with admiration and devotion.

Jessie Bernard, the eminent sociologist and feminist, was a close friend during the Washington years. She pointed out that I was actually a victim of sexism in that I was qualified for employment at far higher government levels–far more qualified, in fact, than many men in top management. However, I didn't want to be in top management since I was already stressed by overwork, and I did want to have time and energy for my family. I wanted job flexibility that allowed me to drop all work responsibilities for a while if Bill or the children really needed me.

Family was, and still is, first, though my scholarly work was, and is, extremely important to me. For virtually my entire career, I have struggled with the conflict between job and family, work responsibilities and personal loves. This continues to be true, even though I am now retired (officially at least) and my children, all middle aged, are also struggling with careers vs. responsibilities for their children. Of course, this continuing life-long tug-of-war gives me deep empathy for all employed, or wanting to be employed, mothers.

A number of women with whom I worked in the government were special inspirations to me, and their influence remains. They were outstanding in their work, devoted to public service, and wondrously supportive of my endeavors.

Despite the tragedies of the mid and late 1960s, I rejoiced in the positive programs of the Great Society and my small part in them. After all, I was there during an exciting resuscitation of some of the splendid New Deal programs of the 1930s when I had come in as a new professional. I was there in a period of extraordinary hope that racism and poverty could finally be conquered. I was there, with others, to push for Civil Rights legislation, public support of family planning programs, the establishment of Head Start, the demand for high quality child care centers, the astonishing community action programs, enhanced job training for welfare recipients, enriched social services, a vast proliferation of research projects aimed at better understanding and help for poor families–and all the rest.

It is seriously wrong to accept the generally groundless conservative attacks on Great Society programs as failures that only embodied "throwing money at problems." Most of the antipoverty programs were carefully devised. Many (such as Head Start, family planning services, and participation of the poor in program development and implementation) were based on large bodies of research. Admittedly, these programs did not cure poverty, but they reduced it and improved the life chances of thousands of citizens. It was a mistake to think we could abolish poverty. Its roots are far too deep in our social, economic, and political structures and in the severe handicaps of some people for this to occur. But we did ameliorate poverty and make more real a democratic society–at least for a time. These are issues I continue to study, speak, and write about to this day.

During the '60s, I became more and more active in the National Council on Family Relations (NCFR) and the National Groves Conference on Marriage and the Family. In my government job, I was supposed to make links with selected national professional organizations in order to "educate" them on various federal policy issues and learn from them and mobilize their support for some of our programs. Different staff people in our social welfare research division chose different organizations for our linking efforts. I chose NCFR and Groves because of my strong interest in families and the example of the earlier work of my mother. I greatly enjoyed participating in these organizations, especially in meeting leaders in the fields of family related social sciences. Many of these people became respected friends. They were also extremely valuable in making me a member of social science networks. I soon was serving on organization boards, giving papers at national conferences, and planning these conferences.

In the mid-1970s, I was (I think) the first woman president of the Groves Conference. By now, we have had a number of women presidents of both the Groves Conference and NCFR and women constitute the majority of members of both of these professional organizations. I find the meetings far more egalitarian, and certainly on just as high a level of scholarship as they were earlier.

As to my government job, my mind still staggers as I recall the merciless driving force of President Johnson, who seemed to be convinced that federal workers could accomplish anything for the Great Society if he just pushed us hard enough. Despite the impossibly hard tasks he imposed on us, I, and other staff people, didn't mind too much since we agreed with his program goals. The final blow was struck by the election of President Nixon and the resultant growing politicization and undermining of the intellectual integrity of the federal government. Nixon's destructive force made me and many others physically and emotionally ill. By 1969 I decided that I had to get out.

My final major effort as a part of the federal government came in 1969. The Senate had appointed a huge "blue ribbon" commission on the mental health of children and youths. This commission was to study the problem nationwide and report back to Congress about their findings and recommendations for future prevention and treatment. The many committees of consultants outside of government had met for several years under the staffing of a group from the National Institute of Mental Health (NIMH). The goal was to prepare a report with recommendations for prevention and treatment of emotional problems and mental illness in children and youths. The report suffered from conflicts between the "experts" (psychiatrists, psychoanalysts, psychologists, sociologists, social workers, and educators), a plethora of advocacy groups, and the professional writer who had prepared it.

The deadline for publication was coming up, the report was in meltdown, staff people were in despair, and the mental health of virtually everybody involved was in tatters. I was thrilled when I was asked to undertake the important task of rewriting this report. My dearly loved Wilbur Cohen, HEW's Secretary, arranged for me to go on paid leave for this mental health endeavor. I attended many deeply moving meetings of such groups as welfare mothers, civil rights advocates, and the parents of autistic children. I attended committee meetings of the experts. I read reams of research articles about the probable causes and cures of mental illness. I took cartons and cartons of the technical reports home with me, making outlines of their contents, analyzing and summarizing the findings, and adding some ideas of my own.

I dictated tapes for chapter after chapter. Interestingly, no committee had really tackled a range of issues concerning families and mental health other than to produce essays by psychoanalysts with the familiar theme of blaming parents, especially mothers, for the mental health disorders of their children. The research, though scanty at the time, didn't really support this conviction of the all-male committees. Listening to parent advocate groups, I had become impressed with the case evidence they gave which suggested that having a mentally disturbed child in the family caused parental reactions that made the deeply involved mothers seem overly-protective and the less involved, harassed fathers seem "weak." These parental reactions seemed to have a feedback effect, enhancing, at times, the problems of the children.

At the request of the commission's executive committee, I wrote my own chapter on families and mental health, including the "family system" viewpoint. This led to a brutal battle with the psychiatric-psychoanalytic group, so they wrote their own chapter on children's emotional disorders, but I didn't back down. It included an emphasis on the mental health stresses imposed on families by both poverty and racism as well as by the birth of children with mental defects. I worked seven days a week, fourteen hours a day to finish this report on time. Through all the attendant stress, I had very little staff support other than that given by the women workers who all had clerical jobs. The men of the staff seemed to fade into the woodwork. This report, of course, had large political and career implications; only a hardy few dared to stick their necks out and make clear statements.

Finally the report was done on time (Joint Commission on Mental Health of Children, 1970). A celebration was staged with the Commission's Executive Committee, in all their male pomp and glory, presenting the document to an all male Senate Committee in the presence of a large assemblage of TV and newspaper reporters. As an afterthought, the Chair of the commission invited me to attend as a humble member of the throng. He even indulged me by inscribing a copy of the report with his name. He pledged that, henceforward, I would be honored as the most knowledgeable person in the country on the subject of mental health. He said he would see to it that I would be a keynote speaker at national mental health conferences. Nothing ever came of his promises. Would this have happened to a man? I strongly doubt it.

On the Home Front

Before I discuss further career adventure, I must return to life within my own family where tragedies concerning Bill accumulated. I realized ever more clearly, and still reluctantly, that he and I were engaged in a complex power struggle. Following the help I received in psychotherapy, I mustered the strength to say, for the first time, that I wanted some control over what happened to my paycheck, the central resource in our family finances. I also insisted that we move from our big nine-room house with its backbreaking acre of gardens, shrubs, and enormous trees to a much smaller, manageable, cheaper home.

All of this self-expression on my part was extremely difficult for both Bill and me. I was keenly aware of his many sufferings, of his miserable slide into illness from being a highly acclaimed career man and a centrally important and active member of our family. I knew of the multiple frustrations he experienced every day as he tried with his poor, damaged body to conquer his environment. He had become demanding, filled with rage, controlling of me and the children. What a change from his earlier calm, loving, kind personality. I realized that my own physical and mental health were in peril and that I must survive with the strength for the well-being of us all.

Eventually, in rage and desperation, Bill attempted suicide while I was at work. When I came home, I found him unconscious. The doctors said he probably wouldn't live and that if he did, he would be a vegetable. I found a note from Bill, written in advance, indicating he would come back home with nursing help if he survived. I felt that *I* wouldn't survive if this happened. Doctors assured me that if he lived, nursing care would be essential. So I rented our house and found a small apartment for myself on Capitol Hill near my job. This was a bold, desperate, semi-liberating step.

Then one day Bill "came to." I was called to see him. He opened his eyes and said, "Did you remember to get our furnace cleaned for the winter?" Bill was certainly no vegetable, but he was terribly weak and handicapped. After weeks, he went to a nursing home with the help of my father and myself. After a few months, he decided he didn't need to be in a nursing home. It was terribly hard for me to stand firm to the effect that I now had my own apartment and that we would have to live separately. Surely this was devastating to Bill, but both sadly for him and fortunately for me he had no choice. I found him a first floor quiet apartment in a suburb near my parents' home and helped him move in. From then on, we lived separately, but I visited him several times a week, bringing groceries, cooking good meals, cleaning, and trying to cheer him. I also was his major financial support, though he also had Social Security as a disabled person.

In time, the above events had some positive outcomes for both of us. Bill was desperate for a sense of function and purpose in his life. He felt out of communication with everyone and as if he were being reduced to nothingness. I suggested that he write about his childhood as a way of communicating with his children since he had such severe speech problems. I brought him a copy of Proust's *Remembrance of Things Past* and an electric typewriter to facilitate his typing. And lo! Bill wrote beautiful essay after essay about his Maine childhood. Although he had not written much before, his superior intelligence, strong aesthetic feelings, and determination to do well resulted in magnificent literary productions, far more splendid than I, the presumed writer, will ever produce. Most of these essays were sold to such magazines as *Yankee* and *Old Sturbridge Village,* both New England journals. Bill has left an enduring, priceless heritage to his entire family and to countless others, many of whom wrote him fan letters. He continued his writing for over ten years. These essays are especially moving because they reveal an extraordinarily talented perceptive person–a person who was so tragically struck down in his youth, but whose writings reveal none of these sorrows–only his multiple talents.

Our separation also had many positives for me. I luxuriated in my Capitol Hill apartment–a three room romantic hideaway on the third floor of an old building where my windows overlooked the Capitol and Washington Monument. I reveled in my new freedoms, including the freedom to entertain friends in my home, an activity that had been forbidden by Bill. There was also the freedom to work long hours on my job with no housework interruptions. It was dangerous to live on Capitol Hill at that time with its high crime rate and paucity of services. It was also noisy and dirty, but, as a friend said, I was rejoicing in being a "Hippy Emeritus."

By 1970, when I left my federal job, I had reached a relative learning plateau. Looking back over the years, I realize I reached a transition point. I ran out of role models to which I could aspire and became a role model, myself. I moved belatedly from being a junior professional to being a senior one. Well, it was about time; after all, I was in my fifties, but, then, I had started late. Thus I will just give a few career highlights regarding the next fifteen years.

ACADEMIC ROLES

Becoming an Academic Dean

From 1969 to 1971, I was academic Dean of a small, conservative liberal arts college for women. Misreading the actual, dubious meaning of academic freedom at the college, responding to the academic and youth revolution of that period as well as to the rapidly declining student enrollment at that school, I foolishly took the lead in all sorts of "radical" innovations for the college. I promoted a mental health service for students and supported student participation in peace demonstrations. I also took leadership in reducing numerous heavy course requirements in the curriculum and approved of student pleas to have smoking permitted in dormitories. I gave permission for students to seek family planning services if they so desired. Then, too, I sponsored faculty and student "focus" groups for participation in many aspects of curriculum planning and also pushed for full racial integration within the college. I also argued for a shift to coeducation and, with the cooperation of some faculty members and state officials, launched a graduate program in the human sciences for human services. This program still flourishes. I foolishly and far too independently "did the right as I saw the right," and to my shocked amazement I was fired from my job.

I should have learned to be more cautious in respect to faculty, alumni, and community politics in all of these undertakings, but caution has never been my strength. I did learn the excruciating agony of being fired, of knowing the overwhelming pangs of severe economic insecurity, and of wallowing in guilt for the disasters I had brought to my family. This vastly increased my empathy with poor and unemployed people.

When all the dust finally settled on the academic revolution of this small college, I was fired for being too radical and the President was fired for being hopelessly out-of-date–a kind of uneasy balance that was hard on everybody.

An International Project

Within three months of this debacle, I was saved by a federal grant from the Agency for International Development to the School of Public Health and School of Social Work of the University of Michigan. I was asked to be the curriculum coordinator for a project that was to develop population education programs in many schools of social work around the world. Part of my assignment was to consult for three weeks with the Dean of the School of Social Work in Teheran, Iran! This assignment afforded a profound experience in working in this amazing country. Most of Iran was hardly ready for modern concepts and programs for family planning. I did the best I could within the limits of the situation. I left with vivid memories of the brave faculty members of the school of social work, of sublimely beautiful mosques and gardens, of camel caravans, of tent encampments of wandering tribes, of vast stretches of arid lands, and of mystic visions of the ancient ruins of Persepolis–once the thriving center of the long-ago Persian Empire.

I eventually realized that I was not on the tenure track at the University of Michigan, contrary to verbal assurance given me when I was employed. (More learning–be sure you get job contracts in writing; don't trust anyone. I should have known this by age fifty-seven, but my ignorance about practical matters was appalling and isn't real sharp even today.) Since I was on "soft money," my job was at peril when the grant expired. Reluctantly, tardily, I took job-seeking action and most fortunately ended with a full *tenured* professorship in the School of Social Welfare at the University of Wisconsin in Milwaukee (UWM) where I went in 1972 and stayed until 1989.

The University of Wisconsin Milwaukee

By and large, I had a wonderful time in this job. I learned to love "squeaky clean," almost socialist, heavily Germanic Milwaukee. I also loved the natural glories of Wisconsin with its generous cornucopia of marvelously planned and administered state and county parks. I enjoyed tremendous freedom on my job; the state university system of Wisconsin is admirably strong on principles of academic freedom and faculty governance. Much to my delight, I obtained a number of federal and state research and program development grants. Two were my favorites: a state grant supported a sizeable study of parent satisfactions and dissatisfactions and their correlates (1980b, 1980d); a federal grant provided for an analytic overview of all US research on adolescent sex behaviors (Chilman, 1979a, 1979b, 1980a, 1980d, 1980e). This resulted in two books: *Adolescent Sexuality in a Changing American Society: Social and Psychological Perspectives* (1979c), and a second edition, in 1983, which added chapters on programs and practice guidelines for human service professionals.

NICHD, my granting agency, widely distributed the 1979 book to a host of social and behavioral science research scholars in the population planning and adolescent sexuality fields. I had worked extremely hard on this book and brought much of my previous professional experiences to it. However, the backing and distribution by NICHD helped immensely in bringing considerable recognition to both the report and myself. I continued studying and writing in this field until 1989 or so and practically paraded under the pseudonym of Ms. Adolescent Sexuality–a bit embarrassing for an old woman in her seventies Chilman, 1974, 1983, 1985, 1986, 1988, 1989, 1990a, 1990b). I finally quit studying, writing, and lecturing on this topic–I felt I had learned about as much about it as I truly could or actually wanted to.

More recently, I have returned to studying and writing about an earlier deep concern: the problems of families in poverty (Chilman, 1973a, 1973b, 1973c, 1975a, 1991, 1992a, 1992b, 1993, 1995). This is not actually a big shift from the adolescent sexuality topic since research reveals that poverty and racism are the factors most closely associated with early unprotected, nonmarital intercourse for the majority of teens who become unmarried parents.

My continuing basic concerns about poor and other troubled families led to initiating, writing, and coediting a five volume book series in 1988, *Families in Trouble*. This series, developed in partnership with fellow faculty member Elam Nunnally and our school's Dean, Fred Cox, reflected our joint beliefs that family courses should have a strong research base and should include content on knowledge about families and their problems, together with implications for professional counseling and education plus existing and needed public policies. We garnered a splendid cast of contributors and published a five volume series (Chilman, Cox, & Nunnally, 1988a, 988b, 1988c; Nunnally, Chilman, & Cox, 1988a, 1988b).

The University of Wisconsin social work graduate students were very dear to me, for the most part. The majority of them were middle-aged, married women; relatively few were young recent graduates, and the minority were men. Almost all of these students were working their way through school and commuting from a broad region of the state. UWM chiefly represented part of the great experiment in democracy characteristic of many, but not all, state universities systems of this country. Most of my students came from farm or blue-collar urban families and were children or grandchildren of immigrants who chiefly came from Germany, Scandinavia, or Poland. I saw, as I gazed at them, the process of the American dream in its arduous development. These were special groups of people who were fortunate enough and worked hard enough to be making it.

During these and earlier years, I was lucky to be invited to give lectures and consultations to groups all over the United States. Especially after I went to the University of Wisconsin, I was also asked to speak at international conferences in London, Vancouver, Nairobi (Kenya), Dubrovnik (Yugoslavia), and, very recently, Santiago (Chile). It was wonderful to have my way paid to these meetings, but it was even more splendid to have the opportunity to interact with people from many nations. I learned from all of them and deepened my convictions that we all basically share a universal humanity and that, in a fundamental sense, we are far more alike than we are different.

Particularly in my Wisconsin years, I found I was a role model (disgusting words) not only to my students, but to many faculty members, especially but not exclusively, to the younger women. In turn, I vastly admired them. The young women were a new generation of youthful, outstanding career people. They were attractive, charming, and competent. Gone was the earlier, more usual female PhD image that I hoped I didn't reflect: the frumpy, mannish woman who allegedly had to follow a professional career because no man would want to marry her. Most of our young faculty women reflected a radical shift in our society toward greater gender equity. This was a happy shift, indeed, both for the young women themselves and for the larger society. Generally speaking, knowing these young faculty members was a source of personal enrichment and enjoyment.

Family Affairs

It is now time to backtrack again and shift to my own family scene since the 1960s. Bill and I were proud and relieved to see our three daughters graduate from college. Each followed these achievements by acquiring full scholarships for the Master's degree: Peggy in social work from Bill's and my alma mater, the University of Chicago; Jeanne in Art Museum Curatorship from the University of Michigan; and Cathy, in English Literature from the University of Toronto. Peggy later earned a PhD in Clinical Social work from Simmons University in Boston.

Bill and I also shared joy (and trepidation) in marriages of these dear daughters–two to men from Oberlin and one to a sociology PhD from the University of Michigan. Over the years, we rejoiced with our daughters and their husbands in the arrival of their children–our grandchildren.

From 1976 onward, Bill and I could no longer rejoice together, for in this year, finally totally defeated by ever-worsening health, including encroaching blindness, Bill committed suicide–and this time it was a complete job. He did this on a cold, gray November afternoon when hope drops low for all of us. I found him in the evening when I went to take him dinner. I will never forget or recover from the desolate sight. I understood and basically approved of Bill's euthanasia. If he had gone on living, he would have had to go to a nursing home for the rest of his life–a misery for all. I shall always miss him and meditate on both the great victories as well as deep tragedies of his life. He remains as both an intense joy and sorrow to our children and me.

SEMI-RETIREMENT

So now, in 1999, I am living in Washington where I have been retired from the University of Wisconsin for over ten years. Life, indeed, is far more serene that it once was, though not exactly relaxed. Never that. I live in a condominium amid the treetops overlooking my long-loved Potomac River and close to many of the great Washington institutions: the Capitol, the Museums, Congress, the Library of Congress, the Supreme Court, and the offices of many national organizations.

Professor Emerita Margaret Feldman, a long-term friend and colleague, widow of Professor Harold Feldman, also a dear friend, wonderfully lives near me. In fact, she found me my present apartment. Our roots go back to years before we were born. Amazingly, our mothers were both in a small group of physical education majors in Oberlin's class of 1911! We find we have many similar ideas about such virtues as physical exercise, good nutrition, not wasting a minute of any day, "working for the night is coming" when we will work some more, but we add a pinch of fun.

Margaret and I both got Master's degrees in social work in our early twenties, and PhD's in psychology in our forties. I really didn't know her until she started coming to national conferences with her husband, Harold. We became good friends then and have worked together on projects over the years, especially since I returned to Washington. Margaret is Washington representative for the National Council on Family Relations, and today attends an incredible number of national meetings of all kinds. She is also a leader in numerous national organizations and has involved me in some of them. Although I generally resist deep involvement in organizations, I am seriously interested in some she has led me to. I am grateful for her linkage efforts on my behalf, such as membership in the Washington-based public policy committee of the National Council on Family Relations and the board of the Consortium of Family Organizations (COFO). Moreover, together we developed and carried out the 1992 national Groves Conference annual program. This conference theme was close to our hearts: "Family Issues and Federal Social Policies." So, here we are, in our eighties, originally linked through our mothers who graduated from Oberlin in 1911. What a small, fascinating, and happy world it can be!

I continue to study, lecture, and write on many family-related issues, especially those in the areas of public policies and poverty. I continue to work with a number of national organization, including the National Council on Family Relations and the Groves Conference on Families. Recent reactionary legislation, such as welfare "reform," depresses me mightily, but as my social worker father used to say, "Up and at them; never give in, change is always possible." Looking back over the years, I realize that my life story illustrates the many facets of social and behavioral sciences, especially family social science theory. I, like others, am a product of the interweave of many life strands: genetics, multigenerational family system experiences, my particular age cohort, and the historical periods through which I have lived. I have been shaped by enormous cultural and other changes of the 20th century; my own particular life situation at different times; my friendships, my family, and the numerous important resources to which I have had access–financial, educational, recreational, cultural, and environmental. I have, indeed, been fortunate and continue to feel empathy and responsibility toward those who have not been so blessed. I am a card-carrying, un-tired liberal–a dyed-in-the-family humanist, forever. In short, before I go, I want to say "Thank you."

REFERENCES

Chilman, C. S. (1964a). The crisis and challenge of low-income families of the 1960s: Implications for parent education. *Journal of Marriage and the Family, 26*, 1, 39-43.

Chilman, C. S. (1964b). Economic and social deprivations: Its effects on children and families in the United States–A selected bibliography. *Journal of Marriage and the Family, 26*, 4, 495-498.

Chilman, C. S. (1965). Child-rearing and family relationship patterns of the very poor. *Welfare in Review, 3*, 1, 9-19.

Chilman, C. S. (1966a). *Your child: 612*. Children's Bureau, US Department of Health, Education and Welfare. Washington, DC: US Government Printing Office.

Chilman, C. S. (1966b). *Growing up poor: An overview and analysis of child-rearing and family life patterns associated with poverty*. Washington, DC: US Dept. of Health, Education, and Welfare.

Chilman, C. S. (1966c). *Moving into adolescence*. Children's Bureau, US HEW, US GPO.

Chilman, C. S. (1966d). Marital stability and patterns of status variables: A comment. *Journal of Marriage and the Family, 28*, 4, 446-448.

Chilman, C. S. (1966e). Dating, courtship and engagement behavior of married, compared to single, undergraduates with an analysis of early-marrying and late-marrying students. *Family Coordinator, 15*, 3, 112-118.

Chilman, C. S. (1966f). Social work practice with very poor families: Some implications and suggestions from research. *Welfare in Review, 4*, 1, 13-22.

Chilman, C. S. (1966G). Population dynamics and poverty in the United States: Implications for family planning programs. *Welfare in Review, 4*, 6, 1-13.

Chilman, C. S. (1967). Poverty and family planning in the United States. *Welfare in Review, 5*, 4, 3-15.

Chilman, C. S. (1968a). Fertility and poverty in the United States: Some implications for family-planning programs, evaluations, and research. *Journal of Marriage and the Family, 30*, 2, 207-227.

Chilman, C. S. (1968b). Family at mid-stage in the family life cycle. *Family Coordinator, 17*, 4, 297-312.

Chilman, C. S. (1969a). A philosophy and some principles proposed for family planning programs. *Family Coordinator, 18*, 3, 195-201.

Chilman, C. S. (1969b). Social and psychological research and Family Planning. *Journal of Marriage and the Family, 42*, 4, 793-805.

Chilman, C. S. (1973a). *Some psychological aspects of fertility, family planning and population policy in the US: Psychological perspectives on population*. New York: Basic Books.

Chilman, C. S. (1973b). Public social policy and population problems in the United States. *Social Service Review*, *47*, 4, 411-530.

Chilman, C. S. (1973c). Public social policy and families in the 1970's. *Social Casework*, *54*, 10, 575-585.

Chilman, C. S. (1974). Some psychological aspects of female sexuality. *Family Coordinator*, *23*, 2, 123-131.

Chilman, C. S. (1975a). Families and poverty in the early 1970s: Rates, associated factors, some implications. *Journal of Marriage and the Family*, *37*, 1, 49-60.

Chilman, C. S. (1975). Home: Safe harbor or storm center? Stress, blue cross association, *VXXV*, no 1, 42-48.

Chilman, C. S. (1978). Habitat and American families: A social-psychological overview. *Family Coordinator*, *27*, 2, 105-111.

Chilman, C. S. (1979a). Teenage pregnancy: A research review. *Social Work*, *24*, 6, 492-499.

Chilman, C. S. (1979b). Illegitimate births to adolescents: An overview of social and psychological research. *Marriage and Family Review*, *2*, 4, 3-11.

Chilman, C. S. (1979c). *Adolescent sexuality in a changing American society: Social and psychological perspectives* (1st edition). New York: Wiley (2nd edition 1983).

Chilman, C. S. (1980a). Adolescent sexuality in a changing American society: Social and psychological perspectives: Implications for further research. Washington DC: US GPO, 1978.

Chilman, C. S. (1980b). Parent satisfaction, concerns and goals for their children. *Family Relations*, 29, 3, 339-345.

Chilman, C. S. (1980c). A history of parent education and participation in the United States. National Institute of Education, US HEW.

Chilman, C. S. (1980d). Social and psychological research concerning adolescent childbearing: 1970-1980. *Journal of Marriage and the Family*, *42*, 4, 793-805.

Chilman, C. S. (1980e). Adolescent pregnancy and childbearing: Findings from research. National Institute of Health, Washington DC, US GPO.

Chilman, C. S. (1982). Major trends of families and their mental health in the United States: 1957-1978. *International Journal of Sociology of the Family*, *12*, 2, 217-227.

Chilman, C. S. (1983). *Adolescent sexuality in a changing American society: Social and psychological perspectives for the human services professions*. John Wiley and Sons.

Chilman, C. S. (1985). Feminist issues in teenage parenting. *Child Welfare*, *64*, 3, 225-234.

Chilman, C. S. (1986). Adolescent heterosexual behaviors. In R. Feldman & A. Stiffman (Eds.), *Advances in adolescent mental health*. New York: JAI Press.

Chilman, C. S. (1988). The background of the present abortion controversy. *Affilia: Journal of Women and Social Work*, *3*, 2, 41-54.

Chilman, C. S. (1989). Some major issues regarding adolescent sexuality and childbearing in the United States. *Journal of Social Work and Human Sexuality*, *8*, 1, 3-25.

Chilman, C. S. (1990a). Low-income families and public welfare organization. In D. Unger & M. Sussman (Eds.), *Families in community settings* (pp. 128-143). New York: The Haworth Press.

Chilman, C. S. (1990b). Promoting healthy adolescent sexuality. *Family Relations, 39*, 2, 123-140.
Chilman, C. S. (1991). Working poor families: Trends, causes, effects, and suggested policies. *Family Relations, 40*, 2, 191-198.
Chilman, C. S. (1992a). Welfare reform or revision: The family support act of 1988. *Social Service Review, 66*, 349-377.
Chilman, C. S. (1992b). Hispanic-American families in the United States: A review of research. In H. P. McAdoo (Ed.), *Family ethnicity: Strength in diversity* (pp 141-163). Newbury Park: Sage Publishing Co.
Chilman, C. S. (1993). Parental employment and child care trends: Some critical issues and suggested policies. *Social Work*, 38, 4, 451-460.
Chilman, C. S. (1995). Programs and policies for working poor families: Major trends and some research issues. *Social Service Review, 69*, 3, 516-524.
Chilman, C. S. & Meyer, D. L. (1966). Single and married undergraduates' measured personality needs and self-rated happiness. *Journal of Marriage and the Family, 28*, 1, 67-76.
Chilman, C. S., Cox, F. M., & Nunnally, E. W. (Eds.) (1988a). *Employment and economic problems: Families in trouble series*, Vol. 1. Newbury Park, CA: Sage.
Chilman, C. S., Cox, F. M., & Nunnally, E. W. (Eds.) (1988b). *Chronic illness and disability: Families in trouble series*, Vol. 2. Newbury Park, CA: Sage.
Chilman, C. S., Nunnally, E. W., & Cox, F. M. (1988c). *Variant family forms: Families in trouble series*, Vol. 5. Newbury Park, CA: Sage.
Joint Commission on Mental Health of Children (Chilman, C. S., member) (1970). *Crisis in child mental health: The challenge for the 1970s research findings and policy implications*. Harper and Row, 1970. Co-author.
Nunnally, E. W., Chilman, C. S., & Cox, F. M. (Eds) (1988a). *Troubled relationships: Families in trouble series*, Vol. 3. Newbury Park, CA: Sage.
Nunnally, E. W., Chilman, C. S., & Cox, F. M. (1988b). *Mental illness, delinquency, addictions, and neglect. Families in trouble series*, Vol. 4. Newbury Park, CA: Sage.

A Personal and Intellectual Journey

John Scanzoni

KEYWORDS. Autobiography, family policy, functionalism, religion, gender

FUNDAMENTALISM AND FUNCTIONALISM

The Academic Environment

The 1960s were, in many respects, the most turbulent years of the 20th century. For me, the decade opened in graduate school at the University of Oregon and closed in the sociology department at Indiana University. Not only did the decade transform me, it remade the domain of sociology in general and modified the study of family in particular. Structural-functionalism was, in 1960, the dominant theoretical paradigm throughout sociology, and many of its essential assumptions were woven–albeit tacitly–into the study of "the family," or of "marriage and the family." Although Hill and Hansen's influential 1960 essay documented a variety of competing paradigms, none posed a critique of the underlying functionalist model of the "normal" family to which they all more or less adhered (Parsons, 1955, 1965). Neither did any of those paradigms identify the potentially negative consequences of that model for adults, children, and the larger society. Likewise, virtually all the contributors to the Christensen's landmark anthology (1964a) uncritically incorporated that same model into their thinking.

Accordingly, it should come as no surprise that I began my career imbued with the tenets as well as the spirit of functionalism. The Bell and Vogel (1960) anthology aimed to make functionalism more of an overt presence in the study of family, and it was among the first books I encountered in graduate school. At the same time, William J. Goode was generating a number of significant works that sought to make notions of social and cultural change less foreign to functionalism (1959, 1963). Goode believed that "family sociology" was a low prestige specialty because, among other things, it lacked theoretical sophistication. He argued that its theoretical importance, and thus its prestige, could be upgraded through utilizing the style of functionalism he advocated. Persuaded by Goode's reasoning, I designed my dissertation as a study of the consequences of religious ideology for clergy marriages (Scanzoni, 1965a, b, c). One of the study's central themes was that family cannot be analyzed apart from an understanding of its environment. That might include economic and political structures, its community setting, as well as its cultural context–the beliefs, values, and norms enfolding the household. Accordingly, by comparing and contrasting the consequences of religious ideology (conservative vs. liberal) for marriages, I was studying family in its cultural context.

Family Environment

It was not by chance that I possessed a keen interest in studying religious ideology. Although I was baptized a Roman Catholic, my mother converted to Protestant fundamentalism when I was 5 years old. She then became an active member of a fundamentalist church close by our tiny flat on Chicago's near north side where we lived with my father. He was employed as a baker–a skilled trade to which he had been apprenticed as a boy in the Tyrol of northern Italy. Shortly after World War I (spent on the Russian front as a conscript in the Austrian army), he migrated to and became a citizen of the U.S. Although born in the U.S., at the age of 3 my mother was taken back to the Tyrol by her father. He knew my father, and, when my mother was 19, he shipped her back to America and arranged a match between the two of them. Our flat was located in a largely Catholic working-class neighborhood, comprised predominantly of Irish, German, and Italian families, alongside a sprinkling of Jewish families. Because almost every boy in the neighborhood expected to follow his father's example of getting a skilled or semi-skilled blue collar occupation, most perceived school as an odious though unavoidable encumbrance. As a result, there was enormous peer pressure to submerge any academic talents and interests one might possess. For whatever set of reasons, I chose instead to express and develop my abilities. Hence, I became a stigmatized outsider, and on more than one occasion was roughed up by some of the more aggressive bullies. I quickly learned to make friends with several of the less hostile boys, and they frequently defended me against my nemeses. Among the saddest memories of my mid-adolescence was going with my friends to the nearby Firestone company distribution center and applying for part-time work. They asked for and got "blue collar" jobs on the loading dock that paid better than the "white collar" office jobs. I, nonetheless, went the latter route, and it struck me quite painfully that suddenly I was an outsider even to the friends I liked so well and to whom I owed so much.

While becoming gradually dislodged from my working-class roots, I got increasingly active in my mother's rather huge fundamentalist church. Although sited on the furthest possible boundary of the neighborhood, it was in no sense a part of it, and very few "locals" attended. It was comprised instead of a middle class clientele drawn from the entire north side of the city and several of its bordering suburbs. It was, in fact, a wholly different world than anything else I knew, but I was welcomed into it with great cordiality. Not only was I totally committed to its beliefs, values, and norms, but I also volunteered my talents and energies to serve in every way possible. Eventually, both my peers and the adults recognized me as being among the leaders of the church's youths. That was quite remarkable, because not only were my peers middle and upper-middle class, many also belonged to prestigious families that were influential in the broader national subculture of which our church was a very important part. Among other things, religious fundamentalism paved my entry into secular functionalism: Both shared a fidelity to "cultural determinism." In both settings, "good values" and "right thinking" are said to result in "good behavior." Ergo, "good behavior" leads to family stability and social order. Moreover, that entire "social system" was said to be orchestrated by a predetermined cultural script.

It took me some years to conceptualize my church experiences as a vehicle for social mobility. The adults and my peers were role models of middle class life, and thus operated as a type of "fictive kin." They showed me what goals to strive for and supplied me with a wide range of intangible resources–including a good deal of personal encouragement that expedited the achievement of those goals. Because further education was deemed essential, I entered and was graduated from Wheaton College (IL), a college that was "evangelical" and, for that reason, less parochial than my fundamentalist church had been. I should note that although the difference in religious doctrine may seem arcane to outsiders, the subtle distinctions in ideology are exceedingly vital to the insiders. Thus began my pilgrimage away from a highly constricted understanding of Christianity to the much broader and inclusive view that I now embrace. The chief mission of the college faculty as a whole was to inspire intellectually sheltered youths such as myself to develop our critical thinking skills. That aim was pursued quite vigorously by the sociology professors who counted me among their more promising majors. So much so in fact that, upon graduation, they urged me to pursue a PhD in sociology. Although strongly inclined to do just that, I chose instead to become a religious worker in the evangelical tradition. My wife Letha and I (along with our 18 month old son) were assigned to rural western Oregon where we served for three years. Among other things, that experience convinced me that teaching sociology was not such a bad idea after all and that I might do more to help families through research and teaching, then through religion and so I (along with Letha and now two sons–Steve and Dave) left religious work to become a full-time student at the University of Oregon.

RESEARCH INTERESTS

Although the first major research project that I pursued at Indiana was grounded in functionalist theory, I nonetheless modified my analyses by blending them with Gouldner's (1960) modest version of social exchange theory. "Family order" sprang, I argued, not solely from role conformity, but also from role reciprocity (Scanzoni, 1970). Based on the results of a 1967 Indianapolis household survey, the study tested the notion that marital satisfactions and stability emerged from the husband's "effective" participation in the occupational system. Next, I utilized that same blend of functionalism and Gouldner's exchange theory in a study of African-American husband-wife households (Scanzoni, 1971). My aim was to demonstrate that family patterns and processes depended more on economic access than on race per se. Accordingly, I argued that as black men gained the same access as white men to the "opportunity structure," the more their family patterns and processes would be comparable.

Feminism and Families

By 1970, functionalism was deposed throughout the discipline as a whole. It was impotent when it came to making sense of the convulsive societal struggles occurring during the 1960s. Within the study of family, however, the functionalist model maintained a sub rosa influence. Nevertheless, it now came under siege from several related directions–none of which had ever mattered very much in the study of family.

First and foremost were issues of gender equity raised by proponents of what was then called "Women's Liberation." Their aim was to renew and redirect the 19th century feminism that slumped into dormancy after passage of the 1920 suffrage amendment. My apostasy from functionalism began by reading a 1967 Margaret Mead essay appearing in an anthology forecasting a wide range of social trends stretching ahead to the year 2000. Mead did a scorching critique of the nuclear family–something I had never seen done before. She argued that gender inequity was fashioned into its very warp and woof–much to the detriment of women, men, and children, to say nothing of the larger society. She believed, however, that by 2000 family patterns would change significantly, resulting in less gender inequity. At the same time, Mead uncannily predicted that if the changes were not executed in a "socially responsible" manner, a counter-revolution would ensue. And indeed as she anticipated, today's conservatives–both secular and religious–aim to reverse the changes of the past 30 years by turning back the clock and limiting the freedoms that women and their male allies have struggled to gain.

Stimulated by Mead, I immersed myself in the gender literature being produced in immense quantities on both sides of the Atlantic. In 1970, I taught the first ever "sex roles" class in our department, and one of the first on "women's issues" at Indiana University. I was, at the same time, devouring the literature on post-Emancipation African-American household patterns, as background for my 1971 book. While doing so, it struck me that several issues being raised by feminists had been matters of everyday life among black households for decades. Perhaps chief among those issues was what Jeanne Noble (1966) called the black woman's identity as "worker"–an identity relatively uncommon among white women of post-World War II America. The feminist literature addressed the broader issue in terms of "economic self-sufficiency," and described it as a woman's capabilities of supporting herself and any children, and apart from a man if need be. Owing to decades of economic discrimination against black men, many black women had been forced–contrary to their religious upbringing–to adopt this identity. In any event, the theme of black women's *struggles* (to provide for themselves and their children, and against white racism, and sometimes against black men) resonated with the notion of struggle central to feminist thinking in general, and to the conflict theories that informed it. From then onward, I made gender struggle a central theme of my research and writing. I completely abandoned the consensus model of functionalism–a model that Seeley et al. (1956) had in any case shown to be largely mythical even in the 1950s "Golden Age" of the suburban nuclear family.

Other researchers were treading the same path, as demonstrated by, among other events, an entire 1971 issue of *Journal of Marriage and Family* (August) devoted to "Sexism in Family Studies." That was a first, as was the very next issue of *JMF* dedicated to "Violence and the Family." This November 1971 issue on violence also included a section containing additional articles on "Sexism in Family Studies." Previously, that signal indicator of male oppression had rarely been noted in family studies. Fortified by the realization that the sociology of family was being reinvigorated both theoretically and substantively, I undertook a book project that was quite different from the two preceding it. Rather than being limited to survey data that I myself had collected, I drew on the extant literature from a variety of disciplines (Scanzoni, 1972). My chief aim was to expand the work of a number of theorists who sought to reconceptualize marriage in egalitarian terms (e.g., Rapoport & Rapoport, 1971). Although acknowledging that the majority of marriages were indeed described by functionalist notions of role specialization, I argued that a tiny but growing minority could be described in terms of role *interchangeability*.

The Equal-Partner Marriage

Given the abatement of assigned roles, relentless decision-making became the central feature of the "equal-partner" (EP) marriage. Following Blau (1964), Simmel (Levine et al., 1976), and Waller (1938), I utilized a conceptual model in which a dynamic version of exchange theory became indistinguishable from conflict theory. Moving beyond mere reciprocity per se, the model postulated that bargaining and negotiation were now mandatory to manage the inevitable struggles between wife and husband. Furthermore, EP marriages required that the woman's commitment to labor force participation be just as strong and as solid as the man's commitment. At the same time, a model based on interchangeability demanded that *his* commitment to children and to domestic chores be just as firm as hers. In that regard, I shared the optimism of many feminists that men would surely perceive the justice of women's equity, and would gradually come to embrace the cause as their own. I also concurred with advocates arguing that political and economic structures would eventually adapt to, and thus become more supportive of, EP marriages. I concurred further that the EP marriage was socially responsible in Mead's sense. Indeed, it appeared that children would be a great deal better off than they had been under the functionalist model, because now they would enjoy a higher level of intangible inputs from men. Men likewise would profit from greater involvement in the lives of children.

Values and Science

Asserting that adults and children were "better off" in one kind of marriage than another speaks to the issue of values. Christensen's (1964b:970) essay, "The intrusion of values," captured how most social scientists at the time, including me, felt about the place of values within the scientific enterprise: "Science seeks to discover *what is* rather than what ought to be: it looks for *truth,* not proof; it cuts new trails, letting the chips fall where they may, rather than defending old ones or catering to vested interests." Heady words indeed, and he added that although the same person might be a researcher and an advocate, the two roles must be kept sharply distinct. Accordingly, I could fit my evangelical belief that the husband should be the head of the wife into one pigeonhole, while my scholarship regarding gender equity could fit neatly into another. Alas, the more I read and thought about personal freedom, human development, and individual growth, the more untenable that partitioning became. Gradually, I was forced to relinquish my evangelical beliefs about male authority and family order. My final effort to bridge evangelical with contemporary thought about marriage was in a book aimed at evangelical laypersons (Scanzoni, 1974d). Equally significant, I began to comprehend how unworkable it was to separate my research efforts from my policy agenda. By way of illustration, the biologist does cancer research in order to uncover and understand *what is.* But that is merely the initial step in the research process. The requisite next step in his or her ongoing investigation is to discover if it is possible to *change* that reality into a different empirical reality–a reality more in line with what he or she believes *should be.* (See Greenwood & Levin, 1998, for an elaboration of this strategy that they call action research.) Understanding and explanation of that particular phenomenon are considered incomplete unless and until empirical efforts are made to change existing reality. In a like, though obviously not identical, manner, I was investigating marriages, not merely to describe them, but ultimately to try to help reconfigure them in more egalitarian terms.

The Pivotal Role of Negotiation

That objective drove my next major research effort–a regional household survey aimed at uncovering links between gender "roles" and fertility control (Scanzoni, 1975). Most demographers argued that it was in the national interest to reduce the then high levels of unintended pregnancies and unwanted births. My study suggested that within age, educational, employment, and racial categories, the more egalitarian (less "traditional"/more "modern") women's own gender role preferences were, the fewer children they intended to bear and the more effectual were their contraceptive practices. Consequently, if I were to configure egalitarian marriages, I must, first of all, advocate that women should internalize less conventional gender role preferences. The outcome should be fewer children, thus enabling the woman to participate more actively in the labor force. Second, if she were to behave in that nonconventional fashion, I must correspondingly assert that she would need to carry on vigorous and effective negotiation with her husband.

Those negotiation themes were explored extensively in my next book based on a follow-up household survey of the younger wives from the prior fertility control study (Scanzoni, 1978). My growing interest in husband-wife negotiation was the basis for an essay on "power" in families (1979a), published in the Burr et al. volumes–the successor to the Christensen *Handbook.* The latter saw no need for such a chapter because in the 1950s and early 1960s, "marital power" was simply not the pivotal issue it became by the late 1970s. My concern with gender-based conflict and negotiation was further elaborated in two additional essays (Scanzoni, 1979b, 1979c) in a book with Maximiliane Szinovacz (1980) and in an essay with Greer Litton Fox (1980).

Those several works sought to explore how marital decision-making was being significantly influenced by differences in men's and women's access to economic resources, by their gender role preferences, and by gender distinctions in negotiating styles. Importantly, the matter of dyadic negotiation was no longer circumscribed by marriage per se. The 1980 book recognized the increasing presence of cohabiting unions (both straight and gay/lesbian) and identified the major theoretical difference between formal and informal status: The social legitimation bestowed solely on heterosexual marriage was bound to have profound implications for dyadic decision-making. Furthermore, given that decision-making *processes* are the central nexus of today's dyadic love relationship (regardless of its legal status or sexual orientation), I added that researchers were well advised to focus primarily on those processes, and secondarily on the dyadic patterns that they generate and continually modify (Kingsbury & Scanzoni, 1973). Following my own counsel, Deborah Godwin and I expanded those notions in a series of articles (Godwin & Scanzoni, 1989a, b; Scanzoni & Godwin, 1990). Our aim was to conceptualize and measure the decision making *interaction* between spouses and to show how those processes were linked to ongoing marital patterns.

Public Policies

Concurrently, I pursued my growing interest in public policy via several articles and a book (Scanzoni, 1979e, 1981, 1982, 1983, 1987, 1989, 1991). Common to each effort were two themes: One was that policy and theory were flip sides of the same coin. As we shifted our conceptualization of family away from a static, or functionalist, model to a dynamic process-oriented model, our understanding of what makes "good families" should undergo a corresponding change. Policy, I argued, should aim explicitly to promote gender egalitarianism, and specific programs ought to be designed to further that goal as illustrated in Shehan and Scanzoni (1988). Those programs would focus on internal household processes (e.g., facilitating effective and creative decision-making), as well as on external issues including (but not limited to) high quality childcare, alongside equal opportunities for women in school and marketplace. A second theme pervading those policy works was my critique of the 1980s' conservative counter-revolution that, unfortunately, came to pass as Mead said it would. Although it was and is spearheaded by those of an evangelical bent, the movement also includes secular conservatives. Given my own roots, I could *feel* what the religious right was and is up to, in a way that perhaps eluded colleagues who had never been caught up in the fervent passions of the evangelical tradition. Whether secular or religious, what the conservatives seek is *family order* above all else. As Mead warned, the fact that their policy objective would come chiefly at the expense of women appears merely incidental.

PERSONAL FLUIDITY

While developing a change-centered model of family, fluidity became a feature of my own life. In 1978, I moved from Indiana University to the University of North Carolina-Greensboro, and in 1987 I went to the University of Florida. I became divorced in 1982, followed by a period in which I quickly ascertained for myself how vastly altered the "dating" and sexual scenes had become. My colleague Mary Joyce (Jo) Hasell and I began to live together in 1986 and were married in 1988.

My own experiences, to say nothing of the research literature, highlighted a construct first identified by Bernard Farber in 1964. He asserted that there was a metamorphosis in Western culture away from the functionalist notion that "orderly replacement" based on marital permanence was the foundation of the "institution" of family. In its place, he said, was the emerging notion that every adult, *regardless of current marital and/or parenting status,* has the right to form a(nother) relationship. This term was further elaborated by Swidler (1980). Farber coined the term "permanent availability" to describe the alleged shift away from the virtue of stability to the conception that change was equally meritorious. But the instant rejoinder to his controversial thesis was a deafening silence, perhaps because no one wished to believe him. I did, however, adapt his ideas for two empirical pieces (Scanzoni, 1968; Morgan & Scanzoni, 1987). Nonetheless, by the 1990s, the literature vindicated his acumen: People now want a "good" dyadic love relationship to last indefinitely precisely because it is *good.* However, people are no longer willing to drag out a "bad" relationship (including marriage) any longer than forced to.

So fundamental a transformation in the very essence of marriage led several colleagues and me to think about recasting our understanding of the contemporary dyadic love relationship (Scanzoni, Polonko, Teachman, & Thompson, 1989). We argued that within the cultural imagination, marriage retained its mystical qualities. Wedding rituals were (and are) believed to transmute persons, and thus to confer on them a unique and esteemed status, marked by alleged parental dependability in which children presumably flourish (Freese, 1991). But, on the other hand, in the real world of everyday life, marriage was being demystified: Marriage rates were going down, while rates of divorce, cohabitation, singleness, and solo-parenting were going up. Over time, the goal of getting and staying married was being forced to share its formerly unrivaled status with the equally salient goal of human and personal development. It was becoming just as vital for a woman or a man to be a "growing" person as it was to be formally married. The upshot was that marriage was more appropriately characterized by Farber's than by Parsons' laws.

The Generic Components of Dyadic Love

Furthermore, given the evidence showing that many of the everyday behaviors (e.g., decision-making, household chores, parenting, sexual patterns) of formal and informal unions (straight or gay/lesbian) were virtually indistinguishable, my colleagues and I searched for an overarching construct that might subsume the dyadic love relationship in general. We conceived of the dyadic union as a specific instance of Faris's (1937) primary group. The German sociologist Lerke Gravenhorst (1988) supplied one such construct. She used the admittedly awkward tag *erotic friendship* to conceptualize the contemporary dyadic union, whether formal or informal. The next step was to ask if the "erotic friendship"–whether formal or informal–possesses certain identifiable *generic* components. This was similar to the quest taken by Spiro (1963:119) in the context of the post-World War II Kibbutzim. If we visualize the dyadic love relationship as analogous to an organic cell, then we may say that its generic components are two in number. First, its lining or boundary is the partners' shared commitment to sexual monogamy. Second, its nucleus is the partners' mutual participation in emotional intimacy. To those core generic components, the partners may or may not choose to add certain features that raise the magnitude of their interdependence (Scanzoni & Marsiglio, 1993). Coresidence is a vital feature and, increasingly, that implies co-parenting because one or both partners may convey children to their union. And whether children are present or not, the partners (straight or gay/lesbian) may seek to bear and/or adopt (more) children together. Despite the fact that they may choose *not* to add the feature of formal marriage, most heterosexual couples eventually marry. The belief that marriage is a unique, esteemed, and elevated status–though under siege–remains quite potent. Recently, David Popenoe's research institute captured media attention because its nation survey concluded that not only are Americans less likely to marry than ever before, but fewer people who do marry report being "very happy" in the marriages (Flectcher, 1999).

The Preeminence of Process

The upshot is that in 30 years I have progressed from advocating *structure* (permanent heterosexual marriage, governed by role specialization) to promoting *process:* Throughout their entire life course people should exercise their right *and* their duty to make wise and responsible choices regarding love-partners, children, and employment. At certain periods of one's life course, one may in fact choose marriage, but at other points something else. No one pattern (i.e., the typical nuclear arrangement) is ever intrinsically superior to any other. Nevertheless, what is superior or inferior is the wisdom of the choices made, how "effectively" they were negotiated if a partner was involved, and how accountable one is for the outcomes of her or his choices (Scanzoni &

Godwin, 1990). For brazenly expounding that *process* thesis to undergraduates (Scanzoni, 1995), I was taken to task for allegedly corrupting their minds and morals (Glenn, 1997; Scanzoni, 1997).

Glenn's ill-tempered attack on me and Popenoe's (1996) proposed neo-functionalist model of marriage reflect their proclivity to face today's challenges using yesterday's strategies. By contrast, Mead (1967) anticipated today's challenges when she declared that the quest for the holy grail–freedom and independence–must be balanced with responsibility by and for all the parties involved. Children, she cautioned, could easily fall through the cracks of adult individualism. Today, for example, I, along with many others, celebrate household *diversity*. We are gratified that adults are increasingly free to compose their own household in ways that seem best to them at a specific juncture of their life course. Furthermore, we applaud the new household *homogeneity*. We now recognize that all dyadic love relationships are generically alike in terms of their core components. And they are equivalent insofar as the route to constructing a rich love relationship is bound up in the dynamics of effective negotiation. We are, in essence, creating micro-level democracies in which everything is negotiable except the principle that everything is negotiable (Scanzoni, 1983).

Reconstructing Childhood and Adolescence

But how do children fit into the new household? In many academic departments there are courses about family and separate courses about children and their development. However, little attention is paid to a theoretical and substantive synthesis of the lives of adults and children. *The American Sociological Association* has a section on family, and a section on children, but there is no section devoted to the syntheses of the lives of adults and of children–the closest would be the "Aging and Life Course" section. Over the years, I followed the practice of keeping the two spheres relatively distinct and, as a result, failed to reflect very much on the lives of children. However, given that the everyday lives of children and of adults are inextricable, it seems, in hindsight, that I was remiss. It now occurs to me that the absence of a theoretical and substantive synthesis of their lives is *one* reason why conservatives were able to curb the feminist movement. Progressives have thus far been unable to develop a coherent and compelling rejoinder to the prevailing conservative preachment that today's children are the victims of adult individualism and that the chief means to ameliorate their suffering is for adults (women in particular) to cut back on self-fulfillment.

While searching for the high moral ground that might place conservatives on the defensive, I have been learning about an innovative approach to childhood that reconstructs it in a manner analogous, though not identical, to the contemporary reorganization of adulthood (Blitzer, 1991; Corsaro, 1997). Rather than obsessing with role conformity as the functionalists did, we now view adults as agents of their own destiny: They are exercising choices within a set of social constraints and enablings (Scanzoni & Marsiglio, 1993). Hence, why not view children in that same light? As fitting as that may sound, what does it truly mean to conceive of children and youths as "capable of partnership with adults for social change" (Boulding, 1996:590)? My response stems from one of Mead's insights. When I first read it in 1967, I was utterly oblivious to its implications–perhaps because it was so far ahead of its time. She advocated the invention of contemporary social networks analogous to the nonmodern kin networks she analyzed with great acuity. Another anthropologist, Carol Stack (1974), later applied the label "fictive kin" to describe the non-blood support networks she studied in the Chicago area (cf. Rivers & Scanzoni, 1997). My first empirical foray into the thicket of trying to build and study fictive kin networks came at the urging of a colleague from the college of architecture–a designer who, as I noted above, is also my spouse (Hasell & Scanzoni, 2000). Jo argued that "household" is just as much a spatial as a social phenomenon. She added that understanding the household requires a grasp of both its social and its spatial connections to its immediate environment–its neighborhood. This perspective was squarely in the tradition of the "Chicago School," one of the pioneering movements in the early 20th century.

The Household Embedded Within Its Neighborhood

Conceiving of an "embedded" rather than an "isolated" household was not entirely foreign to my earliest work. Back then, the environmental factors were religious ideology, followed soon after by the husband's fit with the economic system. Unfortunately, however, I viewed both the household and its environment in static terms. The principal conceptual issue was how the consensus, order, and stability of the household were influenced by its milieu. Today, the conceptual issues are drastically different. Specifically, how might the neighborhood constitute a structural means to facilitate the new household diversity and homogeneity? Similarly, how might the household help to structure its own neighborhood (Scanzoni, 2000)? At the very same time, how would it expedite responsibility for children? Could the neighborhood, in both its social and its spatial dimensions, somehow be the instrument to develop a body of literature in which the confluence of the lives of children and of adults would become the principal focus? And could it also help to position the feminist movement once again at the forefront of progressive social change?

I soon discovered that a number of scholars from several countries and a range of disciplines (e.g., Weisman, 1992; Andrew & Milroy, 1988; Spain, 1992, 1993) were already pondering those profound and bewildering issues. Horelli and Vespa (1994), for instance, concluded that, despite a half-century commitment to gender equity and to facilitative social programs, it cannot be said that Scandinavian women and men have yet achieved equivalent status. Moreover, the lack of gender equivalence is even more unmistakable in other parts of Europe as well as in North America. Horelli and Vespa ruefully acknowledged that the optimism felt by 1970s' progressives (myself included) regarding gender equity has not materialized. They got even more gloomy by suggesting, as did Mead, that the "isolated," i.e., nonconnected, household is a "structurally challenged" phenomenon. In 1953, Nisbet argued, that we were asking far too many things of the isolated nuclear family; requiring it to now demonstrate a full measure of gender equity may simply be asking too much. Consequently, Horelli and Vespa asserted that in *addition* to striving for economic self-sufficiency based on education, occupation, and income, women together with men should endeavor to construct household "connectedness" in both its social *and* its spatial senses. They portrayed their schema as a "Nordic Feminist Vision" and coined the label "The New Everyday Life" (NEL) to apprehend their conception of the embeddedness of the household within its neighborhood

The Historical Elaboration of Families

I became fascinated with NEL for all the reasons just cited, plus an overarching one. In my life as a functionalist, I never mistrusted Parsons' evolutionary wisdom. He asserted that the post-World War II nuclear family, after more than two hundred years of trying, had finally "reached the maximum level of isolation [independence, autonomy], just as American society has reached the maximum level of industrialization" (Pitts, 1964:88). Intriguingly, it seems never to have occurred to Parsons that the economic system of Western societies would keep on evolving into what today we call the post-industrial age. In a like manner, it never appeared to him that American households would keep on developing beyond the model he championed. It is indisputable that citizens are reinventing the internal structure of the household. At the same time, how far can those efforts continue without also tampering a bit with its external structure–in short, modifying its isolation, i.e., nonconnectedness? That was the issue I explored in my most recent book (Scanzoni, 2000), and I probed it by elaborating the notion of the NEL community.

Among other things, I indicated that the NEL neighborhood might establish itself to be a zone of "safety"–a sanctuary within which women and children would face a considerably reduced threat of domestic aggression–the seeds of this idea can be found in Durfee (1993), and Waldfogel (1998). In addition, building on the seeds of an idea proposed by Coleman (1990), I proposed that the NEL neighborhood might designate itself to be a zone of "productivity." Such a zone implies that the community creation of children's social capital and human capital might somehow provide both men and women with a high degree of personal gratification and a strong sense of moral worth. That kind of arrangement could perhaps be one means to help wean men away from the ethos of "productivism," and thereby facilitate a level of gender equity that has so far eluded us. This arrangement would become the structural basis for community participation in the lives of children and youths and, in turn, for their participation in the life of the community. Constructing a zone of productivity implies that the lives of children and of neighborhood adults would become commingled in ways that are quite different from what is typical today. The study of their confluence would give rise to a body of knowledge in which their interdependence is the pivotal focus of our attention. Furthermore, *diversity* of household composition, of age (mature citizens would play an integral role), of racial/ethnic background, and of economic status would be a principal hallmark of NEL. The two latter dimensions are particularly vital if the neighborhood is to establish and maintain the sort of partnership with the government envisioned by Coleman (1990).

New Action Theory and Action Research

And that is where I am just now. I recently applied for external funding to study a "cohousing" community.[1] My objective is to determine the conditions under which that neighborhood might, or might not, be willing and/or able to refashion itself into a "Prevention Zone" aimed at reducing the likelihood of domestic aggression. I proposed to utilize the methodology called "action research" in which the professional plays the role of "friendly outsider," and is thereby a "co-researcher" with the group members, or "insiders." This particular research schema presumes that the scientific goals of understanding and explanation are inextricable from the participants' own objectives–whether those are group change or maintenance (or some blend thereof) or dissolution. I view action research as the empirical arm of new action theory (Alexander, 1988). As I see it, persons have been actively reinventing *internal* household patterns for many decades. We are discarding static role specialization in favor of a dynamic negotiation model. At the same time, however, we are loathe to relinquish the household autonomy that was strongly associated with role specialization. Nonetheless, as we keep on inventing ways to expand personal *in*dependence will we, paradoxically enough, gradually begin to devise means to increase household *inter*dependence? Will that occur because we discover by degrees that those seemingly contradictory yearnings may in some enigmatic way reinforce one another? That question intrigues me, and, at first glance, it appears eons away from the concerns that first drew me into social science. But in fact it is not. I have always felt that freedom is the highest human good, and I have consistently looked for ways to facilitate it. I am still looking.

NOTE

1. A copy of my research proposal is available on request. "Cohousing" refers to a network of presently existing neighborhoods in Scandinavia, Holland, and North America. Each neighborhood contains an established degree of spatial and social connectedness, but does not typically seek to supplement that connectedness with distinctive NEL features (see, e.g., Fromm, 1991; Hanson, 1996; Hasell & Scanzoni, 2000; Meltzer, 2000). The web site of *The Cohousing Network* is <www.cohousing.org>.

REFERENCES

Alexander, J. C. (1988). The new theoretical movement. In Neil J. Smelser (Ed.), *Handbook of sociology* (pp. 77-102). Newbury Park, CA: Sage.

Andrew, C. & Milroy, B. M. (Eds.) (1988). Life spaces: Gender, households, employment. Vancouver: University of British Columbia Press.

Bell, N. W. & Vogel, E. F. (1960). Toward a framework for functional analysis of family behavior. In N. W. Bell & E. F. Vogel (Eds.), *A modern introduction to the family* (pp. 1-33). New York: Free Press.

Bernard, J. (1964). The adjustments of married mates. In H. T. Christensen (Ed.) *Handbook of marriage and the family* (pp. 675-739). Chicago: Rand McNally.
Bernard, J. (1972). *The future of marriage*. New York: World Books.
Billingsley, A. (1968). *Black families in white America*. Englewood Cliffs, NJ: Prentice-Hall.
Blake, J. & Davis, K. (1964). Norms, values, and sanctions. In R. E. L. Faris (Ed.), *Handbook of modern sociology* (pp. 456-484). Chicago: Rand McNally.
Blankenhorn, D. (1995). *Fatherless America: Confronting our most urgent social problems*. New York: Basic Books.
Blau, P. M. (1964). *Exchange and power in social life*, New York: Wiley.
Blitzer, S. (1991). They are only children, what do they know? A look at current ideologies of childhood. In S. E. Cahill (Ed.), *Sociological studies of child development, Vol. 4, Perspectives on and of children* (pp. 11-28). Greenwich, CT: Jai Press.
Boulding, E. (1996). Book Review. *Contemporary Sociology, 25*, 5, 589-590.
Bulmer, M. (1984). *The Chicago school of sociology: Institutionalization, Diversity and the issue of sociological research*. Chicago: The University of Chicago Press.
Christensen, H. T. (Ed.) (1964a). *Handbook of marriage and the family*. Chicago: Rand McNally.
Christensen, H. T. (1964b). The intrusion of values. In H. T. Christensen (Ed.), *Handbook of marriage and the family* (pp. 969-1006). Chicago: Rand McNally
Coleman, J. S. (1990). *Foundations of social theory*. Cambridge: Harvard University Press.
Corsaro, W. A. (1997). *The sociology of childhood*. Thousand Oaks, CA: Pine Forge Press.
Dizard, J. E. & Gadlin, H. (1990). *The minimal family*. Amherst: University of Massachusetts Press.
Durfee, D. T. (Chair). (1993). U.S. Advisory Board on Child Abuse & Neglect. (September), *Neighbors helping Neighbors: A new national strategy for the protection of children*. Washington DC: Department of Health & Human Services, Administration for Children and Families.
Farber, B. (1964). *Family: Organization and interaction*. San Francisco: Chandler.
Faris. E. (1937). The primary group: Essence and accident. In L.A. Coser & B. Rosenberg (Eds.), *Sociological theory* (pp. 298-303). New York: Macmillan.
Freese, P. (1991). The union of nature and culture: gender symbolism in the American wedding ritual. In P. Freese & J. M. Coggeshall (Eds.), *Transcending boundaries: Multi-disciplinary approaches to the study of gender* (pp. 97-112). New York: Bergin & Garvey.
Fromm, D. (1991). *Collaborative communities: Cohousing central living, and other new forms of housing with shared facilities*. New York: Van Nostrand Reinhold.
Gans, H. J. (1991). Urbanism and suburbanism as ways of life: A reevaluation of defintions. In H. J. Gans (Ed.) *People, plans, and policies: Essays on poverty, racism, and other national urban problems* (pp. 51-69). New York: Russell Sage.
Giddens, A. (1994). *Beyond left and right: The future of radical politics*. Stanford, CA: Stanford University Press.
Glenn, N. D. (1997). A critique of twenty family and marriage and the family textbooks. *Family Relations: Journal of Applied Family and Child Studies, 46*, 3, 197-208.

Godwin, D. D. & Scanzoni, J. (1989a). Couple consensus during marital joint decision-making: A context, process, outcome model. *Journal of Marriage and Family*, 51, 4, 43-956.

Godwin, D. D. & Scanzoni, J. (1989b). Couple decision-making: Commonalities and differences across issues and spouses. *Journal of Family Issues*, 10, 3, 291-310.

Goode, W . J. (1959). The sociology of the family. In R. K. Merton, L. Broom, L. S. Cottrell, Jr. (Eds.), *Sociology today: Problems and prospects* (pp. 178-196). New York: Basic.

Goode, W. J. (1963). *World Revolution and Family Patterns*. New York: The Free Press.

Gouldner, A. W. (1960). The norm of reciprocity: A preliminary statement. *American Sociological Review*, *25*, 2, 161-178.

Gravenhorst, L. (1988). A Feminist looks at Family Development Theory. In D. Klein & J. Aldous. (Eds.), *Social stress and family development* (pp. 79-101). New York: Guilford.

Greenwood, D.J. & Levin, M. (1998). *Introduction to action research: Social research for social change*. Thousand Oaks, CA: Sage.

Hanson, C. (1996). *The cohousing handbook: Building a place for community*. Point Roberts, WA: Hartley & Marks Press.

Hasell, M. J. & Scanzoni, J. (2000). Cohousing in HUD housing: Prospects and problems. *Journal of Architectural and Planning Research*, 17, 1, 133-145.

Hayden, D. (1981). *The grand domestic revolution: A history of feminist designs for American Homes, Neighborhoods, and Cities*. Cambridge, MA: MIT Press.

Hill, R. & Hansen, D. A. (1960). The identification of conceptual frameworks utilized in family study. *Journal of Marriage and Family*, *22*, 4, 299-311.

Horelli, L. & Vespa, K. (1994). In search of supportive structures for everyday life. In I. Altman & A. Churchman (Eds.), *Women and the environment* (pp. 201-226). New York: Plenum.

Kingsbury, N. & Scanzoni, J. (1993). Structural-Functionalism. In P. Boss, W. Doherty, R. LaRossa, W. Schumm, & S. K. Steinmetz (Eds.), *Sourcebook of family theories and methods* (pp. 195-217). New York: Plenum.

Levine, D. N., Carter, E. B., & Miller, E. (1976). Simmel's influence on American sociology-I. *American Journal of Sociology*, *81*, 1, 813-845.

Mead, M. (1967). The life cycle and its variations: The division of roles. *Daedalus*, *96*, 3, 871-875.

Meltzer, G. (2000). Cohousing: Verifying the importance of social context in the application of environmentalism. *Journal of Architecture and Planning Research*, *17*, 1, 110-134.

Morgan, M. Y. & Scanzoni, J. (1987). Assessing variation in permanence/pragmatism orientations. *Journal of Divorce*, *11*, 1, 1-23.

Nisbet, R. A. (1953). *The quest for community: A study in the ethics of order and freedom*. New York: Oxford University Press.

Noble, J. L. (1966). The American Negro woman. In J. P. Davis (Ed.), *The American Negro reference book* (pp. 501-559). Englewood Cliffs, NJ: Prentice-Hall.

Olson, D. H., McCubbin, H., Barnes, H., Larsen, A. Muxen, M., & Wilson, M. (1983). *Families: What makes them work*. Beverly Hills, CA: Sage.

Parsons, T. (1955). The American family: Its relations to personality and to the social structure. In T. Parsons & R. F. Bales (Eds.), *Family, socialization and interaction process* (pp. 3-33). New York: The Free Press.
Parsons, T. (1965). The normal American family. In S. M. Farber, P. Mustacchi, & R. H. L. Wilson (Eds.), *Man and civilization: The family's search for survival* (pp. 31-50). New York: McGraw-Hill.
Pitts, J. R. (1964). The Structural-functional approach. In H. T. Christensen (Ed.), *Handbook of marriage and the family* (pp. 51-124). Chicago: Rand McNally.
Popenoe, D. (1996). Modern marriage: Revising the cultural script. In D. Popenoe, J. B. Elshtain, & D. Blankenhorn (Eds) *Promises to keep: Decline and renewal of marriage in America* (pp. 247-270). Lanham, MD: Rowman & Littlefield.
Rapoport, R. & Rapoport, R. N. (1971). *Sex, career, and family*. Beverly Hills: Sage.
Research Group. (1991). *The New everyday life: Ways and means*. Stockholm: The Nordic Council.
Risman, B. J., & Johnson-Sumerford, D. (1998). Doing it fairly: A study of post-gender marriages. *Journal of Marriage and Family*, *60*, 1, 23-40.
Rivers, R. M. & Scanzoni, J. (1997). Social families among African-Americans: Policy implications for children. In H. P. McAdoo (Ed.), *Black families* (pp. 333-348). Newbury Park CA: Sage.
Scanzoni, J. (1965a). Resolution of occupational-conjugal role conflict in clergy marriage. *Journal of Marriage and Family*, *27*, 3, 396-402.
Scanzoni, J. (1965b). Innovation and constancy in the church-sect typology. *American Journal of Sociology*, *71*, 3, 320-327.
Scanzoni, J. (1965c). A note on method for the church-sect typology. *Sociological Analysis*, 26, 4, 189-203.
Scanzoni, J. (1970). *Opportunity and the family*. New York: The Free Press.
Scanzoni, J. (1971). *The black family in modern society: Patterns of stability and security*. Boston: Allyn & Bacon. Rev. 1977, Chicago: University of Chicago Press.
Scanzoni, J. (1972). *Sexual bargaining: Power politics in American marriage*. Englewood Cliffs, NJ: Prentice-Hall. Rev. 1982, Chicago: University of Chicago Press.
Scanzoni, J. (1975). *Sex roles, life-styles and childbearing: Changing patterns of marriage and family*. New York: The Free Press.
Scanzoni, J. (1978). *Sex roles, women's work and marital conflict: A study of family change*. Lexington, MA: D.C. Heath/Lexington.
Scanzoni, J. (1979a). Social processes and power in families. In W. R. Burr, R. Hill, F. I. Nye, & I. L. Reiss. (Eds.), *Contemporary theories about the family, Volume I* (pp. 295-316). New York: The Free Press.
Scanzoni, J. (1979b). Social exchange and behavioral interdependence. In T. L. Huston & R. L. Burgess (Eds.), *Social exchange and developing relationships* (pp. 61-98). New York: Academic Press.
Scanzoni, J. (1979c). An historical perspective on husband-wife bargaining power and marital dissolution. In G. Levinger and O.C. Moles (Eds.) *Divorce and separation* (pp. 20-36). New York: Basic Books.
Scanzoni, J. (1979d). *Love and negotiate: Creative conflict in marriage*. Waco, TX: Word Books.

Scanzoni, J. (1979e). Strategies for changing male family roles: Research and practice implications. *Family Relations: Journal of Applied Family and Child Studies*, *28*, 4, 435-442.
Scanzoni, J. (1981). Family dyamics. In M. E. Olsen & M. Micklin (Eds.), *Handbook of applied sociology* (pp. 115-133). New York: Praeger.
Scanzoni, J. (1982). Reconsidering family policy: Status quo or force for change? *Journal of Family Issues*, 3, 3, 277-300.
Scanzoni, J. (1983). *Shaping tomorrow's family: Theory and policy for the twenty-first century*. (Foreword by Jessie Bernard). Newbury Park, CA: Sage.
Scanzoni, J. (1987). Families of the 1980s: Time to refocus our thinking. *Journal of Family Issues*, *8*, 4, 394-421.
Scanzoni, J. (1989). Alternative images for public policy: Family structure versus families struggling. *Policy Studies Review*, *8*, 3, 599-609.
Scanzoni, J. (1991). Balancing the policy interests of children and adults. In E. A. Anderson & R. C. Hula (Eds.), *The reconstruction of family policy* (pp. 11-22). New York: Greenwood.
Scanzoni, J. (1995). *Contemporary families and relationships: Reinventing responsibility*. New York: McGraw-Hill.
Scanzoni, J. (1997). Fashioning families and policies for the future–not the past. *Family Relations: Journal of Applied Family and Child Studies*, *46*, 3, 213-217.
Scanzoni, J. (2000). *Designing families: The search for self and community in the information age*. Thousand Oaks, CA: Pine Forge.
Scanzoni, J. & Fox, G. L. (1980). Sex roles, family and society: The seventies and beyond. *Journal of Marriage and Family*, *42*, 4, 743-756.
Scanzoni, J. & Godwin, D. D. (1990). Negotiation effectiveness and acceptable outcomes. *Social Psychology Quarterly*, *53*, 3, 239-251.
Scanzoni, J. & Marsiglio, W. (1993). New action theory and contemporary families. *Journal of Family Issues*, *14*, 1, 105-132.
Scanzoni, J. and Polonko, K., Teachman, J., & Thompson, L. (1989). *The sexual bond: Rethinking families and close relationships*. Newbury Park, CA: Sage.
Scanzoni, J. & Szinovacz. M. (1980). *Family decision-making: A developmental sex role model*. Newbury Park CA: Sage.
Scanzoni, J. (1998b). Rethinking the paradigm for child protection. In *The future of children: Protecting children from abuse and neglect*. Los Altos, CA: The David & Lucile Packard Foundation, Center for the Future of Children, *8*, 1, 104-119.
Schwartz, P. (1994). *Peer Marriage: How love between equals really works*. New York: The Free Press.
Seeley, J. R., Sim, R. A., & Loosley, E. W. (1956). *Crestwood Heights*. New York: Basic Books.
Shehan, C. L. & Scanzoni, J. (1988). Gender patterns in the United States: Demographic trends and policy prospects. *Family Relations: Journal of Applied Family and Child Studies*, *37*, 4, 444-450.
Spain, D. (1992). *Gendered spaces*. Chapel Hill: University of North Carolina Press.
Spain, D. (1993). Gendered spaces and women's status. *Sociological theory*, *11*, 1, 137-151.
Spiro, M. E. (1963). *Kibbutz: Venture in utopia*. New York: Shocken Books.
Stack, C. (1974). *All our Kin: Strategies for survival in a black community*. New York: Harper & Row.

Stoller, F. H. (1970). The intimate network of families as a new structure. In H. A. Otto (Ed.) *The family in search of a future* (pp. 145-160). New York: Appleton-Century-Crofts.
Swidler, A. (1980). Love and adulthood in American culture. In N. J. Smelser & E. H. Erikson (Eds.), *Themes of love and work in adulthood* (pp. 120-150). Cambridge, MA: Harvard University Press.
Trent, J.W. (1987). A decade of declining involvement: American sociology in the field of child development, the 1920s. In P. A. Adler, P. Adler, & N. Mandell (Eds.), *Sociological studies of child development, Vol II* (pp. 11-37). Greenwich, CT: JAI.
Waldfogel, J. (1998). *The future of child protection.* Cambridge, MA: Harvard University Press.
Waller, W. (1938). *The family: A dynamic interpretation.* New York: Dryden.
Weisman, L. K. (1992). *Discrimination by design: A feminist critique of the man-made environment.* Urbana: University of Illinois Press.
Westoff, L. A. & Westoff, C. F. (1971). *From now to zero.* Boston: Little, Brown.
Wharton, A. S. (1993). Book Review. *Contemporary Sociology, 22*, 3, 172-173.
Yankelovich, D. (1981). *New rules: Searching for self-fulfillment in a world turned upside down.* New York: Random House.

My Life Story: Reflections of an Early Family Scholar

Harold T. Christensen

KEYWORDS. Autobiography, marriage, research, religion, handbook

EARLY YEARS

I began life as a disappointment. My father's journal entry for March 10, 1909 consisted of one sentence: "Our second baby boy was born at 9 p.m." That was all; no more, no less. While father's writing style typically leaned toward the sparse, factual statement, with little embellishment, I cannot, as I now examine the record, help but notice a difference in tone between this entry and those for my two brothers immediately preceding and following me. Father referred to the advent of his first-born as a "very welcome visitor in our home" and described his third-born as being "a sweet little fellow." Not that I am envious. Indeed, as measured by subsequent events, I have enjoyed every bit as much love and respect and parental pride in later years as have any of the others. I sometimes even think that I may have had more than my share. But there is good reason for the initial parental shock, which I now know accompanied my arrival into this world.

I was born with a cleft lip. My upper lip was split near its center and pulled grotesquely toward either side. The upper gum was open as well, and my nose lay flat against the right cheek. I must have looked a sight. Being totally unprepared for anything like this, my parents were at first both frightened and puzzled. I have been told that they even wondered, momentarily, if this might be a punishment for something they may have neglected or done. Fortunately, they soon regained their composure and perspective and preceded to do everything they could to meet the situation head on, with only my welfare in mind. A crude but state-of-the-art surgery at the time saw me through my infancy and childhood periods. At about age twelve, I was placed in the hands of a pioneering specialist in lip surgery who was traveling through from the east coast and was able to reshape my appearance so that, from that time on, one could scarcely tell if anything were amiss.

Quite honestly, I never have felt any handicap from this accident of nature, throughout either the sensitive years of adolescence or the highly competitive years of adulthood. Had I been female, of course, that might have been different, for society is more inclined to judge physical appearance in women than in men. But even as a male, if the original repair job had been allowed to stand, I most certainly would have suffered from feeling different than others and being self-conscious over it. Furthermore, if my birth deformity had included a cleft palate as well, as sometimes happens, this could have left me with the severe handicap of having to deal with a speech impediment. I guess I was just lucky.

I was reared in a typically large and conforming Mormon family. My childhood and adolescent years were spent in southeastern Idaho, first in Preston and then Rexburg, not far from Utah's northern border. Both of these communities were predominantly Latter-day Saint (Mormon) with respect to both population and culture, so I grew up not knowing much else. I regularly participated in church and local school activities, absorbing most of the values and life goals to which I was exposed. And yet, from the very beginning, there was a streak of independence within me that kept pushing to come out. I wanted to do my own thinking–to be my own person.

I had six brothers, no sisters. My next younger brother, Cornell, who of all my siblings I felt closest to, closest with respect to temperament and outlook as well as age, proved to have a profound influence upon my life; and I think I did upon his as well. As young men, we shared many heart-to-heart conversations. Cornell was a deep and honest thinker. There were times during his youth and young adulthood when he found himself struggling fiercely against what he considered unreasonable conventions and pressures upon him to conform. At one time, he told me, head tilted back, "I care not what others think; it is to myself alone that I am responsible." Later, he succinctly summed up these and related feelings in a highly reflective journal he had started keeping, in these words: *"I refuse to be standardized!"*

After a lingering illness and at the relatively young age of twenty-six, Cornell died. For a time prior to his passing, he was free in declaring himself to be an agnostic, occasionally even an avowed atheist. His ordeal and rebellion caused our parents great anguish, every bit as much for his mental/emotional struggle and loss of faith as for his physical suffering and loss of life. Although my own inner rebellion did not go so far as his, I clearly understood what Cornell meant by his stand against institutional pressures, by his disinclination to let himself become "standardized." I empathized with his struggle.

Earlier, during the summer of 1928, I joined Cornell and our father in a most rewarding mountain-climbing experience: an ascent up the Grand Teton of western Wyoming. This magnificent peak stands some 13,766 feet above sea level. According to official records, only twenty-two earlier climbing parties had been successful in scaling it. Some had tried and failed, and a few climbers had died in the attempt. Space here will not permit any detailed accounting of our climb. But it included such hair-raising adventures as these: ice-chipping for footholds on an outward-sloping ledge that had to be crossed, with nothing below to catch us had we slipped; hanging by our fingers while accomplishing a hand-over-hand maneuver across a portion of a high cliff, where a mistake would have meant falling for the rest of our lives; and much, much more. On several occasions we felt sorely tempted to give up. But we did not turn back, and the awe-inspiring views afforded us from the top, once we had achieved it, made us ever so thankful that we had not.

The experience just related produced a profound impact upon my young, impressionable, still-to-be-fully-defined personality. For one thing, it seemed to stimulate within me a creative urge that pressed for poetic expression. This was something new, and it surprised me, but I let myself go. Here are two stanzas lifted from one such attempt:

HORIZON'S BEYOND

The heights above us beckon on
Until we reach the top
And then our vision lifts to more
We climb and never stop
But the higher up in life we go
(As on a mountain trail)
The more we see and understand
And beauties more unveil

Ah, dreams of happiness!
May you lead me true

May you teach me how to wait
And how to work life through
For I want to live as a man should live
And I want to play my part
So teach me to work and to love and to give
And to fight life through from the start–
To Horizon's Beyond.

Early School Honors

I used this same theme, "Horizon's Beyond," for my valedictory address at the 1928-29 graduation exercises at Ricks College, where I had been enrolled. Ricks was, and remains, a Mormon-operated junior college located in Rexburg, Idaho. In addition to being chosen valedictorian that year, I also had served as Student Body President, had been a member of the debate team, and was featured in the annual yearbook as the Most Prominent Male Student of the Sophomore Class.

Incidentally, being chosen valedictorian was the third such honor to eventually come my way. Earlier ones had been at grade school and high school graduations, and there was to be a fourth–at my yet-to-be-reached graduation from Brigham Young University in 1935.

Obtaining good grades in school has always been my lot. I attribute this more to hard work than anything else, more to plodding than to superior intelligence. From my earliest days, the notions of having a purpose, seriously applying oneself, and assuming responsibility had been drilled into me by my parents, religious leaders, teachers, and close associates. I always have been, and remain, an extremely conscientious person. Even *too* conscientious at times, I sometimes think. For while this characteristic is basically a positive trait, as most would agree, it inclines me to be overly serious on occasions when what may be needed most is some frivolity.

At least three major life-goals were drilled into me during my formative years by the family and the religious culture into which I had been born: (1) to marry compatibly and rear a worthy family; (2) to be "successful" in life, defined less in terms of acquiring wealth and more in making a "mark" in the world via higher education; and (3) to serve a full time Mission for my Church. I was molded and shaped by the culture to accept each of these goals and to work toward their fulfillment. Nevertheless, as is common in Mormondom, the first two of these goals were expected to wait until the third one had been accomplished.

While I had some dating experience as an adolescent and even, on a couple of occasions, had become involved in fairly serious romantic attachments, I did not feel myself ready, or would not permit myself, to make any kind of life commitment until the mission expectation had been completed. To be sure, not every young pre-mission Mormon caught up in the emotions of courtship remains this firm to Church commitment. But I felt almost compelled; it was putting "duty" first. Similarly, I already had made a good start toward the educational goal. This process, I felt, could be interrupted without causing harm. My drives toward higher academic degrees could be held back until after the mission was over, a view encouraged both by my parents and Church. Conscientious Harold!

Mission Years

So, a Mormon mission it was. I left for New Zealand in late 1929 and served there for a period of nearly four years, working mainly with the native Maori people. The usual term for a foreign mission at that time was two-and-one-half years. Mine turned out to be longer due to receiving an exceptional appointment as Acting Mission President. The regular president, who was elderly, had been forced by illness to return home. Furthermore, this was at a time when a number of missionaries located there had been greatly reduced due to The Great Depression.

On the whole, I found my mission experience both challenging and rewarding. There were some discouragements and inner struggles to contend with. However, in total, and in perspective, I tend to give it a strong plus. My firsthand exposure to a new and vastly different culture brought with it an enlarged understanding of people, their life ways, and their problems. Mission work at such a young age, added maturity, which in turn has helped shape and advance my professional career.

I can recognize in my missionary experience an early attraction to sociology as a field for study and of marriage and the family as a specialty within that field. Throughout my New Zealand stay, I found myself to be an atypical missionary. I followed an approach that was not so much scriptural as it was observational and analytic. More than trying to convert, I tried to reason with people and, when opportunity presented itself, to help them work through their personal and interactional problems. There were numerous occasions, for example, when I found myself faced with the task of trying to help solve a marital or family difficulty. And, while realizing that I probably was of some help, I, nevertheless, frequently felt inadequate in the attempt. This made me want to learn more about these things. Later on, upon returning to academic studies, I quite naturally found myself inclined to focus upon sociology and family as fields of study.

Continuing My Education

I enrolled at Brigham Young University soon after returning from New Zealand in the fall of 1933. I started out as a junior, having completed the freshman and sophomore levels at Ricks College some four years earlier. Wanting to make sure that my choice of a major was a good one, I took my time. This meant that most of that first year was filling group requirements, plus trying out elective courses that attracted me and seemed to offer promising career opportunities. I even, at one time or another, considered such diverse options as Physics and Political Science. But my eventual selection, not made final until the beginning of my senior year, was Sociology, a decision I have never regretted.

On June 5, 1935, I graduated with a Bachelor of Science degree. Alice and I entered our marriage on that very same day. My academic record as an undergraduate had been sufficiently outstanding, along with active participation in extracurricular events, such as serving as Senior Class President, being on the debate team, and giving Assembly talks, that I was invited to join the Sociology Faculty in the coming fall. I readily accepted. By arrangement, my first two years on the faculty had me teaching only half time in order to permit me to meet requirements for BYU's Master of Science degree. This was awarded in the spring of 1937. Then one year later, I was granted an extended leave-of-absence to enable me to accept a Fellowship and pursue graduate studies at the University of Wisconsin. It was not until the fall of 1940 that I returned to my duties at Brigham Young University. But since my dissertation was only part way along by then, I found it necessary to undertake part-time teaching duty for a year, pushing to complete my graduate work. Once the writing was out of the way, I returned to the Wisconsin campus for the final defense of the dissertation. In August of 1941, I was awarded the Doctor of Philosophy degree.

MY YEARS AT BRIGHAM YOUNG

It was during my tenure at Brigham Young University, two years as an undergraduate and twelve on the faculty, that my career as a sociologist, most especially as a *Family Sociologist,* took shape. But before getting into that, I will discuss my years as a neophyte-professor and thus help set the stage for describing the accomplishments of my career.

At Brigham Young University, I was recognized and functioned as Sociology Department Head from the time of my return from Wisconsin in 1940. But there had been no formal listing of this role until the 1944-45 catalogue appeared. As administrator, I was able, over the years, with others, to both enlarge and strengthen the department in most of its aspects: the faculty, curriculum, class enrollments, and our core of majors and minors. A very important part of this strengthening was the permanent establishment of a Master's Degree program. Just a few years prior to this, I had been the recipient of the first Master of Sociology degree.

As a teacher, I was required, as were all Brigham Young University instructors, to handle a section of offerings sponsored by the Division of Religion. My particular assignment, which was a fortunate one I thought, for it fit my interests and strengthened my emerging specialty in family studies, was a section of a course titled "Courtship and Marriage." Within the Sociology Department, I handled my full share of the large introductory classes, plus several advanced and/or new courses which I felt sufficiently qualified to teach. Representative titles were "Sociology of the Family," "Population Problems," "Cultural Anthropology," "Social Statistics," and "Research Methodology."

In addition to carrying out my administrative and teaching responsibilities, I felt driven to give serious time and effort to research. So, I worked long hours, sometimes returning to my office on an evening or on weekends. I tried out little survey projects using students as subjects. And I would share the results with my classes as well as other relevant research, including aspects of my own completed Master's thesis and Doctoral dissertation, all of which enriched the instructional process. Thus, I saw myself developing as a research-oriented professor.

My ambition to develop myself professionally and to get ahead in my field led me to publish. By the time I left Brigham Young University in 1947, I had in print, mostly in standard sociological journals, nine articles (Christensen, 1938a, 1938b, 1939, 1942, 1946a, 1947; Christensen & Green, 1942; Christensen & Hill, 1942, 1943) with three additional ones scheduled to appear in 1948 (Christensen, 1948a, 1948b 1948c). Of these twelve, three were based upon aspects of my Master's thesis, which had pioneered the record-linkage approach for measuring patterns of child-spacing; two were based upon aspects of my Doctoral dissertation, titled "Population Pressure Among Wisconsin Farmers"; five based upon responses in the student surveys that I had conducted; and the remaining two upon social-psychological and sociological aspects of World War II.

The War

From the early-to-middle 1940s, all of America was being profoundly affected by Pearl Harbor, and the events that followed. Brigham Young University and the Provo community were no exceptions. I was a part of the in-between-wars generation, too young to be drafted in World War I and too old for World War II. What is more, being married and having children only added to my deferment potential. While feeling greatly relieved overall, I, at the same time, occasionally had to fight against an annoying sense of guilt. So I tried to do what I could to help out. For example, during two of the summers and the academic year in between, I moonlighted as a carpenter in the construction of the Geneva Steel Plant, near Provo, which was being rushed to completion as part of the war effort.

At the University, I planned and taught a new course titled "War and Society." I also organized and participated in a publicly held faculty panel discussion called "War, Philosophy, and Atrocity." In addition, I found myself growing in demand as a public speaker within the larger community, the usual request being that I treat some aspect of the war theme. Here are a few examples of that activity: "Social Aspects of American Defense," given as a Founder's Day address at Ricks College; "Youth, War, and the Future," given at a meeting of the Provo Women's Literary League; and "The Social Impact of War on Utah," delivered at Weber College in Ogden at the concluding symposium session of the Utah Academy of Arts and Sciences.

In September of 1943, Mayor Harding appointed a nine-member Provo Civic Welfare Committee, with me as its chairman, to "study the problems, determine facts, and make recommendations for improvements to the City Commission." We met biweekly, or more frequently as needed. The Committee readily achieved the respect of the community and of city officials and was given good press.

About one year prior to that appointment, I had the privilege, together with four other faculty members, of making an on-sight study-visit to one of the wartime relocation camps set up for Japanese Americans. This one was called Topaz and was located just a short distance from Delta, Utah. We saw the guard towers, the barbed-wire fences, and the row upon row of plain and crowded barrack-life buildings sitting on dry dusty ground, with very little vegetation in evidence. What we saw depressed us. But along with the dark side, we also observed occasional American flags hanging above some of the apartment front doors and attempts at starting small gardens in the dry soil. We observed neatness in housekeeping despite the plainness and the crowding. Even more important, perhaps, we saw smiles and detected in the manners of many what appeared to be a resolve to make the best of their forced detainment.

The work of our Provo Civic Welfare Committee had barely started when a most unfortunate racial incident took place right within our own community. At the request of Utah County, a group of Japanese internees had been temporarily moved from Topaz to a makeshift farm labor camp near Provo to help with the harvesting of crops. One Saturday night a small group of Provo youth terrorized the camp by firing several shots into the tents. Fortunately, no one was hit. The federal government responded quickly by requesting Mayor Harding to call a public meeting for determining if the Japanese could be protected or should be removed. I attended that meeting. And I was the one who put the resolution that asked for the apprehension and punishment of the terrorists, for the protection of the community's guest laborers, and for the discouragement of all forms of racial antagonism and discrimination. The resolution passed easily.

The Mayor responded the very next day, declaring that armed guards would be placed at the camp and assuring its inhabitants that they would have full protection from the city. Soon afterward, the local newspaper carried a story reporting on a special meeting of our Provo Civic Welfare Committee in which discrimination against any minority was declared to be "un-American, unscientific, and unnecessary."

My Interest in Family Studies

My penchant for family studies started early and expanded dramatically throughout my stay at Brigham Young University. I remember an occasion during the early 1940s when I brought a radio to one of my family classes and adjusted it so students could listen to a special national broadcast featuring Evelyn Millis Duvall. Duvall, with Reuben Hill, was the author of *When You Marry,* one of the first college textbooks on the subject (Duvall & Hill, 1967). She was giving a series of public radio talks, which was attracting wide attention. Predictably, this radio airing before my class captured strong student attention and the discussion was lively.

Evelyn Millis Duvall was also the Administrative Secretary and the real power behind a newly formed (1938) National Council on Family Relations, which was experiencing rapid growth and was pushing for the formation of State Councils to function as affiliates.

Within Utah, interest in this new movement crystallized in the mid 1940s, largely brought about through a series of meetings initiated by sociologist Joseph A. Geddes of Utah State Agricultural College. These small gatherings involved a dozen or so educational, civic, and religious leaders who mainly represented organizations interested in finding ways to strengthen family life within the state. It was during the fall of 1946 that a Utah Council on Family Relations was formally organized, linked to the National Council. I was elected the group's first President.

As part of the Church's 1947 Centennial Celebration of the arrival of Mormon pioneers into the Salt Lake valley, I organized a special series of family related events to take place on the Brigham Young University campus. An attractive brochure was prepared and given wide advance distribution. It listed the following: eight different college courses covering a wide range of family phenomena to be offered during the first and second sessions of Summer School; five separate evening forum presentations spread out over five weeks. Each panel was to be composed of a chairman, two faculty members, and two students; a week-long Family Life Institute involving, principally, five lectures by a visiting specialist from Dr. Paul Popenoe's popular Los Angeles-based American Institute of Family Relations; and the initial annual meeting of our newly organized Utah Council on Family Relations. This latter was to include a general session, a business luncheon, and a public symposium titled "What is Wrong with Modern Marriage?" For the most part, each event went off smoothly and interest proved to be high.

I was privileged to serve as moderator for the above-mentioned public symposium. This, held in the new, large Joseph Fielding Smith Auditorium, attracted an overflow audience. The four panel members were: Mrs. C. Brooks Fry, the visiting specialist who was conducting our Family Life Institute; Doctor Lawrence Bee, who was Director of Marriage Counseling at Utah State Agricultural College; Doctor Virginia Cutler, who was Head of Home Economics at the University of Utah; and Doctor John A. Widtsoe, who was a highly vocal and respected General Church Authority, a member of the Quorum of Twelve Apostles. Our approach was basically positive, yet, at times, politely critical. For, among the topics covered, we included open and frank discussions of such controversial concerns as birth control and family size, sensitive topics in Mormon culture.

Despite being regarded as somewhat controversial, perhaps even dangerous, by some of the more conservative Mormons, I was viewed by a significantly large number of others as being just interesting, challenging, and, at the same time, constructive. And because of this apparent "vote of confidence," there was, for me, an abundance of growth-promoting and image-building opportunities. One category involved public speaking, both on and off campus. Another involved publishing. Earlier mention was made of my breaking into some of the professional journals. That, for the most part, resulted from my own initiative. I also turned to publishing opportunities afforded by standard Church outlets, which came about mostly by way of invitation.

Three articles were published in *The Improvement Era*, now titled *The Ensign*, undoubtedly the most central of Latter Day Saints magazines. Four additional ones appeared in *The Relief Society Magazine*, which served the women's auxiliary of the Church. While several of these seven articles gave focus to family matters, it was my three additional series of invited *lesson materials* that really helped me to blossom as a family scholar. Perhaps least significant of the series was a three-lesson mimeographed packet used for a while by some of the adult Special Interest Groups of the "Mutual Improvement Association, the Church" auxiliary for youths and young adults. It was titled "Home Cooperation Between Parents and Children."

My second experience with authoring lesson materials for the Church came in preparing social service lessons for the Relief Society. Eventually, there were twenty-one covering a three-year period. They were published in *The Relief Society Magazine*. The first year's set of seven, called "Foundations of Successful Marriage," was so well received that I was invited to continue with another fourteen to cover the next two years. This second set dealt with aspects of social ethics. Despite the hard work involved, I found the job both challenging and particularly satisfying. Some illustrative lesson titles are: "Freedom and Responsibility"; "Honesty, the Core of Character"; and "Brotherhood, the Key to Greatness."

While most of my writing for the Relief Society went through the committee review process with little editing and few requests for changes, I do well remember one controversy, which eventually and fortunately reached a "happy ending." Belle S. Spafford, then-chairman of the Social Service Committee and later President of the entire organization, had written me that in one of my lessons ". . . the paragraph

'Sterile Orthodoxy' came in for some very lively discussion and difference of opinion." I had used the phrase "sterile orthodoxy" to emphasize the thought that too much emphasis upon mechanical conformity alone can leave one on the mere "fringe of righteousness." Here is part of what I said:

> . . . mechanical conformity alone . . . stifles the divine spark in man, the creative urge, and makes of him a mere robot or puppet that can be pushed around. Sometimes people lose the real spirit and substance of religion by overstressing mechanical adherence to its forms alone. (The letter killeth, but the spirit giveth life. II Corinthians 3:6.)

After further Committee discussion and receiving the backing of Belle S. Spafford, the paragraph remained.

My most extensive and most rewarding lesson-writing project for the Church was a section of the General Sunday School manual published in 1946 titled *The Latter-day Saint Family.* I wrote the first thirty-six lessons, subtitled "The Church and Modern Marriage," and Archibald F. Bennett wrote the last twelve dealing with genealogy. In my section, the central approach was sociological and, to some extent, research-based within the general framework of Church values. Here is a listing of some of my chapter titles: "The Family in Trouble"; "Cultivating the Graces of Courtship"; "The Start and the Art of Marriage"; "When Children Come"; "Adjustment Problems of the Modern Woman"; "Making Marriage Succeed"; and "New Horizons for the Family."

Several thousand copies of my own one-hundred-forty-three page portion of this manual were reprinted separately and, for a number of years, used as the textbook for existing sections of the Brigham Young University religion class in courtship and marriage. The cover, of course, carried my name as author and *The Church and Modern Marriage* as its title (Christensen, 1946b). This was my first published book. [A later text (1950) had subsequent editions in 1958 and 1971.]

PURDUE UNIVERSITY

In the late summer of 1947 I moved my family to West Lafayette, Indiana, subsequent to accepting a position at Purdue University, which appeared to offer me new challenges and greater opportunities for professional development. It was with mixed feelings that we left the familiar surroundings of Mormon culture. The years that followed gave ample proof that this decision, difficult at the time, was a good one. Never have I had regrets concerning this move.

I remained at Purdue for twenty-eight years before retiring and being named Professor Emeritus. Then, one year after that, and with all of our children launched, Alice and I moved westward again, this time to La Jolla, California, where we now reside.

My appointment at Purdue carried a dual title: Head of the Sociology Section of the Division of Education and Applied Psychology, and Professor in the Department of Child Development and Family Life, which was a part of the School of Home Economics. The expectations of my appointment were that I would: first, build up the sociology discipline to a respectable academic level; and second, coordinate and strengthen the then rival family-life courses being offered by both the sociology and child development units. This last-named goal was achieved rather satisfactorily, to the point of attracting wide attention from other campuses experiencing similar problems of interdepartmental rivalry over the then emerging field of marriage and family life education. We accomplished coordination and harmony by carefully planning together and by cross listing selected catalogue offerings. This meant that class instruction for these courses was supplied by *both* departmental units, with students coming from both sides of the isle, so to speak. Class registration and academic credit, however, went according to the respective unit from which each student came.

I continued in this dual role until about the mid 1950s, at which time I dropped my official connection with Home Economics, while at the same time remaining cooperative and collaborative, for the simple reason that our sociology program was developing so rapidly that it required my full attention.

As to my role in the building of a sociology program at Purdue, here is a brief overview. At the time of my arrival in 1947 there was no sociology department as such, and there were very few sociology courses. Furthermore, the courses that did exist had been set up mainly as service offerings to other departments. Also, graduate work within the field was nonexistent. But by the time I relinquished administrative duties some fifteen years later to enable me to function as a full time teaching and research scholar, sociology had been given departmental status, the faculty had been strengthened and enlarged, the curriculum reworked and greatly expanded, and graduate programs leading to the MS and the PhD had been formally established. By that time, the Department could claim approximately thirty full-time faculty members who served some fifty to sixty graduate students, plus significant numbers of undergraduate majors and minors. Our program had become known and recognized far and wide; sociology at Purdue had attained both a national and international reputation.

An important complement to this department was my own work within the family field. I had maintained a strong interest in family matters almost since childhood and had gained visibility as a family scholar during my years at Brigham Young University. Furthermore, my initial Purdue assignment was in part to help develop family studies at that campus. Thus, maintaining a professional interest in family matters came to me quite naturally. It was at Purdue that my lifelong career took off and my reputation as a sociologist, particularly family sociologist, blossomed.

Any listing of my lifelong professional activities relating to the family field would include the following:

1. Teaching regular university classes on the subject, adding new courses as appropriate, and adjusting the content of existing ones in order to stay at the forefront of ever-expanding knowledge.
2. Working with both undergraduate and graduate students, but especially the latter when their academic focus became family studies. In the role of Major Professor, I mentored over a dozen Master and/or Doctoral candidates to the completion of their degrees.
3. Bringing to the Purdue campus for public lectures or for temporary teaching assignments, a number of eminent scholars whose work was related to the family field including Ernest W. Burgess, William F. Ogburn, Kingsley Davis, John Money, Alfred C. Kinsey, and Margaret Mead.
4. Responding to numerous lecture and/or committee or workshop invitations. They covered a wide range of audiences–PTA groups and schoolteachers or administrators on the local level, and on the national, such as discussing aspects of my premarital sex research at an annual session of the American Medical Association held in Florida.
5. Pursuing my own research and publication interests, which frequently meant extra hours of work during some of the evenings, early mornings, or weekends. Lifetime publications of mine include six books, nineteen chapters within other books, sixty-seven articles in professional journals, fifteen articles in popular or semi-professional sources, four pamphlets or bulletins, and thirty-

two book reviews. The majority of these–but not all–were focused upon family studies.

6. Participating in meetings of relevant professional organizations, such as those of the American Sociological Association, were seldom missed. I participated in other national and international programs as well. In a few of these associations, I held office and read papers at the meetings. I was President of the National Council on Family Relations during 1960-61 and was just prior to that elected to the office of Editor for a three-year term, of its primary journal, *Marriage and Family Living*. It was mostly through my efforts that two meetings of NCFR and Groves were brought to the Purdue campus: the Groves Conference in 1954 and an annual NCFR conference in 1957. Also, I frequently attended meetings of the prestigious groups conference on marriage and the family and, at times, presented papers.

Furthermore, I attended and participated in: (1) Meetings of the International Union of Family Organizations held in Paris, France, 1958; in Rio de Janeiro, Brazil, 1963; and in Liege, Belgium, 1973; (2) Meetings of the International Sociological Association held in Stresa, Italy, 1959; Washington, D.C., 1962; Evian, France, 1966; Varna, Bulgaria, 1970; Toronto, Canada, 1974; and Uppsala, Sweden, 1978; (3) Meetings of the International Seminar on Family Research, some of which took place in conjunction with the ISA gatherings, but also two held separately–in Wageninen, Holland, 1957 and Moscow, USSR, 1971; and (4) a meeting of the Third International Seminar on Gender Identity held in Dubrovnik, Yugoslavia, 1973. At these gatherings I presented papers.

Purdue granted me three official sabbatical leaves of absence: first, for 1957-58 to accept a Fulbright Research Fellowship at the University of Copenhagen to study Scandinavian family culture; second, for the first semester of 1964-65 to visit various countries around the world, primarily for the purpose of examining different government programs touching upon family welfare. Also during this leave, I served as Visiting Professor for a semester at the University of Hawaii; and third, for the second semester of 1971-72 to accept a Visiting Scholar appointment at the University of California, Irvine, California, pursuing my own research and writing interests.

Finally, I had the privilege of accepting some six separate summertime Visiting Professorships, which gave me experience on other campuses: the Pennsylvania State University in 1949; the University of Utah in 1951; the University of California, Berkeley, in 1956; Brigham

Young University in 1961, and again in 1967; and Northern Michigan University in 1971. In addition, I served as Visiting Professor at San Diego State University, California, during the first semester of 1976-77, which followed my retirement. Each of these off-campus appointments–except the first-named where my assignment was to teach Rural Sociology–found me teaching classes on family life education and/or family sociology.

Although the above listing is long, much too long for any detailing here, it does perhaps give insight into some of the major thrusts and accomplishments of my professional career. Yet even this listing is full of gaps; it entirely misses certain other items that could have been, perhaps should have been, included for the picture to be complete. Because of space limitations, however, they must be ignored. So my plan is to conclude the discussion by pointing up just two areas of accomplishment, areas that seem of primary importance and for which I would most like to be remembered: (1) my cross-cultural research and (2) my editing of the *Handbook of Marriage and the Family* (Christensen, 1964).

Cross-Cultural Research

Broadly speaking, the term research refers to systematic inquiry into the nature of any phenomenon. It is through a particular kind of research, however–*scientific* research–that modern man has achieved his greatest feats. Science requires that investigation be based upon empirical and measurable data, that it be as objective or value-free as possible, and that its findings be subject to verification. Social Science, perhaps mainly because of the so-called "soft" nature of its data, has advanced more slowly than have the physical and biological sciences. But it *has* advanced. And I am among those who believe that it will continue to do so insofar as it follows the rigors of the scientific method.

I view myself as a social scientist, more narrowly as a sociologist, and *most* narrowly as a family sociologist. My chief focus as a family scholar has been along lines of cross-cultural research. This focusing began soon after my arrival at Purdue, at which time I became interested in comparing certain of my earlier Utah findings with comparable family data that could be gathered in Indiana. Olive Bowden, a Master's candidate at Purdue, worked with me and we completed the project (Christensen & Bowden, 1953). Then, approximately one decade later, I was granted a Fulbright Research Fellowship to study comparable aspects of the Danish family system. So I spent the 1957-58 academic year attached to the University of Copenhagen, gathering data and laying groundwork for making on-going comparisons across three vastly different cultures: sexually restrictive Mormon culture within America's intermountain west; sexually moderate midwestern culture within America's heartland; and sexually permissive Danish culture which is more or less typical of all of Scandinavia.

This spread across cultures has enabled me to test important hypotheses and to make theoretical statements that have proven helpful in the building of family theory. Since first launching the cross-cultural project, I tended to research premarital sex over the life course of my career. Half of my subsequently published articles have drawn upon this earlier work. The substantive focus of this research, as already indicated, was premarital sex. Not sex in any popular or sensational sense, but only in a statistical or comparative or, one might say, sociological sense. In other words, sex without titillation. I was interested in determining both the attitudes and the behaviors that surround premarital sex; and, what is even more important, in relating those findings to the differing cultural norms, and further relating any discrepancies between actual behavior and their beliefs, which are related to possible effects or consequences that these discrepancies seem to provide.

Two methods were employed: (1) record linkage and (2) use of the questionnaire. Interviews were conducted to establish reliability and to reach deeper into meanings and interpretations. I gathered the Danish record-linkage data and then did comparisons between them and comparable data. George R. Carpenter, a PhD candidate at Purdue, administered and collected questionnaires for the two American samples. By using *two* methods instead of just one, each complementing and supplementing the other, I was able to double-check and thus reinforce my findings and generalizations (Christensen, 1958a, 1958b, 1959, 1960, 1961a, 1961b, 1962, 1963a, 1966, 1973; Christensen & Carpenter, 1962a, 1962b; Christensen & Gregg, 1970).

It was at Brigham Young University during the late 1930s, while working on my Master's thesis, that I first explored record-linkage as a method for research. I began by extracting names, dates, and other data from official marriage and birth records for Utah County, Utah. Then I matched and cross-referenced the separate record sets to produce new information (Christensen,1938b, 1939, 1948b). For example, I was able to measure patterns of spacing of first child from time of marriage and to relate these patterns to factors such as age at marriage and civil versus religious ceremony (Christensen, 1953a, 1953b, 1968; Christensen & Bowden, 1953; Christensen, Andrews, & Freiser, 1953; Christensen, Leslie, & Pearman, 1955). Subsequently, I added divorce records to the matching process, using divorce as an index of marriage failure (Christensen, 1963b; Christensen & Meissner, 1953, 1956; Christensen & Rubenstein, 1956).

The record-linkage approach was applied to each of the three samples studied. The method has the advantage of avoiding the refusal to respond and possible falsification of response, a problem in research using questionnaires.

I have been credited with doing pioneer work in record-linkage, an approach which, especially since the ushering in of the computer age, has been expanding in both usage and in type and number of records utilized, especially by government agencies.

In our cross-cultural research, the questionnaire approach supplemented and complemented record-linkage by obtaining attitudes and behavior not accessible in marriage, birth, and divorce records. Administration of these instruments took place within selected, but essentially comparable, classes found within three universities, one each from the cultures studied. Extreme care was taken at every stage: formulating questions that appeared meaningful; wording them to avoid ambiguity; revising as needed, after pretesting on both sides of the Atlantic; explaining to prospective respondents the scientific nature of the study as well as the intended anonymity of response; and then asking for cooperation to insure success–while at the same time making it clear that anyone was privileged to quietly leave the room should he or she not care to respond. Overall response turned out to be almost one-hundred percent. Detailed explanations of methodological issues and procedures are to be found in several of the published articles.

Samples were selected from three widely differing areas: Utah, Indiana, and Denmark. The research was carried out during 1958. The questionnaire portion of the 1958 study was repeated in 1968 and again in 1978. This has enabled both longitudinal and cross-cultural analyses. Several published articles have reported on both aspects. For the replications, the questionnaire remained unchanged; with reliance upon others for administering it. There were numerous "findings" from the cross-cultural research. One is most salient to the development of family theory. Briefly, while virtually all of both my attitudinal and behavioral measures pictured the Utah culture to be most conservative and the Danish culture most permissive, with Indiana in a middle position, it was in the highly restrictive Utah/Mormon culture where the negative *effects and consequences* of premarital sex were the greatest. This took the form of feelings of guilt accompanying premarital coitus (questionnaire date) and subsequent divorce following premarital pregnancy (record-linkage date) (Christensen, 1958a, 1958b, 1959, 1960, 1961a, 1962, 1963, 1966; Christensen & Carpenter, 1962a; 1962b; Christensen & Gregg, 1970).

It appears that while a culture's restrictive sex norms can reduce a disapproved behavior, it is done at a price. It is when one's values are violated that negative consequences tend to be most pronounced. I have called this proposition *"The Principle of Value."*

Of the special professional recognitions that have come to me during my career, the one most pleasurable was receiving the prestigious Burgess Research Award. This honor was given to me by the National Council on Family Relations at its 1967 meeting. It included a certificate which read, "Presented to Harold T. Christensen, in recognition of continuous and meritorious contributions to theory and research in the family field." The award carried with it an expectation that I would prepare and deliver a paper at NCFR's next annual meeting. That paper, titled "Normative Theory Derived from Cross-Cultural Family Research," was later published in the *Journal of Marriage and the Family* (Christensen, 1969).

Editing the Handbook

The recognition just described came about, in part at least, because of my ongoing, systematic, comparative research. But another important consideration grew out of my role in the production of the *Handbook of Marriage and the Family* (Christensen, 1964). It was sometime during the early 1960s that Edgar F. Borgotta, sociologist and Editor of Rand McNally's Sociology Series, approached me and asked that I take on the editing of a projected handbook covering the marriage and family field. At first I was reluctant, because of pressures I then was under and because I could see that the job, as he defined it, would require considerable time and dedication. So I suggested other names. But he persisted. Eventually, I consented, realizing the importance of such a project and feeling a little flattered to have been invited.

The undertaking required a great deal of time and dedication, although eventually it came to an end. The new and first ever *Handbook on Marriage and the Family* came off the press during the late summer of 1964. It involved twenty-five authors and added up to twenty-four separate chapters for a total of 1,028 pages. The chapters were organized into five major divisions or sections: I–Theoretical Orientations; II–Methodological Developments; III–The Family in Its Social Setting; IV–Member Roles and Internal Processes; and V–Applied and Normative Interests. Each chapter was followed by an exhaustive bibliography covering the subject it treated. I authored the first chapter, titled "Development of the Family Field of Study," and also the last, titled "The Intrusion of Values."

In the Preface I attempted to explain what the book is all about–why the need and how it is approached:

> This book was not intended to have popular appeal: it is not a how-to-do-it manual for the layman explaining the way to success in ten easy lessons, or anything like that. Rather, it was a serious, systematic analysis of the subject under treatment, aimed at the professional worker in the field. Although family phenomena have been exposed to serious study for approximately a century, it is only in recent years that the rigors of the scientific method have come to be applied to them, and it is only now that scholars are starting to concern themselves with the integration of disjointed materials and with systematic theory building. We have wanted to know where we have been, where we are, where we are going, and how to get there–as a profession. Honest self-examination, such as this, is a prerequisite to any coming of age of the field.

The editing process included these steps: (1) preparing a prospectus which spelled out the purpose, gave a tentative outline, and stated the proposed approach; (2) circulating this to a few leaders in the field for their reactions and suggestions, and revising it accordingly; (3) selecting top scholars in the field as prospective authors and sending them the prospectus, along with inviting participation and requesting that their proposed outlines be sent back to me; (4) reconciling the submitted outlines with one another, then revising my overall outline and returning it to the authors so that each could see how his own writing would fit in with what others would be doing; (5) receiving and carefully editing the manuscripts; and (6) following up in the few cases where a person might decide to pull out, or where there were excessive delays in meeting deadlines, or where there was need for extensive changes and/or a rewrite. All in all, I came to realize that the process was demanding an inordinate amount of correspondence from me, involving some of the authors more than others, of course, not only to follow through on corrections but also to iron out gaps and overlaps and to insure minimum uniformity as well as systematic coverage.

More than anything else, perhaps, it was the *Handbook* that did the most to build my reputation as a student of the family institution. This was a pioneer undertaking in theory building, and it became widely used, especially by university graduate students starting to specialize within the field and more seasoned scholars as well. There even were a few copies known to have turned up in faraway places throughout the world. I was told by a few users that they regarded it as the "Bible" of family studies.

At the time of my Purdue retirement in 1975, a prominent fellow family scholar wrote to me as follows:

> Although I cannot be present at the banquet I want you to know that in my opinion you are one of two or three giants who were responsible for bringing family sociology to its maturity. More than any other influence the *Handbook* established the field as a viable, cohesive scholarly domain. Every subsequent effort must date from this foundation and I feel confident that future historians of the field will cite its publication as marking the ending of one era and the beginning of another. Your work, more than anyone else's introduced social theory into the chaotic field of sex research which, prior to your contributions was virtually limited to descriptive studies. In this area you have set a standard, which every subsequent scholar must find difficult to achieve.

SUMMING UP

Well, okay. The statement does impress me as a bit much, but, okay. It now is April, 1993, as I end this somewhat brief account of my life's work. At eighty-four years of age, I find myself still living with Alice, my original partner, who, with her intellect, cooperative spirit, energy, and cheerfulness, continues to lift my spirits and to feed me in ways that reach beyond the realm of physical needs alone. So I guess one could say, and rightly so, that we still are in love, after all of these years. I should point out too that, as a bonus, Alice and I now revel in the blessings of five married children, three daughters-in-law, two sons-in-law, and eighteen grandchildren.

As I see it, my professional and personal family interests have, for the most part, been mutually reinforcing. I believe that I have been a more effective marriage and family teacher, researcher, and–to some extent–theory builder than could otherwise have been possible without the practical experience of being a husband, father, and even grandfather to draw upon and with which to test myself against. And conversely, I believe that I have been a better family man than I otherwise would have been had I functioned without the insights of my profession. All in all, I consider myself fortunate indeed. I have enjoyed a lifetime of satisfactions, both personal and professional. There have been mistakes along the way, to be sure, and an occasional disappointment. But I have enjoyed my share of successes too. Life has been good to me.

EDITORS' NOTE

We are indebted to Carolyn C. Perruci, Professor and Head, Department of Sociology and Anthropology, Purdue University for providing us with Harold Christensen's curriculum vita, newspaper clippings and the Department's Spring, 2000 newsletter. The latter noted that Harold and Alice celebrated their 65th anniversary June, 1999 and Harold celebrated his 91st birthday in March, 2000.

REFERENCES

Christensen, H. T. (1938a). Heterogeneity in age and residence of married couples. *Mental Health, 5*, 4, 1-2.

Christensen, H. T. (1938b). Rural-urban differences in the time-interval between the marriage of parents and the birth of their first child, Utah County, Utah. *Rural Sociology, 3*, 2, 172-176.

Christensen, H. T. (1939). The time-interval between marriage of parents and the birth of their first child in Utah County, Utah. *American Journal of Sociology*, 44, 518-525.

Christensen, H. T. (1942). The family and mental health in wartime. *Mental Health, 10*, 1, 13-16.

Christensen, H. T. (1946a). Factors in the size and sex composition of families; A survey of student opinion. *Proceedings-Utah Academy of Sciences*, 23, 107-113.

Christensen, H. T. (1946b). *The church and modern marriages*. Provo, UT: Brigham Young University.

Christensen, H. T. (1947). Student view on mate selection. *Marriage and Family Living*, 9, 4, 5-88.

Christensen, H. T. (1948a). Mormon fertility: A survey of student opinion. *American Journal of Sociology, 53*, 4, 270-75.

Christensen, H. T. (1948b). An experiment in honesty. *Social Forces, 26*, 3, 298-302.

Christensen, H. T. (1948c). Courtship conduct as viewed by youth. *Journal of Home Economics, 40*, 4, 187-188.

Christensen, H. T. (1950). *Marriage analysis: Foundations for successful family life*. New York: Ronald Press Co. (2nd edition, 1958; 3rd edition with Kathryn P. Johnson, renamed *Marriage and the Family*, 1971)

Christensen, H. T. (1953a). Rural-urban differences in the spacing of the first birth from marriage: A repeat study. *Rural Sociology, 18*, 1, 60.

Christensen, H. T. (1953b). Studies in child spacing: I-Premarital pregnancy as measured by the spacing of the first birth from marriage. *American Sociological Review, 18*, 1, 53-59.

Christensen, H. T. (1958a). The method of record linkage applied to family data. *Marriage and Family Living, 20*, 1, 38-43.

Christensen, H. T. (1958b). Report of University of Copenhagen students survey on sex. *Stud. Med., 16*, 6, 12-13. (Danish Medical Journal).

Christensen, H. T. (1959). Selected aspects of child spacing in Denmark. *Acta Sociologica, 4*, 2, 35-45.

Christensen, H. T. (1960). Cultural relativism and premarital sex norms. *American Sociological Review, 25*, 1, 31-39.

Christensen, H. T. (1961a). Consequences of premarital sexual freedom: A cross-cultural view. *Review of Research and Reflection, 1*, 3, 35-37.

Christensen, H. T. (1961b). Pregnant bride's record linkage studies. In E. M. Duvall & S. M. Duvall (Eds.), *Sex Ways in Fact and Faith* (pp. 129-139). New York: Association Press.

Christensen, H. T. (1962). A cross-cultural comparison of attitudes towards marital infidelity. *International Journal of Comparative Sociology, 3*, 1, 124-137.

Christensen, H. T. (1963a). Child spacing analysis via record linkage: New data plus summing up from earlier reports. *Marriage and Family Living*, 25, 3, 272-280.

Christensen, H. T. (1963b). Timing of first pregnancy as a factor in divorce: A cross-cultural analysis. *Eugenics Quarterly, 10*, 3, 119-130.

Christensen, H. T. (Ed.) (1964). *Handbook of Marriage and the Family* (pp. 969-1006). Chicago: Rand McNally & Co.

Christensen, H. T. (1966). Scandinavian and American sex norms: Some comparisons, with sociological implications. *Journal of Social Issues, 22*, 2, 60-75.

Christensen, H. T. (1968). Children in the family: Relationship of number and spacing to marital success. *Journal of Marriage and the Family*, 30, 2, 283-289.

Christensen, H. T. (1969). Normative theory derived from cross-cultural family research. *Journal of Marriage and the Family, 31*, 2, 209-222.

Christensen, H. T. (1973). Attitudes Toward Marital Infidelity: A Nine-Culture Sampling of University Student Opinion. *Journal of Comparative Family Studies, 4*, 2, 197-214.

Christensen, H. T., Andrews. R., & Freiser, S. (1953). Falsification at age of marriage. *Marriage and Family Living, 15*, 4, 301-304.

Christensen, H. T. & Boden, O. P. (1953). Studies in child spacing: II. The time-interval between marriage of parents and birth of their first child, Tippecanoe County, Indiana. *Social Forces, 31*, 4, 346-351.

Christensen, H. T. & Carpenter, G. R. (1962a). Timing patterns in premarital sexual intimacy: A attitudinal report on three modern western societies. *Marriage and Family Living, 24*, 1, 30-35.

Christensen, H. T. & Carpenter, G. B. (1962b). Value-behavior discrepancies regarding premarital coitus in three western cultures. *American Sociological Review*, 27, 1, 66-74.

Christensen, H. T. & Green, D. L. (1942). The commercialization of patriotism in World War II. *Sociology and Social Research, 27*, 6, 447-452.

Christensen, H. T. & Gregg, C. F. (1970). Changing sex norms in America and Scandinavia. *Journal of Marriage and the Family, 32*, 4, 616-627.

Christensen, H. T. & Hill, G. W. (1942a). Some cultural factors related to occupational mobility among Wisconsin farmers. *Rural Sociology, 7*, 2, 193-201.

Christensen, H. T. & Hill, G. W. (1942b). Some factors in family fertility among selected Wisconsin farmers. *American Sociological Review*, *7*, 4, 498-504.
Christensen, H. T., Leslie, G. R., & Pearman, G. L. (1955). Studies in child spacing: IV–The time interval separating all children in completed family of Purdue university graduates. *Social Forces*, *34*, 1, 77-82.
Christensen, H. T. & Meissner, H. H. (1953a). Studies in child spacing: III–Premarital pregnancy as a factor in divorce. *American Sociological Review*, *18*, 6, 641-644.
Christensen, H. T. & Meissner, H. H. (1956). An analysis of divorce in Tippecanoe Country, Indiana. *Sociology and Social Research*, *40*, 247-252.
Christensen, H. T. & Rubenstein, B. B. (1956). Premarital Pregnancy and Divorce: A Follow-up Study by the Interview Method. *Marriage and Family Living*, *18*, 2, 114-123.
Duvall, E. M. & Hill, R. (1967). *When You Marry*. Boston: Heath.

Families, Social Change, and Individual Lives

Glen H. Elder, Jr.

KEYWORDS. Autobiography, adolescent development, employment, longitudinal research, socialization

INTRODUCTION

The 20th century is marked by one large-scale event after another and their human consequences. As a child of World War II, these consequences have long intrigued me. They also directed my attention to the family. Whether expressed in terms of long-run trends or an economic depression and world war, social change has profound implications for people through its impact on family relationships, structures, and interactions. In this research problem, family life becomes a bridge between the macro-changes of society and the experiences and life chances of individuals. A second type of research problem has focused my attention on the family as a matrix of relationships, a matrix in which members' lives are embedded and regulated across the life span and generations. Individual lives are linked to other lives through family and intergenerational ties.

Across the 1960s and early 1970s, I viewed these questions from a perspective on socialization. But like much of social psychology, this theoretical framework captures influences at a point in time. It does not address the changes that take place in society, in community and family, and in the lives of individuals. From this point to the mid-1970s, I gradually shifted my theoretical perspective toward the life course.[1] This conceptual transition coincided with the theoretical and empirical tasks of following children from the early 1930s to mid-life. Publication of *Children of the Great Depression* (Elder, 1974, 1999) marked the beginning of this new stage of work, as later expressed in *Life Course Dy-*

namics (Elder, 1985a), *Children in Time and Place* (Elder, Modell, & Parke, 1993), and *Children of the Land* (Elder & Conger, 2000).

Time, process, and context are analytic themes that join the two problem foci (on linking social change and individuals, and on linked lives over time) in a framework that has become known as life course theory (Elder, 1992, 1998a). Life course ideas and theory emerged during the 1960s and 70s as longitudinal studies addressed three challenging questions. As they followed children out of childhood and into the adult years (the 1960s), they had to come up with ways of thinking about the evolution of lives over the life span and generations. How are individual lives socially organized, and how do they change? The study of people over time raised the question of how changes in society made a difference in one's life trajectory. The realities of changing lives in changing times called for a way of connecting the two sets of changes. A third task centered on the formulation of developmental or aging concepts and mechanisms that apply across the life span. These include concepts of cumulative advantage and disadvantage, turning points, life trajectory, and transition.

I have organized this short autobiographical essay around four themes, beginning with "Early Influences" and my initial preoccupation with socialization. This is followed by "Observing Families and Lives Over Time," a life stage devoted to the development of *Children of the Great Depression* and the project's influence on my thinking about family and the life course. This work became a platform from which to launch new studies of family and life course in changing times. I underscore distinctive features of this professional stage under the theme "Studying Social Change in the Life Course" and close with "Reflections."

EARLY INFLUENCES

My undergraduate years at Penn State University (1952-57) involved an intellectual journey from the biological sciences and agriculture through philosophy to the social sciences. Though born and reared in Cleveland, Ohio, I ended up on a dairy farm in northeastern Pennsylvania at the beginning of high school after my father had carried out a life-long dream–acquiring his own farm. A fascination with this new world of agriculture led me to Penn State University and its School of Agriculture, though issues of social science eventually captured my attention.

I remember meeting with the kindly Dean of Agriculture about my "smorgasbord" curriculum, and he suggested that I call it "general agriculture." Jessie Bernard taught the only class I had in sociology, and she encouraged my interest in family studies. Other courses at the graduate-undergraduate level were in social psychology, as taught by psychologists. The influence of Theodore Newcomb and Muzafir Sherif prompted me to think about links between people and their groups, such as reference group attachments and orientations. Social and personal change are vividly expressed in these experiences and in my early years in the fully mobilized city of Cleveland during World War II.

Curricular changes during college left me uncertain about future directions, but I pursued an interim assignment on the Dean of Men's staff at Kent State University in Kent, located just below Cleveland and its suburbs. The Dean of Men, Glen Nygreen, had received his PhD in Sociology at the University of Washington under Charles Bowerman, a family sociologist who was trained by Ernest Burgess at the University of Chicago. With the Dean's encouragement, I chose to work on an MA thesis concerning social change and family ties, the changing reference orientations of students who enter college from large and small towns. This research and my indirect ties to Charles Bowerman made the University of North Carolina especially attractive to me as a program for doctoral work. Bowerman had just accepted an appointment as chair of the Department of Sociology (1958–in the family field, Bowerman replaced Reuben Hill, who had taken a position at the University of Minnesota), and he had received a large NIMH grant to study the parent-peer orientations of adolescents. I enthusiastically accepted Bowerman's offer of a research assistantship in the summer of 1958.

In many respects, the ideas in this project reflected postwar developments that segregated children from adults and established fertile ground for the peer group as a countervailing influence to the family. After World War II, an increasing proportion of youths from all strata were enrolled in high school. And demographic forces transformed the landscape of schooling as the "baby boom" became a student surplus. With school time and peers gaining prominence in the lives of youths, the family's role became more problematic to many. This theme appears in David Riesman's *The Lonely Crowd* (1950) and in James Coleman's *The Adolescent Society* (1961). Many of the questions used in Coleman's 1957 study were included in the Bowerman project, despite a substantial difference in perspective and objectives. Coleman interpreted his data as providing support for a view of the peer group as isolated from the adult community and as an adversarial force vis-à-vis the family in the lives of young people.

The parent-peer study established an "intellectual and social community" across my five years of doctoral and postdoctoral work (the latter supported by an NIMH fellowship), with an emphasis on socialization as a link between social structure and personality. The survey was planned as a school-based study of adolescent parent-peer orientations from the 7th through the 12th grade. During the spring of 1960, survey data were collected from 20,000 adolescents in Ohio and in the Piedmont region of North Carolina. The design called for the study of three orientations (affectional, associational, and value) using the adolescent's report on relations to mother, father, and best friends (see Bowerman & Kinch, 1959). This approach enabled Bowerman to assess the potential differentiation of adolescent parent-peer orientations. In this manner, the adolescent project challenged the "either-or" account of transitions to adulthood–that youths develop an oppositional culture *or* follow a pathway of normative continuity into adulthood.

My dissertation focused on the interrelationship of family structure, interactive processes, and adolescent orientations. Well before Diana Baumrind (1975) investigated authoritarian, authoritative, and democratic patterns of childrearing, Bowerman's project collected information on these social structures, as perceived by adolescents (see Elder, 1962a, 1962b, 1963; Bowerman & Elder, 1964). The unidirectional structures (autocratic and authoritarian) were associated with low levels of perceived parental warmth, the lack of explanation, and weak adolescent orientations toward parents. These young people were more likely to be involved in peer groups of an adversarial type. More democratic and permissive structures were associated with greater perceived support from parents and explanation. Consistent with Baumrind's authoritative control, adolescent self-direction under parental control became less restrictive over time, and parental explorations defined a pattern of independence socialization that produced high levels of orientation toward parents in affection, values, and activities. Parents and peers were more often allies in this family environment. The dissertation and post-doctoral studies were published under the title of *Family Structure and Socialization* (Elder, 1980) in an Arno Press series under the direction of Robert K. Merton.

A preoccupation with issues of change represents a defining theme of The Adolescent Project. The changing social position of youths shaped many of the study's concerns; the separation of young people from parental influence, and the accentuation of separate worlds as youths move toward the adult years. However, the study did not address relevant aspects of historical or developmental change, or their interrelationship. Available theory and research models were largely ahistorical, and the cross-sectional design did not permit actual study of family relationships and individual development over time.

As I completed my dissertation and moved into a one-year postdoctoral fellowship, sociologists were beginning to think about such matters. I encountered a little book with a very big message. In *The Sociological Imagination,* C. Wright Mills proposed the "study of biography, of history, and of the problems of their intersection within social structure" as an orienting concept in the behavioral sciences (1959, p. 149). However, we were still years away from working models that would bring this kind of study to life. Little did I know that my first career appointment, at the University of California-Berkeley, would give me a chance to work on such problems.

During my search for job opportunities (1961-62), Bowerman arranged an interview at Chapel Hill with John Clausen, a distinguished sociologist who had just become the new director of the Institute of Human Development at Berkeley. Bowerman and Clausen were longtime friends, dating back to prewar graduate studies at the University of Chicago. In retrospect, the job interview ensured a lasting imprint of the early Chicago School of Sociology on my work (see Abbott, 1999). As mentor, Bowerman strengthened my investment in family studies with a Burgess perspective on the family, as a "unity of interacting personalities." After I accepted Clausen's offer (a joint appointment in the Department of Sociology and the Institute of Human Development), I began to value the study of individual lives, as John had from research at the Chicago Institute of Juvenile Research. Even more importantly, the longitudinal samples at the Institute challenged me to think of families and individuals over time. With rich archival data over nearly 30 years, I could see family life in the experience of individuals, and the role of individual lives in family experience. These impressions had a lasting imprint on my studies of families and the life course.

OBSERVING FAMILIES AND LIVES OVER TIME

My transition to Berkeley, the Institute of Human Development and the Department of Sociology at the University of California, occurred at a momentous time for the social and behavioral sciences on the campus and more generally. And it placed me on a new life trajectory based on a deeper consideration of the large-scale changes in human society and the longitudinal study of people over many years in changing worlds.

Established in the 1950s under the leadership of Herbert Blumer, the Berkeley Department of Sociology quickly became a magnet for distinguished senior faculty. When I arrived in the late summer of 1962, this faculty included Kingsley Davis, Reinhard Bendix, Seymour Martin Lipset, Philip Selznick, Erving Goffman, Neil Smelser, John Clausen, Herbert Blumer, Martin Trow, Charles Glock, David Matza, and Hanan Selvin, among others. Harold Wilensky joined the faculty a year later and became an important source of ideas in my thinking about families and lives over time. Psychology was likewise staffed with many leading figures in the field, and the Institute of Human Development had become a pioneering institution in the study of human development from early childhood into the middle years with its three long-term longitudinal studies.

With a joint appointment in Sociology and at the Institute, I had a rare opportunity to bring both sociological and psychological models to my research. My assignment at the Institute entailed the coding of life history interview data on all members of the Oakland Growth Study (members born in 1920-21). At the time, I did not fully anticipate the dramatic contrast between the cross-sectional Adolescent Study (resembling the storied Platte River, "a mile wide and an inch deep") and 30 years or more of data on families and lives. Survey work blinded me to the temporal thinking and questions that are appropriate for longitudinal research. The three studies at the Institute (in addition to Oakland, the Berkeley Guidance Study, and the Berkeley Growth Study) amounted to a sample of more than 500 people (Eichorn, Clausen, Haan, Honzik, & Mussen, 1981). The Oakland Study (N = 167) obtained annual information from Study members, mothers, and peers from 1931-32 through 1936-38, and then in the mid-1950s, 1960, and 1965. Observational data were available on peer interactions. Building upon these waves of data, I worked with staff to construct life records in different areas, such as family, career, and health.

My experience with the Oakland archive was shaped by observations that reinforced a more temporal approach to families and lives. The most dramatic example had to do with the ever-changing circumstances of families in the Great Depression. I soon realized that static concepts of family SES and the division of labor would not capture the realities of changing families. This is when I began to think of the division of labor in a processual family economy. Family adaptations to income loss became a process by which families constructed their own life course. One set of adaptations entailed a shift in the family economy from capital to labor-intensive activity.

These conceptual changes were the initial steps in launching a study of "Children of the Great Depression." The observation of family patterns over time also provided insights concerning the underlying economic forces that prompted new adaptations and structures. Such observations also prompted more thought about how to conceptualize individual lives. Two perspectives were available at the time, career and life cycle, and neither proved satisfactory (Elder, 1998a, 1998b). The career model dealt with single careers and thus oversimplified the lives of people who were coping with multiple roles at the same time. The concept of life cycle proved a role theoretical account of role sequences and linked lives, but it did not locate people according to their life stage or historical context. And it did not view roles in terms of their time of entry and exit.

To correct these limitations, I added to the life cycle model of role relationships the varied meanings of age, historical and social, in developing an approach to the Oakland study. Neither perspective was adequate by itself. Linked relationships in the life cycle enabled me to understand how economic hardship influenced children through the family. And it proved helpful in thinking about socialization and the sequential roles of adult life. But age distinctions were required to place families in history and to mark the transitions of adult life. The meanings of age brought temporality to the project.

In the late 1960s, I was invited to return to the University of North Carolina at Chapel Hill, and I brought with me a draft of *Children of the Great Depression* as well as essential data files. Following additional editorial work, the book was accepted for publication by the University of Chicago Press, with publication scheduled for 1974. Four theoretical principles of life course theory emerged from the study (Elder, 1998a).

Born in 1920-21, the Oakland study members entered childhood during this prosperous time, and then encountered family hardships as young adolescents through the misfortunes of their parents and relatives. Their historical time placed them at risk of this deprivational event. Some were exposed to severe deprivations through the family, whereas others managed to avoid them altogether. These contrasting experiences, deprived and nondeprived, produced an "experiment in nature" with empirical findings that affirm *the principle of (1) historical time and place: that the life course of individuals is embedded in and shaped by the historical times and places they experience over their lifetime.*

Within their lifetime, the Oakland Study members encountered differences in the temporal order of major events. Some married early and others late. Early marriage tended to generate a cumulation of life disadvantages, such as economic difficulties and the loss of advanced education. Whether early or late, the timing of life transitions proved to have long-term consequences through their effects on subsequent events and choices. *The principle of (2) timing in lives asserts that: the developmental antecedents and consequences of life transitions, events, and behavior patterns vary according to their timing in a person's life.*

Historical and individual experiences are connected through the family and the interdependent fates of its members. Fates are shared through family relationships. For example, economic hardship tended to increase the explosiveness of men who were inclined toward irritability. Thus, the more explosive they became under mounting economic pressures, the more adversely it affected the quality of marital relations and parenting. These observations support *the principle of (3) linked lives: individual lives are lived interdependently, and social-historical influences are expressed through this network of shared relationships.*

Lastly, the economic collapse of the 30s brings to mind a "world out of control," and the Oakland families often worked out successful responses in dire circumstances. Parents and their children made choices and many engaged in effective survival strategies within available options and limitations. These behaviors are expressions of human agency. *The principle of (4) human agency states that: individuals construct their own life course through the choices and actions they take within the opportunities and constraints of history and social circumstances.*

In this manner, empirical observations from the study illustrate core principles of life course theory. I use the term "theory" to refer to a theoretical orientation and framework (see Merton, 1968). Life course theory defines a common field of inquiry by providing a framework on matters of problem identification and conceptual development. In terms of theory, the empirical findings of this work did not support a life outcome of cumulative disadvantage from Depression hardship. Whether deprived in the middle or working class, the Oakland men and women typically fared well in their adult years. The concept of turning point better fits their life course. Three influences played a role in this turnaround–advanced education, marriage, and, especially, military service.

This next phase of my career moved beyond *Children of the Great Depression* in a number of respects. First, responses to the book called for clarifications and elaborations of life course distinctions, and broadened my cross-disciplinary contacts in history (Elder, 1977, 1978; Hareven, 1978) and developmental psychology (Elder, 1998b). Second, questions of generality arose. Are the findings from this study likely to generalize to other birth cohorts, and to other times and places? Theories of cohort differentiation led me to expect little generalization across time and place. The issue of generalizability was addressed by comparing the Oakland cohort with a younger cohort, the Berkeley Guidance sample, with birth years of 1928-29; and by exploring the impact of economic hardship in the contemporary world of inner-city Philadelphia (Furstenberg, Cook, Eccles, Elder, & Sameroff, 1999) and rural Iowa (Conger & Elder, 1994). Third, we had to explain how so many men and women from the Oakland cohort fared as well as they did in life, given their economic disadvantage. What were the key turning points?

STUDYING SOCIAL CHANGE IN THE LIFE COURSE

Children of the Great Depression generated considerable interest among developmental psychologists and social historians. Psychologists saw the work as an effort to place developmental processes in context (see Bronfenbrenner, 1977, 1979), while a small group of young social historians found the perspective of life course an appealing alternative to that of the life cycle. I met with some historians in Boston during the winter of 1975, and this meeting (organized by Tamara Hareven of Clark University) led to a series of workshops and a full week conference on the life course during the summer of 1976 at Williams College. Hareven and her colleagues saw the life course as a more dynamic theory of family change and adaptation than family cycle models, largely through its attention to historical time and social timing. The Williams College conference applied life course theory to 1880 census data on Essex County, Massachusetts. The resulting papers have been published in Hareven's *Transitions: The Family and Life Course in Historical Perspective* (1978). In 1976, Hareven became the first editor of the *Journal of Family History* and actively encouraged the publication of life course studies.

Another important step to elaborate and apply life course theory to families and individual lives occurred in 1977 when I was invited to join the new Social Science Research Council Committee on Life Course Perspectives on Human Development, with its multidisciplinary membership (including psychologists Paul Baltes and M. Brewster Smith–see

Elder, 1985). This committee, initially chaired by Matilda Riley, continued into the mid-1980s with a shift toward child development (psychologists included Mavis Hetherington, Ross Parke, Judy Dunn, and Martin Seligman). The meetings were frequently organized around the investigation of life course questions with longitudinal data sets, such as the Panel Study of Income Dynamics and the Framingham Study.

In the 1980s, an important project sponsored by the Committee brought historians and developmentalists together around life course themes by pairing them on individual studies. Each discipline had something different to offer. Historians brought a contextual understanding to the endeavor; whereas, developmentalists shed light on biobehavioral processes across the life span, something historians knew little about. The project was published as *Children in Time and Place* (Elder, Modell, & Parke, 1993). Legacies of the Committee's labors included a greater appreciation of the developmental and aging implications of the life course, and of historical constraints on development.

In the course of working on *Children of the Great Depression,* I became increasingly aware of the need for a comparative cohort in order to place the empirical results in context. After the book was published, this necessity gained more importance in my mind, as did the need to ascertain how the Second World War affected the men and women who grew up in the Great Depression. *Children* told the story of this Depression childhood and its legacy, but it completely failed to explore the implications of World War II and the Korean War. Over 90 percent of the Oakland men served in World War II, and nearly three-fourths of the Berkeley Guidance Study men also served in the military. After exploring the comparative cohort plan, I settled on the Berkeley Guidance sample as the very best option. The sample included 214 boys and girls who were born in 1928-29. The study members were followed up across childhood, adolescent years, and the middle years.

Work on the Berkeley Guidance Study archive occurred during a sabbatical year in 1972-73, and it led to the unsurprising finding that members of this younger birth cohort were more adversely influenced by prolonged exposure to the Depression's hardship, than members of the Oakland cohort. This negative impact was most evident among the boys. Yet despite this disadvantage, it did not persist beyond the age of 40 or so, owing largely to turning point experiences in the military, especially during the Second World War. In both cohorts, men who entered the military at an early stage were most likely to benefit, more so than men who entered late (Elder, 1986, 1987). Early entry minimized life disruption and opened up the opportunity for educational benefits on the GI bill. Later entry (32 years or more) tended to increase life disadvantage, such as the risk of divorce and worklife disruptions, as revealed in another California cohort (Pavalko & Elder, 1990; Elder, Shanahan, & Clipp, 1994). Other samples and analyses have produced comparable findings (Sampson & Laub, 1996). The Second World War also opened up job and educational opportunities for young women who had grown up in the 30s, and, when coupled with marriage, they frequently defined an escape route from Depression hard times.

Military duty and wartime service illustrate the role of the state in shaping the life course through manpower policies (Mayer, 1986). Another effort to examine this role took me to Shanghai and a life course study of the Cultural Revolution in the People's Republic of China, just prior to the crisis of Tiananmen Square (Elder, Wu, & Yuan, 1993). In collaboration with the Institute of Sociology (Shanghai University) and the Carolina Population Center at Chapel Hill, we used retrospective life history methods in a survey of 1,300 adults in Shanghai during the winter and spring of 1987-88. Among urban young people who were sent to peasant communities, the disruptive forces and sanctions of the forced migration led to the postponement of family events and to some losses of education and career prospects. Since longitudinal samples are not available in developing societies, this study demonstrated the potential of using retrospective life history techniques for recovering knowledge about the enduring effects of prior events.

Each of these studies enabled men to apply life course theory to different types of social change and to use the results to refine the conceptual approach. I continued this method of extending life course theory through different applications when I returned to the University of North Carolina at Chapel Hill in 1984 as the Howard W. Odum Distinguished Professor of Sociology. I had just spent several years at the new Boys Town Center for Studies of Youth and Families (Omaha, Nebraska), and five years as Urie Bronfenbrenner's colleague at Cornell University.

Entirely new projects captured my attention. When hard times visited the rural midwest in the 80s with a sudden collapse of land values, I joined an Iowa State research team headed by Rand Conger on a panel study of economic hardship and its effects with over 450 farm and nonfarm families. Focused on the north central region of the state, the study drew upon elements of my earlier Depression study to trace economic hardship through families processes to the lives of parents and children (Conger & Elder, 1994). Indebtedness, income loss, and unstable work increased the felt economic pressures of Iowa families, and also increased the likelihood of parental emotional distress and marital negativity. These conditions tended to undermine effective parenting and the developmental competence of young people.

But many factors countered such cumulative adversities, including a web of social relationships linking family members and the household to community institutions. These social connections are most evident among families with some ties to agriculture, despite their economic distress. The developmental and protective influence of these "connections" is reported in a forthcoming book, *Children of the Land* (Elder & Conger, in press), along with insights gained from the ways these families managed the risks and options of their children beyond the household. This life course study over seven years (from 7th grade to completion of high school) underscored the importance of investigating whether and how families are linked to the outside world.

Paired with the Iowa Youth and Families Project was a project in inner-city Philadelphia, also focused on how parents manage the risks and options of their children (ages 11-14), this time in dangerous environments. Directed by Frank Furstenberg (with Cook, Eccles, Elder, & Sameroff, 1999), this study found that family resources and strategies proved to be more potent in fostering successful outcomes in young people (in academic achievement, social involvement, emotional health, and the avoidance of problem behavior). There were greater differences within particular neighborhoods, among families and children, than there were between them. As in the Iowa study, involved parents tended to have children who were actively engaged in school clubs and sports. They were also likely to do better academically.

The MacArthur Network on Successful Adolescent Development among Youth in High-Risk Settings supported both the Iowa and Philadelphia studies and enabled us to investigate similar family processes in these different settings. Thus, we found community ties and their developmental benefits in both rural communities and in the inner city. However, such ties are more common in a rural community, and they are more supported by other social forces. Both studies affirm the developmental influence of "linked lives" between the family and other groups in the community. The social ecology of families represents a powerful force in the lives of children, whatever the external danger or risk.

REFLECTIONS

The last half of the 20th century has witnessed a number of intellectual transitions that are expressed in the path I have followed in sociology and the behavioral sciences. These include the increasing tendency to view behavior and collective life in context; to bring an historical perspective to all problems; and to appreciate the temporality of families and of people's lives. For reasons that are not easy to identify, I have always been challenged by the powerful implications of a changing society for people's lives, a topic that was neglected at the time I entered graduate school. Sociologists had little to contribute to an understanding of social change.

Nevertheless, a changeful time should direct at least some attention to the consequences in people's lives, especially with the advantage of longitudinal data. I began to discover valuable insights about these effects by focusing on the family in the Great Depression, drawing from the tradition of social interactionism and socialization studies. Hard times were expressed in different ways through family adaptations, such as changing the family economy to a more labor intensive system. By studying changing lives in changing times, I gradually assembled elements of a life course framework or theoretical orientation, incorporating socialization issues within this broader frame. With the assistance of talented colleagues and students, my studies of other social changes also fostered an elaboration of this perspective, such as manpower mobilization in World War II and rural economic change.

My professional journey in the study of families and lives might well have taken a different course without access to the pioneering longitudinal studies. The growth of longitudinal data archives is truly remarkable in the social and behavioral sciences, and studies based on them have profoundly influenced my thinking about families and their members. In many cases, I have taken longitudinal data that were collected for other purposes and recast them to fit the new questions I wanted to address.[2] In other cases I collected data explicitly for the purposes of assessing these questions. In either case, new data collection methods (such as retrospective life calendars) were needed to address life course questions on family dynamics and continuity.

Today life course studies are helping to locate people in a matrix of age-graded, family relationships, and to place families in the social structures, cultures, and populations of time and place.[3] The studies have brought time and temporality to an understanding of individual lives and families. In various ways, both large and small, this line of work is serving to counter what Robert Nisbet (1969, ch. 8) once called the "timeless realm of the abstract."

NOTES

1. This transition is discussed in my Ernest Burgess lecture (Elder, 1981a), in an essay critical of the temporal limitations of the social structure and personality framework (Elder, 1981b), and most extensively in my Cooley-Mead address published in 1994. A biographical account of the longitudinal studies and their influences on my thinking is reported in a paper for the Landmark Studies Conference of the Henry Murray Research Center (Elder, in press).

2. Our methods for "recasting" data archives to meet the needs of a new type of question are reported by Elder, Pavalko, and Clipp (1993) in *Working with Archival Data.* A general anthology of life course methods has been edited by Giele and Elder (1998).

3. Anne Colby (Giele and Elder, 1998, p. viii) refers to "the tremendous impact on social science that the life course approach has had in the past three decades." She concludes that "the establishment of this approach . . . is one of the most important achievements of social science in the second half of the 20th century" (p. x).

REFERENCES

Abbott, A. (1999). The Continuing Relevance of the Chicago School. In A. Abbott (Ed.), *Department and discipline: Chicago sociology at one hundred.* Chicago: University of Chicago Press.

Baumrind, D. (1975). Early socialization and adolescent competence. In S. E. Dragastin & G. H. Elder, Jr. (Eds.), *Adolescence in the life cycle* (pp. 117-143). Washington, DC: Hemisphere/Halsted Press.

Bowerman, C.E. & Elder, G. H., Jr. (1964). Variations in adolescent perception of family power structure. *American Sociological Review, 29*, 4, 551-567.

Bowerman, C. E. & Kinch, J. W. (1959). Changes in family and peer orientation of children between the fourth and tenth grades. *Social Forces, 37*, 1, 206-211.

Bronfenbrenner, U. (1977). Toward an experimental ecology of human development. *American Psychologist, 32*, 7, 513-531.

Bronfenbrenner, U. (1979). *The ecology of human development: Experiments by nature and design.* Cambridge, MA: Harvard University Press.

Colby, A. (1998). Forward: Crafting life course studies. In J. Z. Giele & G. H. Elder, Jr. (Eds.), *Methods of life course research: Qualitative and quantitative approaches* (pp. viii-xii). Thousand Oaks, CA: Sage.

Coleman, J. S., with the assistance of Johnstone, J. W. C. & Jonassohn, K. (1961). *The adolescent society; The social life of the teenager and its impact on education.* New York: Free Press of Glencoe.

Conger, R. D., & Elder, G. H., Jr. in collaboration with Lorenz, F. O., Simons, R. L., & Whitbeck, L. B. (1994). *Families in troubled times: Adapting to change in rural America.* Hawthorne, NY: Aldine DeGruyter.

Eichorn, D. H., Clausen, J. A., Haan, N., Honzik, M., & Paul H. Mussen, P. H. (Eds.) (1981). *Present and past in middle life.* New York: Academic Press.

Elder, G. H., Jr. (1962a). *Adolescent achievement and mobility aspirations.* Chapel Hill, NC: Monograph of the Institute for Research in Social Science.

Elder, G. H., Jr. (1962b). Structural variations in the child rearing relationship. *Sociometry, 25*, 3, 241-262.
Elder, G. H., Jr. (1963). Parental power legitimation and its effect on the adolescent. *Sociometry, 26*, 1, 50-65.
Elder, G. H., Jr. (1974). *Children of the great depression: Social change in life experience*. Chicago: University of Chicago Press. (Reissued as 25th Anniversary Edition, Boulder, CO: Westview Press, 1999).
Elder, G. H., Jr. (1977). Family history and the life course. *Journal of Family History, 2*, 4, 279-304.
Elder, G. H., Jr. (1978). Family history and the life course. In T. K. Haraven (Ed.), *Transitions* (pp. 17-64). New York: Academic Press.
Elder, G. H., Jr. (1980). *Family structure and socialization*. New York: Arno Press.
Elder, G. H., Jr. (1981a). History and the family: The discovery of complexity. *Journal of Marriage and the Family, 43*, 3, 489-519. Ernest Burgess Lecture.
Elder, G. H., Jr. (1981b). Social history and life experience. In D. H. Eichorn, J. A.Clausen, J. Haan, M. P. Honzik, & P. H. Mussen (Eds.), *Present and past in middle life* (pp. 3-31). New York: Academic Press.
Elder, G. H., Jr. (Ed.) (1985). *Life course dynamics: Trajectories and transitions, 1968-1980*. Ithaca, NY: Cornell University Press.
Elder, G. H., Jr. (1985). Perspectives on the life course. In G. H. Elder, Jr. (Ed.), *Life course dynamics: Trajectories and transitions, 1968-1980* (pp. 23-49). Ithaca, NY: Cornell University Press.
Elder, G. H., Jr. (1986). Military times and turning points in men's lives. *Developmental Psychology, 22*, 2, 233-245.
Elder, G. H., Jr. (1987). War mobilization and the life course: A cohort of World War II veterans. *Sociological Forum, 2*, 3, 449-472.
Elder, G. H., Jr. (1992). Life course. In E. Borgatta & M. Borgatta (Eds.), *The encyclopedia of sociology* (pp. 1120-1130). New York: Macmillan.
Elder, G. H., Jr. (1994). Time, human agency, and social change: Perspectives on the life course. *Social Psychology Quarterly, 57*, 1, 4-15.
Elder, G. H., Jr. (1998a). The life course as developmental theory. *Child Development, 69*, 1, 1-12.
Elder, G. H., Jr (1998b). The life course and human development. In R. M. Lerner (Ed.) *Handbook of child psychology, volume 1: Theoretical models of human development*. 5th Edition (pp. 939-991), William Damon (General Ed.). New York: Wiley.
Elder, G. H., Jr (2000). Historical times and lives: A journey through time and space. *Landmark Studies of the 20th Century Conference*. Henry A. Murray Center for the Study of Lives, Cambridge, MA, April 1999.
Elder, G. H., Jr. & Conger, R. D. (in press). *Children of the land: Adversity and success at century's end*. Chicago: University of Chicago Press.
Elder, G. H., Jr., Modell, J. M., & Parke, R. D. (Eds.). (1993). *Children in time and place: Developmental and historical insights*. New York: Cambridge University Press.
Elder, G. H., Jr., Pavalko, E. K., & Clipp, E. C. (1993). *Working with archival data: Studying lives*. Newbury Park, CA: Sage Publications.

Elder, G. H., Jr., Shanahan, M. J., & Clipp, E. C. (1994). When war comes to men's lives: Life course patterns in family, work, and health. *Psychology and aging* (special issue), *9*, 1, 5-16.

Elder, G, Jr., Wu, W., & Yuan, J. (1993). State-initiated change and the life course in Shanghai, China. Unpublished project report.

Furstenberg, F. F., Jr., Cook, T. D., Eccles, J., Elder, G. H., Jr., & Sameroff, A. (1999). *Managing to make it: Urban families and adolescent success*. Chicago, IL: University of Chicago Press.

Giele, J. A. & Elder, G. H., Jr. (Ed.). (1998). *Methods of life course research: Qualitative and quantitative approaches*. Thousand Oaks, CA: Sage.

Hareven, T. K. (1978). *Transitions: The family and the life course in historical perspective*. New York: Academic.

Mayer, K. U. (1986). Structural constraints on the life course. *Human Development*, *29*, 3, 163-170.

Merton, R. K. (1968). *Social theory and social structure*. New York: Free Press.

Mills, C. W. (1959). *The sociological imagination*. New York: Oxford University Press.

Nisbet, R. A. (1969). *Social change and history: Aspects of the western theory development*. New York: Oxford University Press.

Pavalko, E. K. & Elder, G. H., Jr. (1990). World War II and divorce: A life course perspective. *The American Journal of Sociology*, *95*, 5, 1213-1234.

Riesman, D. in collaboration with Denney, R. & Glazer, N. (1950). *The lonely crowd: A study of the changing American character*. New Haven, CT: Yale University Press.

Sampson, R. J. & Laub, J. H. (1996). Socioeconomic achievement in the life course of disadvantaged men: Military service as a turning point, circa 1940-1965. *American Sociological Review*, *61*, 3, 347-367.

Making the World Safe for Difference

Katherine R. Allen

KEYWORDS. Autobiography, feminism, oppression, sexuality, qualitative research

EARLY BEGINNINGS

Born in 1954, I grew up in a row house in a primarily Irish and Italian Catholic neighborhood in Baltimore in the post-war baby boom era. I was the second child of five, born to young parents, whose tenacious commitment to family bonds kept them together despite many obstacles. My childhood experiences set the tone for a lifelong concern with making the world around me safe for difference. My intellectual goal has been to deconstruct marginalization and reconstruct social arrangements to reflect and respect diversity. Life has also taught me that the head and heart are not separate entities. Feeling and being are as important as thinking and doing (Allen, 2000). Allowing my private and professional experiences to inform each other, I practice a social science that integrates multiple perspectives, contradictions, tensions, and the variability of context and time.

Growing Up a White Girl

Early family life was chaotic, with too few adults to tend to too many children. The children in my neighborhood played in the alley, divided into groups according to who went to public school and who went to Catholic school. In these packs of unsupervised neighborhood kids, I learned such things as what the private parts of other people's bodies looked like as well as how to smoke cigarettes. I witnessed the impact of child abuse as older children took out their anger and victimization from harsh parental discipline on younger children. So much for the security and innocence of childhood in the 1950s. As other feminist scholars have observed (Coontz, 1992; Skolnick, 1991; Stacey, 1996), I saw no golden age of family life that was depicted on television shows and is currently promoted by politicians, clergy, talk show hosts, and many family scholars. Although I felt sorry for the families who were unlike my own–those with only one or two children, those with divorced parents, or those whose parents were talked about as queer–I was still aware that diversity existed all around me and that children were not as safe as they were supposed to be.

Life was racially segregated as well. Whites could go to the local amusement park six days of the week, but blacks could only go on Thursdays. My parents did not allow derogatory remarks about other racial groups, unlike the households of most of our neighbors and extended kin, but their teaching about tolerance did not extend beyond stating the value that everyone was equal. There were few people who were not white in my neighborhood, church, or school. I did not have a teacher who was black until I entered junior high school.

Life was also gendered. I learned to adhere to a double standard that restricted my own self-worth and aspirations. Girls were to be quiet and cute; we couldn't even wear pants to school. After witnessing a first grade teacher grab a girl who had misbehaved and swing her around by the hair until she crashed into a wall, I knew enough to keep as quiet as possible so no one would notice me and hurt me like that. I dreamed of becoming an airline stewardess or a hairdresser when I grew up. Like the Barbie dolls I played with, they had some glamour and flexibility in their lives, and at least they got paid for what they did.

I spent those formative years observing the contradictory messages about race, class, gender, and heterosexuality that positioned me for a life of service and second class status. These messages were so disturbing to my emerging sense of justice that I developed a corresponding urge to rebel against systematically unfair restrictions. Even as a young child, I connected head and heart. I understood the social hierarchy in the major institutions–family, school, and church–structuring my world. I knew about class distinctions, ducking my head when driving in my mother's old car, so friends from school wouldn't see me in such a wreck. But the racism and sexism that were taken for granted in my community offended me the most. Once, in the second grade, when I was walking down the street with my best friend, she told me to hold my breath and cross the street so we wouldn't walk past and catch the germs of a black woman coming in the other direction. I thought she was wrong and stupid to believe such a thing, but I still did as she said. My incredulity wasn't enough to keep me from conforming to peer pressure by obeying the thoughts and actions of adults parroted by my young friend. Little did I know then that we were being socialized into the systems of domination–racism, sexism, heterosexism, and classism–that served to keep most of us in our places.

By the late 1960s, *Life Magazine* was my most reliable teacher. Reading about heterosexual cohabitation in a college dorm brought a mixture of shock and excitement about this brave new world that I would soon enter. I watched the film *Bonnie and Clyde*, which glamorized violence and sexuality in bold, unsettling images, and I got the feeling that Clyde disappointed Bonnie when they were in bed together. I don't know what shocked me more, the fact that they were shown in bed together in the middle of the day, or the hint that he couldn't "act like a man." I had a vague feeling that the filmmakers were depicting him as homosexual, a word I'd heard whispered around my house about a friend's mother (a woman who had very short hair and dressed like a man). Whatever was going on in the film, at 13, I knew it wasn't considered "normal," but it intrigued me anyway. Then I saw *Romeo and Juliet* and was again shocked that two young teenagers were having sex–from what I could gather, people didn't have sex until marriage. Thus, media images from print and film provided an external framework for the confusion I felt as I was coming of age.

At 15, I moved with my family to the west coast, and I tried to fit my own life into the stylized image of being a teenager in southern California. I took incredible risks, hitchhiking or riding my bike to the beach some 15 miles away from my home in nothing more than a bathing suit. Still I managed to stay relatively centered and out of harm's way by active involvement in the United Methodist Church. I played out the competing scripts of an obedient good girl and a wild bad girl without much interference from my family. It was quite possible to live a double life and not raise suspicion about the adult activities in which I was experimenting. Years later, in reading, writing, and teaching about sexuality in women's lives, I came to understand the tension between pleasure and danger (Vance, 1984) that layered the coming of age process for women in my peer group (Baber & Allen, 1992; Fine, 1992; Thompson, 1995).

FINDING FEMINISM, FINDING FAMILY STUDIES

I entered college in 1972, when women's studies courses began to be offered on college campuses. In taking these courses, I found a discourse and practice that captured the tensions I felt and the duality I lived. Feminism gave me the words to describe what I was experiencing. I learned to critique the status quo by attending consciousness-raising groups throughout my college and graduate school years and by taking classes that incorporated an awareness of the intersections of gender, race, and class. Feminism helped me find my voice, muted long before in threats of violence for misbehavior. I started using it to describe the proverbial elephant in the living room that I was able to see but few others in my world were willing to acknowledge.

At the same time that I found a home in women's studies, I was also drawn to classes in family studies, child development, and sociology. As an undergraduate at the University of Connecticut, I majored in child development and family relations, and, as a graduate student at Syracuse University, I chose a similar major (child and family studies, with a certificate in gerontology). Discovering that there was a worldview that placed family structures and processes over the life course in the center of vision was an exhilarating push toward my future career. The multiple languages spoken in the interdisciplinary study of families (verbal, conceptual, empirical, reflexive, and interpersonal) coincided with the way I viewed the world.

One of the reasons I was attracted to family studies was because there were actually women professors in the field, whereas there were no women faculty members in my minor area of sociology. In both universities I attended, family studies was housed in a College of Home Economics, a place where women were faculty and administrative leaders. For many years, Colleges of Home Economics (and subsequent manifestations such as Human Development, Human Resources, Human Ecology, and the like) were the only schools that taught and employed a majority of women. Paradoxically, the liberatory education I hoped to find in family studies was only partial, as Colleges of Home Economics have not been bastions of feminist thought and practice. The historic vision of families promoted in my chosen field has uncritically adopted a functionalist status quo. It has taken the critique of feminist and critical scholars to shake up this placid foundation that undergirded the family studies I was taught (e.g., Allen & Demo, 1995; Baber & Allen, 1992; Cheal, 1991; Collins, 1990; Ferree, 1990; Hare-Mustin & Marecek, 1988; Okin, 1989; Sprey, 1988; Thorne, 1982; Thompson & Walker, 1989, 1995).

Seeing the Invisible

Perhaps because family studies was a discipline that made room for women and families, I still found it a hospitable academic home for studying topics that are denigrated, ignored, falsified, distorted, and linked to the tensions of belonging versus being an outsider. My life's work has been to expose the cultural silence about what is clearly visible to me, but what is treated as invisible by others. When I was an undergraduate student in the 1970s, I did an independent study on feminist women and their male partners. This student project was the first qualitative study I conducted, and I did it before I had systematically studied how to plan and execute a research project. My professor, Robert Ryder, who had previously worked at the National Institute of Mental Health, taught me how to pursue this project based on the method he had used to conduct open-ended interviews with couples in the early years of marriage (Ryder, Kafka, & Olson, 1971). He recommended I find some people who matched my criteria of being a heterosexual couple who identified with feminism, ask them questions and talk with them in a conversational manner, take notes during the interview, and immediately after the interview, write down every detail and comment I could remember. I thought, "I want to do this! This method fits with the way I see the world." I interviewed 11 couples and analyzed the data intuitively, pulling ideas from some of the books I'd read in my classes. One that particularly influenced me was Cuber and Harroff's (1965) *The Significant Americans*. Doing this study demystified the research process for me and gave me the confidence to apply to graduate school. As a graduate student at Syracuse University, I took advanced courses on research methods, and I learned that this intuitive, conceptual, empirical, and reflexive way of analyzing social trends had a long-standing tradition in the social sciences. I learned to name my research practice as qualitative, and I've relied upon that methodology my entire career.

The desire to study the invisible and the contradictory has shaped my academic career. I am more comfortable challenging, rather than defending, the status quo. For my dissertation research, I studied older women who never married. My advisor and mentor was Robert Pickett, a family historian whose passionate integration of the history of Western family systems with the contemporary life course framework inspired my work. I found that contrary to stereotypic notions of "spinsters" as bereft of family that I had read about in the literature, these women were highly engaged with their families of origin. In contrast to the women in the study who had extended their families through marriage, motherhood, and grandmotherhood, the never-married women's lives were about maintaining family bonds across the generations (Allen, 1989; Allen & Pickett, 1987).

Studying Marginalization in Families

Since my professional career began, I have taught in human development and family studies programs (at Texas Woman's University from 1984 to 1989, and at Virginia Tech since 1989), continuing this theme of studying marginalized family experience. These projects include a reconstruction of women's experiences in families from a feminist postmodern perspective (Baber & Allen, 1992) and an examination of older adults' experiences of structural diversity across three generations in their families (Allen, Blieszner, Roberto, Farnsworth, & Wilcox, 1999). Many of the graduate students whose dissertations I've advised investigated marginalized family experience, and we have published their results in family-related journals: older black women's work and leisure experiences (Allen & Chin-Sang, 1990); feminist couples and egalitarian marriage (Blaisure & Allen, 1995); African American midlife couples (Carolan & Allen, 1999); and mothers who have lost a young child to death (Farnsworth & Allen, 1996).

I have also written about the intersection of my private life on my experiences as a teacher, researcher, and citizen in publications dealing with lesbian parenting (Allen, 1997; Stone & Allen, 1998), being an out lesbian teacher in a family studies classroom (Allen, 1995), and ways in which my own transformation from married to lesbian mother has led to deeper understandings of the in-depth interview data I've collected on lifelong single women (Allen, 1994) and older parents of adult lesbian and gay children (Allen, 1999). Recently, I co-edited a text on family diversity in which prominent scholars in the interdisciplinary family field addressed how family experiences vary according to race, class, gender, sexual orientation, and other forms of family structural diversity (Demo, Allen, & Fine, 2000). I was motivated to collaborate on editing this volume because I wanted a text to use in my senior level course, Gender and Family Diversity, that not only presents the most comprehensive analysis of diversity in family studies but also demonstrates the connectedness of scholarship to personal experience.

Understanding the Outsider Within

Teaching about and studying diversity as well as living in a diverse family has put me in an ironic position that is both unsettling and intriguing. A major irony associated with building a reputation as a person who challenges the status quo is that by being a voice for diversity, I've had opportunities to serve as a leader in my field, sitting at the table with others whose perspectives and power I sometimes challenge. I am an officer in professional associations, an editor for mainstream journals, a professor at a major research university, and a keynote speaker at conferences, but, at the same time, due to my association with second class–or even vilified–groups (e.g., woman, lesbian, family scholar, qualitative methodologist), I am also a critic of the very status quo that rewards me. Sitting at the leaders' table confers the opportunity and the power to shape discourse and set policy, but it also brings the danger of co-opting the critical or radical vision that landed me there in the first place (Zwiegenhaft & Domhoff, 1998). This dilemma brings with it the double consciousness of insider/outsider status, described by DuBois and elaborated in Collins (1990), as a standpoint that comes from experiencing the competing realities of occupying privileged and denigrated statuses at the same time.

Again connecting the head and heart, the ironic position in which I find myself has opened a new interest in unmasking the dynamics of leadership and power, particularly for women and those in marginalized groups. Like other feminist and critical scholars, I am intrigued by the dilemma that leadership requires the very power that also degrades one's position as a renegade. Currently, I've been studying ways in which women use power, finding that power can corrupt, because a leader must balance changing with maintaining the status quo. Yet, power also protects. What if those who view the world from the margins never got to the table? My current investigation of women in leadership positions suggests that the very fact of female gender can undermine even the most competent and intelligent of women leaders. Being a woman and a leader still exacts a huge toll. Being a respected woman leader, then, is a heroic achievement because of the structural and personal barriers women are forced to overcome.

Creating Safe Spaces Through Reflexive Practice

My current interest in women, power, and leadership is an outgrowth of a career-long fascination with marginalization. Unless people who live with some kind of difference come forward and allow themselves to be scrutinized, the complexion, gender, and marital status, among other things, of those sitting at the table will remain as uniform as it has historically been (Heifetz, 1994; Hesselbein, Goldsmith, & Beckhard, 1996; Jamieson, 1995; Kanter, 1977; Kolodny, 1998; Zweigenhaft & Domhoff, 1998). Wanting different voices to be heard entails being willing to take the risk of studying, critiquing, and understanding my own lived experience.

Feminist theorist and activist Gloria Steinem (1992) said that our revolutions are both within and without–internal to our own lives and external to the world beyond ourselves. The valued and devalued statuses that comprise my life affect my ability to understand how marginalization impacts others. Self-reflection, which I define as the vulnerable process of grappling with the contradictions and connections in private and public experience, is a method for studying marginalization that is grounded in the real world. What goes on in my personal life informs my research and teaching practice, making me aware of the systems of oppression and opportunity that structure life chances for each of us.

As a reflexive practitioner, I try to make my values and assumptions, growth process and foibles, known to myself and to others. I have kept a reflective diary since I was 15 years old and have been in numerous consciousness groups, from a black and white women's group to a lesbian mothers group. Because of the intense nature of the information I teach (e.g., human sexualities, gender and family diversity, reflexive qualitative methods), checking my own biases and prejudices, lest I impose them on others, is a necessary part of my professional practice. Taking responsibility for my own thoughts, feelings, and actions is a strategy for self-understanding that also informs my social science practice. In the past few years, like others of my generation, I've returned to the meditation practices I learned as a young woman. Choosing to be silent and listen from within is a private discipline that helps me as a family scholar.

In my academic writing, I want to avoid the bluff of couching an argument in something intellectual by writing in plain and transparent ways. My hunch is that some of our discourse about families hides scholars' own unresolved problems or value conflicts. Reflexivity adds clarity by encouraging us to be aware of our private investments in academic disagreements. This way of thinking provides us with the ability to say without fear of ridicule, "What you are doing threatens me because it challenges my way of thinking, or ignores the kind of family in which I live." The writers, teachers, and scholars I admire are willing to admit their vulnerability and demonstrate their strength without degrading others or devaluing feelings and personal experiences.

CONCLUSION

I remind myself that this narrative is just a temporary portrait of my life and work. I know full well that my life is in progress, and lived experiences in the future and reflections on the past will alter this account.

By way of conclusion, the thread that connects my past, present, and future is a desire to live in a world that is a safe and understanding place for self and others. I want more time for human relationships, more forgiveness for false starts and transgressions, and more understanding of difference. I am a family scholar because our discipline offers a worldview comprehensive enough to hold this vision with care and elasticity, without freezing or exploiting an image of the family that caters only to the most powerful. The possibilities for change in our discipline are as infinite and varied as the families we study, and I am motivated by the rewards of deeper understanding that come with the passing of time.

REFERENCES

Allen, K. R. (1989). *Single women/family ties: Life histories of older women.* Thousand Oaks, CA: Sage.

Allen, K. R. (1994). Feminist reflections on lifelong single women. In D. L. Sollie & L. A. Leslie (Eds.), *Gender, families, and close relationships: Feminist research journeys* (pp. 97-119). Thousand Oaks, CA: Sage.

Allen, K. R. (1995). Opening the classroom closet: Sexual orientation and self-disclosure. *Family Relations, 44*, 2, 136-141.

Allen, K. R. (1997). Lesbian and gay families. In T. Arendell (Ed.), *Contemporary parenting: Issues and challenges* (pp. 196-218). Thousand Oaks, CA: Sage.

Allen, K. R. (1999). Reflexivity in qualitative analysis: Toward an understanding of resiliency among older parents with adult gay children. In H. I. McCubbin, E. A. Thompson, A. I. Thompson, & J. A. Futrell (Eds.), *The dynamics of resilient families* (pp. 71-93). Thousand Oaks, CA: Sage.

Allen, K. R. (2000). A conscious and inclusive family studies. *Journal of Marriage and the Family, 62*, 1, 79-92.

Allen, K. R., Blieszner, R., Roberto, K. A., Farnsworth, E. B, & Wilcox, K. L. (1999). Older adults and their children: Family patterns of structural diversity. *Family Relations, 48*, 2, 151-157.

Allen, K. R., & Chin-Sang, V. (1990). A lifetime of work: The context and meanings of leisure for aging black women. *The Gerontologist, 30*, 6, 734-740.

Allen, K. R., & Demo, D. H. (1995). The families of lesbians and gay men: A new frontier in family research. *Journal of Marriage and the Family, 57*, 1, 111-127.

Allen, K. R., & Pickett, R. S. (1987). Forgotten streams in the family life course: Utilization of qualitative retrospective interviews in the analysis of lifelong single women's family careers. *Journal of Marriage and the Family, 49*, 3, 517-526.

Baber, K. M., & Allen, K. R. (1992). *Women and families: Feminist reconstructions.* New York: Guilford.

Blaisure, K. R., & Allen, K. R. (1995). Feminists and the ideology and practice of marital equality. *Journal of Marriage and the Family, 57*, 1, 5-19.

Carolan, M. T., & Allen, K. R. (1999). Commitments and constraints to intimacy for African American couples at midlife. *Journal of Family Issues, 20*, 1, 3-24.

Cheal, D. (1991). *Family and the state of theory*. Toronto, Canada: University of Toronto Press.

Collins, P. H. (1990). *Black feminist thought: Knowledge, consciousness and the politics of empowerment*. Boston: Unwin Hyman.

Coontz, S. (1992). *The way we never were: American families and the nostalgia trap*. New York: Basic.

Cuber, J. F., & Harroff, P. B. (1965). *The significant Americans*. New York: Appleton-Century.

Demo, D. H., Allen, K. R., & Fine, M. A. (Eds.). (2000). *Handbook of family diversity*. New York: Oxford University Press.

Farnsworth, E. B., & Allen, K. R. (1996). Mothers' bereavement: Experiences of marginalization, stories of change. *Family Relations, 45*, 4, 360-367.

Ferree, M. M. (1990). Beyond separate spheres: Feminism and family research. *Journal of Marriage and the Family, 52*, 4, 866-884.

Fine, M. (1992). Sexuality, schooling, and adolescent females: The missing discourse of desire. In M. Fine (Ed.), *Disruptive voices: The possibilities of feminist research* (pp. 31-59). Ann Arbor: University of Michigan Press.

Hare-Mustin, R. T., & Marecek, J. (1988). The meaning of difference: Gender theory, postmodernism, and psychology. *American Psychologist, 43*, 6, 455-464.

Heifetz, R. A. (1994). *Leadership without easy answers*. Cambridge, MA: Harvard University Press.

Hesselbein, R., Goldsmith, M., & Beckhard, R. (Eds.). (1996). *The leader of the future*. San Francisco, CA: Jossey-Bass.

Jamieson, K. H. (1995). *Beyond the double bind: Women and leadership*. New York: Oxford University Press.

Kanter, R. M. (1977). *Men and women of the corporation*. New York: Basic.

Kolodny, A. (1998). *Failing the future: A dean looks at higher education in the twenty-first century*. Durham, NC: Duke University Press.

Okin, S. M. (1989). *Justice, gender, and the family*. New York: Basic.

Ryder, R. G. (1987). *The realistic therapist: Modesty and relativism in therapy and research*. Newbury Park, CA: Sage.

Skolnick, A. (1991). *Embattled paradise: The American family in an age of uncertainty*. New York: Basic.

Sprey, J. (1988). Current theorizing on the family: An appraisal. *Journal of Marriage and the Family, 50*, 4, 875-890.

Stacey, J. (1996). *In the name of the family: Rethinking family values in the postmodern age*. Boston: Beacon Press.

Steinem, G. (1992). *Revolution from within*. Boston, MA: Little, Brown.

Stone, T. J., & Allen, K. R. (1998). Parenthood and pregnancy: The journey of a lesbian couple and their children. In V. R. Fu & A. J. Stremmel (Eds.), *Affirming diversity through democratic conversations* (pp. 171-185). Upper Saddle River, NJ: Prentice Hall.

Thompson, L., & Walker, A. J. (1989). Gender in families: Women and men in marriage, work, and parenthood. *Journal of Marriage and the Family, 51*, 4, 845-871.

Thompson, L., & Walker, A. J. (1995). The place of feminism in family studies. *Journal of Marriage and the Family, 57*, 4, 847-865.
Thompson, S. (1995). *Going all the way: Teenage girls' tales of sex, romance, and pregnancy*. New York: Hill and Wang.
Thorne, B., with Yalom, M. (Eds.). (1982). *Rethinking the family: Some feminist questions*. New York: Longman.
Vance, C. (1984). *Pleasure and danger: Exploring female sexuality*. Boston: Routledge & Kegan Paul.
Zweigenhaft, R. L., & Domhoff, G. W. (1998). *Diversity in the power elite: Have women and minorities reached the top?* New Haven, CT: Yale University Press.

PART IV: INTERSECTIONS: UNIQUE CAREER PATHS TO STUDYING FAMILIES

Intersections: Unique Career Paths to Studying Families

Suzanne K. Steinmetz
Gary W. Peterson

Intersections, points at which divergent roads come together, is a common theme in this collection of essays. Perhaps a more descriptive title for these essays, however, might be "How did I get HERE from THERE?!!" That is, the authors, in a number of these essays, seem amazed at how their choices, often seemingly at odds with previous academic experiences, resulted in academic careers in which they now study individuals and families. Reading these essays allows one to understand how fortuitous or unpredictable experiences and relationships helped to shape their lives and careers. As one reads these accounts, the authors often seem to be trying to make sense of the important "intersections" that provided incremental and successively new directions to their lives. Specifically, the concept of "life intersection" refers to points in life when specific directions were taken, some involving serendipity, sudden obstacles, or based on advice that was given. Different directions were taken by these authors at these intersections due largely to disconnected events, unanticipated happenings, forced circumstances, and fortunate contacts with friends or mentors. These individuals often pursued new pathways when they came to successive intersections in their lives, a process that eventually led them HERE.

The pathways these authors pursued did not emerge from single-minded purposes, but were governed more by unanticipated circumstances. The stories that these individuals tell do not proceed according to clearly defined plots or some sense of purpose conveyed by more conventional novels about progress in life. Instead, the very process of telling their stories encourages them to assign meaning to their life experiences, communicate their identities more clearly, and socially construct what they believe has led them to where they are today.

Many of these authors note that the foundation of their interest in families was structured during their formative years, though they were not aware of this as a "cause" of career direction at the time. Gerald Handel, for example, describes how he grew up listening to the University of Chicago's *Roundtable* radio show and how his fascination with this particular academic institution grew during his youth. William Doherty, in turn, always liked to explore new ideas, and during his youth, the pursuit of fieldwork as a pastor helped him to clarify his interest in families from a secular perspective. Suzanne Steinmetz engaged in volunteer work as a youth and only later in her career obtained the necessary credentials to pursue this work as a professional. Trying different majors in college was also a prevalent theme for several authors. Ralph LaRossa, for example, considered English, psychology, and philosophy before selecting sociology. Hal Grotevant had to decide between chemistry and psychology; Mark Fine's major in economics was transformed into economics *and* psychology. Sheldon Stryker initially pursued social work, but found sociology courses more to his liking. Although Gary Peterson's undergraduate and MA work prepared him to teach history, family studies and sociology became his choice for doctoral work.

Other authors of these essays became disenchanted with alternative career goals and "somehow" ended up in family studies, human development or closely allied fields. For Laurence Steinberg, pragmatics, the need for a back-up plan when acceptance into medical school appeared questionable, resulted in entering graduate school in Human Development. Similarly, Schumm notes that he applied to both VISTA and Kansas State for graduate school; when VISTA failed to come through, he went to graduate school.

A common thread in all of these essays is the tendency for some of these scholars to go beyond traditional ideas in theory, research, and application. Doherty, for example, explored ideas in theology and philosophy and as a 14-year-old youth attempted to refute St. Thomas Aquinas's proofs about the existence of God. For both Schumm and Steinmetz, reviewing articles or papers by established scholars in a manner that questioned their findings helped to shape the family topics they eventually studied.

Gerald Handel, in his essay "Towards Understanding Families as Groups," notes that he entered the University of Chicago where he eventually received both his undergraduate and graduate degrees. Chicago's unique academic environment was expressed formally through a broad-based interdisciplinary PhD program provided through the Committee on Human Development in the College of Social Sciences. Although the only required course on the family was taken the semester that Ernest Burgess was on leave, Handel explored the theoretical linkages among Burgess's concept of 'family as a unity of interacting personalities,' Mead's concept of 'self,' and Cooley's concept of the 'family as a primary group.' The intersection of these diverse intellectual traditions provided by the vast interdisciplinary faculty at Chicago, combined with Burgess', Cooley's and Mead's concepts of family, eventually became evident in Handel's classic study *The Psychosocial Interior of the Family* (1967).

In "The Importance of Serendipity," Laurence Steinberg's essay, chance happenings are a major theme in his education and career. He entered Johns Hopkins University as an English major with a goal of becoming a writer but a course in personality during the second semester of his freshman year turned his interests toward psychology. After leaving Hopkins and continuing his undergraduate education at Vassar, however, he decided on pre-med, noting that medicine and law were the "two appropriate professions for a nice Jewish boy." However, he had no interest in becoming a lawyer. Completing pre-med with a major in psychology, the obligatory tours of the teaching hospitals during medical school interviews (and the greenish hue that appeared from the grim prospect of dealing with actual physical maladies in the future) resulted in rejection letters. On the advice of one of his apartment mates he applied to two graduate schools as a backup plan: Cornell University (where one of his roommates, Jay Belsky, would be attending), and Florida (where his other roommate's father was a professor). Admitted to both, he selected Cornell's Human Development and Family Studies program simply because of geography!

William Doherty's autobiography, "Continuities and Diversities," describes Doherty's academic life beginning as a Catholic seminarian with the goal of becoming a priest. Contrasting with his original career and life direction, Doherty is a practicing Unitarian-Universalist, married and a father of two adult children, and working in a secular university. The complicated path to this career emerged from his love of ideas when, with a friend, he read St. Thomas Aquinas's proofs about the existence of God and tried to refute them. Moreover, when a physics instructor broke the news that light was both a wave and a particle, depending on how you measured it, he had to recognize that, contrary to his early beliefs about the veracity of a single "right answer," this evidence of uncertainty in the world was both a shock and revelation. Like several of the authors in this collection, Bill's undergraduate and MA coursework was based in disciplines not immediately associated with the study of families (i.e., philosophy and theology). However, his pastoral fieldwork reinforced his desire to help families. He left the seminary and entered the PhD program in the Department of Child Development and Family Studies at the University of Connecticut.

In "Coming Full Circle: From Volunteer to Professional," Suzanne Steinmetz notes that during her youth she was a volunteer helper, researcher and writer. The life intersections she experienced involved a number of pragmatic decisions and eventually resulted in her becoming a professional in these areas. Although vocational testing indicated that she should pursue careers in healing, the ministry or engineering, elementary education was selected because it fit the needs of a divorced mother with three children more effectively. Subsequently she entered graduate school in sociology because a career in education had become less appealing to her. Illustrative of how unplanned experiences can be important influences are her reasons for choosing sociology over psychology–the strange, undesirable noises that emanated from the Psychology Department Laboratories were aversive to her. Having completed her undergraduate education on a vocational rehabilitation scholarship, her goal was to study vocational rehabilitation at Case Western Reserve University. Because fellowships were available in sociology but not in vocational rehabilitation, pragmatics dictated her decision to join the ranks of family sociologists.

In his essay, "The Social Construction of a Family Sociologist," Ralph LaRossa notes that he began his academic career with an interest either in becoming a lawyer (because he enjoyed watching Perry Mason) or a teacher. Teaching won out–but the subject matter changed over time. First English, then psychology, followed by philosophy (considered but discarded because it was "too philosophical") were considered–but a single fascinating sociology course sealed his fate. The New School for Social Research was selected for graduate work, primarily because Peter Berger taught there and his book *Invitation to Sociology* had been a major influence on LaRossa. LaRossa notes that, in selecting the methodology for his dissertation, a qualitative approach to the "social construction of reality" was easy. He also knew he wanted to study marriage based on conjoint in-depth interviews. However, he lacked a topic that would enable him to do a longitudinal study. He scanned family textbooks and got a crash course on pregnancy from his wife Maureen, who was a nurse. Thus, his entire career, in which he has studied transitions to motherhood and fatherhood, resulted from "a seemingly haphazard decision, made on a summer evening in 1974."

Since his elementary school days, Harold Grotevant had considered becoming a teacher. In his essay, "Orchestrating Differences: The Making of a Family Psychologist," he notes that he entered the University of Texas, Austin, with a career in teaching and research as a goal. However, the subject matter, either chemistry or psychology, was up for grabs. His choice was made easier by an inspiring teacher in his psychology course at the same time that a chemistry class became deadly boring for him. Following his undergraduate years, however, he also had to face the reality that deferments for marriage and graduate school had been cancelled and his draft number was very low. Consequently, he enlisted in the Naval Reserves, recognizing that, although his eyesight was too poor to become an officer, it was not bad enough to prevent him from being drafted. After two years of active duty, he enrolled in the graduate school at the University of Minnesota's Institute of Child Development. Reflecting on self and others, he notes that two experiences: the first as a minority youth (a Roman Catholic,Yankee outsider in a world of Southern Protestants in Texas) and the second, the diversity he experienced while in the Navy, influenced his interest in the development of identity–which became a lifelong career objective.

In "Reflections of a Psychologist Turned Relationship/Family Scientist," Mark Fine notes that he began in a single discipline (psychology) and gradually made a transition to multidisciplinary work, followed by interdisciplinary research, and, in rare moments, to transdisciplinary scholarships. While completing a major in economics, with plans to go to law school, he took a course in "The Helping Relationship" in the College of Human Ecology at Cornell University. The content of the course and the enthusiastic manner in which the course was taught was a turning point that motivated him to take as many psychology courses as possible and to graduate with majors in both economics and psychology. An interest in clinical psychology during his graduate work with an interest in intervention at the community and societal levels (rather than focusing on interventions with individuals) was fulfilled at The Ohio State University. His early years of graduate education were characterized by skepticism about the value of empirical research, and feelings that scientific research had often been used "against" those who participated in it. By his third and fourth year of graduate school, however, he became challenged to make a unique contribution through scholarly publications. The role of a scholar had firmly taken root.

Sheldon Stryker's essay, "Soft Ideas and Hard Methods: Family Sociologist or Social Psychologist?," specifically identifies a common theme found in several of these selections. "I became a sociologist in part by accident." Stryker draws this conclusion while describing how he entered the University of Minnesota assuming that he would become a "real doctor." Although poor eyesight resulted in his service records being stamped "limited service" and "no overseas duty," he subsequently spent three years as a company medic in a combat engineers outfit in France and Germany during World War II. This experience persuaded him that he was not cut out for medicine and he tried creative writing–but failed to impress his teachers. Stryker next considered social work because he had a friend who planned to do this and also because he recalled the suggestion that he "work with people," after he took a vocational test during his undergraduate years. Consequently he entered the Department of Sociology, where the social work program was located. Since he was a disabled veteran, he was eligible for an additional year of free education (5 instead of 4) and a larger stipend. Although neither becoming a sociologist nor entering graduate school was in his initial career plans, pragmatism suggested that "5 years of free education was obviously better than four," and the die was cast.

In his essay, "The Admiral's Son with an Independent Spirit," Walter Schumm notes that his initial career goal was to get a PhD in psychology, but his father dissuaded him, suggesting "any jerk can get a PhD in psychology." Deciding that a career in oceanography or astronomy would be a good choice, he entered The College of William and Mary because of its good physics and oceanography programs. He experienced roadblocks in these career goals–he easily became seasick and nearly flunked out of physics–but a new pathway opened when he flourished in the social science courses that he was taking. The selection of a graduate school and discipline was decided because Schumm "met some college girls who really liked the Family and Child Development Department at Kansas State University." Although K-State offered the best assistantship for a PhD, he declined this offer because this would make him ineligible to teach there. Purdue was selected for a PhD, and provided an opportunity to study methodology in depth and gain proficiency in teaching, research, and publishing.

The final essay in this collection, "Trying to Make Sense of Self: A Work in Progress," by Gary Peterson, is by another author who became a family scientist through the intersection of a unique set of events and people. John DeFrain, a childhood friend, initially got him interested in college and then influenced him to choose a particular doctoral program. A love of studying history resulted in both an undergraduate degree and a master's degree with the goal of teaching history. Although his initial goal for college was to just get Cs and occasional Bs, he also was determined to actually study what was assigned, not just what he enjoyed. The results were straight As, academic scholarships, and graduation with highest distinction. Following the completion of a master's degree, Peterson spent two years as an Army Officer, where he managed the post Officer's Club and related recreational facilities, and then taught at a junior high school in the Washington, D.C. area. Deciding that he needed a career change, he sought and took DeFrain's advice and entered the doctoral program in the Department of Child and Family Studies, University of Wisconsin-Madison. A year later, with the Madison program in major turmoil, this secularly oriented, politically liberal individual transferred to the doctoral program at Brigham Young University based primarily on a friendship with Randy Day and having heard Reuben Hill's lecture.

These contributors, therefore, seem to have "gotten here" through rather circuitous routes, driven by talents and ambitions, and highly influenced by intersecting paths or alternatives created by a specific course, book, lecture, scholarship, friend's advice, moment of failure, or a notable obstacle. The common theme is that the careers of these scholars were largely developed independently–a specific and integrated "plot" in their narratives that could not have been anticipated in advance. Perhaps this uncertainty in career avenues is actually the force that drew them to the study of families, a domain that is often stereotyped as one of constancy and stability. Instead of such homeostatic qualities, however, the compelling aspect of family life for these scholars may be that of constant change, uncertainty, and most of all, the mystery that is so evident within the realm of families.

Toward Understanding Families as Groups

Gerald Handel

KEYWORDS. Autobiography, family worlds, social psychology of family, sibling relations

INTRODUCTION

I am interested in the different ways that families can be families, the ways in which the members construct a family life. My approach to families is based on two assumptions:

- First, that families are consequential for their members.
- Second, that families function as groups, and the consequences of family membership derive from the way the family group functions.

My own work and research have focused on intact two-parent American families with their own biological children during the child-rearing years, but the concepts I have developed are applicable to other kinds of families and to families in at least some other societies as well. Adopted children, remarried parents, step- and half-siblings, two-job or two-career parents, gay or lesbian parents–all of these characteristics introduce variations different from the families I studied, but all of these kinds of families constitute groups and therefore the two assumptions apply. (A childless couple is not a group but a dyad, and the study of childless couples therefore belongs to a neighboring domain. However, the birth or adoption of a first child changes a couple into a three-person group. As Theodore Caplow [1968], building on ideas of Georg Simmel, emphasized, this change is a very significant one. Although there has been research on the impact of a first birth on the parents, there have been, to my knowledge, few, if any, studies of how these three-person family groups develop their structures and cultures following the arrival of a child.)

The kind of family unit that has been the focus of my research and writing begins with two people deciding that they mean something to each other, joining together, having children, and creating a distinctive group. The family generates its own local culture, even as the members are creating their patterns of interaction, of mutual involvement, of affection and antagonism, conflict and support. I arrived at this view of families late in my graduate studies, but I think there were probably some factors in my background that may have predisposed me to think this way.

SOME PERSONAL BACKGROUND

Differences Among Families

I became aware of differences among families when I was five or six years old. I had a chum who lived across the street in the neighborhood of small houses in Cleveland, Ohio, where I was born and grew up. He and I were both the same age, but whereas I was the older of two children, he was the younger of two. What to me was unusual, however, was that his older brother was about 14 or 15 years older than he was. His brother was a man who went to work, and I remember thinking then that it was odd that a kid has a brother who's a grown man. Another difference between us was that he had an uncle, aunt and cousin who lived a few houses away from us on our street. My nearest aunt, uncle, and cousins lived in Dayton, a city 200 or so miles away. A third difference became apparent in this way: sometimes we would sit on our front stoop, be a little bored, not know what to do, and one of us would suggest to the other, "Let's trade foods." Each would go into his own house and come out with two of something. I usually came out with items such as two bunches of grapes, two cookies, or two apples. He often came out with something that was totally unknown in our household–two pieces of white buttered bread sprinkled with sugar. In our house, white bread was used only for toast in the morning. When we ate bread at other times we ate rye bread baked in a neighborhood bakery. In fact, in our house, my mother never used the term white bread; she always referred to it as toast bread. My recollection is that I was very fond of peanut butter and jelly sandwiches, but they were always made on toasted bread. And there was a fourth difference, and that was that my friend, Howard, had a Christmas tree and an electric train that was set up around it, and I would be invited in at the Christmas season to see his electric train. In our Jewish household, we did not have a Christmas tree, and I did not have an electric train. So these differences between our two families made me vividly aware of the differences among families.

Howard and I lived across the street from each other. We were in the same grade, often walked to school together, walked home from school together, and yet there were these differences. I recall a feeling, I don't know how to label it exactly, when he and I would be playing in the street after school and look up and there would be his older brother, mustached, smoking a pipe, walking home from work at his factory job. I still remember that he worked at the Eaton Axle Company (now the Eaton Corporation). I did not think much about these differences over the years, and yet I feel certain that my awareness of them at an early age probably contributed something to my understanding of the world and sensitized me to the different ways that families can be families.

Relatives

Let me elaborate on a point about my aunt, uncle, and cousins who lived 200 or so miles away. This was the period before we had super highways and before air travel was commonplace. We visited them or they visited us, about once a year; it was a seven-hour train trip or seven-hour automobile trip on the two-lane highways of that time. In the Cleveland area, in distant neighborhoods, there were some relatives of my father, cousins of his generation, but they were not first cousins. We might visit them once or twice a year or they might visit us infrequently. They had children who would have been, perhaps, my second or third cousins. The visiting was between my parents and their parents. The children almost never came and were seldom home when I accompanied my parents; and there was never any personal relationship among us. While technically they were kin in our metropolitan area, I was scarcely acquainted with these cousins.

I grew up with a sense of our family as a relatively self-contained unit, what I later learned was called an isolated nuclear family. I did not grow up with a strong sense of kinship. While I was always extremely fond of my aunt and uncle and cousins in Dayton, and always delighted to visit them or have them visit us, it was a once-a-year celebratory occasion, not a matter of daily life or weekly routine. I also had some cousins in New York on my mother's side (the Dayton family were my father's relatives). I was also very fond of them but we saw them no more than once a year, at most. Again, such trips were special occasions, not part of ordinary life. For me, then, family living was household based. I never had a sense of being part of a vital and interactive kinship system as a personal experience, although I was aware of kinship ties in another way.

My father had had a brother in Europe who died. That brother had five children. At some point during my childhood or adolescence I learned that my father, who in the 1920s was a moderately successful entrepreneur, part owner of a small business that he had built up, had sent boat tickets to these five children to bring them to the United States. One of the five returned the ticket and did not come to this country, choosing to remain because he had been admitted to the University of Cracow in Poland, something which was extremely rare for a Jew because of stringent admissions quotas. The other four, three girls and a boy, did come. The boy, the youngest of the four, who was ten or so years older than I, lived in our house for a couple years when I was about seven, before going to live with our aunt in Dayton. One of the girls developed tuberculosis and died; I never met her. One lived in Dayton and I saw her briefly every other year or so. The third I met only once when I was an adult. So I was a little envious of my friend Howard who could go in and out of his aunt and I uncle's house on the same block, and had a cousin–their daughter–who occasionally played with us. He had another house that he could go in and out of at will, whereas I did not grow up with a sense of a closely connected kinship system. Relatives were geographically distant, we saw them occasionally, and for me my family was my father, my mother, my younger brother, and myself.

My grandparents all died in Europe. I never met them so I never knew any grandparents. I was never told much about them, and I never knew anything about relatives earlier in time than my own grandparents. We were a two-generation family in my experience. My parents were born and grew up in the Austro-Hungarian Empire, in the province known as Galicia. When I was growing up, that was part of Poland, the Austro-Hungarian Empire having been destroyed after its defeat in World War I.

My father had a younger brother who still lived with his wife and children in the village my father emigrated from. I recall my father receiving an occasional letter from him in the late '30s. The family was murdered during the Holocaust, Hitler's program to exterminate the Jews. On a visit to Yad Vashem, the memorial center for victims of the

Holocaust in Jerusalem, Israel, I discovered a document that identified the extermination year as 1942. The cousin who returned the boat ticket also perished in the Holocaust.

My mother had an older brother who lived in Vienna, Austria, with his wife and son. In 1934, when I was 10 years old, we were supposed to pay them a visit. I recall that my uncle sent my parents a cable saying that we should not come because of the turmoil in the streets. The Chancellor of Austria had just been assassinated by rising Nazi groups, and my uncle indicated that he could hear shooting in the street outside their apartment. So we never went.

I still remember vividly March 12 or 13, 1938. When I came home from school, my mother was glued to the radio listening to an eyewitness news account describing Adolf Hitler's Nazi army marching into Austria (on the 12th) and into Vienna, the capital (on the 13th), wildly cheered by crowds as he incorporated Austria into the rising Nazi state. The anxiety on my mother's face was evident.

My parents made efforts to rescue my uncle and his family. My parents were able to get my cousin out of Austria and into the United States in the fall of 1938. I do not know why they could not bring his parents, who made plans to escape to Shanghai, China, the only place that would grant them asylum. My aunt died before they could leave. My uncle did manage to escape to Shanghai, where there was a colony of about 20,000 European Jews who found refuge there during World War II. My uncle came to the U.S. after the war in 1946, and he died two years later at the age of 82.

My father had moved to Cleveland from New York soon after the end of World War I. With a partner he opened a delicatessen; they prospered sufficiently that they left the retail business and established a firm that manufactured and distributed delicatessen products. This business was moderately successful. It managed to survive the initial impacts of the Depression which began in 1929, but in 1935, due to a variety of circumstances, my father lost the business.

One of the contributing factors was my father's illness, which had begun in 1934 and despite treatment was not getting better. He lost faith in his doctor and decided that he had to seek other help, selecting the Mayo Clinic in Rochester, Minnesota, where his illness was diagnosed and he had surgery. He later explained to me that at the time of his illness his business was the target of a hostile takeover. His illness prevented him from doing battle as he would have wanted. He felt compelled to sell his interest for a fraction of its worth because he was concerned that he might not survive his trip to the Mayo Clinic. If this were to happen, and the issue was not settled, my mother, brother, and I would have been left with almost no financial resources. To salvage something, he got what he could for his share to make sure that there would be something for the family to live on. He recovered from his illness and started, in succession, a couple of businesses that did not succeed. From 1935, when I was 11 years old, until 1945, when my father died, the family was in considerably reduced economic circumstances. We experienced what I would later come to understand as some downward mobility. My parents always did manage to have some income, but they had to struggle for it. Some of the strain was evident to me. Fortunately, our house was paid for, so that was not in jeopardy. My father always managed to have a car, but whereas he had always bought new cars when I was very young, the two cars that he bought after 1935 were both used cars.

STUDY AND WORK AT THE UNIVERSITY OF CHICAGO

The University

During the years I was in high school, The University of Chicago used to broadcast every Sunday on an NBC national radio network a half-hour program called "The University of Chicago Roundtable." I listened to it quite regularly. Week after week, two or three professors, with an occasional outside guest–a statesman or other public figure–would discuss a topic of the day. I found these discussions fascinating, became intrigued with The University of Chicago, and developed a strong desire to enroll. I was admitted, earned an AB from The College and stayed on to earn AM and PhD from the Committee on Human Development. At that time, Chicago was organized somewhat differently from most universities, and its organization–and atmosphere–influenced the kind of work I have done.

Under Robert Hutchins, who became its president in 1930 at the age of 29 after having become Dean of the Yale Law School at 27, the bachelor's degree was normally awarded to students who entered as high school graduates after two years instead of four, as at other colleges. (Students could enter The College after two years of high school, but only a small number did.) The academic year was divided into four quarters; courses designed as year-long courses were usually given as a sequence in the Autumn, Winter, and Spring Quarters. The curriculum was largely prescribed.

In addition to a course in English Composition, the student took four year-long courses the first year, one each in the social sciences, humanities, biological sciences, and physical sciences, The next year, the student took follow-up courses in three of those subjects, plus a philosophy of science course. Grades of record were based not on quarterly exams, which were advisory, but on a 6-hour comprehensive examination at the end of the year. These were designed by a Board of Examiners and graded anonymously. Normally, one took four "comps" at the end of each year. The undergraduate courses were designed by a staff for each course, and all were interdisciplinary. While some segments of each course and the associated readings were specified as offering a particular discipline's perspective, the focus in social science was on looking at problems from the perspectives of several disciplines.

For example, the second-year social science course dealt with the problem of freedom and order in society, and we looked at this problem from the perspectives of sociology, psychology, economics, political science and history. One of the features that had attracted me to Chicago was that class attendance was optional. I still remember then Dean of Students Norman Maclean (decades later celebrated for his novella *A River Runs Through It,* and the film based on it) saying at a freshman orientation lecture, "We invite you to drop in on some of our classes and meet some of our professors, but if you prefer to stay in your room and read the Encyclopedia Britannica, published by The University of Chicago, you are free to do so."

The Courses

The teaching was generally so good, however, that I almost never cut class. Also, in the social sciences and humanities, no textbooks were used, and learning to think about the relationships among diverse original sources was greatly facilitated by class discussion and the weekly lectures. The College Social Sciences faculty at that time included a number of young instructors and assistant and associate professors who went on to distinguished careers, including Daniel Bell, Reinhard Bendix, Sebastian de Grazia, Morton Grodzins, Joseph Gusfield, Bert Hoselitz, Morris Janowitz, Philip Rieff, David Riesman, Edward Shils, Milton Singer. All of them have written notable works.

Possibly the most erudite in this very erudite cluster was a man who never published much, Gerhard Emil Otto Meyer. While some students were put off by the combination of his stammer and thick German accent, he was widely admired and beloved for his erudition, gentleness, patience, and wisdom. Trained as an economist, his explanations drew easily and unostentatiously on history, sociology, psychology, philosophy, and literature. Although students were assigned at registration to a particular discussion section for a course, they were at liberty to attend any they wished.

I felt fortunate to be assigned to his section for three successive quarters, and there were many auditors. After class, he could stand for half an hour or longer in the corridor or outside the building continuing a class discussion with a student pursuing an issue, and many did. I once asked him a question and he said "I'll bring you some books," and next time he came with an armful of his books from home. At a time when science and scholarship were widely thought of as the pursuit of truth, I heard from Gerhard Meyer that our goal should be the pursuit of truthfulness rather than truth. (Indeed, engraved in gothic letters on the outside wall of Bond Chapel, across the courtyard from Cobb Hall where our class met, was "Ye shall know the truth and the truth shall make you free," a sentiment that I found inspirational, but Meyer held out a more complex view. The juxtaposition here is mine; I don't think that Meyer was speaking directly to this religious aphorism but rather to an issue of arrogant truth claims in some classroom context that I do not recall.)

Graduate Years: The Committee on Human Development

As I was approaching my bachelor's degree I had to consider what to do next. I certainly wanted to stay at Chicago and work for a Master's degree, usually a three-year program for those who graduated from The College. I was most interested in both psychology and sociology but was not disposed to commit myself to one department over the other. There was a third way. Chicago had a unique program that joined those two fields together with parts of anthropology, biology, and education. I applied to and was accepted by the Committee on Human Development, the oldest of several interdepartmental degree-granting committees at Chicago. Its focus was the social, psychological, and biological factors influencing the growth and development of the human person, and that's what I wanted to understand.

It had begun in 1930 as the Committee on Child Development and changed its name in 1940 as it broadened its attention to the entire life course and life cycle. It was established by professors of sociology, psychology, anthropology, biology, education, and home economics. (Child development in the early days was located in the Department of Home Economics.) By enrolling in H.D., as it was known, I was continuing the interdisciplinary approach to education that I received in the College, but there was a difference. Unlike the College curriculum, which was closely prescribed, in the H.D. curriculum the only prescribed courses were one each in physiology, genetics, and statistics.

The Committee had no courses of its own when I began, although a year or so later it initiated a three-quarter sequence that covered infancy and childhood the first quarter, adolescence during the second, and adulthood and aging the third. Otherwise, the student prepared for an MA Qualifying Examination by taking a judicious selection of courses from a suggested list in psychology, sociology, anthropology, education, and home economics. The fields of knowledge covered by the exam were published in an Outline of Topics in Human Development. Each student was responsible for developing his or her own integration of the diverse material.

All the departments and committees in the Division of the Social Sciences collaborated to organize a three-quarter sequence entitled "The Scope and Methods of the Social Sciences," under the chairmanship of Bert Hoselitz, a sociologically minded economist. I took this course but do not recall whether it was required by the Committee. Hoselitz was a wonderful person who was brilliant, unpretentious, accessible, delightful to talk to, and charming with flashes of merry wit.

When I began my studies in H.D., there was only one course on the family in the Sociology Department and it was usually taught by Ernest W. Burgess, who was also a member of the Executive Committee of the Committee on Human Development. He was widely respected and his eminence was established. However, I had heard him give a lecture or two and did not find him very stimulating, so I took the course during a summer quarter, when it was taught by Svend Riemer, a Visiting Professor from the University of Wisconsin.

We used the Burgess and Locke textbook, *The Family,* published in 1945. In checking through this volume, which I still have, I found, to my surprise, that the book does not cite Burgess's 1926 paper, " The Family as a Unity of Interacting Personalities." I presume that I encountered this paper and the concept embodied in its title in the family course, but I cannot be certain. In any event, at some point in my studies the title and concept registered firmly with me. I became aware that the concept made a lot of sense, was congruent with Cooley's concept of the family as a primary group and George Herbert Mead's concept of the self as produced through interaction. But I also became aware that while it received great respect and reiteration, no research that I read was based on it. The research studies that I read in various courses seemed to split the family; a study dealt either with marriage or with mother-child relationships.

I can't recall a study that put children in their families with fathers, mothers and siblings except Allison Davis and John Dollard's (1940) *Children of Bondage*. The concept of the family as a unity of interacting personalities became a fundamental idea in my own thinking. It influenced my subsequent work which resulted in the book called *Family Worlds*, co-authored with Robert D. Hess (1959); my edited anthology, *The Psychosocial Interior of the Family* (1967b); and a paper that I included in it, "The Analysis of Correlative Meaning: The TAT in the Study of Whole Families" (1967a).

I encountered the ideas of Cooley and Mead in a social psychology course taught in the sociology department. It was usually taught by Herbert Blumer, who had been Mead's student, and coined the term symbolic interactionism. However, in a couple of lectures he had given in the Hoselitz course and others I formed an impression that he was hypercritical of everybody else's work, and he insisted we should do better, without making clear how one could do better. On the basis of that youthful judgment I avoided studying with a man who was already considered a major thinker. Instead, when Blumer left for a year, I took the course with Guy Swanson who at that time was either working on or had just finished his PhD. I remember his course as one of the best that I took–thoughtful, lucid, well organized, a solid introduction to the subject and to the ideas of Cooley and Mead that also later entered into the way I think about families. I emphasize "later," because at this time, my third or fourth year in college, I had not yet developed a focused interest in families, much less had any notion about how the ideas of Cooley and Mead could be used in studying them.

A number of other teachers stand out in various ways. Although he was not a member of the Committee, I particularly admired anthropologist Robert Redfield, with whom I took two courses. He was skillful and challenging, without being alienating, in leading discussions. His lectures were carefully crafted and he spoke with a crisp conciseness in sentences of crystal clarity.

W. Lloyd Warner, who held a triple appointment in Anthropology, Sociology and H.D., was widely influential in the Committee's work. His research and teaching on the importance of social class in all aspects of American life influenced many H.D. students. Hess and I used social class as an important criterion in selecting families for our study. Warner wrote an Introduction to *Workingman's Wife: Her Personality,*

World, and Life Style (1959), co-authored by Lee Rainwater, Richard P. Coleman and myself, all of us Warner students.

William E. Henry, who had been the third person to receive a Human Development PhD, was an assistant professor in the Committee and was doing exciting work with the TAT, taking this projective technique that had been invented for individual personality assessment and showing how it could be used to understand groups. TAT stories were part of the data gathered from the families that Hess and I studied. Later, building on Henry's work, I developed the concept of the analysis of correlative meaning and published "The Analysis of Correlative Meaning: The TAT in the Study of Whole Families" in my anthology, *The Psychosocial Interior of the Family* (Handel, 1967b).

Robert Havighurst, a formidably productive scholar, was the chief administrator of the Committee and although he was reserved I felt that he was very supportive of me. I obtained my first substantial research experience as one of his many research assistants on a project studying moral character development in adolescence.

One of the compelling teachers in the Committee was Bruno Bettelheim, a psychoanalyst who directed the Orthogenic School, a treatment center for severely disturbed children. He had an intimidating, confrontational style, but he was brilliant, original, and provocative. I took two courses with him. I found myself then grappling with the tension between the psychoanalytic way of thinking, which saw early experience as very influential throughout the course of life and the symbolic interactionist perspective, particularly as embodied in George Herbert Mead's concept of emergence (now commonly designated the social constructionist perspective), which understands human activity as arising from and shaped by interactions in the current situation.

At first, I was very inclined to the strong version of determinism that early psychoanalysis offered. I began to move away from it, pulled not only by Mead, but also by the appearance in 1950 of Erik Erikson's *Childhood and Society*. This was a new version of psychoanalysis, one that recognized the importance of culture and social structure, and comprised the entire life course and the key inflection points at life stages beyond childhood. Whatever its limitations, Erikson's theory is still, to the best of my knowledge, the only substantial theory of the entire life course.

It is clear that people do change throughout the course of their lives. Socialization is a lifelong process. Nevertheless, I do not think that we are yet able to formulate with any clarity concepts which explain great degrees of change or the limits of change. There is an open-endedness to the life course, but there are also constraints. Some of them are situational, but some of them are interior constraints, interior to the person and based on that person's experiences and interpretation of those experiences. Yet to be adequately described and understood are the ways in which constraint and option are genetically encoded in DNA.

While working toward my master's degree, I decided that I wanted to train in clinical psychology, which was offered through the Department of Psychology and was available to H.D. students. First, I took a year-long proseminar in general psychology and then went through the clinical training program. I had two internships in clinical psychology, a 6-month internship at the Institute for Juvenile Research (IJR), a long-established child guidance clinic, and then later a year's internship at Michael Reese Hospital in Chicago. During my last year of study toward the PhD, I was becoming more interested in the family field and during the Autumn Quarter of that last year I took a course on family interaction with Professor Nelson Foote who had come to the University a year or so earlier. While I enjoyed my clinical training, which consisted entirely of psychological testing and analysis of the results, since only psychiatrists then did therapy in Chicago, I decided that I was not interested in a clinical career. I had wanted the training primarily to gain understanding of personality, although such a career was also in my mind as a possible option.

During my year at Reese I had some conversations with Robert D. Hess, who had been a couple years ahead of me in the H.D. program and had been appointed an Instructor in the Committee. I went to him in his capacity as advisor to doctoral students to explore what I might do after finishing my doctoral course work. Both at IJR and at Reese I had sometimes been part of clinical teams that analyzed the personalities of several members of a family. (This was before the invention of family therapy.) That experience, my interest in child development and personality, Cooley's concept of families as primary groups, Burgess's concept of the family as a unity of interacting personalities together influenced my conversations with Hess, who was then working primarily on problems of cognitive development with Allison Davis, an anthropologist on the Committee and in the Department of Education. After a couple of conversations, Hess and I agreed to study child development in the context of whole families. We wrote a grant proposal to the National Institute of Mental Health to study how parents influence their children. Hess was principal investigator and I was co-principal investigator. When the grant came through, I was appointed Research Associate in Human Development. We intended to develop a new methodology.

To understand how parents influence their children, we needed to obtain data from each parent and each child and to understand them as a family. This was a departure from the prevailing practice of studying families by interviewing wives only or understanding child development by gathering data from one child in a family and its mother.

We proposed to study "ordinary families" selected from the community. We also referred to them as "non-clinical families." Neither Hess nor I was prepared to study children under age six. Thus, we selected families with either two or three children between the ages of six and 18. We believed that at age six children could be interviewed. We were trying to understand child development in the context of family functioning. Based on work of Robert J. Havighurst and Allison Davis, as well as others, we knew that there tended to be social class differences in the ways that parents socialize their children. We were also aware of ways in which children resist parental guidance and direction and the many cross-currents and conflicts in families.

We were trying to find some way to integrate the many relevant considerations and to grasp this complex of family functioning. We experienced many frustrations regarding our methodology, an entirely novel strategy, with no guidelines in the literature. Cooley, Mead, and Burgess provided sensitizing concepts but no procedures for applying them to actual data from actual families. Fortunately, the Committee on Human Development was an institutional setting in which working on novel ideas and novel approaches was expected and encouraged. There was no pressure or institutional norm to use well established methodologies.

FAMILY WORLDS

While Hess and I experienced a fair bit of anguish as we struggled with our material, eventually we came to some closure. The first products of our work were two papers: Hess was the primary analyst and author of one (Hess & Handel, 1956), and I was the main author of a much briefer one (Handel & Hess, 1956). The latter was originally presented in 1955 at the Annual Symposium of the Committee on Human Development. It was a first groping toward a qualitative analysis, and it became the first publication to bear my name. The major fruit of our work was a book called *Family Worlds*. The manuscript was submitted to The University of Chicago Press, which sent it to two anonymous readers. We later discovered that one was Reuben Hill, already one of the leading family sociologists, and the other was M. Robert Gomberg, a social worker who was associated with Nathan Ackerman who was in the early stages of developing the new field of family therapy. Both recommended that the work be accepted for publication, and it was (Hess & Handel, 1959). Hill suggested some revisions, which we made. We found out that he was one of the readers when the book came out because the dust jacket carried a quotation from his review: "Breaks new ground in the social psychology of the family." This was a most heartening evaluation.

The book was generally well reviewed (Gould, 1959; Henry, 1961; Jackson, 1962; Kerchoff, 1959; Komarovsky, 1959; Maretzki, 1959; Osborn, 1960; Schroeder, 1960). Although there were no negative reviews, we received a very lukewarm review from Harvey Locke (1959) in the *American Sociological Review*. A paperback edition with a new preface was published by The University of Chicago Press in 1974. With these two editions, the book stayed in print for 30 years, until January of 1990. A German translation was published in 1975, with a 20-page analytic epilogue written by the translators. In 1995, the 1974 edition was reissued by University Press of America.

Recently, I attempted to itemize the ways in which our book broke new ground in the social psychology of the family, and I list them here.

1. Building on Cooley's, Mead's, and Burgess's prefigurative ideas, we conceptualized five processes of family functioning that constituted new social psychological theory of the family. While not a complete theory nor aspiring to be, these processes were a notable advance in showing how families construct their lives.

2. We showed the efficacy and importance to families of Mead's concept that individual members of a group each have their own perspective. The individually obtained data made it possible to demonstrate that family members–each child and each parent–have individual perspectives.

3. The study was one of the first to include fathers as socializing agents. It also was the very first to include both fathers and mothers in the same study, and to indicate how their relationship as husband and wife influenced the socialization of their children.

4. The study's data and theoretical formulations incorporated sibling relationships into the socializing process within families.

5. Children were considered as active interactants in their families, as agents, and not simply as recipients of parental actions. We documented initiatives that their parents disapproved as well as their conformity and resistance to parental initiatives.

6. Families were conceptualized concurrently in psychological, sociological, and social psychological terms. All families studied were of northwest European ancestry. This was purposeful because we wanted to control for ethnic variation, that is, to understand variation within a population that was not ethnically diverse. We also selected families of working-class, middle-class, and upper-middle-class status because we were interested in social class variation. But we did not operate with a concept of *the* working-class or *the* middle-class family. We were cognizant of variation within status levels. We considered that each member of a family had personality distinctiveness as well as resemblances to other members and that each family had to construct its own life partly by negotiating these differences and similarities.

7. We formulated five social psychological processes that are constitutive of family life:

a. Establishing a pattern of separateness and connectedness.
b. Establishing a satisfactory congruence of images through the exchange of suitable testimony.
c. Evolving modes of interaction into central family concerns or themes.
d. Establishing the boundaries of the family's world of experience.
e. Dealing with significant biosocial issues of family life, as in the family's disposition to evolve definitions of male and female and of older and younger.

8. In a departure from the prevailing view of culture as a property only of a society or a major segment of it, *Family Worlds* introduced and documented the idea that each family can be regarded as having its own local culture.

9. The data collection procedures included projective tests, specifically the Thematic Apperception Test and sentence completion tests. These instruments reflected our view that some aspects of one's beliefs about oneself and others are more easily communicated indirectly than by interview.

10. *Family Worlds* illustrated the importance of qualitative methodology, and, more specifically, the value of case study methodology in family research. The value has at least two aspects:

a. Growth of knowledge is not simply a matter of accumulating generalizations but also of careful specification, knowing what significant phenomena are lost in the process of generalization;

b. What we need to know cannot adequately be encompassed in a framework of relating dissected variables to each other; we require studies of functioning units which try to capture and comprehend the nature of the unit in its operating complexity.

SUBSEQUENT WORK

Workingman's Wife

After I completed my work with Hess, I wanted to stay in Chicago. I joined Social Research, Inc., a small consulting firm that had been established some years earlier by Professors W. Lloyd Warner, William E. Henry, and Burleigh B. Gardner. Gardner was an anthropologist who had been on the faculty of The University of Chicago School of Business. One of the senior staff members in the firm was Lee Rainwater, who recognized that some of our projects for clients yielded data that, with permission, could form the basis of books written for a social science audience. He took the lead in seeking to utilize some of our work in this way.

The first result of this effort was a book by Rainwater, Richard P. Coleman, and myself entitled *Workingman's Wife* (1959), a study of working-class housewives that grew out of research we did for Macfadden Publications, publisher of *True Story* magazine. Their readers included several million working-class housewives, whose lives they wanted to understand better. After submitting our reports to the sponsor, they allowed us to use the data for a book which we addressed to the social science community.

While working at Social Research, Inc., on my own time I continued my efforts to develop a concept of a social psychology of families, based on two premises:

1. Conceptualizing families as groups of interacting members,
2. Obtaining data from each member of the families studied.

In my student days, I had never heard anyone refer to the social psychology of families; indeed, the term is not much used even now. Nonetheless, I felt that Cooley's concept of families as primary groups and Burgess's concept of the family as a unity of interacting personalities had foreshadowed such a discipline or field or area, and I was gratified by Reuben Hill's use of the term to characterize *Family Worlds*.

After finishing my dissertation and getting my PhD in 1962, I took two steps while still at Social Research, Inc. I wrote a paper entitled "Psychological Study of Whole Families," which was an attempt at a comprehensive critical review of the extant literature–psychological, sociological, anthropological, psychiatric–that could be construed as contributory to such a field. In January 1965 it was published in *Psychological Bulletin,* one of the official journals of the American Psychological Association (Handel, 1965). The response to that paper was staggering; I received more than 300 requests for reprints from readers in 12 countries. Eventually, it was reprinted in seven anthologies, including one in Japanese.

The Anthology

My next challenge was to prepare an anthology of writings that would present this new field, the social psychology of families, to a larger audience of professionals and students. In 1967, Aldine published *The Psychosocial Interior of the Family: A Sourcebook for the Study of Whole Families,* which included selections from sociology, psychology, child development, psychiatry, and anthropology (Handel, 1967a). In my introductory essay and introductions to the various sections, I tried to indicate the nature of this interdisciplinary field. A third edition was published in 1985; a fourth edition, co-edited with Gail Whitchurch, was published in 1994. Of course, the family as an institution has greatly changed in the years since I began my work.

There are more forms of family today than there were in the 1950s, or at least the varieties are more noticeable. Although some modifications of procedure may be required, the facts that nuclear families are now more likely to have two employed spouse-parents or that divorce and remarriage have increased do not, in my view, render obsolete the approach to the social psychology of families that I have promulgated over the years. For example, in the case of children of divorced and remarried parents who divide their time between two new parental households, it may be necessary to study both new families in order to understand the children's family membership and participation. The goal remains always to understand families as groups by taking account of the perspectives and impact of all the members. Who is included in "all" varies with the family composition and with the research problem. In families with two parents, whether they are together or separated, and with more than one child the methodological requirement is to study and consider spousal, parent-child, and sibling relationships concurrently as mutually relevant.

To a significant extent, the study of families today remains divided between a spousal axis and a parent-child axis. Researchers interested in child development for a long time studied it in terms of mother-child relationships. Some years ago they added what I call a parallel science of father-child relationships because such studies were not conducted in the same families as mother-child studies. More recently there have been a few studies in which mother-child and father-child relationships in the same family are considered, but not much attention is paid to the marriage as an influence on children. On the other hand, researchers interested in marriage show little interest in the relation of marriage to parent-child relationships. The fact that husbands and wives who are also parents of young children inhabit a shared household over an extended period of time and constitute a small group has become the foundation of the new field of family therapy that began about the same time that Hess and I began our work in 1952, but has had only modest impact in family studies outside family therapy.

Despite the fact that Cooley's concept of primary groups is discussed in virtually every introductory text in sociology, it has not been used as a basis for sustained sociological study of families. Moreover, it has no currency in the child development field, which seems unable as yet to utilize the concept of family group.

MOVING ON

After I had been at Social Research, Inc. for several years, the three people I worked with most closely left within a short time. Sidney Levy, whom I had known since our undergraduate days together in The College as well as later in H.D., went to Northwestern University as Professor of Behavioral Science in Marketing. Lee Rainwater went to Washington University in St. Louis as Professor of Sociology and director of a huge project studying black families living in public housing. Ira Glick decided he did not want to run an organization and set up shop as an independent consultant. The work had begun to be stale for me and, although I had become a Vice President, the organization lost much attraction after these three departures. After some casting about, I joined the Center for Urban Education, a federally sponsored educational research laboratory in New York City. Before a year was out, I was invited to join the faculty of the Sociology Department at The City College of the City University of New York, and I accepted. Two years later I was elected to the faculty of the PhD Program in Sociology in the City University's Graduate School.

Studying Siblings

I had retained a full set of all the interviews from my project with Hess, and there was one more paper I wanted to write if I could. I wanted to arrive at a better understanding of sibling relationships. My relationship with my own brother had, since childhood, not been good. In middle age I worked hard to repair damage for which I felt some responsibility, and in time our mutual comfort level rose substantially. My personal experience convinced me that sibling relationships are far more important in family life than family researchers, with a few exceptions, then recognized. I asked myself the question: Why do siblings in some families grow up to be friends while in other families they do not? Looking for clues, I studied the interviews from all the parents and all the children in the 33 families of the Hess-Handel cluster.

My analysis of this material led me to identify four sibling issues on which families work, which I called equity, maturity, loyalty, and individuality. I discussed these issues in some detail and proposed that the answer to my question could be found in how families deal with them over an extended period of time. Since I did not have information on adult outcomes, my proposal can only be a hypothesis for future research. I hope that someone reading my sibling paper (which I wrote in two slightly different versions) will want to take up where I left off and pursue this topic. Although marriage and family have never been major areas of concentration in the CUNY doctoral program in Sociology, I did offer courses in family interaction for several years, and they did stimulate some dissertation work.

Colleagues' Use the Whole Family Methodology

The first dissertation I directed was by Juan-Luis Recio, a student from Spain, now a Professor of Sociology in the Universidad Complutense in Madrid. He used the Hess-Handel methodology, which I have since come to call "whole family methodology," and produced a substantial dissertation entitled " Family as a Unit and the Larger Society: Adaptation of Puerto Rican Migrant Families to a Suburban Mainland Setting." By interviewing both parents and all the children in many families he showed how the different community involvements (women with church, men with employers, children with school and peer group) resulted in different reactions to migration and consequent conflictful family interactions regarding initial hopes of returning to Puerto Rico with enough money saved to buy a house. Recio did a very thorough review of the migration literature and found that studies such as his which obtained the migration experiences of children and parents in their family units are very rare.

Edward Speedling, a medical sociology student, took my course, then followed with an independent reading course with me, and asked me to be on his dissertation committee. He studied the families of men who had suffered a heart attack, interviewing and observing family members both at the bedside and in their homes. His dissertation became a fascinating book, *Heart Attack: The Family Response at Home and in the Hospital* (Speedling, 1982).

Perhaps the greatest satisfaction for a researcher is knowing that one's work is useful for others in theirs. Studies such as Recio's and Speedling's, as well as Piotrkowski's *Work and the Family System* (1979), and Clark's *Family Life and School Achievement* (1982), have utilized the social psychological perspective that I have been discussing. All of them took the concepts and methods into new realms. In recent years I have been gratified by invitations to contribute discussions of my work to volumes devoted to these issues (Handel, 1991; 1996).

My hope is that the fruitfulness of this social psychological approach will become more widely recognized by researchers and that it will be more widely used.

AUTHOR NOTE

Gerald Handel, PhD, is Professor of Sociology, The City College and The Graduate Center, City University of New York.

I thank Marvin Sussman for inviting me to contribute to this volume, and Sue Steinmetz and Gary Peterson for carrying forward the project. My wife, Ruth, has been most helpful both in facilitating my computer use and in suggestions for improving my chapter.

REFERENCES

Burgess, E. W. (1926). The family as a unity of interacting personalities. *Family*, 7 (1), 3-9.

Caplow, T. (1968). *Two against one*. Englewood Cliffs, NJ: Prentice-Hall.

Clark, R. (1983). *Family life and school achievement*. Chicago: University of Chicago Press.

Davis, A. & Dollard, J. (1940). *Children of bondage*. Washington, DC: American Council on Education.

Erikson, E. (1950). *Childhood and society*. New York: W. W. Norton.

Gould, F. (1959). Review of Family Worlds. *Merrill-Palmer Quarterly*, 5, 4, 198-199.

Handel, G. (1965). Psychological study of whole families. *Psychological Bulletin*, 63 (1), 19-41.

Handel, G. (1967a). Analysis of correlative meaning: The TAT in the study of whole families. In G. Handel (Ed.) *The psychosocial interior of the family* (pp. 104-124). Chicago Aldine.

Handel, G. (Ed.) (1967b). *The psychosocial interior of the family*. Chicago: Aldine.

Handel, G. (1985). Central issues in the construction of sibling relationships. In G. Handel (Ed.). *The psychosocial interior of the family*, 3rd Ed (pp. 367-396). Hawthorne, NY: Aldine de Gruyter.

Handel, G. (1986). Beyond sibling rivalry: An empirically grounded theory of sibling relationships (pp. 105-122) in P. A. Adler & P. Adler (Eds.), *Sociological studies of child development*, Vol. 1. Greenwich, CT: JAI Press.

Handel, G. (1991). Case study in family research. In J. R. Feagin, A. M. Orum, & G. Sjoberg (Eds.), *A case for the case study* (pp. 244-268). Chapel Hill: University of North Carolina Press.

Handel, G. (1996). Family worlds and qualitative family research: Emergence and prospects of whole-family methodology. In J. F. Gilgun & M. B. Sussman (Eds.) *The methods and methodologies of qualitative family research* (pp. 335-348). New York: The Haworth Press, Inc.

Handel, G. & Hess, R. D. (1956). The family as an emotional organization. *Marriage and Family Living*, 18 (2) 99-101.

Henry, W.E. (1956). *The analysis of fantasy: The thematic apperception technique in the study of personality*. New York: Wiley.

Henry, J. (1961). Review of Family Worlds. *Harvard Educational Review*, 31, 3, 361-362.

Hess, R. D. & Handel, G. (1956). Patterns of aggression in parents and their children. *Journal of Genetic Psychology*.

Hess, R. D. & Handel, G. (1959). *Family Worlds*. University of Chicago Press. Paperback edition with new Preface 1974. Reissued 1995: Lanham, MD: University Press of America.

Hess, R. D. & Handel, G. (1975). *Familienwelten*. Dusseldorf, West Germany: Padagogischer Verlag Schwann. Translated by W. Loch, H. Paschen, & G. Priesemann.

Jackson, D.D. (1962). Review of *Family worlds. Journal of Nervous and Mental Disease*.

Kerchoff, A. C. (1959). Review of *Family worlds. Social Forces*, *38*, 2, 168-169.

Komarovsky, M. (1959). Review of *Family worlds. Marriage and Family Living*, *21*, 4, 399-400.

Locke, H. J. (1959). Review of *Family worlds. American Sociological Review*, *24*, 6, 904-905.

Maretzki, T. (1959). Review of *Family worlds. American Anthropologist*, *61*, 6,1105-1106.

Osborn, H. (1960). Review of *Family worlds. Social Work*, *5*, 1, 116-117.

Piotrkowski, C. (1979). *Work and the family system*. New York: Free Press.

Rainwater, L., Coleman, R. P., & Handel, G. (1959). *Workingman's wife: Her personality, world, and life style*. New York: Oceana.

Recio, J-L. (1975). Family as a unit and the larger society: *Adaptation of Puerto Rican migrant families to a suburban mainland setting*. PhD Dissertation, Graduate School, City University of New York.

Schroeder, D. (1960). Review of *Family Worlds. American Journal of Orthopsychiatry, 30*, 4, 845-846.

Speedling, E. J. (1982). *Heart attack: The family response at home and in the hospital*. New York: Tavistock.

The Importance of Serendipity

Laurence Steinberg

KEYWORDS. Autobiography, adolescence, parenting, serendipity, puberty

INTRODUCTION

I have no idea where my interest in the parent-adolescent relationship came from. Despite what you may think, it is certainly not an attempt to understand my own adolescence, because there is little there that requires any in-depth interpretation. I grew up in the 1950s and '60s in the affluent suburbs outside New York City, in a conventional Jewish middle-class household, the firstborn son of a business executive and housewife. My parents loved me, pushed me, nagged me, and, from the looks of old photographs, overfed me. I am told that my younger brother Andy and I fought constantly, but I cannot recall over what. Most of what I remember from my teenage years involves not my family, but my friends–driving around Westchester County, listening to "progressive rock" on WNEW-FM, playing poker during study hall, arguing about the relative value of various members of the New York Knicks, and laughing a lot, drinking and getting high at the home of whichever friend had parents who were out of town for the weekend. In the late 1960s, this is what Jewish middle-class suburban boys in New York did.

I have surprisingly few memories of family life during this time or, for that matter, during any of my childhood, which makes my interest in studying family relationships seem odd, when you think about it. A psychologist might be inclined to attribute my lack of childhood memories to some sort of massive repression, but I'm sure this is not the case. My lack of memories about my family life growing up is due to the simple fact that there is very little to remember. Life in our household was very routine, and little changed from one day to the next, except for what we ate for dinner, and even that didn't change all that much. Most of my friends who, as middle-aged adults, have vivid recollections of their family life had either a very wonderful or very terrible childhood. I had neither. Perhaps this is why I ended up specializing in the study of normal family relationships, rather than dysfunctional ones. My own adolescence was disgustingly normal.

I do remember that my mother and I went through a difficult period during my teenage years, where we seemed to be at each other's throat much of the time, but few of our conflicts ever escalated into anything worthy of detailed description. It was more the regularity of our bickering than the intensity of the fighting that bears comment. Our conflicts followed a highly structured routine: We would argue almost every afternoon at 5:00 or 5:30, usually about something having to do with dirt. (My mother's insistence on keeping the house clean had the quality of a crazed obsession, and one of my few vivid memories is of her inspecting our walls for finger smudges, with a bottle of something called Carbona Wall-Wipe and a rag in hand.) My father would come home from work at around 7:00 and listen to my mother's exaggerated complaints, whereupon I would receive an unemotional lecture from him in private on why it was more important to apologize to my mother than to be right. I would then offer an unfelt apology, which my mother would begrudgingly accept, and things would settle down in time for dinner. The next day, though, the cycle would begin again. It all makes perfect sense now that my doctoral dissertation examined the normative nature of mother-son conflict. My mother actually accused me of doing the study in order to get back at her. I think she was kidding, but you know what Freud said about jokes and the unconscious.

Getting Interested in Psychology

I did not enter college in 1970 intending to become either a psychologist or a professor. As a freshman at Johns Hopkins, I majored in English and had hopes of becoming a writer. The fact that I was terrible at it was only a minor impediment. I started to become interested in psychology during the second semester of my first year, because of a course in personality theory taught by Bob Hogan. Our final assignment in the course was to analyze Dick and Perry, the psychopathic killers in Truman Capote's *In Cold Blood,* and Hogan, in his comments on my paper, was very complimentary about my psychoanalytic skills. Hogan was an exceptionally charismatic and popular instructor, who bore a striking resemblance to one of the Smothers Brothers, in both physical appearance and comedic skill. I cannot recall whether it was his manner, the course content, his ten written words of encouragement at the bottom of my paper, or the combination of all three that hooked me. However, by the end of the semester I was ready to abandon the study of Victorian literature and Romantic poetry.

Hogan's class was one of the few high points in an otherwise miserable year at Hopkins. I transferred to Vassar as a sophomore in 1971. This was an enormously important turning point in my life, for Vassar was where I was introduced to academics as a profession. In much the same way as I was drawn to psychology because of my fascination with Bob Hogan as a person, I was drawn to a career in academics because of the personal relationships I formed with several of my professors there, most importantly, Anne Constantinople and Vicki Raeburn. I had never known college professors before–growing up, none of my friends' parents nor any of my parents' friends were professors–and I envied the life they led, or at least the life I thought they led. To be sure, much of what I imagined the professorial life to be was my own romanticized version of how professors lived. But as a naive and impressionable 20-year-old, I identified intensely with what I imagined the academic life to be. I started smoking a pipe and wearing a lot of tweed.

My interest in a career in academic psychology conflicted with my upbringing, which was decidedly polyester, and not tweedy. Which is why, shortly after arriving at Vassar, I decided to go pre-med. I can only explain this by saying that I was raised to believe that there were simply two professions that were appropriate for nice Jewish boys, and I had no interest in becoming a lawyer. The truth of the matter was that I had no real interest in becoming a doctor either. Still, I completed the pre-med curriculum while majoring in psychology, and at the beginning of my senior year, I applied to about a dozen medical schools. I started going on interviews for admission, which I came to dread. My ambivalence about a career in medicine must have been apparent to the people interviewing me, because, despite a strong academic record and respectable test scores, I was repeatedly turned down. Maybe the interview committees could tell from the greenish hue my face would take on during the obligatory tour of the teaching hospital that the idea of coming into contact with actual physical maladies made me nauseous. The rejection letters rolled in, and I began to worry about my future, or the lack of one. I used the letters to wallpaper our apartment's bathroom.

At the time I was sharing an apartment with three other Vassar students, one of whom was Jay Belsky. (Jay would go on to become one of the leading psychologists in the study of infant development.) Jay suggested that I consider applying to graduate school in psychology as a fall-back position, since I majored in it, enjoyed it, and seemed to have some talent for it. And, of course, there was my interest in living the life of a professor. I applied to just two programs: one at Cornell, and one at Florida. The logic behind these choices was impeccable. I applied to Cornell because Jay was applying there, and he told me that it was a good department. I applied to Florida because one of my other apartment-mates was the son of a psychology professor there, which was reason enough for me. I was admitted to both schools and selected Cornell because I had no desire to live in Florida. Late that spring I was also admitted, finally, to medical school, but, against my relatives' advice–or perhaps in spite of it–turned down the offer and went off to graduate school in Human Development and Family Studies. Had I been accepted into med school earlier in the year, I would probably be practicing medicine today.

GRADUATE SCHOOL

Cornell in the mid-1970s was an exciting place to be for those interested in human development. Urie Bronfenbrenner–who would later become a close friend and mentor, but only after I left Cornell–was just then developing the "ecological perspective," a movement, of sorts, that would dramatically change the field of developmental psychology over the next decade. All of us, even those of us who did not work with Urie, were influenced by his point of view, whether we knew it or not.

When I arrived at Cornell in the fall of 1974 I knew little about what I wanted to study other than the fact that I was still interested in personality, an interest left over from my Dick and Perry days. The closest match on the faculty was John Hill, the department chair. I was assigned to John as his advisee, and began attending his research meetings. It was this bit of serendipity that got me involved n the study of adolescence. It also got me my first job.

At the time, John was one of the only scholars in the field of developmental psychology who specialized in adolescence. It is hard to believe, but as recently as 1974, there was virtually no literature on adolescent development to speak of. Most of what was written at the time was based on clinical anecdote, and any serious scholar of development looked upon the study of adolescence as an empirical wasteland, which it more or less was. John had been asked by the National Institute of Education to develop a research framework for studying adolescence, and he had finished a draft of this the summer before I got to Cornell. He handed it to me during our first meeting, and I more or less memorized it.

John's own research at the time was on the development of social cognition in adolescence. I could not think of anything less interesting. I wanted to study personality development, and although I didn't tell John, I was flirting with the idea of becoming a family therapist and combining an academic career with one in clinical psychology. Family therapy was all the rage at this time. Cornell did not have a clinical program, though, and there was no way for me to gain any expertise in clinical psychology through my graduate program. I contacted a family therapist at a local clinic who had studied with Minuchin, the family therapy guru of the moment, explained my situation, and convinced him to take me on as an apprentice. My first case was a married couple that was having sexual problems. During our first session, the husband said to me, "She doesn't like it when I kiss her cupcakes." I decided I wasn't cut out to be a family therapist.

Although I was not interested in John's research on person perception, I remained in his research group because he was a great advisor. To John's credit, he permitted me to branch off on my own and pursue my interest in family systems theory. I began to think about taking some of the procedures used to study family interaction in the therapeutic context and using them to study "normal" families. Given John's interest in adolescence, it made sense for me to focus my interest in family dynamics on this age period.

Serendipity struck again during my second semester of school. My girlfriend at the time was studying abroad for the year, and I didn't have much of a social life. Every Friday afternoon, to kill time, I would go to the library for a couple of hours and read through the abstracts of a variety of psychology and sociology journals. One afternoon, during my second semester of graduate school, I came across a study by Ted Jacob, comparing patterns of interaction in families with 11- versus 16-year-olds from working- and middle-class households. As I read and reread the article, I began to envision a similar study that bridged this work with John's conceptual framework. Although it was not presented this way, Jacob's study was, in essence, a study of changes in family dynamics during the transition from childhood into adolescence. I thought it would be interesting to see if the changes in family interaction that took place at this time were linked somehow to changes in the child.

Rather than look at interaction patterns as a function of age, though, like Jacob did, I decided to look at them as a function of the adolescent's biological, cognitive, and social maturation. That night, I began designing a study to look at changes in family interaction as children entered puberty, developed formal operations, and moved from elementary to secondary school, a study that eventually became my dissertation. It is the little random events, like discovering Jacob's study at a time I was ready to assimilate it, that make individual careers what they are.

I started the study during my second year of graduate school, although it took some persuading on my part to do so. John was a bit skeptical of a second-semester graduate student's plan to start his dissertation research this early in grad school. I made a deal with John: I would analyze the first wave of cross-sectional data for my predissertation project. If the results looked promising, I would conduct more data collection and analyze the longitudinal data for my dissertation. After recruiting a team of Cornell undergraduates to help–we were doing 30 home observations and microcoding audiotapes of mother-father-son interaction–I started collecting data in the fall of 1975. The cross-sectional analyses proved interesting, and I conducted observations of the same families the next spring and again the following fall.

I found that family interaction patterns were closely linked not to the child's chronological age, school grade, or cognitive maturation, but to his pubertal status (Steinberg, 1981). It appeared as if conflict between adolescents and their mother intensifies as boys begin to mature, peaks during the apex of their growth spurt, and then subsides somewhat as their physical maturation is completed. Up until this point, almost all that had been written about puberty and adolescent development examined the effects of early or late maturation. My dissertation demonstrated that puberty played an important role in the adolescent's social relationships even when it occurred on time.

ACADEMIC POSITIONS

UC Irvine, and a Break from Family Research

Although I finished my doctorate in three years–in part because John was leaving Cornell in 1977 and I did not want to have to get a new advisor–I had no job offer in hand as late as May of my last year. I had traveled to Washington to interview for a position as a researcher at a nonprofit organization with a government contract to study day care centers, which was not what I wanted to do. I then returned to Ithaca late one night after a long drive home during which I became depressed over the fact that I wasn't going to get to be a professor after all. At my office, a message was waiting for me to call someone at the University of California, Irvine. I had never heard of Irvine. It turned out that they were looking at the last minute for someone who could teach developmental psychology, and the head of their search committee had placed calls to the department chairs of three or four well-known graduate programs. Because John was Cornell's department chair at the time, he got the search committee's call, and he suggested that they contact me. I called the search committee chair back the next day and was interviewed and offered the job over the phone. After I accepted the offer, I looked on a map to see where Irvine was. I defended my dissertation in August, 1977 and drove that next week across the country to take a faculty position at UC Irvine on a one-year replacement position that turned into a tenure-track job in the Program in Social Ecology.

I would return to the study of family relations later in my career, but by the time I left Cornell, in 1977, I was ready for a change. The one-year position at Irvine turned into a tenure-track Assistant Professorship and five years later, a tenured Associate Professorship. My years at UC Irvine were dominated by my involvement in a large-scale research project that Ellen Greenberger and I launched, on the impact of employment on adolescent development and adjustment (Steinberg, Greenberger, Garduque, Ruggerio, & Vaux, 1982). This research had little to say about family relations and adolescent development, but it was an important component of my career, for through my collaboration with Ellen, I learned how to write grant proposals, manage large-scale field research, and develop and carry out policy-relevant research.

The Madison Study

In 1983, I left Irvine to take a faculty position at the University of Wisconsin–Madison. The year before I had gotten married, and my wife, Wendy, and I decided that we wanted to try living outside of California. Wendy had been born and raised in Southern California, and she had never lived outside the state. I knew the East and West Coasts, but had never lived in between. We both wanted a change, and Wisconsin offered me a huge raise and a promotion to Full Professor.

Our years in Madison were good ones. Our son, Ben, was born there in 1984, and life was calm and simple. I was able to work at home often, and even when I had to go in to the office, my "commute" was a 10-minute bike ride. I was able to be much more involved in caring for Ben than would have been the case had we been living in Southern California and fighting the constant freeway traffic.

Ellen and I continued to write up pieces of the adolescent work study. We decided to write *When Teenagers Work* (1986), in which we were able to take the time and space we needed to really flesh out our ideas about adolescent employment in detail. By now I had enjoyed enough of a break from family research to revisit some of the issues I had explored in my dissertation. In 1984, I started a new study of family relationships at adolescence that extended my earlier work in several ways. In addition to studying how family relationships changed during adolescence, I was also interested in understanding how different approaches to parenting affected adolescent development.

At the time I began working on the research design, I took on Susan Silverberg as a graduate advisee. I had supervised a couple of graduate students while at Irvine, but Sue was really the first doctoral student I worked with who shared my specific interests in family relations in adolescence. Sue was especially interested in looking at the transition into adolescence from the parents' point of view, which had not been done before. Although I had planned on collecting data from parents, the questions I intended to ask concerned child-rearing. Sue thought we were missing an important opportunity to learn about parents' psychological development and how this was affected during the transition. What we learned from Sue's portion of the study turned out to be far more interesting than what we learned from the part that I had designed.

My collaboration with Sue was the first in what would become a series of fabulous working relationships with graduate students, at Wisconsin and, later, at Temple. I realized throughout the course of these collaborations how much I had learned, unconsciously, from my relationship with John about the importance of the mentor-student relationship. John knew when to be supportive and when to be critical. (I can still recall, in its entirety, his written reaction to the first draft of my dissertation proposal: "This is not good enough for me to comment on.") He was able to balance my dependence on him as an advisor with my growing needs for autonomy as an independent investigator. I've tried to model John in the way in which I supervise my students. Working with graduate students has been, and probably will always be, my favorite part of the job.

The Madison study revitalized my interest in studying adolescent family relationships. My students and I were enormously productive, and we published numerous articles on the impact of parents on adolescent development (Steinberg, Elmen, & Mounts, 1989), on the development of autonomy (Steinberg & Silverberg, 1986), on parents' mental health during the adolescent transition (Silverberg & Steinberg, 1990), and, of course, on the impact of puberty on family relationships (Steinberg, 1987).

I noted earlier that serendipity has played a major role in my development as a researcher, and something that happened at this point in my career is a perfect illustration. I got a call from John asking me to pinch-hit for him as a speaker on a panel examining similarities and differences between the social relations of humans and other primates. Jane Goodall, the eminent primatologist, was going to be the featured speaker, and two other scholars (one of whom was to have been John) were asked to contribute to the symposium. In John's place, I was supposed to give a talk on parent-adolescent relationships in humans and nonhuman primates. Not knowing the first thing about primate development, I made an appointment with the director of the Wisconsin Primate Center (where Harry Harlow had done his famous studies of infant monkeys and surrogate mothers), who was able to point me to the relevant literature. I steeped myself in this work for the next week, and came away with enough of an understanding of family relations among monkeys and apes to at the very least avoid embarrassing myself in front of Goodall. I started to think about parent-adolescent relationships in an evolutionary perspective.

Around this same time, I was visiting my old college apartment-mate, Jay Belsky, at Penn State, where he was on the faculty. One afternoon, while driving around the Pennsylvania countryside, we started discussing my findings on puberty and parent-child conflict. Jay asked how I was so sure that it was puberty that was causing the increase in conflict, rather than the reverse; perhaps, he suggested with characteristic audacity, conflict between parents and adolescents stimulated pubertal maturation. My initial reaction was to laugh, but I said that it was easy enough to look at with our data, since we had assessed both puberty and parent-child conflict among all of our Madison families twice over a one-year period. I ran the analyses as soon as I got home.

Sure enough, the analyses suggested that pubertal maturation seemed to be stimulated by conflict and distance in the parent-child relationship, at least among girls. I published an article showing that preadolescent girls who fought with their parents were more likely to begin puberty earlier than girls whose family relationships were not as conflicted (Steinberg, 1988). Most other researchers were highly skeptical of the finding–I can remember giving a talk at Stanford University and having

Eleanor Maccoby approach me afterwards to tell me how much she liked the talk and how doubtful she was of the finding–but I had drawn enough attention to the issue to stimulate other researchers to examine their data in similar ways. The finding has now been replicated at least a half dozen times.

Intrigued by the finding, I made another appointment with the Wisconsin Primate Center director to ask if what we had found in our study made sense in terms of what we knew about puberty among primates. He informed me that the timing of pubertal maturation in many species of monkeys and apes was linked to the quality of the juvenile's family relationships, in exactly the same way as we had found among humans. Closeness between parents and offspring inhibited pubertal maturation, whereas distance accelerated it. I developed an evolutionary model of adolescent family relationships to try to explain these findings, in which I suggested that parent-adolescent conflict was an adaptive mechanism that had evolved to avoid inbreeding within family groups (Steinberg, 1989). I sent a draft of the paper to John, who called late one night to tell me how proud he was of the work I was doing, which meant the world to me. Later, with Jay, I expanded this into a broader, sociobiological theory of socialization and adolescent psychopathology (Steinberg & Belsky, 1996).

Most of my work during my tenure at Madison focused on variations in parenting practices and their impact on adolescent development and adjustment. Since graduate school, I had maintained a strong interest in the work of Berkeley psychologist Diana Baumrind, and I was especially interested in looking at her notions about "authoritative" parenting in samples of families with adolescents. Baumrind's work had focused mainly on development during early and middle childhood, and I was eager to see if the psychological benefits she had found to be associated during childhood with parenting that was warm yet firm were present among teenagers as well. In a series of papers, we showed that this was indeed the case (Steinberg, Elmen, & Mounts, 1989).

As I began to publish more in the area of adolescent-family relationships, and, more specifically, on effective parenting during the adolescent years, I began to receive phone calls from journalists interested in writing about family life with teenagers. It seemed that the public's desire for information about raising teenagers was tremendous. One day, on a lark, I dropped in to the local bookstore to see what had been written on the subject that was aimed at parents of teenagers. I was shocked to discover that there was very little on the shelves, and that what was there was almost always in contradiction to the scientific literature. I had not written for popular audiences before–the closest I had come was authoring a college textbook on adolescence (Steinberg, 1985)–but I felt confident that, if paired with the right person, I could produce a useful book for parents. I called Ann Levine, an acquaintance who was an accomplished social science writer, and asked if she was interested in working together on an advice book for parents of adolescents. Our collaboration resulted in *You and Your Adolescent* (Steinberg & Levine, 1990).

In 1987, serendipity struck again. Out of the blue I received a call from Fred Newmann, a colleague at Wisconsin's School of Education, who invited me to join a team of researchers studying high school reform, at a newly formed research center established at Wisconsin by the federal government. Fred had experts at the Center who specialized in secondary education, but there was no one at the Center with special expertise in the study of adolescent development. Fred invited me to play this role and join the Center's team. In return for my time and input, I would have access to a portion of the Center's budget, which I could use to support my work on adolescent family relationships. The only catch was that the work had to have relevance for the study of high school reform.

One of the fabulous things about being on the faculty of a top-notch university like Wisconsin is the access one has to the best scholars in their respective fields. I knew that Brad Brown, who was in the department of Educational Psychology, was one of the leading experts in the study of peer relationships in adolescence. I called Brad and asked if he would be interested in collaborating on a new project, one designed to look at the joint influences of parents and peers on adolescent achievement. Brad was enthusiastic, and we agreed to spend the next few months reading and discussing the relevant literature. It looked to us as if this was an area that was ripe for empirical attention, and we set about designing a study. I would take primary responsibility for the family component, and Brad would lead up the portion of the study on peers.

I was in my office one day when one of my graduate students came in with an unpublished paper by a sociologist at Stanford named Sanford Dornbusch, who had been studying the impact of parents on adolescent achievement. From the looks of the paper, it appeared as if he had already done exactly what I had hoped to do in the new study with Brad. My first reaction was that it was more or less pointless to do what someone had already done, and I called Brad with the bad news. Later that day, though, I decided to call this Dornbusch fellow and ask a few detailed questions about what he had studied. I introduced myself over the phone and explained what Brad and I were interested in doing.

Sandy could not have been happier. He suggested that we pool our efforts and our funding and work together. I hung up the phone and called Brad, who agreed that it was worth looking into. The next day I flew out to California to meet with Sandy in person.

I don't think I've ever met a more generous colleague than Sandy–or one who talked faster. We sat in his office and discussed what a collaboration might look like. By the end of the day, we had drafted a written understanding of the proposed collaboration and planned a series of meetings to bring the Stanford and Wisconsin research teams together. Over the next year, Sandy, Brad, and I, along with our research staffs, met several times and designed an enormous study–one that ultimately would involve three years of data collection and more than 20,000 adolescents in Wisconsin and Northern California. We were able to take the measures of parent-adolescent relationships that had been employed in smaller scale studies and use them to test hypotheses in a large, ethnically-diverse sample.

New Directions at Temple

In 1988, we moved from Madison to Philadelphia, where I joined the Psychology Department at Temple University. Although I had been exceptionally happy at Wisconsin, as a family, we had grown tired of small-town Midwestern living. Wendy wanted to return to graduate study in creative writing, and whereas Temple had a graduate program in writing Wisconsin did not. By this time, Brad, Sandy, and I had started data collection, and the research teams were up and running. We had hired postdoctoral fellows at both Stanford and Wisconsin to manage the day-to-day workings of the project, and this made it possible (if not ideal) for me to move to Philadelphia and co-direct the project from a distance.

Because I was not intimately involved in the actual data collection for this study, I had time during my first years at Temple to take on another writing project. Having successfully co-authored *You and Your Adolescent,* I felt emboldened enough to try writing another book for the general public. My intent was to write a book on the parent-adolescent relationship based on the Madison study, but as I sifted through the questionnaire data we had collected as well as transcripts of the hundreds of interviews we had conducted with teenagers and their parents, I drew a blank, literally. I stared at an empty computer screen for the better part of a year. It was the first extended writing block that I had ever experienced.

Part of my block stemmed from some awful news I had received. John Hill had become very ill, and late in 1988, he died. I felt as if I had lost a father, an older brother, and a best friend, all folded into one person. Every time I tried to read or write anything about adolescence, I thought of John. I began to feel the sort of irrational guilt that one feels when a parent dies. Had he known how much I was influenced by him? Had he known how important a role he had played in my development? It was an eerie feeling, and one that was far more powerful than I could ever have expected.

Eventually, I came out of my funk. It occurred to me that what was most interesting about the study we had done in Madison was the parents' perspective on the transition of the family into adolescence. Perhaps this realization had something to do with my own development as a father. Although Ben was still a young child, I could already feel how profoundly his own development was affecting the way that Wendy and I saw ourselves. I returned to the data and the interviews with an eye toward using them to tell the "story" of adolescence from the parents' point of view. Building on the ideas that Sue Silverberg and I had developed when we first designed the project, I began to sketch out an outline for a book that would examine the intersection of adolescence and midlife. After struggling for many months to find the right "voice" for the book, I turned to Wendy for help. Together we wrote *Crossing Paths* (Steinberg, 1994), an exploration of the ways in which the child's entry into adolescence affects the mental health, social relationships, and self-conceptions of mothers and fathers as they negotiated their own transition into midlife.

Once the manuscript for *Crossing Paths* was handed over to our publisher, I turned my attention to the tidal wave of data that was coming in from our California and Wisconsin samples. I became very interested in exploring ethnic differences in parenting and its relation to adolescent adjustment. Our Madison study, which produced numerous papers on the benefits of authoritative parenting, had been almost exclusively white. With the demography of American adolescence changing as rapidly as it was, many social scientists began asking whether the "truths" about parenting derived from studies of white adolescents generalized to other populations as well. The massive data set we had collected allowed us to look at this in detail. I was asked to give an invited address at the 1990 meetings of the American Psychological Association, and I decided to focus on ethnic differences in family socialization.

This work proved to be extremely interesting. Although there were important exceptions to the rule, overall, our findings suggested that authoritative parenting was beneficial for all teenagers, regardless of their race, family structure, or socioeconomic status (Steinberg, Mounts, Lamborn, & Dornbusch, 1991). The most important exception to this pattern concerned academic achievement, though, where we found that authoritative parenting did not seem to have the same advantages for Black or Asian youngsters as it did for Whites or Hispanics. Subsequent analyses of the data indicated that this was probably the case because of different levels of peer group support for achievement in different ethnic groups, a finding that served to remind me that one could not study parenting without taking the other aspects of adolescents' lives into account (Steinberg, Dornbusch, & Brown, 1992). Bronfenbrenner's ecological perspective, to which I had been exposed in my early days of graduate school, proved invaluable in helping me to make sense out of our findings.

Drawing heavily on Urie's perspective, and consulting with him frequently as I looked at our data, I began to look at "parenting in context." I asked Nancy Darling, a former student of Urie's, to come to Temple to work as my postdoctoral fellow, analyzing the large data set. We wrote several empirical papers based on these data as well as a long conceptual piece on socialization in the family (Darling & Steinberg, 1993; Lamborn, Mounts, Steinberg, & Dornbusch, 1991; Steinberg, Lamborn, Dornbusch, & Darling, 1992; Steinberg, Lamborn, Darling, Mounts, & Dornbusch, 1994). In 1993, I had a chance to pay tribute to Urie, as a speaker and contributor to a festschrift honoring his career. I also tried pulling together a lot of what I had been thinking about concerning families, peer groups, neighborhoods, and ethnic differences in adolescent development (Steinberg, Darling, Fletcher, Brown, & Dornbusch, 1995). In 1996, with the assistance of Sandy and Brad, I fleshed out these thoughts in *Beyond the Classroom* (1996), probably the piece of work of which I am the proudest.

After I finished *Beyond the Classroom,* I went through a period of feeling directionless. Nothing seemed interesting. I had no idea what I wanted to work on. I was totally burned out. I went to see a therapist who specialized in stress reduction and did a lot of work with people who had to create things for a living: writers, scientists, musicians, artists. I told him I was afraid that I would never find anything interesting to work on again. He told me that I should stop pushing so hard and try just *being*. He said something would surely come along and that the key was waiting for it, rather than seeking it. He prescribed golf. I said that I was worried that when colleagues asked me what I was working on, I wouldn't be able to answer. He said that I should say that I was working on my golf game and not worry what people thought. I took up golf and discovered that it's a lot harder than academics.

Several months later my therapist's prediction came true. I got a call from an old friend, John Monahan, a former colleague of mine from my early days at Irvine. John was directing a research network for the MacArthur Foundation, on mental health and the law. We hadn't spoken in years. John called to ask if I was interested in writing a piece on adolescent judgment and decision-making, especially with regard to the treatment of adolescents under the law. I wasn't particularly interested, but I wasn't working on anything else at the time, so I agreed and asked Beth Cauffman, one of my graduate students at the time who became a close collaborator, to help write the piece (Steinberg & Cauffman, 1996). I went to one of John's network meetings and discussed some of these ideas with the group. Soon, I was invited to join one of the foundation's other research networks, on psychopathology and development, headed by David Kupfer. And later that year, I got a call from the MacArthur Foundation asking if I would head up a new research network for the foundation in 1996. Since then, I've been concentrating in my work on psychopathology and on juvenile justice issues.

SUMMING UP

A couple of weeks ago, I was having dinner with an old friend from our days in Madison. He asked me what I thought I'd be working on ten years from now (I'm now 47). I thought about it and realized that I haven't a clue.

When I teach graduate seminars, I often ask students to look at an individual scholar's career and try to make sense of it. I'm not sure what I would say about my own. As I've looked back by writing this essay, what is most striking to me is to realize how much of my career was formed by events that could not have been predicted, by good fortune, and by just being in the right place at the right time. It's like Woody Allen once said: "Eighty percent of success is just showing up." It's a hard thing to explain to someone just starting out, but despite all of the things we do to try to make things happen, many of the best things that happen to us are things we have no control over. Like golf.

AUTHOR NOTE

Laurence Steinberg, PhD, is Distinguished University Professor of Psychology, Department of Psychology, Temple University, Philadelphia, PA 19122.

REFERENCES

Darling, N. & Steinberg, L. (1993). Parenting style as context: An integrative model. *Psychological Bulletin, 113* (3), 487-496.

Greenberger, E. & Steinberg, L. (1986). *When teenagers work: The psychological and social costs of adolescent employment.* New York: Basic Books.

Lamborn, S., Mounts, N., Steinberg, L., & Dornbusch, S. (1991). Patterns of competence and adjustment among adolescents from authoritative, authoritarian, indulgent, and neglectful homes. *Child Development*, 62 (5), 1049-1065.

Silverberg, S. & Steinberg, L. (1990). Psychological well-being of parents at midlife: The impact of early adolescent children. *Developmental Psychology*, 26, 4, 658-666.

Steinberg, L. (1981). Transformations in family relations at puberty. *Developmental Psychology, 17* 6, 833-840.

Steinberg, L. (1985). *Adolescence.* New York: Knopf.

Steinberg, L. (1987). The impact of puberty on family relations: Effects of pubertal status and pubertal timing. *Developmental Psychology, 23*, 3, 451-460.

Steinberg, L. (1988). Reciprocal relation between parent-child distance and pubertal maturation. *Developmental Psychology, 24*, 1, 122-128.

Steinberg, L. (1989). Pubertal maturation and parent-adolescent distance: An evolutionary perspective. In G. Adams, R. Montemayor, and T. Gulotta (Eds.), *Advances in adolescent development* (*Volume 1*) (pp. 71-97). Beverly Hills, CA: Sage.

Steinberg, L. (with W. Steinberg). (1994). *Crossing paths: How your child's adolescence triggers your own crisis.* New York: Simon & Schuster.

Steinberg, L. (in collaboration with B. Brown & S. Dornbusch) (1996). *Beyond the classroom: Why school reform has failed and what parents need to do.* New York: Simon & Schuster.

Steinberg, L. (1999). *Adolescence* (*5th edition*). New York: McGraw-Hill.

Steinberg, L. & Belsky, J. (1996). A sociobiological perspective on psychopathology in adolescence. In D. Cicchetti and S. Toth (Eds.), *Rochester Symposium on Developmental Psychopathology* (*Volume 7*), pp. 93-124.

Steinberg, L. & Cauffman, E. (1996). Maturity of judgment in adolescence: Psychosocial factors in adolescent decisionmaking. *Law and Human Behavior, 20* (2), 249-272.

Steinberg, L., Darling, N., Fletcher, A., Brown, B., & Dornbusch, S. (1995). Authoritative parenting and adolescent adjustment: An ecological journey. In P. Moen, G. Elder, Jr., and K. Luscher (Eds.), *Examining lives in context: Perspectives on the ecology of human development.* (pp. 223-266). Washington: American Psychological Association.

Steinberg, L., Dornbusch, S., & Brown, B. (1992). Ethnic differences in adolescent achievement: An ecological perspective. *American Psychologist, 47* (6), 723-729.

Steinberg, L., Elmen, J, & Mounts, N. (1989). Authoritative parenting, psychosocial maturity, and academic success among adolescents. *Child Development, 60* (6),1424-1436.

Steinberg, L., Greenberger, E., Garduque, L., Ruggiero, M., & Vaux, A. (1982). Effects of working on adolescent development. *Developmental Psychology, 18* (3), 385-395.

Steinberg, L., Lamborn, S., Darling, N., Mounts, N., & Dornbusch, S. (1994). Over-time changes in adjustment and competence among adolescents from authoritative, authoritarian, indulgent, and neglectful families. *Child Development, 65* (3), 754-770.

Steinberg, L., Lamborn, S., Dornbusch, S., & Darling, N. (1992). Impact of parenting practices on adolescent achievement: Authoritative parenting, school involvement, and encouragement to succeed. *Child Development, 63* (5) 1266-1281.

Steinberg, L., & Levine, A. (1990). *You and your adolescent: A parent's guide for ages 10 to 20.* New York: Harper & Row.

Steinberg, L., Mounts, N., Lamborn, S., & Dornbusch, S. (1991). Authoritative parenting and adolescent adjustment across various ecological niches. *Journal of Research on Adolescence, 1* (1), 19-36.

Steinberg, L. & Silverberg, S. (1986). The vicissitudes of autonomy in early adolescence. *Child Development, 57* (4), 841-851.

Continuities and Diversities

William J. Doherty

KEYWORDS. Autobiography, fatherhood, spirituality, community, therapy

INTRODUCTION

As I drove the long road to the main building of the Paulist Fathers Novitiate in Oak Ridge, New Jersey, where I was to attend a reunion of my Catholic seminary class of 1966, I was aware mainly of the discontinuities in my life between 1966 and 1999. I was no longer a Catholic, let alone a Catholic seminarian intending to be a priest. As a Unitarian-Universalist, my religious views fell outside of mainstream Christianity. I had married in 1971 and recently had launched two adult children. I work in a "secular" University teaching family social science and marriage and family therapy. When I first greeted my classmates in the dining hall of the novitiate, the distance between the man at age 21 and the man age 54 seemed great indeed.

The reunion reoriented me like an earthquake re-shuffling the tectonic plates. I came to see the closeness, not just the distance, between myself then and myself now–the continuities, not just the discontinuities. It was like meeting myself again in a time warp with people who knew me then and were eager to know me now. In addition to powerful personal and spiritual discoveries, I found a new sense of the weaving of the threads of my current academic and professional career back to my developmental years. It is those threads that I would like to share with you under several major headings, writing chronologically within each of six quite diverse themes that have characterized my professional life story.

THE WORLD OF THEORY

I have loved ideas since I was age 14, when I discovered philosophical questions through conversations with a 17-year-old friend. We would actually read St. Thomas Aquinas's proofs for the existence of God and try to refute them! (This hubris has probably never left me, but I hope it is now tempered by a sense of humor.) Flash forward to the mid-1980s, when I wrote an article for *Family Process* titled "Quanta, Quarks, and Families: Implications of Quantum Physics for Family Research" (Doherty, 1986). This paper, which laid out a philosophical basis for post-positivist family science based on the theories behind quantum physics, had its roots in a single science class in seminary. I clearly remember the day when the physics instructor broke the news that light was both a wave and a particle, depending on how you measured it. During this course, we had re-conducted the experiments underlying the original debate about the wave theory versus the particle theory of light. First it was clear to me that light comes in waves, but then the particle experiments led me to reject wave theory in favor of particle theory. In the last class period of the semester, the instructor, Father Justin McCormick, pulled the intellectual floor out from under me by declaring that the "truth" in this case was both/and–both particle and wave, depending on how you chose to measure it. I was a 19-year-old Catholic lad who believed there was one right answer for every important question in life. I think I never recovered from the shock. My quantum physics paper, published 22 years later, allowed me to make some sense for my work of my first intellectual experience of non-sense.

In my college years in seminary, I did not a take single course in psychology or the social sciences. But I had a good dose of philosophy–medieval philosophy through the early 20th century–followed by two years of graduate work (and an MA) in theology. Even in theological studies, I was attracted to philosophers because they dealt with first principles. In 1969-70, I did my master's thesis on Alfred North Whitehead's philosophy of God, a pretty bold project since Whitehead was not even a Christian thinker. But the Catholic Church and the Paulist Fathers were more far more open-minded in 1970, following the Vatican Council, than when I had entered seminary in 1963.

My study of Whitehead in seminary influenced my later theoretical work in family science, not only in the quantum physics article but also in the contextual approach of the first chapter of the *Sourcebook of Family Theories and Methods: A Contextual Approach* (Doherty, Boss, LaRossa, Schumm, Steinmetz, 1993). Whitehead stressed the interdependence of everything in the universe and the processual flow of these influences over time. Conceptualizing anything outside of its process and context was to commit the "fallacy of misplaced concreteness." In my work on the *Sourcebook,* I was committed to exploring the sociohistorical and cultural forces that have shaped the family field, not for the purpose of debunking but for the purpose of understanding. Before the *Sourcebook,* most forays into the historical context of a theory in our field were aimed at showing how its flaws stemmed from its historical biases (as with Structural-Functional theory in the 1950s). The problem with this approach in practice is that it assumes that the critic does not also stand in a particular historical context that shapes the critique–a context that in turn will be used to explain and critique the work of the critic!

Thus emerges an intellectual thread going back to my Catholic adolescence and young adulthood: ideas and theories are very important, to be taken fully seriously, but they are context-dependent. Hardly any family scholar would disagree with this in principle, but the contextual approach is quite difficult to make part of one's everyday work as a researcher and teacher. Mostly our writing reflects what I term the "Olympian perspective," that is, the author who proposes, explicates, and critiques from the mountain top without acknowledging the context out of which this work emerges–the mountain of personal, gendered, ethnic, philosophical, theological, historical, cultural, and other contexts. For example, scholars criticize the structural-functionalists of the 1950s for their emphasis on social conformity but generally do not acknowledge how the social revolutions of the 1960s and 1970s have shaped the current generation's distrust of social conformity in favor of individuality. Another example: most scholars who write about religion and the family, or about spiritual issues in family therapy, do not mention their own religious context. Rarer still is the ability not only to acknowledge contextual factors in one's work but also to explore how these factors create lenses through which we ourselves see some family and other social phenomena, and how the same lenses may limit what we can see. I'm not sure I am very good at this myself, but I do hold it as a scholarly ideal in an era of complexity. In any event, I am a committed theoretician with a contextual twist.

THE WORLD OF PRACTICE

At the same time as I was a young teen pondering Aquinas' proofs for God's existence, I was doing volunteer work in the community.

Through a Catholic organization called the Legion of Mary, I visited shut-ins and old people in nursing homes, among other activities. I wanted to be a priest not so much to be a scholar as to be a pastor. My Irish Catholic family (two parents, four siblings) supported my ideals quietly but without cheerleading or pressuring. It was clear to me that I was choosing a life that my parents would be proud of, but my parents also had a pragmatic Catholicism that was a bit skittish about too much overt piety. Wanting to serve people in my life, I felt I had a calling to the priesthood as my place to serve. I was attracted to the Paulist Fathers, a progressive American-born religious order, because of their history of innovative pastoral practice and outreach to the American culture, and their commitment to fostering individual initiative among their priests. I wanted to serve, but I also wanted to make a difference by not following the traditional paths.

The thread of working with families started in 1967 when I began to do pastoral field work as a seminarian at St. Martin's Church in a mostly African-American community in Washington, D.C. I did home visits to get to know the parents of the children I was working with, and I organized neighborhood groups of parents to meet with teachers. Looking back, I see how little I understood then, as a celibate young Catholic seminarian, about raising children, but I could offer my interest and support. For the first time I had glimpses inside families other than my own, and I was hooked on their fascinating relationships and dynamics. But beyond any intellectual interest, through my home visits, I received the gift of people opening their hearts and stories to me, especially their stories of pain and hope. For an intellectually oriented and fairly self-contained young man, these were powerful shaping experiences. I began to write poems about my experiences with these families. Following is one I saved. It is about an elderly African-American woman who opened up to me with her story. But it's also about the revelation that I could be a caring presence for someone who is hurting without having to interpose my own story or to share the air time. Old Mrs. Brown helped propel me out of my 22-year-old self-centeredness.

Old Mrs. Brown

Old Mrs. Brown, don't be so sad,
and don't talk on so long, with wet eyes.
(Why can't you relate, equate
like strong people do?)

You say you've lost your husband and your sister and your son–in one year?
(Why can't you relate, equate?
Don't talk on so, you're not giving me a chance.)
You say your daughter deserted her infant son
and you've mothered and fathered him these nine years,
and you're old.
(It's my turn to talk, Mrs. Brown, can't you see?)
You say that your husband was adrift on a strange ocean those last six years,
a solitary senile stranger who you scarcely knew.
And you kept and cared for him because he always used to say,
in those happy years,
that he'd rather turn to ashes than finish his life in some foundation.
(Perhaps you'd be interested in an experience I had recently.)
And when he died at last, you collapsed with grief.
You went to your daughter's farm (doctor's orders)
and you wept when alone.
For, you said, even when his spirit was not with you,
You could still put your hand on him–your firm, creased, soft hand.
One day, you tell me, your daughter squeezed your arm and said
"I'm sadder than you, Ma. I've lost a father and a mother too."
And then your strength ebbed back.
Tell me more, Mrs. Brown, I am listening.

There have been many other teachers like Mrs. Brown in my life as a practitioner. Having discovered the world of families in seminary, I knew I wanted to be a family professional when I left seminary in 1970. But I had never heard of the field of family studies, and I thought marriage and family therapy was taught only in psychology and social work departments. Graduate school in psychology would have required me to take a year or more of undergraduate course work to be eligible, and I was unwilling. So I filled out applications to social work master's programs in the New York City area, where my wife and I had moved after we married in 1971. By happenstance, I visited a friend who was in a PhD program in the Department of Child Development and Family Studies at the University of Connecticut. Once I discovered that this kind of program existed, where I could study and learn to work with families as my main emphasis, I tore up the social work applications and applied to the Connecticut program. There I worked with and was mentored by Eleanore Lucky and Robert Ryder. From Eleanore I learned to see families humanistically, not just as systems. From Robert I learned a cool-eyed skepticism about inflated claims and covert value positions. And with two mentors who integrated and valued both research and practice in their careers, I never looked back from choosing a career doing the same.

My contributions to the world of practice have fallen in four areas, which I will describe briefly: the Family FIRO Model, medical family therapy, the Levels of Family Involvement Model, and my work on morality and therapy (which I address in a later section of this chapter). I came to the Family FIRO Model from my concurrent study in graduate school of family systems and small group development. Along with my colleague Nicholas Colangelo, I adapted Will Schutz's Fundamental Interpersonal Relations Orientation model of group develop to family development and family therapy (Doherty & Colangelo, 1984; Doherty, Colangelo, & Hovander, 1991; Doherty & Hovander, 1990; Horst & Doherty, 1995). The model includes three core dimensions of family interaction–inclusion, control, and intimacy–and proposes that these three constitute a hierarchical, developmental sequence when families undergo structural and other major changes. In other words, the first developmental task of families is to reformulate inclusion processes such as role re-definition, boundary setting, everyday connecting, and creating shared meanings. The success of this inclusion work influences how they manage control issues that arise in family conflict. Lack of clarity about roles in a new stepfamily, for example, leads to non-resolvable family control problems. Intimacy interactions, defined as close emotional interactions involving mutual self-disclosure, in turn are compromised by negative control dynamics and facilitated by positive control dynamics. Besides this developmental proposition, the other major proposition of the Family FIRO Model is that the three sequential dimensions can be viewed as a priority sequence to guide clinical intervention: inclusion issues take first priority, followed by control issues, and then by intimacy issues. Facing a couple with uncertain commitment to the marriage (an inclusion issue), negative conflict patterns, and a lack of emotional intimacy, the therapist should focus first on the commitment issue to determine whether there is enough "glue" in the relationship to work on the control issues, which in turn would have to improve for the relationship to be safe enough to work directly on intimacy. This model, which seems to tap an implicit clinical decision-making used by many experienced therapists, has been useful in training family therapists who are dealing with a wide range of problems simultaneously at the beginning of therapy.

My second contribution to the practice of marriage and family therapy derived from my work as a faculty member in the Department of Family Practice (1979-83) at the University of Iowa and later the University of Oklahoma (1983-86). (My first two years as an academic, 1977-79, were in the Department of Home Economics at the University of Iowa.) Working full time in a family practice medical residency program was another ground shifting experience. Prior to that position, my main contact with the medical world was through my wife, Leah, who is a nurse. In family medicine, I learned how limited my perspective on families had been to the psychosocial side, ignoring the biological, and how much I had focused on intra-familial dynamics to the exclusion of families' relations with broader systems such as health care systems. These experiences led to a series of collaborative books with physician and family therapist colleagues that helped to launch the field of family systems medicine and medical family therapy (in sequential order: Doherty & Baird, 1983; Doherty & Baird, 1987; Doherty, Christianson & Sussman, 1987; Doherty & Campbell, 1978; McDaniel, Hepworth & Doherty, 1992, 1997). I believe that the principal contributions of this work have been in two areas: theoretically, a biopsychosocial/family systems model that transcends the limitations of traditional family systems theory; and clinically, a collaborative, multidisciplinary way to work with families experiencing serious medical problems. It continues to be one of my passions.

The third area of contribution started in family medicine and extended to one of my original practice areas that I had strayed from: family life education. A core issue for professionals who work with families outside of therapy settings–providers such as physicians, nurses, medical social workers, and parent educators–is how far to wade into the personal and family problems of their clients or their clients' families. In the mid-1980s, my colleague Mac Baird and I developed a model of five levels of involvement with families, beginning with minimal involvement (level 1) and then moving hierarchically through collaboration and information (level 2), emotional support (level 3), brief focused intervention (level 4), and family therapy (level 5). This model has proved useful in the training of family physicians to do mid-range work with families–a combination of level two information and collaboration with level three emotional support (Doherty & Baird, 1986, 1987). And it has led to a variety of research studies spearheaded by Kim Marvel documenting that the levels can be reliably and validly measured in everyday medical practice (Marvel, Doherty & Weiner, 1998; Marvel, Schilling, Doherty & Baird, 1994). More recently, I have applied the levels model to the work of parent and family educators, where it has proved useful in helping these family professionals define what they do and do not do with families (Doherty, 1995a). Specifically, most parent educators aspire to level three competency, and some parent educators develop level four skills (brief focused intervention) under the supervision of a level five family therapist. The model has helped to address the decades old question of the difference between family education and therapy.

In reflecting on this varied body of work in the domain of practice with families and other professionals, I now can see more clearly the influence of my Catholic roots on my desire to be of service to others. Of particular importance has been the influence of the Paulist Fathers on my efforts to think creatively about serving in ways outside the mainstream of current practice. This has been modified somewhat by more recent influences of Unitarian-Universalism toward more open-mindedness and respect for human and professional diversities than I would have been able to accept earlier.

THE MORAL WORLD

Throughout the first three decades of my life, I was very interested in moral issues. This changed when I started my PhD work in 1974, as I began to take on the value-neutral approach of social science and therapy. I came to reject both the traditional moral theologies of my Catholic past and developmental moral frameworks such as Kohlberg's, on which I had done a master's thesis in 1973 (Doherty & Corsini, 1974). No longer a believing Catholic, and yet not deeply into Unitarian-Universalism, I became a moral relativist: because different people in different social and cultural conditions value some behaviors more than others, there is no clear way to decide what is right and wrong, and therefore people should be free to follow their own values unless their behavior clearly infringes on someone else's rights. I rejected Kohlberg's moral stage theory when Gilligan and others pointed out its bias towards rational, individualistic reasoning, and when I saw an arrogance in defining the "highest" moral stage to coincide with Kohlberg's own moral positions. I became a moral critic and skeptic who believed that the goal of social science and therapy were to be as a value-free as possible, and that the chief threats to family science and family therapy were covert values that encouraged conformity to traditional social values. Having ascended Mount Olympus, I was largely unaware of what I was bringing to the moral table. I stayed there for the next ten formative professional years.

I still remember where I was sitting, in the spring of 1985, as I started reading the book *Habits of the Heart: Individualism and Commitment in American Life* (Bellah et al., 1985). It was my first confrontation with how the skeptical, value-free stance I had taken towards family science and family therapy was deeply flawed. I had assumed I had transcended most culturally-based values in favor of a scientific and clinical worldview, when I was actually swimming in the mainstream current of American individualism, with its emphasis on self-interest and avoidance, especially by professionals, of any language that smacked of moral discourse. The key chapter was the one presenting an interview with a California therapist who was asked why she was committed to her children. Her responses were entirely self-oriented: commitment was a personal value to her, and she would feel terribly guilty if she abandoned her children. Absent, despite probing questions, was any articulation that parental commitment is a broader ethical principle than a strictly self-chosen value. The therapist made it clear that she could not speak for what anyone else's values should be, just her own idiosyncratic value stance. I was disturbed to acknowledge that, if I were the one interviewed, I would probably have demonstrated the same impoverished moral discourse. It was a wake up call.

What followed was another 10-year period of exploration of the moral domain in family science and in family therapy, culminating in my choice of the theme for the 1993 National Council on Family Relations Annual Conference, "Moral Discourse About Families," and then the 1995 book *Soul Searching: Why Psychotherapy Must Promote Moral Responsibility* (Doherty, 1995b). The principal themes of my work in this area are as follows: (a) being value-free and morally-neutral about families and therapy is impossible; (b) the so-called "value-free" stance generally means that one embraces uncritically the mainstream cultural assumptions about values and morality–which in the case of the U.S. means an ethic of individual self-interest; and (c) it is possible to engage in moral consultation in therapy that both reflects the therapist's moral sensibilities and respects the autonomy and the diversity of contemporary clients and families. For example, the decision to divorce or to stay married is, in part, a moral decision because it affects so many stakeholders in the marriage and family. Neither rational choice theory in social science nor therapists' attempts to be neutral and value free about this decision does adequate justice to the domain of moral responsibility in this often-torturous decision. *Soul Searching* brought together a critique of mainstream psychotherapy, an alternative view of the moral sense from symbolic-interactional theory, and a hands-on treatment of the craft of engaging in moral conversation with clients.

This interest in issues of moral responsibility in families led directly to my current work on fatherhood. The pivotal clinical case in my career, in 1987, was a recently-separated father who was about to abandon his children. That case was where I translated, for the first time, the *Habits of the Heart* critique into my practice. And it sparked an ongoing professional interest in fathers and father-child relations, no doubt also strongly influenced by the transforming personal experience of being a father to children born in 1973 and 1975. This early interest in fatherhood bore fruit in the mid-1990s in a report on responsible fatherhood commissioned by the Department of Health and Human Services, which was later published by the *Journal of Marriage and the Family* (Doherty, Kouneski, & Erickson, 1998). In 1999, I became Principal Investigator on a federally funded research study to test the efficacy of a transition to fatherhood intervention in promoting closer father-child ties and better father-mother collaboration.

My work on the moral domain of families and therapy reflects the "both/and" stance I now try to integrate in my professional life. That is, it reflects an important element of Catholicism–that moral issues are highly important and must be taken seriously in private and professional life–and a dimension of Unitarian-Universalism–that moral sensibilities and values arise best from respectful dialogue among equal citizens and must continually be adapted over time. It also reflects an element common to both of these disparate religious traditions: that morality is not just a private matter but also a public one. Much of my current development is in the area of families and community.

My interest in community, combined with the both/and philosophy, leads me to seek ways of speaking and writing that emphasize points of convergence among rival positions rather than contributing to further polarization. I see writing as having similarities with therapy: language can be used to connect and open up possibilities for understanding, or it can be used to obfuscate and take one-up positions. I am particularly proud that two individuals with very different perspectives have publicly endorsed *Soul Searching*: pioneering feminist family therapist Rachel Hare-Mustin and radio talk show host Laura Schlesinger!

THE RESEARCH WORLD

I went to graduate school to become a practitioner–first, a family life educator and then a marriage and family therapist. But after doing a master's thesis, I was hooked on research. My first study was not in the family area but in the human development, with a thesis on intelligence and creativity as predictors of moral development in college women. Getting it published (Doherty & Corsini, 1976) was the reinforcement I needed to believe that I could write for publication and have an academic career.

As I look back at my research publications, I see several areas that interested me for a while, to be succeeded by new interests. No single topic has captured me for more than five years or so. I started out with dissertation and follow up work on personality and marriage (Doherty & Ryder, 1979). Then I became interested in the application of cognitive social psychology, especially attribution theory, to the study of the family (Doherty, 1981a,b,c). Once I moved to teaching at medical schools, my research interests turned to family and health topics, including the family dynamics of health behaviors such as smoking, obesity, and cooperation with medical regimens (Doherty & Allen, 1994; Doherty & Whitehead, 1986; Whitehead & Doherty, 1989; Doherty & Harkaway, 1990; Doherty, Schrott, Metcalf & Vailas, 1983).

One content thread connecting my pre-medical school and post-medical school research is divorce, which I have studied from both adult and child perspectives and which has connected with my interests in the moral underpinnings of marriage (Doherty, 1980, 1983; Doherty & Burge, 1989; Doherty & Needle, 1991). Another thread through the years has been an interest in what happens to families in the community when they are involved with family professionals or family education programs. Back in graduate school, I became concerned about the cult-like features of Marriage Encounter weekends (Doherty, McCabe, & Ryder, 1978). This concern led to a series of studies documenting patterns of negative effects of these weekend experiences on certain couples (Doherty, Lester & Leigh, 1986; Lester & Doherty, 1983). In the 1990s, my "real world" research interests surfaced in work on the professional practice patterns of marriage and family therapists and the satisfaction and outcomes of their clients (Doherty & Simmons, 1995; Simmons & Doherty, 1998). This research was the first in the family field to reflect the new national emphasis on health services research in community settings, as distinguished from university or laboratory based studies with unknown generalizability to the community of practitioners and clients.

My current research focus is on fathering. I got into this issue after being invited to head up a U.S. Department of Health and Human Services contract project to write an overview and conceptual framework on responsible fathering. I had been interested in fatherhood from a clinical perspective for many years (Doherty, 1981), and more recently, from the perspective of their moral responsibilities to their children (Doherty, 1995b). But now I immersed myself in the research on fatherhood and first authored the HHS report and subsequent journal article (Doherty et al., 1998). This work in turn influenced the funding priorities of the federal grant agencies, and my colleagues Marti Erickson and Ralph LaRossa and I applied for, and won, a grant to test an educational intervention on the transition to fatherhood. This project began in the fall of 1999, and I expect to stay in the fatherhood research area, if my past record repeats itself, for about five years.

THE WORLD OF MAINSTREAM CULTURE

My interest in context, morality, practice, and community have moved me to become a student of mainstream U.S. culture and how it affects families and those of us who study and work with families. I now keep files with articles and clippings on contemporary popular culture and especially the market culture which has come to dominate the U.S. and the rest of the Western World. I have been struck by how, in the family field's interest in cultural and ethnic factors affecting families, we have tended to focus appropriately on the issue of specific racial and ethnic groups, but then ignore the larger culture that sweeps along almost all families in its powerful current.

This interest in cultural movements spurred my fascination with the development of modernist culture in the early and mid-twentieth century and the more recent emergence of postmodernism, subjects I have written about for both family therapy (Doherty, 1991) and family science audiences (Doherty, 1999). The issues are too complex to explicate briefly here, but my view is that family science was born as a modernist social science with a belief in the pursuit of knowledge by methods that strive to be as objective as possible. Postmodernism, with its profound skepticism about professional knowledge, and even the Enlightenment idea of progress, has challenged the foundations of modernist assumptions in a way that the field is just beginning to come to grips with. But postmodernism, itself, embraces no explicit value system (implicitly the value seems to be one of liberation from oppressive systems), and is thus not capable of providing the kind of synthesis the family field now needs. We are increasingly caught between paradigms, not only modernism versus postmodernism, but the related polarity between positivism versus postpositivism. Established scholars feel the strain less acutely than graduate students and new scholars because we launched our careers in a single modernist, positivist tradition, where many of us succeeded and won tenure before the grand critiques arrived on the scene. The next generation has absorbed both the earlier tradition and its critiques at the same time. Most cannot be the true believers we were in the old paradigm, but as yet there is no new consensus about how to operate with the new paradigm. Like it or not, they are the first generation of postmodern family scholars.

My most recent work in the area of culture has focused on the analysis of the consumer culture as it has invaded family life and the professions. I have been mentored in this area by Harry Boyte and Nancy Kari, from the Center for Democracy and Citizenship at the University of Minnesota (Boyte & Kari, 1996). Boyte, Kari, and their colleagues, coming mostly from political science and social activist perspectives, argue that Americans are increasingly becoming a nation of consumers as opposed to productive citizens. I have used this work to develop a critique of how therapists and other family professionals, through an allegiance to a top-down expert model, unintentionally perpetuate a professional versus consumer dichotomy with families. Knowledge and resources are centered in the professions whose job is to get out the word to families. Families' job is to listen well and practice what we preach. This approach is endemic in twentieth century professions, not just in the family field. I am beginning to write and speak about an alternative model for family/professional/community partnerships that aim to unleash the expertise of families in community, with professionals serving as consultants and catalysts instead of just service providers.

My second approach to consumer culture is reflected in a new book on the consumer culture of childhood and the therapeutic culture of parenthood (Doherty, 2000). Written for parents, this book argues that the consumer culture's invasion of family life has led many parents to see themselves mainly as providers of services to entitled children. Children's responsibilities as citizens of families and communities become invisible, and parents lose confidence in their ability to set limits and create expectations for their children. Associated with the consumer model of childhood is the trend for contemporary families to be hyperactive in filling children's schedules, which leads to a decrease in commitment to family rituals (Doherty, 1997). On top of these problems with the consumer model is the influence of a cultural therapeutic model of parenting that stresses the fragility of children and the importance of parents not showing anger or expecting social conformity. My most recent book on the theme of the consumer culture and the family deals with what I have termed "consumer marriage" (Doherty, 2001).

I am currently working on community activation around the theme of family time, which is threatened by the consumer culture, and leads families to lose their rituals and their mindfulness about family bonds (Doherty, 1997). Following is a statement I drafted with a community group working on a mission of taking back family time. It gives the flavor of this work that blends the themes of family, mainstream culture, social responsibility, and community. The title of the statement is "Families' Civic Work: Family Life First."

> Family Life First is a group of citizens in suburban Minneapolis who are committed to building a community in which family life has *first* priority in an over-busy and over-scheduled world. The group is committed to reversing the deleterious effects of the consumer culture on childhood. Today, parents see themselves as competitive providers of services to children, while children are overscheduled in a frantic pursuit of experiences and opportunities for personal enrichment and advantage over peers.
>
> Family Life First was created out of a town meeting in Wayzata, Minnesota, attended by parents and community leaders concerned with this social problem that "has no name." It consists of parents, community leaders, clergy, teachers, and other professionals. Family Life First is based on the premise that the family can only be a seedbed for current and future citizens if it has the central authority for raising children. This means achieving balance between internal bonds and external activities. It also highlights the fact that this balance has become gravely out of whack for many families of all social classes, and that strengthening family life requires a grass roots movement led by families themselves.

The exaggerated emphasis on athletics is a case in point for change. One participant in the town meeting reported that she feels "terrorized" by coaches who insist on practicing on Mother's Day and Thanksgiving Day. Another was told by the soccer coach that her family could take vacation only during a two-week period in August. Most social, educational, and religious programs are aimed at individuals who are pulled out of their families. In one town, the coaches and clergy met in a "summit meeting" to divide up families' times so as to avoid competition between church and sports. Ironically, despite the over-abundance of community activities available (in one community there are 14 organized activities for three-year-olds), there are few chances for whole families to participate in common, intergenerational activities. There are even fewer opportunities for families to engage in citizenship activities that build the commonwealth. We are a hyper-individualistic, consumer-oriented society that values families as a political icon and marketing target, but does not take family seriously as a place for growing productive citizens.

"Family Life First" has generated a vision of a desired future for families. It has begun a series of stakeholder interviews to better understand the problem and to solicit allies. We want to inspire a broad community discussion about an unspoken problem. We are committed to a "no-villains" approach that does not blame parents, coaches, clergy, or any others. But we aim to have political clout through publicly recognizing community activity groups that support families in making their time a priority, in part through generating media attention for public events. A specific work in progress is to develop along with community activity groups, youth, and families, a set of working policies that acknowledge, support and respect families' decisions to make family time a priority. One program director in a prominent agency has stated that a "Family Life First Seal of Approval" would give them the political leverage to make programmatic changes in his agency.

We are also thinking beyond Wayzata. We aim to stimulate a national movement of families taking back their lives through democratic public work. We are committed to reversing the encroachment of the consumer culture on the world's smallest democracy–the family.

THE WORLD OF PROFESSIONAL ORGANIZATIONS

Being a Catholic seminarian made me an ultimate organization man. It has never left me. I see myself as a first-generation family scientist and marriage and family therapist who is committed to the future of the family field. I am first generation because my teachers and trainers came from the original disciplines of psychology and sociology, but I identify with the newer family field rather than these root disciplines. I have been committed to the professions of family scientist, family life educator, and marriage and family therapist. As mentioned before, my professionally-oriented research, funded by the American Association for Marriage and Family Therapy, has focused on the practice patterns and client outcomes of marriage and family therapists across the country (Doherty & Simmons, 1996). The professional contribution of this work has been to promote the viability of marriage and family therapists in the health care system.

In NCFR, I have served in a number of organizational roles, including co-founder of the Families and Health Section, Program Vice-President for the conference on moral discourse on families, co-founder of the Men in Families focus group, and President in 1998-99. I suspect that my most lasting contribution to NCFR will be the leadership I provided (along with Greer Fox and Mary Jo Czaplewski) in shifting the NCFR Board's governance process from a stultifying, reactive non-model to the Carver Policy Governance model. The Carver model emphasizes that the Board's job is not to micro-manage the staff but to generate vision and set priorities for the association, based on input from members. Staying the course for this necessary change, while dealing constructively with the anxiety of many NCFR members about the change from a familiar but flawed governance model, was the most difficult professional leadership experience of my career. And the most satisfying.

THE WORLD OF TEACHING

Because every brief autobiography has to set limits in scope, I will confine myself to three pointed comments on my role as a teacher. Teaching is where my identities as scholar and practitioner come together as nowhere else. Teaching for me is a fusion of academic science and interpersonal art. And I have been blessed with outstanding students, some of whom have become cherished colleagues, friends, and teachers.

PARALLEL PATHS, CONTINUITIES, AND DIVERSITIES

One of the surprises of the Paulist novice reunion in June 1999 was the discovery of a parallel path that I have been taking along with the Paulist community, despite little contact for many years. The Paulists also lost some of their moral and spiritual footing during the 1970s and early 1980s, leaning too strongly towards an individualistic model that lacked enough depth and accountability. In letting "a thousand flowers bloom," the Paulists, like the mainstream social science and therapy worlds that I occupied, had trouble articulating their moral and spiritual grounding as a community. Interestingly, the Unitarian-Universalist faith, where I settled after leaving the Catholic Church, is now facing the same dilemma: how to be true to a founding principle of individual freedom of belief and expression while creating a community of moral and spiritual depth and accountability. I take comfort in these parallel struggles and efforts to find a new synthesis between individual and community, between freedom of choice and responsibility for choices made, between family as a locus of self-interest and a domain of mutual accountability. My public philosophy is now an activist brand of communitarianism.

I continue to work at discovering and forging a coherent identity and a mission from the apparently discontinuous threads of my professional life. Here is my latest attempt: I am a Catholic-Paulist-Unitarian/Universalist-Family Scientist-Family Therapist who loves theory, practice, moral exploration, research, cultural exploration and democratic community building, organizational development, and working with students. Lots of diversity and lots of continuity–that sums it up for now.

AUTHOR NOTE

WIlliam J. Doherty, PhD, is affiliated with the Family Practice in the Family Social Science Department. 1985 Buford Avenue, University of Minnesota, St. Paul, MN 55108.

REFERENCES

Bellah, R. H., Madsen, R., Sullivan, W. M., Swidler, A., & Tipton, S. M. (1985). *Habits of the heart: Individualism and commitment in American life*. Berkeley: University of California Press.

Boyte, H. C. & Kari, N. K. (1996). *Building American: The democratic promise of public work*. Philadelphia: Temple University Press.

Colangelo, N. & Doherty, W. J. (1988). The family FIRO model: The integration of group theory and family theory. *The Journal for Specialists in Group Work, 13*, 4, 194-199.

Doherty, W. J. (1980). Divorce and belief in internal versus external control of one's life: Data from a national probability sample. *Journal of Divorce, 3*, 4, 391-401.

Doherty, W. J. (1981). Cognitive processes in intimate conflict: I. Extending attribution theory. *American Journal of Family Therapy, 9*, 1, 3-13.

Doherty, W. J. (1981). Cognitive processes in intimate conflict: II. Efficacy and learned helplessness. *American Journal of Family Therapy, 9*, 1, 35-44.

Doherty, W. J. (1981). Involving the reluctant father in family therapy. In A. Gurman (Ed.), *Questions and answers in the practice of family therapy* (pp. 167-168). New York: Brunner/Mazel.

Doherty, W. J. (1981). Locus of control differences and marital dissatisfaction. *Journal of Marriage and the Family, 43*, 2, 369-377.

Doherty, W. J. (1983). Impact of divorce on locus of control orientation in adult women. *Journal of Personality and Social Psychology, 44*, 4, 834-840.

Doherty, W. J. (1986). Quanta, quarks, and families: Implications of quantum physics for family research. *Family Process, 25*, 2, 249-264.

Doherty, W. J. (1991). Beyond reactivity and the deficit model of manhood: A commentary on articles by Napier, Pittman, and Gottman. *Journal of Marital and Family Therapy, 17*, 1, 29-32.

Doherty, W. J. (1991). Family therapy goes postmodern. *The Family Therapy Networker, 15*, 5, 36-42.

Doherty, W. J. (1995a). Boundaries between parent and family education and family therapy. *Family Relations, 44*, 4, 353-358.

Doherty, W. J. (1995b). *Soul searching: Why psychotherapy must promote moral responsibility*. New York: Basic Books.

Doherty, W. J. (1996). The best of times and the worst of times: Fathering as a contested arena of academic discourse. In A. J. Hawkins & D. C. Dollahite (Eds.), *Generative fathering: Beyond deficit perspectives*. Newbury Park, CA: Sage Publications.

Doherty, W. J. (1997). *The intentional family*. New York: Addison-Wesley.

Doherty, W.J. (1999). Postmodernism and family theory. In M.B. Sussman, S.K. Steinmetz, & G. W. Peterson (Eds.) *Handbook of marriage and the family* (pp. 205-217). Second edition. New York: Plenum.

Doherty, W. J. (2000). Take back your kids: Confident parenting in turbulent times. South Bend, IN: Sorin Books.

Doherty, W. J. (2001). Take back your marriage: Sticking together in a world that pulls us apart. New York: Guilford.

Doherty, W. J. & Allen, W. (1994). Family functioning and parent smoking as predictors of adolescent cigarette use: A six year prospective study. *Journal of Family Psychology, 8*, 3, 347-353.

Doherty, W. J. & Baird, M. A. (1983). *Family therapy and family medicine: Toward the primary care of families*. New York: Guilford Press.

Doherty, W. J. & Baird, M. A. (1986). Levels of physician involvement with families. *Family Medicine, 18*, 3, 153-156.

Doherty, W. J. & Baird, M. A. (Eds.). (1987). *Family-centered medical care: A clinical casebook*. New York: Guilford Press.

Doherty, W.J., Boss, P., LaRossa, R. Schumm, W., & Steinmetz, S. (1993). *Sourcebook of family theories and methods: A contextual approach* (pp. 3-30). New York: Plenum.

Doherty, W. J., & Burge, S. K. (1989). Divorce among physicians: Comparisons with other occupational groups. *Journal of the American Medical Association, 261*, 16, 2374-2377.

Doherty, W. J., & Campbell, T. (1988). *Families and health*. Newbury Park, CA: Sage Publications.

Doherty, W. J., Christianson, C. E., & Sussman, M. B. (Eds.). (1987). Family medicine: The maturing of a discipline. New York: Haworth Press.

Doherty, W. J., & Colangelo, N. (1984). The Family FIRO Model: A modest proposal for organizing family treatment. *Journal of Marital and Family Therapy, 10*, 1, 19-29.

Doherty, W. J. Colangelo, N., & Hovander, D. (1991). Priority setting in family change and clinical practice: The Family FIRO Model. *Family Process, 30*, 2, 227-240.

Doherty, W. J., & Corsini, D. A. (1976). Creativity and intelligence as predictors of moral development among college women. *Journal of Creative Behavior, 10*, 4, 276-284.

Doherty, E. W., & Doherty, W. J. (1998). Smoke gets in your eyes: Cigarette smoking and divorce in a national sample of adults. *Families, Systems & Health, 16*, 4, 393-400.

Doherty, W. J. & Harkaway, J. E. (1990). Obesity and family systems: A family FIRO approach to assessment and treatment planning. *Journal of Marital and Family Therapy, 16*, 3, 287-298.

Doherty, W. J. & Heinrich, R. L. (1996). Managing the ethics of managed healthcare: A systemic approach. *Families, Systems & Health, 14*, 1, 17-28.

Doherty, W. J. & Hovander, D. (1990). Why don't family measures of cohesion and control behave the way they're supposed to? *American Journal of Family Therapy, 18*, 1, 5-17.

Doherty, W. J., Kouneski, E., & Erickson, M. F. (1998). Responsible fatherhood: A review and conceptual framework. *Journal of Marriage and the Family, 60*, 2, 277-292.

Doherty, W. J., Lester, M. E., & Leigh, G. (1986). Marriage Encounter: Couples who win and couples who lose. *Journal of Marital and Family Therapy, 12*, 1, 49-61.

Doherty, W. J., McCabe, P., & Ryder, R. G. (1978). Marriage Encounter: A critical appraisal. *Journal of Marriage and Family Counseling, 4*, 4, 99-107.

Doherty, W. J., & Needle, R. (1991). Psychological adjustment and substance use before and after a parental divorce. *Child Development, 62*, 2, 328-337.

Doherty, W. J., & Ryder, R. G. (1979). Locus of control, interpersonal trust and assertive behavior among newlyweds. *Journal of Personality and Social Psychology, 37*, 12, 2122-2220.

Doherty, W. J. & Ryder, R. G. (1980). Parent Effectiveness Training (P.E.T.): Criticisms and caveats. *Journal of Marital and Family Therapy, 6*, 4, 409-419.

Doherty, W. J. Schrott, H., Metcalf, L., & Vailas, L. (1983). Effect of spouse support and health belief in medication adherence. *Journal of Family Practice, 17*, 5, 837-841.

Doherty, W. J. & Simmons, D. S. (1996). Clinical practice patterns of marriage and family therapists: A national survey of therapists and their clients. *Journal of Marital and Family Therapy, 22*, 1, 9-25.

Doherty, W. J., Su, S., & Needle, R. (1989). Marital disruption and psychological well-being: A panel study. *Journal of Family Issues, 10*, 1, 72-85.

Doherty, W. J. & Whitehead, D. (1986). The social dynamics of cigarette smoking: A family FIRO analysis. *Family Process, 25*, 3, 453-459.

Horst, E. A., & Doherty, W. J. (1995). Gender, power, and intimacy. *Journal of Feminist Family Therapy, 6*, 2, 63-85.

Lester, M. E., & Doherty, W. J. (1983). Couples' long term evaluations of their Marriage Encounter experience. *Journal of Marital and Family Therapy*, *9*, 2, 183-188.
Marvel, M. K., Doherty, W. J., & Weiner, E. (1998). Medical interviewing by exemplary family physicians. *Journal of Family Practice*, *47*, 5, 343-348.
Marvel, M. K., Schilling, R., Doherty, W. J., & Baird, M. A. (1994). Levels of physician involvement with patients and their families: A model for teaching and research. *Journal of Family Practice*, *39*, 6, 535-544.
McDaniel, S., Hepworth, J., & Doherty, W. J. (1992). *Medical family therapy*. New York: Basic Books.
McDaniel, S. H., Hepworth, J., & Doherty, W. J. (Eds.). (1997). *The shared experience of illness: Stories of patients, families, and therapists*. New York: Basic Books.
Simmons, D. S. & Doherty, W. J. (1995). Defining who we are and what we do: Clinical practice patterns of marriage and family therapists in Minnesota. *Journal of Marital and Family Therapy*, *21*, 1, 3-16.
Simmons, D. S. & Doherty, W. J. (1998). Does academic training make a difference in the practices of marriage and family therapists? *Journal of Marital and Family Therapy*, *24*, 4, 321-336.
Whitehead, D. & Doherty, W. J. (1989). Systems dynamics in cigarette smoking: An exploratory study. *Family Systems Medicine*, *7*, 3, 264-273.

Coming Full Circle: From Volunteer to Professional

Suzanne K. Steinmetz

KEYWORDS. Autobiography, family violence, families at risk, youth, theory

INTRODUCTION

The title of this essay reflects my coming full circle in two distinct ways. The first is in terms of fulfilling what appeared, at the time, to be strange career recommendations (physician, minister or engineer) based on vocational testing–discussed below. However, I have also come full circle in terms of moving from volunteer social worker, involved in providing help to the poor and oppressed, and amateur writer and researcher reporting on community activities for our local weekly newspaper, to a professional therapist and mediator, researcher, and writer.

In many ways, this essay reflects changes over a decade. When Marvin Sussman first asked me to write this essay, I had recently moved from University of Delaware to Indiana University-Purdue University at Indianapolis and a year later had accepted the role of Chair with considerable reluctance. Fortunately, the department flourished–a tribute to the faculty's resilience rather than my skills as Chair. I considered my primary accomplishments during the 3+ years as: (1) moving the faculty into a suite of offices that were considerably larger (and painting them a color that under our florescent lights was not a subdued terra cotta, but hot pink!), and (2) providing considerable assistance (and issuing some minor threats) to assure that two assistant professors, who had not been properly mentored, were promoted. I enjoyed working with the faculty; I hated the forms, endless meetings, and senseless chores that were associated with the role of Chair. This reinforced my own assessment that administration was not my strong suit.

My family has also changed considerably during this time. Two of my children were married and I had three grandchildren when I wrote the first draft of this essay. As the drafts evolved, so did my family. I now have eight grandchildren, have helped my daughter through a divorce, and helped with the wedding arrangements for my son. Sadly, I also was there to support my son and daughter-in-law with funeral arrangements when their daughter was full-term but stillborn. I am no longer in a commuter marriage as my husband took early retirement several years ago to join me in Indianapolis.

Family of Orientation

I was the eldest daughter of two daughters in a two-parent family. My mother, Louise Bertha Tagg, an only child, was very well read although she had only a high school education. Her family was minor German nobility who had immigrated to the U.S. at the turn of the century. The family had money and she many opportunities, such as traveling oversees, that were not common experiences for young women in her generation. Her mother died when she was several months old and her stepmother, her mother's best friend, died during the flu epidemic when my mother was about 4 years old. Her father (Jablensky) placed her in an orphanage when he could no longer care for her. My mother's maternal aunts and uncles removed her from the orphanage and obtained legal guardianship and she adopted their name, Tagg. When I was growing up, talking about my paternal grandfather was a taboo subject. During the fall of 2000 while looking through old albums that my sister had acquired upon my mother's death, I found a photograph of my maternal grandparents taken at the beach about 1904. It had been wrapped in plastic wrap and placed, face down, in an album and in my mother's handwriting labeled "Mother and Father." The irony of protecting it from dampness in storage by wrapping it in plastic wrap, but placing it face down so it could not be observed, suggests that although my mother wished to dismiss this part of her life, but for historical purposes, felt obligated not to destroy it.

Although her family wanted her to observe upper class traditions such as private schooling and making a debut, she resisted because she believed that in America one did not adhere to a class-based system. My mother always pushed the envelope such as smoking in public or wearing a "daring" bathing suit at a time when women covered up on public beaches. One incident that occurred in the mid-1950s remains vivid in my mind. We were rehearsing with the Philadelphia Orchestra, and an African American member of our ballet company was asked to leave the green room. My mother, all 5′2", stood up, put her arm around him and stated that this was HER son and he was not leaving!!!

My father's (Isadore Kurland) parents and older brother immigrated from Russia; my father, an older brother and two younger sisters were born in the U.S. He was a pharmacist and well educated, having completed the equivalent of a Master's degree at the Philadelphia College of Pharmacy and Science. He died about the time I returned to college so he never got to see me graduate. In fact, he died about a month before my sister graduated from college. Knowing how much he valued education, he surely would have been pleased with his daughters' accomplishments.

I have a younger sister, Cyndi Kurland, who moved from New Jersey to Southern California about eight years ago. She has a degree in English and has taken considerable additional college work in art and photography. She has worked in photography, journalism and sales. Her current hobby is performing at local comedy clubs.

Family of Procreation

My husband, Thomas Pickett, who I met on a geology field trip during my second try at undergraduate education, has a doctorate in geology. Unlike my parents, who were relatively recent immigrants, he can trace his family's arrival in America to the early 1600s. I recently discovered (also as a result of my photo project) that my children's birthfather's family (on the maternal side) can document that a forbearer came over on the Mayflower.

Tom was the Associate Director of the Delaware Geological Survey located at the University of Delaware until he took early retirement to join me in Indianapolis after a seven-year commuter marriage. He does some consulting, some part-time teaching, and continues to do research and publish on early American pewterers. He also contributes as a board member and committee member of two local youth organizations and is an active docent for the Historical Landmarks Association. We are both trained as mediators and once a week, for the past four years, we have conducted court-ordered mediations for the Marion County Superior Courts. When addressed as Mr. Steinmetz by unknowing students and associates, he is quick to point out that "He didn't change his name when we married."

My eldest child, George Steinmetz, has a bachelor's degree with honors in automotive engineering and recently completed a master's degree in Information Science. He currently works in Network Operations for Sprint. He met his wife Janet when they were students at Pittsburg State University, in Kansas. They live in Olatha, Kansas, a suburb of Kansas City, with their sons, Sam (11), Charlie (8), Mike (5) and daughter, Rebecca (2). Since his children were born, George has worked a second shift in order to care for their children during the day while his wife teaches school. George has inherited my father's love of cutting-edge technology, which is evident not only in his educational choices but also in his home. Lights go on and off as you move past them (because the children would not turn them off when they left the room), and video cameras enable the parents in the main level of the house to observe the children in the lower-level family room.

My second child, Gregg Steinmetz, has a bachelor's degree in Business Administration with emphasis on marketing and transportation from Ohio State. He has worked in middle- and upper-level management in several transportation companies. He moved from Chicago to Southern California, after a record-breaking cold and equally record-breaking heat wave. Following in the tradition of his own stepfather, when he married Sandra he acquired a stepson, Matt Villalvazo. Matt, who is now 12, is Mexican-American, thus adding some diversity to our family. A son, Jarrett (2), was followed by a daughter, Ciara Rae, in January 2001. As noted earlier, we never got to know Ciara and we are all struggling to deal with this unanticipated loss. As one might expect from the middle child and a redhead, Gregg "marches to the beat of a different drummer." He is the entrepreneur of the family and with his wife is involved in various business opportunities. They live in Orange, California, where he is currently a realtor and in the process of obtaining his Real Estate Broker license. He is contemplating starting his own business.

My youngest child, Singrid Steinmetz Ascani, married Larry who she met while they were students at California State University at Long Beach. Singrid has taken after my mother who was a champion diver and my father who was a gymnast in high school. She is the athlete in the family and won Most Valuable Player on the Delaware softball All-State team during high school. After graduating from college with a bachelor's degree in athletic training, she married and worked for a number of years in the defense industry, which caused her considerable ethical conflicts (payback for the ethical conflicts I felt when she joined a military-type drill team and twirled a rifle in high school). She returned to college and received her RN degree and works in respiratory and critical care units at Long Beach Memorial Hospital. Recently divorced, she lives with her boys, Brian (13) and Sean (11), in Garden Grove, California, where they are very active in Scouts, camping and sports.

The Importance of Science and Research

My parents instilled in me several values that have affected my development as a person and scholar. The first was a strong interest in science and research. My father was a pharmacist from the old school and had developed a number of medicines and special formulas. I remember numerous family discussions revolving around science and questioning of ideas. For a middle-class family living in a rural village in the 1940s and 1950s, we had a fairly large reference library–several sets of encyclopedia, atlases, various scientific handbooks, and volumes of poetry, essays, plays by known literary figures and books by the great western thinkers. My father, whose hobbies were photography and ham radio, was intrigued with the newest technology (we had one of the first, if not the first, TV in our community) and was always building and modifying equipment for photography and ham radio. My father was very active in the local civil defense organization. Like my mother, giving back to the community was very important.

My interest in writing and seeing my work in print started early. In high school I was a "stringer" for the weekly newspaper and wrote a column on the local activities in my community. I found that doing "research" on these activities and adding a sentence or two enhanced not only my column, but also my purse since I was paid on the column inch. I also co-authored our school song (sung to the tune of Loch Lomond–to fit our "Scottish" senior yearbook theme). Corny, but fitting for the times, our class decided that it would be nice to have our own song for graduation so I volunteered to try to write one (and recruited a friend to help). It never occurred to me or my classmate that this might be beyond our capabilities.

We are nearing the end of our happiest days
With joy and sorrow in knowing
We'll soon say good-bye to our Class of '58;
Both our tears and our smiles are glowing
We look toward the past at the work we have done

And the great reward it is bringing–
The friendships we've made and the memories we'll keep–
As our graduation song we are singing (Chorus)
With diplomas in hand we walk down the aisle;
How our hearts and our voices do tremble.
We take one last glance at our friends in cap and gown,
Knowing thus ne'er again we'll assemble.

My parents also firmly believed that it was important to learn to think for myself, not to go along with the crowd. "Be a leader, not a follower." As a young child, this statement was usually followed with "If Sally jumped off the roof, would you also do it?"–or some variation of this theme. This advice was later extended to "don't believe everything you hear or read." However, this stance has the potential of causing conflicts and an early one arose when I was around 12 and was going through classes in order to be confirmed in the Episcopal Church. I quickly discovered that I just couldn't accept some of the teachings and I kept questioning my teacher and my mother about the veracity of the material we were supposed to believe as the "truth." The church's emphasis on form over content and the hypocrisy that I observed made me aware that I did not believe in the Church, the doctrine, or most of the activities of mainstream organized religion.

As a college student and later as an academic, I tend to not accept what I read or hear, but question it. I want to know not only what has happened, and if there are other interpretations of a phenomenon, but more importantly why it happened. This approach has been particularly painful for me when the autopsy of my granddaughter failed to identify any problems. Obviously, everything was NOT normal. My parents' emphasis on not taking anything for granted (in life and in science) and looking beyond the surface to the processes involved has had a lasting impact.

I believe that I have transmitted this value to my children. When my eldest child, George, was in fourth grade, I went into the living room to discover him holding his own in a debate with a Jehovah's Witness over the age of the earth. He kept insisting that the fossil record indicated that the earth was millions of years old, not a few thousand as the Jehovah's Witness stated, using the Bible as evidence. Gregg, during a fifth grade field trip, held a lively debate with a docent at Winterthur Museum who kept insisting that a chair was Queen Ann style, while Gregg kept insisting, correctly so, that it was a Chippendale style. Singrid tested the limit in high school by being the first female student to enroll in a year-long course on auto mechanics–a requirement of all my children before they could own a car. She also began taking college courses at the University of Delaware in her sophomore year in high school, as did Gregg (in his senior year), for pragmatic, financial reasons (it was free, I taught there) rather than because they were honor students–which in high school, they were not.

EARLY ADULTHOOD

Undergraduate Education

It had been expected that I would follow in my father's footsteps and become a pharmacist or scientist, yet I had spent an considerable part of my youth training to be a classical dancer and in the theater. At that time, the life of a ballerina was marginal. Very poor pay, few professional companies and from my observation most dancers did not appear to be pictures of health. Furthermore, I did not find the idea of living out of a suitcase to be desirable. Rather than attending the Philadelphia College of Pharmacy and Science or Julliard, the choices that had been presented throughout my childhood, I entered the University of Delaware, known at that time for both their excellent Theater and Chemistry Departments, and became a double major.

Following the trend of my generation, I married someone I met in college, completed two semesters and then worked for a few years, until our first child was born. However the dual interest–science and theater–continued and I worked at Sun Oil Company in basic research then and opened a dance school and was active in local community theater.

After three children and a divorce, I realized that my limited formal education and few marketable skills required a re-evaluation of my goals. In the mid-1960s re-entering college life as a 26-year-old was still fairly unusual. This was certainly the case at the University of Delaware, a predominately residential college that did not permit women students to wear slacks on campus until 1968. I returned to college with the support of my Vocational Rehabilitation counselor, Robert Rodgers, and a college professor, Dr. Wallace Maw, both met through a mutual acquaintance, feeling more like a grandmother than a college student.

One requirement of Vocational Rehabilitation was to participate in a half-day comprehensive set of IQ, psychological and vocational tests. Recognizing the importance of these tests, I arrived at 9:00 a.m. and applied myself with diligence. Not understanding the goal of the various tests, I made sure that my "draw a house" was perfect. Since I have no artistic talent, and, as I discovered from the tests, virtually no spatial perception, this was a challenge. Likewise, I spent considerable time on the sentence completion tests, making sure that my sentences were comprehensive, grammatically correct and showed creativity. I even provided alternative interpretations for the "arrange a cartoon" test. When, I had finally completed the battery of tests, the test administrator escorted me out of the office. Imagine my surprise when I discovered that the office was empty since it was after 6:00 p.m. I had taken the entire day (9 hours) without a break to complete a set of tests that typically are completed in a 4-hour testing situation.

Fortunately, I passed! My IQ was sufficiently high to support success in college; my psychological tests revealed that I was basically normal and capable of dealing with the stress of returning to college as a divorced mother of three. The vocational testing, however, was puzzling since my tests revealed that I should consider becoming an engineer, minister, or physician. Strange careers choices for a squeamish atheist with limited spatial perception. I was able to convince my rehab counselor that elementary education would be a good choice for a divorced mother of three, since it was the one career in which your schedule matched that of your children.

Interestingly, after student teaching, I realized that I was not cut out to be an elementary school teacher. However, throughout my adult life I have continued to build dams, sea walls, boat launches, room additions, and terraces (an expression of my engineering bent?). In 1994, I completed my MSW and a few years later became a Reiki Master–an energy transfer skill that is a useful healing technique not only for family and friends but also when my students have a variety of broken bones and other injuries (an expression of healing or being a physician?). In 1998, I was ordained as a nondenominational minister in the Order of Melchizedek. Perhaps the vocational tests were right!

Graduate School Years

After I returned to college, I made a "deal" with my rehab counselor. He agreed that I could receive financial support for childcare, transportation and books, for two years of graduate education if I completed my undergraduate degree in two years. By carrying 20-21 credits each semester and going to summer school I was able to graduate in two years. I realized that I loved research and would enjoy teaching at the college level, but not in the field of education. I had particularly enjoyed both my Educational Sociology course and my Educational Psychology courses (I read a book and tested out of the required "Introduction to Sociology" course). However, at the University of Delaware, the Psychology Department was engaged in research with cats. Strange and uncomfortable noises seemed to emanate from the psychology wing. In contrast, the Sociology offices seemed quiet and agreeable. Thus, having never taken an undergraduate Sociology course, I applied to the PhD program in Sociology at Case Western Reserve and was accepted.

I had selected Case Western Reserve University because the Sociology program had a PhD fellowship in Vocational Rehabilitation. I was so impressed with the influence and success that my rehab counselor seemed to enjoy that I wanted to follow in his footsteps. However, when I interviewed at CWRU, the Graduate Coordinator informed me that there were no fellowships left in vocational rehabilitation, but if I was interested in family there was a traineeship in that area. So, being a pragmatist, I thought, "OK, I'm interested in family," applied for and was awarded a NIMH family traineeship. I worked at College of Urban Affairs as a research assistant over the summer, then packed up my house and drove a 28-foot U-Haul to Cleveland.

Moving to Cleveland was quite an adventure. I had lived my entire life in three different states (New Jersey, Delaware, Pennsylvania) but the distance encompassed only about 30 miles. I was moving away from the mideastern coastal states to the Midwest. The sign that greeted you as you crossed the border from Pennsylvania into Ohio noted that you were "Entering the heart of the Midwest" (although as a resident of Indiana, I now recognize that the sign was either considerably out-of-date, or that the Pennsylvania Highway Department was geographically challenged). I was attending a university that until a year earlier reflected its once geographic location–Western Reserve University. My children and I were leaving the rest of our family behind. And I was taking graduate work in a discipline in which my only familiarity was a quick read of an Introductory Sociology textbook.

We found wonderful housing as a token white family in Shaker Heights but bordering on Hough, an area that had seen racial unrest several years earlier. There were 28 white children enrolled in the elementary school–three of the 28 were mine. When I enrolled the children in school I asked about lunch and was informed that all the children go home for lunch. I asked, "What do children do if their parents work?" and, without missing a beat was told, "Their maids make their lunch." Clearly this was a different world–not only in terms of diversity, but also in terms of social class.

I bartered for daycare for my daughter in return for teaching dancing to the different classes. I also taught the children French. For their recital, the children performed some dance numbers and sang "Frere Jacque" and a few other French songs garnered from the text in "music education," a required course for all elementary school majors. The children were accompanied by tape recorded piano music which was quite a challenge since in addition to not speaking French, I also do not play the piano!!!

After receiving my master's degree, I returned to Delaware and married Thomas Pickett, who I first met on a geology field trip as an undergraduate student. I was aware that lots of scholars did not have a PhD and I did not think that this lack would hinder my ability to do research. For about two years I taught and did research at Lincoln University. I also enrolled at Temple University, and taught there as an instructor. At Temple University, I had the opportunity to round out my background with courses in social stratification, social mobility, comparative sociology, socialization, urban, social movements, and criminology–important courses since I lacked an undergraduate degree in sociology and my master's degree consisted of classes in methodology, statistics, theory, and family.

By this time, I had published several papers (Steinmetz, 1971; 1973; Steinmetz & Straus, 1973) and an edited book, and two additional papers were in press (Steinmetz, 1974a; 1974b; Steinmetz & Straus, 1974). But, I lacked a PhD. From my naive perspective, it appeared that I would not need one. After all, I was doing research and teaching classes. At a meeting of the National Council of Family Relations in the fall of 1973, some colleagues who were recruiting to fill a family position approached me. They asked when and where I received my PhD. When I told them that I did not have one, they responded that their University would not consider hiring someone without a PhD (or at least ABD). Reality hit!!! I talked to Jetse Sprey and Marvin Sussman, faculty from CWRU who were attending the meeting, about the possibility of returning to complete my degree in an efficient way (i.e., have my work at Temple University as well as independent research count). I had already passed my theory and methods qualifying exams and completed the residency requirements. I only needed some additional coursework, two specialty exams, and a dissertation to obtain the prize!

The work I had completed at Temple gave me an area in "socialization" as well as my area in "family." This seemed to be the most expedient way to complete the doctorate. Marvin Sussman, Chair of the Department of Sociology at that time, agreed. He arranged things so that I would only need to take a few courses on campus. During the spring of 1974, I flew from Philadelphia to Cleveland once a week. I would arrive around 10:00 a.m. to attend two seminars and be back in Ohio by early evening. In the summer of 1974, I wrote my specialty exams in family and socialization; the latter provided the basis of a chapter on childrearing (Steinmetz, 1978a) in *Contemporary Theories* (Burr, Hill, Nye & Reiss, 1978). I also prepared my dissertation proposal and gathered data in late summer, and fall. That year I was also teaching a full load as a visiting assistant professor at the University of Delaware as a replacement for Barbara Settles, who was on sabbatical. During winter session (a 5-week period between fall and spring semester), I analyzed my data and wrote drafts of my data chapters. I completed the drafts in April and defended in early May.

Fortunately, my committee requested only very minor changes and I was able to make these changes in a few hours and turned in the completed product before leaving for Delaware. I do believe that my committee was extremely kind in requiring so few changes. I, on the other hand, completely tore the work apart, including reanalyzing data, when I prepared the dissertation for the monograph *The Cycle of Violence: Assertive, Aggressive, Abusive Family Interaction*, published by Praeger (Steinmetz, 1977a).

MIDDLE ADULTHOOD

For purposes of this essay, I am considering "Middle Adulthood" to be that period after completing my dissertation until I assumed co-editorship of *Marriage & Family Review*–not based on age, but rather on my career. I consider this period to be my most productive academic years in terms of research publications and grants. Also, my children were completing their education, getting married and starting families during this period.

Questioning Rules and Roles in Publications

I had been interested in childrearing research, specifically the research linking childrearing techniques with specific outcomes, since my undergraduate days. However, my work in family violence began when I questioned Murray Straus about some of the findings he presented in a paper he read at a conference. I had just started my second year as a graduate student, and was not aware that this was not the typical way to interact with an established scholar–especially one I had never met until this conference. Straus challenged me to "prove" my findings. I did, and the resulting article, my first publication, "Occupation and Physical Punishment: A Response to Straus," appeared in the *Journal of Marriage and the Family* (Steinmetz, 1971). A collaborative relationship resulted in several articles and books (Steinmetz & Straus, 1973; 1974; Straus, Gelles & Steinmetz, 1980a; 1980b).

The Gender Bias in Research Studies. Another early publication grew out of a paper for a class in social stratification at Temple University. Upward and downward mobility for men was based on a comparison of the social class of a son's father with his own social class. Women's social class, however, was reckoned by comparing their fathers' social class with that of their husbands'. I wanted to compare the mothers' social class, based on their own educational and occupational achievements, with that of their daughters, based on the educational and occupational achievements of their daughters.

Unfortunately, no data had been collected through research studies or the Census that would enable me to do this. With all of the data collected, funded and disseminated by the government using taxpayers' money, the Census Bureau did not have any data that would allow a researcher to compare mother's status with father's status as head of house. In fact, until 1970, they instructed enumerators to recode as male head, any family that had a male over 18 years of age residing in the home, regardless of that male's employment status or financial contribution to the household.

My anger over the government taxing women's salaries to support the Census Bureau yet refusing to acknowledge that, if an adult male lived in the home, women could still be the head of household, resulted in the article entitled "The Sexual Context of Social Research" (Steinmetz, 1973). The research reviewed for this study also revealed that studies of childrearing were based almost exclusively on data provided by the women on their childrearing practices. This practice was lacking in logic, since the same literature also linked child-rearing practices to social class. The concept social class, in turn, was based entirely on the father's educational level and occupational attainment, which resulted in the extensive body of gender-biased research on childrearing and family studies.

The bias against men in the family and childrearing literature was further explored in an article "Male Liberation: Destroying the Stereotypes" (Steinmetz, 1974b). This article examined not only the phenomenon of ignoring fathers' contribution to childrearing, but also other biases that ridiculed and degraded males such as the "Dagwood

Bumstead" view of males as bumbling idiots; "males as happy bachelors" and "strong males don't cry" (or show any emotions except violence–the manly emotion).

I greatly admired Melvin Kohn's work, especially his classic study *Class and Conformity: A Study in Values* (Kohn, 1969) and other research linking social class values based on the jobs one held to child rearing techniques. However, it appeared to me that (1) differences existed within a job category (e.g., between a theoretical engineer who studied processes in a lab and who interacted on a collegial level with subordinates, versus an engineer in a plant, who supervised workers and expected strict adherence to rules and regulations), and (2) the skills required for a particular job might cut across social class boundaries (e.g., the skills of a dentist being perhaps more similar to those of an auto mechanic or welder). A subsequent article (Steinmetz, 1974a), found a stronger relationship between types of punishments and job-related skills than between types of punishment and social class.

The Battered Husband Controversy. During the next few years, I explored the connection between using physical force to discipline children and subsequent childhood aggression (Steinmetz, 1977b; 1978a), and published a number of articles and chapters on family violence (Steinmetz, 1978b; 1978c; 1978d; 1980a; 1981a; 1982a; 1987b) as well as the book based on my dissertation (Steinmetz, 1977a). Because of the visibility of my work on battered women and children, I was always warmly welcomed as a guest speaker and often treated as a minor hero.

This changed after I published "The Battered Husband Syndrome" (Steinmetz, 1977-78; 1978e). Since I had been interested in family violence, especially intergenerational trends, I had analyzed my data as couple violence rather than husband to wife and wife to husband violence. My colleagues chided me, noting that this couple violence was no doubt primarily husband-to-wife violence. To test their hypothesis, I analyzed the data separately by perpetrator and victim. Although my data were from a small sample, I was astonished to discover that in many categories wives were equally violent or more so than their husbands. Some findings were initially published (Steinmetz, 1976), but it was the 1977-78 publication that drew the fire. The findings occurred not only in several studies in the U.S., but also in Canada, Puerto Rico, Finland, Israel (a large sample of Kibbutz and nuclear families), and a large multi-ethnic sample in Belize (Steinmetz, 1978f; 1980b, 1981b; 1989a; 1994; Steinmetz & Lucca, 1988; Steinmetz & Pelliccario, 1986; Straus, Gelles, & Steinmetz, 1980a; 1980b).

I was the object of considerable discussion and some threats of violence, ironically from angry women because I dared to report that women could also be violent. Subsequently, two national surveys of family violence and countless smaller studies in the United States and dozens of other countries have supported my initial findings on violence between men and women.

The Battered Elderly Are Discovered. I also attracted considerable interest when I presented Congressional Testimony on "Overlooked Aspects of Domestic Violence" (Steinmetz, 1978g). Cronin and Allen (1982) acknowledged my testimony, noting:

> Although the Congressional Hearing was not the first published reference to elder abuse, it was the "first to gain such national prominence, and was the sole portion of the Hearings to earn coverage in the *New York Times*, as well as a mention from Walter Cronkite."

I provided testimony to Congress on elder abuse a year later (Steinmetz, 1979), and explored this topic in a number of journal articles and chapters that resulted from an in-depth study of families caring for an elder (Steinmetz, 1978h; 1981d; 1982b 1983; 1985; 1987a; 1988a; 1989b; 1990a; 1990b; 1993; Steinmetz & Amsden, 1983). My monograph, *Duty Bound: Elder Abuse and Family Care* (Steinmetz, 1988c), was also published.

Organizational Roles. This strong individualistic characteristic has also resulted in crossing boundaries into areas not typically crossed by women or social scientists. When I was at the University of Delaware, I was initiated into Sigma Xi (a national research society) as one of the first social scientists to be initiated, since the Sigma Xi was hard-science oriented. At that time, the spring of 1975, the few "social" science members were psychologists conducting clinical studies. The membership had assumed that only scholars doing research in the physical, natural, or biological sciences would be doing "science." Two years later, I became not only the first woman president of the University of Delaware chapter, but also the first social scientist to hold that office. This artificial dichotomy of "hard" or "soft" science has never made any sense to me and I have striven to straddle that dichotomy. In 1980, I was elected President of the Delaware Academy of Science, thus becoming the first social scientist and first woman to be elected to this post. Sixteen years after serving as the President of the University of Delaware chapter, I served as the President of the Indiana University Medical

Center chapter of Sigma Xi. Although I was not the first woman to hold that post, I was the first social scientist to do so. I admit that I enjoy being first in these areas although as I noted in a public service announcement I taped for National Brotherhood Week, as long as we have to preface successes with "the first" (woman, black, Catholic, etc.), then we have a long way to go before we reach true equality.

Changing Jobs. Possibly one of the greatest challenges that I have taken to date occurred in 1989 when I left the University of Delaware, where I had been employed full-time since completing my doctorate in 1975. I left Delaware to take a position as Professor of Sociology at Indiana University-Purdue University in Indianapolis (known as IUPUI). This is a large urban campus containing the Purdue Schools of Science, Engineering and Technology, and Hotel and Restaurant Management and the Indiana University Schools of Liberal Arts, Social Work, Nursing, Medicine, Dentistry, Journalism, Education, and Business, as well as a number of hospitals that are part of the IUPUI complex.

Not only was I changing disciplinary ties from a Department of Individual and Family Studies in what was once a College of Home Economics to a Sociology Department, but also I would be entering a commuter marriage. These moves are always influenced by a carrot and a stick. The stick was represented by a growing unhappiness with Department politics, general University turmoil, and severe salary compression at the University of Delaware. These circumstances were so upsetting that I resigned from the University BEFORE I had even begun to search for a new job. Magically, I was approached about coming to IUPUI within days of resigning. The carrot was represented by an opportunity to teach classes in my own discipline, Sociology; to do research in a setting with a full complement of professional schools which were not available at the University of Delaware; the opportunity to play a cooperative research role with the government of Indianapolis; a most generous increase in salary with a substantial computer and library allowance; and a substantial amount of money to enable me to establish a family research project.

The decision to leave the University of Delaware was probably one of the best decisions I have ever made. I quickly realized that I had missed being able to teach sociology courses and discuss "sociology" with colleagues. Although there were times when I missed my husband and our visits were never long enough, I found the opportunity to put my career and my own needs first–the only time in adulthood that I had that luxury–to be exciting. My work since coming to Indianapolis has developed along two divergent tracks: one is more applied and focused on adolescents and families at risk (Kinney & Steinmetz, 1994; Steinmetz, 1995; Steinmetz, 1996; Steinmetz, 1999a), the other is a growing interest in sociological and family theory (Adams & Steinmetz, 1993; Peterson & Steinmetz, 1999; Steinmetz, 1999b; Settles, Steinmetz, Peterson & Sussman, 1999). I am currently working with a Sociologist in Japan on the writings of Tongo Takebe, a contemporary of Auguste Comte (1798-1857).

Social Consciousness

Another major influence on my life was the social consciousness that my parents instilled in me. In many small but important ways they demonstrated by their actions the importance of helping others, and doing so in ways that did not result in a loss of pride. Our table was always full of fresh produce and other farm items that had been exchanged for needed medicine. My parents were always active in informal ways to help the needy, as well as the organized forms such as the cancer drive and the local civil defense organization.

Even as a very young child, I visited, entertained and assisted people in mental institutions, nursing homes, and county homes–where the poor and elderly lived. I can remember trudging out to the migrant farms to take food, clothing, and toys to a family that had been identified as needing help. I remember that my mother always made sure that in addition to the necessities of food, clothing, and medicine, there were "luxury" items for each individual "to brighten their day." Unlike the current view that the poor are weak of character and responsible for their current status, my parents viewed the poor as being no different from those with wealth other than having experienced a misfortune. As the more fortunate, it was our obligation to help those who were less fortunate since we could not know whether we might also need assistance at some time in the future. It wasn't something one did for charity; it was our obligation to humanity.

It was instilled, more by role modeling than discussion, that my quality of life could not be separated from the quality of life of others–privileged or oppressed. Possibly this is why I have been so interested in research on those who are oppressed. Only if we understand the processes that lead to oppression can we hope to develop a way to obliterate it.

During this time, I was a member of a professional ballet company, and two to three times a week I would take the bus to Philadelphia (about an hour and a half ride). The company performed with the Philadelphia Orchestra and the Philadelphia Opera Company, and I had experiences, such as eating lunch with Eugene Ormandy, conductor of the Philadelphia Orchestra during the 1950s, which, I'm sure, were atypical for a kid from rural New Jersey. In the summer I studied classical ballet and dance in New York City and lived in a residence hall for women. As we lived in a rural community and television was still relatively rare at this time, I can remember my classmates being astonished that I was able to stand on my toes, as they had never seen this before. During high school, I lived in two worlds. By day I was a typical teenager living in rural Pennsville, New Jersey–a small community with hometown values. In the evenings, weekends, and summer I was an aspiring ballerina studying in Philadelphia and New York. Perhaps this prepared me to feel comfortable in a world characterized by opposites, such as considering myself to be a feminist and a mentor of female students, yet publishing data indicating that husbands might also be victims of domestic violence.

My choice of high school was another important influence in my life. Because there was no high school in my community, I had to select a high school in one of the two neighboring towns. I could have gone to the high school located in Pennsgrove (Pennsgrove Regional High School, or Re High, where Bruce Willis, the television and screen star, attended several years later) or Salem High located in historic Salem, New Jersey.

I chose Salem probably because I sense that my parents preferred this choice and also I because I had friends who lived there. Salem had a heavy Quaker influence, and in the mid-1950s the town and schools were fully integrated in every sense. The Vice President of our class was African American and all of our activities were integrated. At the time I did not fully understand the importance as well as the uniqueness of our high school's tradition of living on a boat during our senior class trip to Washington, DC. This was done because the hotels in Washington were segregated and we could not have stayed together as a class. The Quaker influence was everywhere. Not only were many of my friends Quakers, but the Underground Railroad had operated in Salem and some of my friends actually lived in houses that had served in that capacity.

I do not remember much discussion about race relations or integration–or even that our high school was different. It was not the spoken word, but the acts that dominated and left their impression. I followed this tradition of actions over words. As noted earlier, I lived in a predominately black neighborhood while in graduate school. Following what I had observed in high school, I never mentioned race to my children and it was years later before they remarked that there seemed to be very few white children in their school. I am pleased that my children have absorbed this view of life and have friends representing considerable diversity. As my daughter recently remarked, "We were raised to be color-blind." Thus, in a subtle but important way, my experiences at Salem High School reinforced the social consciousness that was expressed by my parents (e.g., the need to help others and a recognition of the uniqueness and value of all people).

Editing: The Handbooks and Journal

In the mid-1980s, Marvin Sussman asked if I would join him in a project that he had started several years earlier (Sussman & Steinmetz, 1987). Since the last *Handbook on Marriage and the Family* (Christensen, 1964) was considerably out of date, Sussman had obtained a contract from Plenum to produce a new *Handbook.* This provided me with the opportunity to invite colleagues from my cohort–many of whom were women, many who were new assistant professors when first invited (many are now well-known professors who have left their mark on the field). The *Handbook* was the lead review in *Contemporary Sociology* (Adams, 1988). A second edition of the *Handbook* (Sussman, Steinmetz & Peterson, 1999) continued the tradition.

I was also a member of the editorial team selected by the Theories and Methods Workshop, held in conjunction with the National Council on Family Relations, to produce the *Sourcebook of Theories and Methods* (Boss, Doherty, LaRossa, Schumm, & Steinmetz, 1993). A collaborative effort from the beginning, the *Sourcebook* used an historical, contextual approach.

Since 1998, Gary (Pete) Peterson and I have served as Co-Editors of *Marriage & Family Review.* We are members of different academic cohorts and our different backgrounds and experiences complement each other. The autobiography project, of which this essay is a part, was initially proposed by Sussman. However, except for a few essays and some outlines, the project had stalled. When Pete and I took over as co-editors, the essays from the dozen or so individuals (my own included) who were initially contacted by Marvin Sussman were in files. After reading these essays, Pete and I decided not only to continue the project, but also to enlarge and redirect it.

These essays document the family, educational, and social backgrounds of researchers. Thus, we can observe, first hand, how one's life experiences shape one's research. Of major importance, however, is that the autobiographies prepared by the older generation of scholars (e.g., Harold Christensen, Bernard Farber, Marvin Sussman, Margaret Feldman, Catherine Chilman, and Evelyn Duvall) document the earliest academic roots of the field of family. Their personal accounts provide valuable insights into the subject matter and methods of teaching, as well as anecdotal information from our earliest family scholars.

COMING FULL CIRCLE: LATE ADULTHOOD

Considering myself to be in "late adulthood" is based on how I conceptualize myself in academic terms, not age. Having turned 60 in January 2001, I would technically be considered early aging. However, I consider myself to have entered late adulthood when I assumed, with Pete Peterson, the role of Co-Editor of *Marriage & Family Review*. From a family perspective, it is roughly the time when my husband retired and joined me in Indianapolis, and corresponds with my own children having reached middle adulthood, since they are all past 35 years of age, married (and divorced) and are raising their own children.

Following the advice I offer my students–never stop learning–I completed a Master's Degree in Social Work in 1994. This provided me the credentials and the experience necessary for conducting research through intense involvement with families at risk. I also took training to be certified as a civil and family mediator and, with my husband, conduct mediations for Superior Court. I find this activity to be most rewarding because I am able to combine my training in therapy and my research in family and life course development to assist participants in resolving their disputes. I am currently doing *pro bono* work with survivors of satanic ritual abuse, the most violent and cruel intergenerational form of domestic violence. My home has served as a 'safe home' during certain holidays when these individuals would be at most risk for self harm as well as harm from cult members.

Thus, I've come full circle on the two levels discussed in the opening of this essay. Despite my earlier resistance to the results of vocational testing which suggested that my strengths were in healing, ministering and engineering, I now heal through my Reiki and therapy training and have become an ordained nondenominational minister, which assists my work with cult survivors. My "engineering" strength, however, has remained at the amateur, private-purpose level. On a second level, my early interest in helping others has now expressed itself through community involvement at various levels. However, I now have the training and certification to provide therapy and conduct mediations. I have moved from volunteer helper to professional social worker/therapist. I also now have the education and experience to be considered a professional researcher and writer, no longer the high school student who looked up facts in the encyclopedia in order to enhance the information on community activities for the local newspaper.

What Is Success?

When Marvin Sussman, my dissertation chair and lifelong mentor, invited me to prepare this chapter in the early 1990s, he told me I was "considered to be a success." This caused me to reflect on what is success and to realize that it is relative. Obtaining a bachelor's degree after becoming divorced and while caring for three small children seemed an overwhelming obstacle and definitely not the norm at a primarily residential college. Accomplishing that goal was, for me, immensely rewarding; even more than obtaining my MA or PhD. Not only did this represent closure on unfinished business and fulfilling an expectation that my parents had held for me, it meant the potential opening of doors that I had only dreamed could be opened.

Reflecting further on Marvin's statement, I had to question, is success measured by the number and status of one's publications, or number and size of one's research grants? I remember the excitement of seeing my first article in print (Steinmetz, 1971). The first request for a reprint came from Evelyn Duvall. I framed her request and it is prominently displayed in my home office. It was indeed a heady experience to think that someone of her stature would want to read something that I had written!

Reflecting still further on Marvin's use of the word "success" I wondered if success should be measured by the prestige of one's Department and the University where you are employed. Or is success measured by what you have left to society as a result of being on this earth and your own personal feeling of accomplishment?

I believe that I am leaving behind on this earth some worthwhile accomplishments. I am very proud of my children's successes. They are kind, compassionate, bright individuals who in many small ways work to overcome the oppression of others. I take pride in the fact that my research, along with that of others, was instrumental in the development of legislation, social policies, and social services to protect individuals from family violence. I hope that someday all researchers and social activists will recognize that we cannot reduce and eliminate one form of abuse (e.g., wife abuse) until we attempt to reduce and eliminate all forms of family violence, including husband abuse and childhood bullying. Like all scholars, I hope that my research will contribute to a growing body of knowledge about families.

There are several publications of which I am especially proud. The first is an article I published entitled "Wife Beating: A Critique and Reformation of Existing Theory," which questioned the idea that it was the woman's learned helplessness that resulted in her being abused and suggested that the abuse, which shared many similarities with brain washing, resulted in the learned helplessness behavior (Steinmetz, 1978f). This article also suggested that there were two distinct types of wife abuse: the "Saturday Night Brawlers," in which the wife participated in and often initiated the violence, and the "Chronic Battered Syndrome," characterized by terroristic, extremely violent abuse of the women.

I am also proud of the monograph growing out of my dissertation because it was the first study to examine violence between all family members: spousal, parent-child, and, sibling violence (Steinmetz, 1977a). Another favorite is my monograph entitled *Duty-Bound: Elder Abuse and Family Care* (Steinmetz, 1988c), which used a combination of qualitative and quantitative methodology and analysis for understanding the stress, burden and associated violence resulting from caring for an elderly kin. The findings indicated that it was the caregiver's perception of how stressful it was to provide care, not the actual amount of care that needed to be provided, that resulted in conflict and violence.

I consider the book prepared in honor of Marvin Sussman's retirement to be a major accomplishment for different reasons. In addition to a conference held in Sussman's honor, he was presented with the book *Family and Support Systems Across the Life Span* (Steinmetz, 1988b), containing articles contributed by colleagues and former students, most of whom were presenters at the conference. This was possible through an arrangement with Eliot Warner, Editor at Plenum, to publish the book in a few months if I provided camera-ready copy. For nearly a month, I typed, edited, and formatted the articles–typing well into the night, in fact, several times throughout the night. Graduate students and my husband provided help by proofing the chapters. The entire project had been kept a secret; thus, Sussman was really surprised when he was presented with a copy of the book at the beginning of the conference. The production folks at Plenum were so quick in printing the book that the contract for the project arrived several days after the boxes of books arrived. Royalties from the book were contributed to a fund that

Sussman had established at the University of Delaware library. I am pleased to note that as of 2000, a dozen years later, the fund was still collecting royalties.

Finally, I am proud of my contributions to both editions of the *Handbook of Marriage and the Family* (Sussman & Steinmetz, 1987; Sussman, Steinmetz, & Peterson, 1999) and the *Sourcebook of Family Theories and Methods* (Boss et al., 1993), and the chapter that I authored/co-authored (Adams & Steinmetz, 1993; Steinmetz, 1987b; Steinmetz, 1999a).

Show Business

I have been able to indulge my early show biz aspiration through appearances on TV talk shows and newscasts. In addition to local shows in Philadelphia, Baltimore and Indianapolis, I have been on *Donahue* several times, *Oprah*, *Larry King*, *Sonia*, *Hour Magazine*, the *Today Show*, *20/20* and a series on CNN. I have also done on-air commentary for the Mike Tyson trial. One whirlwind tour consisted of testifying in Congress, appearance on a DC panel interview with Ellen Goodman and Claude Pepper, having my research cited by Walter Chronkite during the evening news, and being the featured guest on the *Donahue* show. My celebrity status ended abruptly upon arriving home to four days of dirty dishes and dirty clothes, kids needing help with school projects and a pile of term papers to grade. Well, so much for celebrity status! The glory was short-lived and I was brought quickly down to earth.

Probably the most amusing incident occurred when a syndicated morning show wanted to book me into several markets. Unfortunately, the Baltimore, Maryland, appearance coincided with a deadline to read the final draft of a thesis. Not only was I Chair of the thesis committee, but the student was the wife of the President of the University of Delaware. The dilemma was resolved when the producer agreed to send a limo to the University so that I could review the thesis while being driven to the studio. The limo pulled up about the same time as the Dean, and several staff and faculty arrived. You can imagine the look on their faces when the limo stopped, a uniformed driver opened the door, and I entered offering no explanation.

Alex Haley, the author of *Roots* (1976) and the commencement speaker at the University of Delaware some years ago, noted that when you see a turtle on a fence post you know the turtle did not get there by itself. Clearly I have benefited from mentors who listened to my ideas and challenged me to prove them and mentors who told me not to give up when things looked bleak (especially Wallace Maw, Barbara Settles,

Murray Straus, and Marvin Sussman). I have also benefited greatly from the workers in the trenches–the social service and health care workers who sensitized me to need to examine the phenomena of husband and elder abuse–years before these became popular social issues. I hope that it is one of the qualities that I have instilled in my students–listen, question, and never stop learning–then share your knowledge so that others may learn.

AUTHOR NOTE

Suzanne K. Steinmetz, PhD, MSW, is Professor, Department of Sociology, Indiana University-Purdue University at Indianapolis, 425 University Blvd., Indianapolis, IN 46126.

REFERENCES

Adams, B. (1988). The state of family "art." *Contemporary Sociology, 17*, 5, 578-583.
Adams, B. & Steinmetz, S.K. (1993). The history of family theory. In Boss, P., Doherty, W. J., LaRossa, R., Schumm, W., & Steinmetz, S. K. (Eds.) *Sourcebook of family theories and methods: A contextual approach* (pp. 71-94). NY: Plenum.
Boss, P. G., Doherty, W. J., LaRossa, R. Schumm, W. & Steinmetz, S. K. (Eds.). (1993). *Sourcebook of family theories and methods: A contextual approach.* New York: Plenum.
Burr, W. R., Hill, R., Nye, F. I., & Reiss, I. L. (Eds.) *Contemporary theories about the family (vols. 1 & 2)*. NY: Free Press.
Christensen, H. T. (1964). *Handbook of marriage and the family*. Chicago: Rand McNally & Company.
Cronin, C. & Allen, A. (1982). The use of research sponsored by the Administration on Aging, case study no. 5: Maltreatment and abuse of the elderly. Washington, DE: Gerontological Research Institute.
Haley, A. (1976). *Roots*. New York: Doubleday.
Kinney, E. D. & Steinmetz, S. K. (1994). Notes from insurance underground: How the chronically ill cope. *Journal of Health Politics, Policy and Law, 19*, 3, 633-642.
Kohn, M. (1969). *Class and conformity: A study of values*. Homewood, IL: Dorsey Press.
Peterson, G.W. & Steinmetz, S. K. (1999). Perspective on families as we approach the twenty-first century: Challenges for future Handbook authors. In M.B. Sussman, S.K. Steinmetz, & G. Peterson (Eds.) *Handbook of marriage and the family* (pp.1-10). New York: Plenum.
Settles, B., Steinmetz, S.K., Peterson, G.W., & Sussman, M. B. (Eds.) (1999). *Conceptualizing families: International perspectives*. Binghamton, NY: Haworth Press.

Steinmetz, S. K. (1971). Occupation and physical punishment: A response to Straus. *Journal of Marriage and the Family*, *33*, 4, 664-666.

Steinmetz, S. K. (1973). The sexual context of social research. *The American Sociologist*, *9*, 3, 111-116.

Steinmetz, S. K. (1974a). Occupational environment and its relationship to physical punishment. In Steinmetz & Straus (Eds.) *Violence in the family* (pp.166-172). New York: Harper and Row.

Steinmetz, S.K. (1974b). Male liberation: Destroying the stereotypes. In E. Powers & M. Lee (Eds.) *The process of relationships* (pp. 55-57). (2nd ed., 1976).

Steinmetz, S. K. (1976). Wife beating-husband beating: A comparison of the use of physical violence between spouses. In M. Roy (Ed.) *The battered wife: A socio-psychological study of domestic violence* (pp. 63-72). NY: Van Nostrand Reinhold Co.

Steinmetz, S. K. (1977a). *Cycle of violence: Assertive, aggressive and abuse family interaction*. New York: Praeger.

Steinmetz, S. K. (1977b). The use of force for resolving family conflict: The training ground for abuse. *Family Relations*, *33*, 4, 19-26.

Steinmetz, S. K. (1977-78). The battered husband syndrome. *Victimology*, *2*, 3-4, 499-509.

Steinmetz, S. K. (1978a). Disciplinary techniques and their relationship to aggression, dependency and conscience. In Burr, W. R., Hill, R., Nye, F. I., & Reiss, I. L. (Eds.) *Contemporary theories about the family* (vol. 1, pp. 405-438). NY: Free Press.

Steinmetz, S. K. (1978b). Violence among family members. *Marriage & Family Review*, *1*, 2, 1-16.

Steinmetz, S. K. (1978c). Sibling violence. In J.M. Eekalaar& S.N. Katz (Eds.). *Family violence: An international and interdisciplinary study* (pp. 462-465). Toronto, Canada: Butterworth Publishers.

Steinmetz, S. K. (1978d). Family violence: The silent crisis. *Proceedings of the thirteenth annual interagency workshop*. The Institute of Contemporary Corrections and the Behavioral Sciences, Sam Houston State University, Huntsville, Texas.

Steinmetz, S. K. (1978e). Services to battered women, still our greatest need: A reply to Field & Kirchner. *Victimology*, *3*, 1-2, 222-226.

Steinmetz, S. K. (1978f). Wife beating: A critique and reformulation of existing theory. *Bulletin of the American Academy of Psychiatry and the Law*, *6*, 3, 322-334.

Steinmetz, S. K. (1978g). Overlooked aspects of family violence: Battered husbands, battered siblings and battered elderly. Testimony presented at the U. S. Congress-House Com. on Science and Technology *Research into violent behavior: Domestic violence*. Hearings. 95th Congress (Feb. 15-17).

Steinmetz, S. K. (1978h). Battered parents: The politics of selective inattention. *Society*, *15*, 5, 54-55.

Steinmetz, S. K. (1979). U. S. Congress-House. Select Committee on Aging. *Elder abuse: The hidden problem*. Briefing by the Select Committee on Aging. 96th Congress. (June 23, 1979). pp. 7-10.

Steinmetz, S. K. (1980a). Violence prone families. *Transactions of the New York Academy of Sciences*. Vol. 347, pp. 251-265.

Steinmetz, S. K. (1980b). Women and violence: Victims and perpetrators. *The American Journal of Psychotherapy*, *34*, 3, 334-350.

Steinmetz, S.K. (1981a). Investigating family violence. *Journal of Home Economics*. *72*, 2, 32-36.
Steinmetz, S.K. (1981b). Cross-cultural marital abuse. *Journal of Sociology and Social Welfare*, *8*, 2, 404-414.
Steinmetz, S. K. (1981d). Elder abuse. *Aging*, 315-316, (Jan/Feb), 6-10.
Steinmetz, S. K. (1982a). Cross-cultural comparison of sibling violence. *International Journal of Family Psychiatry*. *2*, 3/4, 337-351.
Steinmetz, S. K. (1982b). Family care of elders: Myths and realities. In Stinnett et al. (Eds) *Family strengths*: *IV* (pp. 213-233) Lincoln: University of Nebraska Press.
Steinmetz, S. K. (1983). Dependency, stress and violence between middle-aged caregivers and their elderly parents. In J. I. Kosberg (Ed.). *Abuse and maltreatment of the elderly* (pp. 134-149). Littleton, Mass: John-Wright, PSG, Inc.
Steinmetz, S. K. (1985). Family violence towards elders. In S. Saunders, A. Anderson, C. Hart, & G. Rubenstein (Eds.) *Violent individuals and families*: *A handbook for practitioners* (pp.137-162). Springfield: Charles C. Thomas, Publisher.
Steinmetz, S. K. (1986). *The violent family*. In M. Lystad (Ed.) The violent home (pp.51-70). New York: Brunner/Mazel.
Steinmetz, S. K. (1987a). Elderly victims of domestic violence. In C. Chambers (Ed.). *The elderly*: *Victims and deviants* (pp. 126-141). Athens: Ohio University Press.
Steinmetz, S. K. (1987b). Family violence: Past, present, future. In M. B. Sussman & S. K. Steinmetz (Eds.) *Handbook of marriage and the family* (pp.725-765). New York: Plenum.
Steinmetz, S. K. (1988a). Parental and filial obligation and support: Myths and reality. In S. K. Steinmetz (Ed.) *Family and support systems across the life span* (pp. 165-182). New York: Plenum.
Steinmetz, S. K. (Ed.) (1988b). *Family and support systems across the life span*. New York: Plenum.
Steinmetz, S. K. (1988c). *Duty bound*: *Elder abuse and family care*. Newbury Park: Sage.
Steinmetz, S. K. (1989a). Women and violence: Victims and perpetrators. *American Journal of Psychotherapy 34*, 3, 334-350.
Steinmetz, S. K. (1989b). Elder abuse by family caregivers: Processes and intervention strategies. *Contemporary Family Therapy*, *10*, 4, 256-271.
Steinmetz, S. K. (1990a). Elder abuse: Myth and reality. In T. Brubaker (Ed.) *Family relationships in later life* (pp. 193-211). Newbury Park, CA: Sage Publication.
Steinmetz, S. K. (1990b). Elder abuse by adult offspring: The relationship of actual vs. perceived dependency. *Journal of Health and Human Resources Administration*, *12*, 4, 434-463.
Steinmetz, S. K. (1993). The relationship between dependency and elder abuse. In R. J. Gelles, & Loeske, D. (Eds.), *Current controversies in family violence* (pp. 222-236), Newbury Park, CA: Sage.
Steinmetz, S. K. (1994). The case of violence against men. In J. Kammer (ed.) *Good Will Towards Men* (pp. 122-132) New York: St Martins.
Steinmetz, S. K. (1995). Violence in families. In R. D. Day, K. R. Gilbert, B. H. Settles, & W. R. Burr (Eds.) *Research and theory in family science* (pp. 255-269). New York: Brooks/Cole Publishing Co.

Steinmetz, S. K. (1996). *Boys' school: A demographic analysis.* Prepared for Marion County Department of Community Corrections, Indianapolis, IN.

Steinmetz, S. K. (1999a). Adolescence in contemporary families. In M.B. Sussman, S.K. Steinmetz, & G. Peterson (Eds.) *Handbook of marriage and the family* (pp. 371-423). New York: Plenum.

Steinmetz, S. K. (1999b). Sociological theories of violence. In V. Van Haslett & M. Hersen (Eds.) *Handbook of psychological approaches with violent criminal offenders: Contemporary strategies and issues* (pp. 13-36). NY: Plenum, 1999.

Steinmetz, S. K. & Amsden, D. (1983). Dependent elders, family stress and abuse. In T. Brubaker (Ed.) *Family relationships in later life* (pp. 173-192). Beverly Hills, CA: Sage Publications.

Steinmetz, S. K. & Lucca, J. (1988). Husband battering (with J. Lucca) in V. Van Hasselt, R. Morrison, Bellack and M. Herson. *Handbook of family violence* (pp. 233-246). New York: Plenum.

Steinmetz, S. K. & Pelliccario, J. (1986). Women, ethnicity, and family violence: Implications for social policy. In W.A. Van Horne & T.V.Tonnesen (Eds.) *Ethnicity and Women* (206-223). Madison, WI: University of Wisconsin Press.

Steinmetz, S. K. & Straus, M. A. (1973). The family as a cradle of violence. *Society.* 10, 6, 50-56.

Steinmetz, S. K. & Straus, M. A. (1974). *Violence in the family.* New York: Harper and Row.

Straus, M.A., Gelles, R., & Steinmetz, S. K. (1980a). Physical violence in a nationally representative sample of American families. In J. Trost (Ed.) *The Family in Change* pp. 149-165). Vasteras, Sweden: International Library.

Straus, M. A., Gelles, R., & Steinmetz, S. K. (1980b). *Behind closed doors: Violence in the American family.* New York: Doubleday.

Sussman, M. B. & Steinmetz, S. K. (Eds.) (1987). *Handbook of marriage and the family.* New York: Plenum.

Sussman, M. B., Steinmetz, S. K., & Peterson, G. W. (Eds.) (1999). *Handbook of marriage and the family* (2nd Edition). New York: Plenum.

The Social Construction of a Family Sociologist

Ralph LaRossa

KEYWORDS. Autobiography, marital conflict, marital power, transition to parenthood, fatherhood, motherhood

I

I was born in Brooklyn in 1947, moved to Queens in 1952, and spent much of my youth watching television, playing stickball, and rooting for the Yankees. I attended the local Catholic grammar school, where I majored in penmanship and "sitting quietly"; then went on to the Jesuit-run high school, Brooklyn Prep, of which my most vivid memories include being subjected to random haircut inspections, taking speech classes to eradicate our "crude" New York accents, and studying Latin for four years.

My father dropped out of high school during the Depression, was in the army air corps during World War II, and eventually became an elevator maintenance supervisor for Rockefeller Center. I loved it when I would visit him on the job and he would take me through the underground maze that allowed him to move from one building to the next without ever seeing daylight. Joseph LaRossa was fascinated with circuitry, knew Manhattan like the back of his hand, and had a sense of humor his friends found endearing. He also was a quiet, caring man who taught by example and lived his life by the rule that as long as he woke up each morning, whatever else followed was easy. The day he failed to wake up changed me forever.

My mother was a seamstress and artist who graduated from high school in 1940 and who, by all rights, should have gone on to college, but was prevented from doing so because her parents simply could not afford it. Frances Maniscalco LaRossa had a thirst for knowledge, loved archeology in particular, and prided herself on the fact that all the kids in the neighborhood liked to hang around our house. Remembering what it was like to be discriminated against just because she happened to be Italian, she would not allow a prejudicial word to be spoken in her home. It was my mother who impressed upon me the value of education and who taught me what it means to sacrifice for your children. She, too, has passed away, but her spirit lives on in everything I do.

In 1964, I entered St. Peter's College (another Jesuit-run school, located just across the Hudson River in Jersey City), with the idea of becoming a lawyer or teacher. My parents were convinced that I would go into law, given how much I enjoyed watching episodes of *Perry Mason* and debating current events. Teaching won out in the end, I think because I fell in love with the whole faculty role model mystique. As a college student, it just seemed to me the greatest thing in the world to have the kind of impact on others that my professors were having on me.

By my sophomore year I had pretty much made the decision to teach at the college level, but had not decided yet on what I was going to teach. Initially, I thought it might be English, but I guessed, probably correctly, that my preference for nonfiction over fiction would be a liability. Next, I declared Psychology as a major, which I might very well have stuck with, were it not for the fact that the whole Psychology faculty at St. Peter's consisted of one person. I also took a number of courses in Philosophy, because it was a required minor, and absorbed a great deal–especially from one soon-to-be priest, James Loughran, S. J., whom I admired very much. But Philosophy was, well . . . too philosophical. I wanted something more concrete. Then, in spring 1966, I took a Sociology course from Robert Stump, S. J. (SO 022, "Social Institutions") and was immediately enthralled. The classroom discussions led by this young instructor seemed so relevant to what was happening in the world then. The same was true for the Sociology courses taught by Stephen Doyle, Arthur LeClaire, and John Schlereth.

The 1960s, I need not point out, were tumultuous years, what with the Civil Rights movement and the Vietnam War being played out in the streets and on the news. In the midst of it all, Sociology came across as a discipline that was earnestly striving to understand what was going on and to help change things for the better. I figured that becoming a Sociology professor would give me the opportunity to contribute positively to social change. Like others in my age cohort, I wanted to "make a difference."

Among the social science books I read as an undergraduate, there was one that made more of an impression on me than any other–Peter Berger's *Invitation to Sociology* (1963). There was just something about the book that I found fascinating. I think much of it had to do with Berger's focus on everyday life and his humanistic perspective. *Invitation to Sociology* has since become a classic and touched many people, I am sure. The most direct influence it had on me, however, was that when the time came to choose a graduate school, I found myself leaning toward attending the New School for Social Research, where Berger was a faculty member.

Berger was not the New School's only draw. The fact that it was close to home was also a plus. A few months before graduation, I dropped by the St. Peter's College coffee house and happened to strike up a conversation with a student from St. Peter's Hospital School of Nursing. To this day, Maureen and I kid each other about who "picked up" whom. We both agree, however, that we started to date in 1968, fell in love soon thereafter, and were married in 1970. I had an inkling that the two of us would become seriously involved, and I was not about to jeopardize the relationship by leaving town. So the New School it was.

During my first year at the Greenwich Village campus, I made it a point to take a course with Peter Berger who had recently completed, with Thomas Luckmann, *The Social Construction of Reality: A Treatise in the Sociology of Knowledge* (1966), a more abstract version of *Invitation to Sociology* (1963) (at least that's how I interpreted it). Berger devoted his lectures to elaborating the basic tenets underlying his and Luckman's new book. His exposition resonated with me; I began to see reality construction all over the place (still do, to some extent).

Other professors at the New School were equally inspiring. Carl Mayer taught an absolutely wonderful course on Max Weber. Robert Perinbanayagam got me excited about symbolic interactionism. Joseph Bensman, Emil Oestereicher, Deborah Offenbacher, and Arthur Vidich made social class and stratification come alive. Mary Henle's course convinced me that I would do well to keep on top of what was happening in the field of Psychology. And Paul Lazarsfeld, who was a Visiting Professor at one point, was flat-out mesmerizing.

When I completed my MA, I had another choice to make–to either continue at the New School for a PhD or go somewhere else. I decided to go somewhere else. The faculty-student ratio at the New School was not ideal (some of my classes had over 60 students) and the heavy New York traffic was starting to get to Maureen and me. We thought it would be interesting to "run away" to the country, so I applied to several schools in New England and eventually opted for the University of New Hampshire, after being offered an assistantship. The year was 1972.

UNH had only recently begun to award PhDs in Sociology, so there wasn't a long list of distinguished alums that one could identify with. But what UNH lacked in tradition, it more than made up for in faculty enthusiasm and student support. Murray Straus had been hired away from the University of Minnesota, and been awarded a National Institute of Mental Health grant to establish a family violence research/training program. Walter Buckley had moved from the University of California in Santa Barbara and was encouraging everyone to think in "systems theory" terms. (Both taught challenging courses, but Murray's research methods seminar was the most useful course I have ever taken.) Several new Assistant Professors–Tom Burns, Loren Cobb, Howard Shapiro–had also come on board and become leaders in the department right away. Unlike at the New School, UNH's graduate classes were small and intimate. The collegiality among the students was warm. I thought the place was electric.

I selected Howie Shapiro to chair my dissertation because of his interest in phenomenology and symbolic interactionism and because I simply enjoyed talking with him. My first inclination was to do something theoretical, but Howie thought I should do an empirical project. (I remember once sticking my head in his office and saying, "I got it! 'The Epistemology of Everyday Life.' " He threw me out.) I also was leaning toward the sociology of deviance and mental illness (Erving Goffman's ideas [1961, 1974] were a draw), but Howie wanted me to become a family sociologist. His reasoning was that family sociology was one of the department's strengths and that I would be better trained if I went in that direction. He was right; students should capitalize on a faculty's expertise. Although I have never lost interest in epistemology or in how humans distinguish what is supposedly "normal" from what is not, I also have never regretted Howie's pushing me into the family field.

By summer 1974, Howie and I had agreed that I would do a qualitative "social construction of reality" study of marriage, based on conjoint in-depth interviews. We thought that interviewing the husband and wife together would provide an opportunity to observe how the couples created "meaning" through social interaction. We also felt that, since the reality construction process occurs over time, the study should be longitudinal. But how could I convince couples to let me into their homes for multiple visits? Wouldn't they think I was prying too much?

I kept delaying "going into the field," until Howie finally said that if I had any hope of graduating in 1975 and going out on the job market, I'd better come up with an entree plan–fast. For some reason, I cannot recall why, I thought that looking through a bunch of undergraduate family textbooks would help. So I grabbed as many editions as I could off Howie's shelf, carted them home in the trunk of my Pontiac, and deposited them on the living room floor. After dinner, I began leafing through the stack. One of the textbooks took a family developmental approach and included a discussion of the transition to parenthood. Scanning the unit on pregnancy, I got an idea. Suppose I interviewed the couples while they were expecting a child? Would it not make sense for me to ask to visit with them more than once, given that it is generally assumed that pregnancy proceeds in "stages"? I turned to Maureen and asked her how long pregnancy lasted. We didn't have any children at the time, but Maureen was a nurse, so she was able to give me a crash course on pregnancy testing (home kits were unavailable then), "quickening" (when the mother feels movement inside the womb), and pre- and postpartum timelines. Working from her answer, I scribbled out a schedule to conduct in-depth interviews with a small sample of couples (ultimately 16) during the 12th, 20th, 28th, and 36th weeks of gestation. The next day I marched into Howie's office, proudly announced what I had come up with, got his okay and eventually the committee's, and within a month was knocking on Couple #1's door. After a year of full-time interviewing, analyzing, and writing, I was done. I defended my dissertation on August 8, 1975, graduated soon thereafter, and by Labor Day was in Atlanta, eagerly anticipating the start of my first academic job as an Assistant Professor in the Department of Sociology at Georgia State University.

II

I like to ask people how they chose their careers because, for me, a seemingly haphazard decision, made on a summer evening in 1974, influenced what I would do for the rest of my life.

Most of my research over the past 25 plus years has focused on the transition to parenthood and on fatherhood and motherhood. Yet, up until the time that I looked through those textbooks, I had not given much thought to those issues. Indeed, Maureen and I had not decided at that point whether to become parents ourselves. (We eventually did decide and now have two sons, Brian and Adam.) Another interest I have long had is qualitative family research. This, too, can be traced to questions that I found myself wrestling with while trying to complete my dissertation.

In the early 1970s, the UNH Sociology department did not offer a qualitative sociology course, so I had to rely on the available how-to guides (e.g., Glaser & Strauss, 1967; Lofland, 1971) and pretty much train myself. I quickly discovered, however, that while these guides were very helpful, they said very little, if anything, about the challenges of qualitatively studying *families*. Finally, my dissertation sensitized me to the importance of gender stratification. While I had taken a lot of courses at the New School and UNH, I had never taken a course in the Sociology of Gender. Hence, I really was not prepared for the power processes that came to the fore during my interviews. I thought I was going to see examples of what, in the "social construction of reality" perspective, was euphemistically called "nomos" building (Berger & Kellner, 1964). What I saw instead was raw family politics. Having been drawn to the discipline of Sociology because of its attention to social inequality, I had come to realize that some of the most ruthless battles over "turf" and for civil rights were being waged inside the home.

I think everyone's life is affected by a multiplicity of factors, not the least of which are events and contingencies that spring up on the side of the road and that get you thinking about something that you might not have otherwise thought about, or get you involved in a project that you might not have otherwise gotten involved in, and the next thing you know you have taken a turn that you really hadn't planned on taking at all, and–surprise, you've become a family specialist, or a fatherhood researcher, or a Yankee fan in the home of the Braves. I am not trying to suggest that human agency or free will (call it what you want) does not play a part in a person's career, for I do believe that we make choices that also influence whom we become. But when I have occasion to reflect on the past, as I have been given the opportunity to do here, I find the concept of "unanticipated consequences" to be a valuable heuristic tool.

As soon as I got to Georgia State University (GSU), I set my mind to trying to get my dissertation published. My committee had convinced me that my study of marriage and pregnancy had the potential to be a book, so I put together a prospectus and promptly sent it to a variety of publishers, and just as promptly got a ton of rejection slips back. I was crushed. The GSU Sociology department was in the midst of developing a PhD program and, from the beginning, I had been told that I was expected to "produce" at a high rate. During my job interview, when the subject of publication came up, I confidently said that I could meet the standard. I already had one article based on a paper that I had written for Walter Buckley's theory course: "Interpreting Hierarchical Message Structure," *Journal of Communication,* 1974. My experience with that article, however, had not taught me how much work it takes for the average person to get something published. I had sent the paper in, and the editor immediately accepted it. (I have never had an editor do that since.) My not-so-hard-won success with "Interpreting Hierarchical Message Structure" had led me to believe that publishing was a cinch. But now I was learning just how difficult it was. My worst fear was that I would never get anything else accepted, be denied tenure, and find myself out of academia altogether.

Then, one day, fortune smiled upon me. I got word from the editor of the National Council on Family Relations' monograph series, Jetse Sprey, that Sage Publications was interested in acquiring the manuscript. Needless to say, I was ecstatic. Revisions were suggested and a new title was proposed: *Conflict and Power in Marriage: Expecting the First Child* (CPM). By July 1977, the book was out.

CPM gave me my first sense that something I wrote might actually be read. As far as I knew, there were only three people in the world who ever bothered to take a look at my communication article: Maureen, and Joe and Fran LaRossa. But with CPM, I had individuals coming up to me at professional meetings to say that they not only had read the book but had assigned it in their classes. I mention this not because I want to make the case that the book was important (CPM sold only about 2,500 copies). Rather, what I am trying to say is that the belief that someone other than my family might be interested in what I had written was a strong motivator for me to *continue* writing.

Knowing that what I had written might be used in classes also changed my perception of the relationship between teaching and research. I went to graduate school because I wanted to be a teacher. I left graduate school with the desire to be *both* a teacher and a researcher. As a newly-minted PhD, I saw teaching and research as competing domains. But after a while, I began to view the two as symbiotic. I found that if I talked about my own research, I could get students excited about doing research. I also observed that as a practicing researcher, I was in a better position to translate the nuances of other people's scholarly efforts. Finally, aware that other professors might be assigning books and articles that I had published in their classes, I grew increasingly sensitive to the responsibilities that researchers have not just to other researchers but to students outside their own universities–and to the community at large.

In time, two other single-authored publications grew out of the results of my dissertation (LaRossa, 1978, 1979). While these were interesting pieces to me, they seemed to make little difference to anybody else. (They are rarely cited.) There was an article, however, stemming in part from my dissertation, but not in the sense of reporting results, that did appear to have some impact on the field–and on me as well. While conducting the interviews with the expectant couples, I wasn't entirely comfortable with what I was doing. The problem wasn't methodological, but ethical. Was it okay to invade people's privacy to the degree that I was? Were my interviews, which sometimes got pretty intense, having an adverse effect on the fathers- and mothers-to-be or on their marriages? What was going to happen when the couples read the dissertation, which used a case study format, and saw their lives translated into "conflict and power" terminology?

These were not unusual questions for a qualitative researcher to ask, but as best I could tell from the methods texts around then, they were questions that revealed special ethical problems for researchers studying families. At the 1978 NCFR meeting, I was talking to Linda Bennett and Richard Gelles who mentioned that they had confronted the same questions, as well as others, while completing their dissertations. Linda, Rich, and I began thinking that it might be worthwhile to write a paper based on our collective experiences, so we went out to lunch, threw around some ideas, and decided to submit something for the Theory Construction and Research Methodology Workshop at the 1979 NCFR meeting. The paper we wrote eventually appeared in the *Journal of Marriage and the Family* under the title "Ethical Dilemmas in Qualitative Family Research" (1981).

The ethical dilemmas paper prompted me to think more about qualitative family research as an entity unto its own (i.e., as "qualitative family research"). I also began to ponder the status of qualitative family research. I could see that most qualitative methods texts ignored families, but I was getting the sense, too, that family studies paid little attention to qualitative work. Qualitative family research appeared to reside in professional limbo, with no established "place" in either the qualitative field or family field. What would happen, I wondered, if we looked at the *Journal of Marriage and the Family*, arguably the premier journal in NCFR's arsenal? How much qualitative family research would we find there? The answer came when, several years later, Jane Wolf and I teamed up to analyze every odd-numbered volume of JMF from 1965 to 1983. The study we did confirmed what many of us suspected but did not want to admit or publicize–that qualitative family research was not being taken seriously by family scholars. Janie and I learned something else, too. Tracing the history of the family field itself, we discovered that qualitative family research had not always been on the outskirts. Indeed, just the opposite was true. Qualitative family research had been instrumental to the development of family social science in the early 20th century.

The results from our study were published in JMF and titled simply, "On Qualitative Family Research" (LaRossa & Wolf, 1985). The story of the study, however, does not end there. Prior to its publication, Janie and I had delivered a draft of the paper at the 1984 NCFR Theory Construction and Research Methodology Workshop. The response from many in the room, a packed house, was heartwarming. But there was also an atmosphere of disappointment, even anger. The consensus among attendees was that JMF, not to mention the whole family field, was operating at half strength. By not taking full advantage of what could be discovered by using qualitative methods, family scholars were, so to speak, blind in one eye. Toward the end of the session, a sign-up sheet was circulated. Anyone interested in pursuing the issue could write their names down. I left the meeting with that list and, for weeks afterward, received letters from others who wanted to be part of the group. I decided to take it a step further and placed notices in several professional newsletters, announcing the formation of a Qualitative Family Research Network. A footnote also was added to Jane's and my JMF article, indicating that a network was being organized and that people could join by writing to me. Then, in October 1985, I mailed a letter to "all interested parties" to say that I had reserved a time slot at the upcoming National Council on Family Relations' meeting for everyone to get together, and that there also would be a session on qualitative family research at the 1986 American Sociological Association meeting. In the letter, I told the group: "Your stories, more than anything else, convinced me that something had to be done." I also communicated my own position on the value of qualitative research: "I am not someone who believes that qualitative research is 'better' than quantitative research. I do not see quantitative methods as intrinsically trivial or dehumanizing or sexist. No, what concerns me is that family scholars, as of late, seem to have forgotten that a multi-method approach is the best way to study families, and that the issue is not qualitative vs. quantitative research but good vs. bad research." Between 1986 and 1988, I sent out more letters and eventually expanded the missives into stenciled-off newsletters with articles written by network members and guest contributors. I also edited a special issue of the *Journal of Contemporary Eth-*

nography on qualitative family research, titling my article in the issue, "Renewing Our Faith in Qualitative Family Research" (1988b).

The Qualitative Family Research Network has grown to some 400 members, thanks in large part to the committed people who have nurtured its development over the years. Among the many who have contributed, two individuals deserve special praise. Katherine Allen served as the network's treasurer during the group's early days, and analyzed the responses from a survey in which members were asked what their thoughts were on the future of the network. Katherine also took over the editorship of the newsletter in 1989, when my active involvement with the network effectively ended, and she continued to be a member of the steering committee for years after that. Jane Gilgun also was a member of the first steering committee, and has been intensively involved in the network since. For more than a decade, Jane has edited the network's newsletter, *Qualitative Family Research,* and is primarily responsible for making it the superior publication that it is.

Although my interest in qualitative research remains strong (I teach the qualitative methods course in my department), I have not written anything directly bearing on the topic for a while. Basically, I ended up getting pulled into other projects. One was a government-sponsored grant on the history of fatherhood. The other was the *Sourcebook of Family Theories and Methods: A Contextual Approach* (1993), which Pauline Boss, William Doherty, Walter Schumm, Suzanne Steinmetz, and I co-edited.

My being on the *Sourcebook* team actually stemmed from my connection with qualitative family research. When it appeared in the mid-1980s that there would be a follow-up text to the *Contemporary Theories* volumes (Burr, Hill, Nye, and Reiss, 1979), I expressed the hope that qualitative family research would be taken seriously. Later on, I learned that the invitation I received to join the editorial board reflected a desire to make the book not only interdisciplinary in scope but also methodologically eclectic.

III

In *Conflict and Power in Marriage: Expecting the First Child,* my interest in the social reality of pregnancy was secondary to my interest in the social reality of marriage. The title of the book prioritized the theoretical processes of conflict and power; the heart of the book could be said to be the model of marital politics presented in Chapter 7. I recall being fascinated with conflict theory and with the challenges of conceptualizing and measuring marital power, and thought for sure that I would be writing more about those topics. As for fatherhood and motherhood, institutions which also had figured significantly in CPM, I didn't know whether I'd have much more to say. But then an opportunity presented itself that prompted me to study parenthood more closely.

Today, the Office of Research and Sponsored Programs at Georgia State University is strongly committed to providing a variety of internal grants to facilitate faculty research. In the 1970s, however, the only kind of internal grant available was one that would support putting on a conference. There was just a little money in pool, generally no more than $7,000 for any given project, but if you could come up with an idea for a study that would be of interest to the community and the press, and be willing to publicize the findings at a campus conference, then you had a pretty good chance of getting funded.

I guessed that the university would be more likely to fund a conference on parenthood than on marital power, so I proposed a study of "husbands, wives, and infants" (i.e., a study of marriage *after* the child arrived). In July 1977, I received an award and quickly initiated a study of 20 couples (10 of whom just had their first child and 10 of whom just had their second child) who would be conjointly interviewed during the 3rd, 6th, and 9th months postpartum. The resemblance to my dissertation was deliberate and essentially pragmatic. The funding period for the grant was only one year, July to June. The conference would have to take place in the spring. I did not have the time to develop an entirely new research design, and thus went with the familiar. I knew the pros and cons of doing conjoint, in-depth interviews, and I knew the kind of analysis that I would have to do in order to stage a credible conference.

The project moved very smoothly. I wasn't able to interview the couples myself, so I hired a Clinical Psychology graduate student, Victor Wagner, and outlined the questions I wanted him to ask. Vic seemed to intuitively know how to establish rapport and his clinical training made him a good quasi-non-directive interviewer. The spring conference ("What Does It Mean to Be a Parent?") went off without a hitch, and all 60 interviews were completed and transcribed by the summer.

Reading the transcripts, I grew increasingly excited over the fact that there seemed to me to be a lot more "going on" after a child arrived, compared to before. Conflict and power issues were thrown into bold relief, and comments about the level of "continuous coverage" demanded by infants appeared on almost every page. Yet another reason the couples' experiences captured my attention was that since the project had begun, Maureen and I had decided to become parents ourselves. Our first child was due in January 1979.

Throughout the data collection phase, I had talked with Maureen about how the project was going. Now with the data in hand and with our own impending parenthood, our nightly conversations became more animated. Would we be transformed as the couples being studied had been transformed? Would we have as much conflict? All sorts of notions were charging around in our heads, and what happened next seemed only logical at the time. I said to Maureen, "Why don't the two of us, working together, systematically analyze the transcripts?" The leverage gained would be substantial, I thought. Maureen and I would be carrying out a "participant informed" study, whereby we would be making sense of the 20 couples' transition to parenthood at the same time that we were trying to make sense of our own. What's more, since Maureen was going to go on a three month maternity leave once the baby came, she would have more time to devote to the analysis. (This statement, I soon discovered, only showed how much I had *not* read the transcripts; for if I had, I surely would have understood the time constraints under which Maureen and I would be operating.)

Maureen was wary of embarking on such a project in her so-called "spare time." At the end of the maternity leave, she would be returning to her job as a child development nurse in the "Developmental Continuity Program" at Grady Memorial Hospital (a job she still holds today). How could she do that and everything else, plus analyze the transcripts? What made the difference in her decision to say yes was the favorable response that we got from Sara Miller McCune, Publisher and President of Sage Publications, during a lunch meeting at the 1978 NCFR meeting. Sara loved the idea of the two of us co-authoring a book and sent us a contract soon after receiving our prospectus.

I still recall the many weekend mornings that Maureen and I would wheel Brian in his stroller around Orme Park, just a few blocks away from where we live, as we talked about this or that couple, or pondered this or that conceptual category and its dimensions. I have never been immersed in a project that has gone as well as that one. The analysis and writing just seemed to flow. It took less than two years from the moment the book was first proposed to the day we sent in the final manuscript. *Transition to Parenthood: How Infants Change Families* was published several months after it was put into production, in 1981.

People seemed to like the book. It sold well while it was still in print, and it continues to be cited today. I think its popularity lies in the attention that it gave to the political machinations surrounding the transition to fatherhood and motherhood, and because of its emphasis on the sociological/structural vs. biological and psychological, factors that go into creating gendered divisions of child care. On a personal level, *Transition to Parenthood,* and the analysis that led to it, made both Maureen and I more introspective about becoming parents.

IV

In 1986, I was at a point where I was trying to decide what to do next. Since the publication of *Transition to Parenthood,* I had written an article on "The Transition to Parenthood and the Social Reality of Time" (1983), gotten involved in the qualitative family research movement, edited a text on using case studies in the classroom, *Family Case Studies: A Sociological Approach* (1984), and written another book on pregnancy, birth, and parenthood, *Becoming a Parent* (1986). I toyed with the idea of doing another in-depth interview study, but couldn't get excited about any of the projects that I had devised. I was deliberately trying to come up with something that was "different," something that would get me charged up.

While I was thinking about the whole thing, the enjoyment I had writing one particular chapter in *Becoming a Parent* kept cropping up in my mind. It was the chapter on birth, which, unlike the others, had taken more of an historical viewpoint. I had become fascinated with the history of birth practices, and with how the medical establishment had wrestled away control of the delivery process from mothers and lay midwives. It wasn't just the content of the battle that intrigued me, but the sociological advantage on the battle that a long-term chronological vision afforded. I knew that good social science required a historical perspective, but I had never written anything that required me to directly apply that perspective to a phenomenon or event. That is, until I wrote the birth chapter.

I started to ask questions to which I before had given only a passing nod. Questions like: What social form did the transition to parenthood take in the United States in the 18th and 19th and early 20th centuries? What did the division of childcare look like then? I found books and articles that tried to answer the question as it applied to motherhood, but could locate only a few that did so with respect to fatherhood. And then something came to me. I realized that although none of the books and articles I had written had the word "fatherhood" or "fathers" in the title,

I had in effect been studying *men as parents* my whole professional life, beginning with my dissertation when I had decided to interview expectant fathers as well as expectant mothers. But I had not studied them historically. Maybe I should now.

After considering several options, I submitted a proposal to the Sociology section of the National Science Foundation to carry out a historical study of fatherhood between World War I and World War II. The project got high marks and was funded (after a "revise and resubmit") in 1988.

The jump start that I was hoping for had come. I discovered that not only did I enjoy reading family history books and journals, but that I absolutely loved going to the National Archives and Library of Congress (and many other repositories since) and poring over old documents. I'd leave town for days on end, go into a "zone" where I would spend hours upon hours essentially "reading other people's mail," and return to Georgia State with a suitcase of text data ready for analysis.

About the same time that I was preparing my NSF grant proposal, the journal *Family Relations* put out a "call for papers" for a special issue on families and change. I wondered whether I might have something to submit. I had not collected much historical data as of yet, but I had made a few trips to Washington, D.C., for my pre-tests. I also thought I might draw on the theoretical sections of the proposal where I talked about the value of examining both the "culture of fatherhood" (i.e., the shared norms, values, and beliefs surrounding men's parenting) and the "conduct of fatherhood" (i.e., what fathers do, their parental behaviors) when assessing change. The culture-conduct distinction is one that Maureen and I had intimated in *Transition to Parenthood,* in our discussion of how excuses and justifications are offered when a family's culture and conduct are not in sync. The article that I sent in and that was eventually accepted for publication was titled "Fatherhood and Social Change" (1988a). Nothing that I have written has been reprinted as much as that article has. It's also one of my favorites.

My dad died three months before "Fatherhood and Social Change" appeared. I know it's not customary to dedicate journal articles, but I wish now that I had dedicated that one to him.

Since receiving the NSF grant, I have devoted most of my effort to plotting the history of fatherhood, both its culture and conduct. Betty Ann Gordon, Ronald Jay Wilson, Annette Bairan, Charles Jaret and I analyzed *Saturday Evening Post* cartoons from the 1920s, 1930s, and 1940s, and found evidence to suggest that the image of the 20th century American father has followed a fluctuating pattern (LaRossa et al.,

1981). In a follow-up study, Charles Jaret, Malati Gadgil, G. Robert Wynn, and I looked at Father's Day and Mother's Day comic strips from 1940 to 1999 and uncovered changes that lend support to the fluctuating image hypothesis (LaRossa, Jaret, Gadgil, & Wynn, 2000). In two other studies, Donald Reitzes and I specified how the culture and conduct of fatherhood in the 1920s and 1930s were intricately connected and how the reliance on women's self-reports can underestimate the level of paternal involvement at various times (LaRossa and Reitzes, 1993; 1995). (Don and I also recently completed a study of childhood in the interwar years [LaRossa & Reitzes, forthcoming].) And in *The Modernization of Fatherhood: A Social and Political History* (1997), I synthesized the data that I had gathered with the NSF grant, essentially arguing that (a) yesterday's fathers were more involved than people today generally given them credit for, hence the widely held claim that the conduct of fatherhood has dramatically improved over the course of the 20th century needs to be tempered; and (b) the social institution of fatherhood is more pluralistic than not (technically speaking, *fatherhoods* is more accurate than *fatherhood*), which means that any serious historical effort must clearly specify which of the many fatherhoods is being studied. (The social construction of reality is kaleidoscopic.)

V

When my children were younger, I used to tease them by saying that I expected them to get PhDs and become college professors. Their response generally was along the lines of, "No way, Dad!" The thought of spending their whole life in school was just too much for them to bear. Brian and Adam are now in college and high school, respectively, and give little indication that they will do anything other than follow their own passions.

And that's precisely what I would want them to do. I consider myself lucky to be in a career that I genuinely enjoy, and I would be thrilled if Brian and Adam ended up in occupations that gave them the same level of satisfaction. I appreciate the gift that my parents gave to me of helping me find my own way. It's a gift that I hope to pass on.

AUTHOR NOTE

Ralph LaRossa, PhD, is Professor of Sociology, Georgia State University, Atlanta, GA 30303.

REFERENCES

Berger, P. L. (1963). *Invitation to sociology: A humanistic perspective*. Garden City, NY: Anchor/Doubleday.

Berger, P. L. & Kellner, H. (1964). Marriage and the construction of reality. *Diogenes*, 46, 1-25.

Berger, P. L. & Luckmann, T. (1966). *The social construction of reality: A treatise in the sociology of knowledge*. Garden City, NY: Anchor/Doubleday.

Boss, P., Doherty, W. J., LaRossa, R., Schumm, W. R., & Steinmetz, S. K. (Eds.) (1993). *Sourcebook of family theories and methods: A contextual approach*. New York: Plenum Press.

Burr, W. R., Hill, R., Nye, F. I., & Reiss, I. L. (Eds.) (1979). *Contemporary theories about the family, Volumes I and II*. New York: Free Press.

Glaser, B. G. & Strauss, A. L. (1967). *The discovery of grounded theory*. Chicago: Aldine.

Goffman, E. (1961). *Asylums: Essays on the social situation of mental patients and other inmates*. Garden City, NY: Anchor/Doubleday.

Goffman, E. (1974). *Frame analysis*. New York: Harper & Row.

LaRossa, R. (1974). Interpreting hierarchical message structure. *Journal of Communication, 24*, 2, 61-68.

LaRossa, R. (1977). *Conflict and power in marriage: Expecting the first child*. Beverly Hills, CA: Sage Publications.

LaRossa, R. (1978). Conjoint marital interviewing as a research strategy. *Case Analysis, 1*, 2, 141-149.

LaRossa, R. (1979). Sex during pregnancy: A symbolic interactionist analysis. *Journal of Sex Research, 15*, 2, 119-128.

LaRossa, R. (1983). The transition to parenthood and the social reality of time. *Journal of Marriage and the Family, 45*, 3, 579-589.

LaRossa, R. (Ed.) (1984). *Family case studies: A sociological perspective*. New York: Free Press.

LaRossa, R. (1986). *Becoming a parent*. Beverly Hills, CA: Sage Publications.

LaRossa, R. (1988). Fatherhood and social change. *Family Relations, 37*, 4, 451-457.

LaRossa, R. (1988). Renewing our faith in qualitative family research. *Journal of Contemporary Ethnography, 17*, 3, 243-260.

LaRossa, R. (1997). *The modernization of fatherhood: A social and political history*. Chicago: University of Chicago Press.

LaRossa, R., Bennett, L. A., & Gelles, R. J. (1981). Ethical dilemmas in qualitative family research. *Journal of Marriage and the Family, 43*, 2, 303-313.

LaRossa, R., Gordon, B. A., Wilson, R. J., Bairan, A., & Jaret, C. (1991). The fluctuating image of the 20th century American father. *Journal of Marriage and the Family, 53*, 4, 987-997. 375-387.

LaRossa, R., Jaret, C., Gadgil, M., Wynn,G.R. (2000). The changing culture of fatherhood in comic-strip families: A six-decade *Journal of Marriage and the Family, 62*, 2, 375-387.

LaRossa, R. & Mulligan LaRossa, M. (1981). *Transition to parenthood: How infants change families*. Beverly Hills, CA: Sage Publications.

LaRossa, R. & Reitzes, D. C. (1993). Continuity and change in middle class families, 1925-1939: The culture-conduct connection. *Journal of Marriage and the Family*, *55*, 2, 455-468.

LaRossa, R. & Reitzes, D. C. (1995). Gendered perceptions of father involvement in early 20th century America. *Journal of Marriage and the Family*, *57*, 1, 223-229.

LaRossa, R. & Reitzes, D. C. (forthcoming). Two? Two and one-half? Thirty months? Chronometrical childhood in early 20th Century America. *Sociological Forum*.

LaRossa, R. & Wolf, J. H. (1985). On qualitative family research. *Journal of Marriage and the Family*, *47*, 3, 531-541.

Lofland, J. (1971). *Analyzing social settings: A guide to qualitative observation and analysis*. Belmont, CA: Wadsworth.

Orchestrating Differences: The Making of a Family Psychologist

Harold D. Grotevant

KEYWORDS. Autobiography, identity, narrative, family psychology

INTRODUCTION

For a social scientist who studies identity and narratives, writing about the significant forces that shaped one's professional life is indeed a daunting task. As a developmental-family psychologist, I am keenly aware of the ways in which rearing, experiences outside the family, genetics, and serendipity together contribute to human development. Narrative psychologists have noted that people reflecting on their lives take their current situation as the end point and then select information about their past in order to construct a coherent narrative ending with the present (Boxer & Cohler, 1989). Thus, the account that follows is one of several possible narratives that might be written about my life.

In this brief autobiography, I first present the narrative of my early years and how I see them laying the foundation for my professional interests. Second, I discuss my research contributions and how they have become interwoven over the course of my career. In this context, I talk about the joys of collaborative relationships I have experienced with colleagues and students. I next discuss ways in which I have adapted to a complex, active career, through music and other non-work activities. I close with the mention of some current challenges and speculations about the future.

EARLY YEARS: EXPERIENCES WITH DIFFERENCE

I am a baby boomer, born in 1948 to parents who married during World War II, while my father was in the Navy and my mother worked to support the soldiers on the front. My ancestry is northern European: my father's ancestry is Dutch (Grotevant) and English (Vincent); my mother's is Irish (Ryan) and German (Wilhelm). My father was raised Baptist and my mother Roman Catholic. Many said this "mixed marriage" would never last, although my parents just celebrated their 55th wedding anniversary.

The first house I remember was in a suburb of Utica, New York, a neighborhood of young, growing families who were working toward the American dream of a peaceful, prosperous life following the trauma of war. It was also a community ambivalent about becoming America's melting pot. Even though neighbors were cordial and helpful to one another, invisible boundaries separated those who spoke only English from those who also spoke Polish or Syrian. Ethnic rivalries were much more among the Polish, Italian, Irish, Germans, and Eastern Europeans than among African Americans, Latinos, and Whites. As a child, I was keenly aware of the ethnic differences that separated families from each other.

My father worked in sales for a company that coupled promotions with involuntary family relocations. When I was 9, my father was promoted and we were transferred to Buffalo, New York. In less than one year, he was promoted again, and we were transferred to Dallas, Texas, where I lived until the end of high school.

What a different world Texas was! One thing such a move meant was that we were separated from our extended family. I think my parents experienced this with a mixture of sadness and relief to be free of the intrusiveness of family life in a small community. Gone were the ethnic worlds of New York where I was in the majority group; now I was the outsider. I was introduced to my fifth grade class as "the Yankee." Not only was I a Yankee, but I was also Roman Catholic, a religion held in great suspicion by my conservative Protestant classmates. Now clearly a minority, I felt most comfortable with other "minority" kids. Of course, this was Texas before the days of desegregated public schools, so the other minority kids were mainly Jewish, Catholic, or nerds. We developed close bonds.

My religious upbringing left me with a hyperactive superego, which my college experiences helped to moderate. Although I remember some religiously painful experiences, I also look back with gratitude for the strong message of social justice that I heard from the church. As an adolescent, I had the following quote from Samuel T. Coleridge on a piece of paper under the glass on my desk: "By what I have effected am I to be judged by my fellow man; what I could have done is a question for my own conscience." It is on the first page of the Commonplace Book I maintain to this day.

COLLEGE TO GRADUATE SCHOOL, BY WAY OF THE NAVY

I always loved school and considered becoming a teacher since my elementary school days. Although I considered other options for myself, I always seemed to return to a career in education. It would allow me to live in the world of ideas and to share them with others to facilitate their growth. Once in college (at the University of Texas at Austin), it was clear that I would be aiming for a career in university teaching and research. I thought I would major in psychology, but wanted to keep my options open during my first year. As an entering freshman, I decided to take both chemistry and psychology and see which resonated the best. There was no contest. Chemistry was deadly boring, not at all as engaging as it was in high school. Psychology was exciting. Even though it was taught in an auditorium of 500 students, the fresh new assistant professor (social psychologist Bob Helmreich) engaged me from the start. By mid-term, my major was set.

My university experience was exhilarating. I finally felt free of the restrictions of home life and could shape my own world, set my own schedule, and engage with friends and activities without parental scrutiny. I loved it! To celebrate my first day of "freedom," I went to a movie my parents had forbidden me to see–*Who's Afraid of Virginia Woolf?* Pretty tame by today's standards. I can remember so many days walking around the campus, being glad to be alive and brimming with spirit. Anything seemed possible. I experienced college life in its fullness, including extracurricular activities, employment, activism, and courtship.

I met my wife, Susan Miskell, at the end of my freshman year at the Catholic Student Center, where I was the vice-president for social action and she was the publicity chair. Together, we tutored people in a low-income neighborhood studying for the GED and responded to other opportunities to channel the idealism of our social consciences. All of this happened during the turbulent late 1960s. The passion of the debate over the Vietnam War was energizing.

I never thought the war would involve me directly. My eyesight is so poor that I always assumed I would not qualify for service. By the middle of my senior year, I was notified that I was likely to be drafted upon graduation. Deferments for marriage and graduate school had been canceled. My cohort was in the first draft lottery, in which birthdates were randomly selected to rank order that year's crop of men for the draft. I still remember that night. My number was 24, so it was certain that I would be drafted after graduation. To reinforce the notion, my draft board sent me notice to report for a physical.

What a quandary. I had already been accepted for graduate school at the University of Minnesota's Institute of Child Development and was very eager to continue my education through to the PhD. Susan and I were planning to marry the day after graduation. I was against the war, but did not have a sufficient paper trail to merit conscientious objector status. Neither did I want to spent the rest of my adult life in exile in Canada or maim my body to become ineligible. I learned that my eyesight was too bad to allow me to qualify for officer rank, but not bad enough to prevent me from being drafted. So with trepidation and reluctance, I enlisted in the Navy Reserves for a commitment of two years' active duty and a total of six years' reserve duty. As an ex-Navy man, my father was proud of my enlisting. I simply saw it as the best among a number of undesirable alternatives.

By some miracle, I was the only recruit from my unit who was not sent on sea duty to the Pacific or to Vietnam; I was stationed in an office at Mare Island Naval Shipyard, north of San Francisco. The two years were full ones: I lived and worked with types of people I had never been exposed to before, including zombies and bikers, and learned a lot about myself and others in the process. After some months, Susan was able to join me there, and the experience became a sweeter one. Our first son, Paul, was born at Travis Air Force Base in 1972. At the same time, I mourned the time I felt I was wasting, and I impatiently longed to begin graduate school. There were many weekends I walked introspectively around the Berkeley campus, wishing time would pass more quickly.

We headed for Minnesota after our two years passed. Neither of us had ever been there before, but we knew the university had the best graduate program in the country, and that was enough. The Institute of Child Development was an incredibly exciting place to be. I had written in my graduate school application that I was interested in individual differences: Why do some people have a greater capacity for change than others? And how do families contribute to these differences? In today's parlance, one could say I was interested in resiliency.

At the beginning of my second year, I had the opportunity to join a new research project being headed by Sandra Scarr and Richard Weinberg. The studies to be undertaken were behavior genetic investigations into the malleability of intellectual and personality development. What an exciting opportunity and a good match for my interests. I frequently look back on my time with Sandra and Rich with gratitude, because I feel that my experience on their projects instilled in me an "internal working model" of relationships between faculty and graduate students that has given me many satisfying experiences as a faculty mentor. They had faith in me, even when I had less confidence in myself. They were generous with opportunities to learn all those things that are rarely taught in class–how to review manuscripts and write grant proposals, how to handle rejection, how to treat graduate students well, how to organize a large research project, how to treat research participants with respect, how to deal with contentious colleagues, how to hold to one's principles in the face of controversy, and most importantly, how to be passionately in love with your work.

As a graduate student, I visited the homes of many adoptive families and interviewed parents and adolescents about their experiences. Although the primary purpose of the study was to make behavior genetic comparisons on standardized cognitive and personality measures, our lengthy interview afforded the opportunity to learn a great deal about adoptive family life, especially about the management of "difference" in adoptive families. My dissertation examined genetic and environmental contributions to the development of interests and personality, and several components of it focused on family process contributions.

I completed the doctoral program in four years, on a fast track because I was eager to stop being a student and have a job. Unlike most of my fellow graduate students, I was married and had a young child. Susan had just completed her MBA, and we were eager to settle into "real life." I applied for positions all over the U.S. but was especially attracted to an opportunity to return to the University of Texas, a university I loved in a great city that was my wife's hometown. We had planned to visit Austin over Christmas break (1976), and I wrote the department ahead of time to see if I could drop by and meet some of the faculty. They responded by sending me an agenda for a formal interview. After my interview, the budget council convened. At the end of the afternoon, the department chair offered me a position as Assistant Professor!

One of the attractions of coming to the Child Development and Family Relationships division (in the Department of Home Economics) was that it was transforming itself from a program that focused primarily on young children to one focusing on development through adolescence in the family context. There was a commitment to hire more research-focused faculty (Catherine Cooper and I were among the first) and to create a doctoral program. It was also a real pleasure to return home. I eagerly agreed to teach a course on Family Relationships in my first semester, knowing that this would be an opportunity to stretch in some new ways, since I had not had formal course work specifically on families in graduate school.

IDENTITY AND RELATIONSHIPS: RESEARCH PURSUITS AND THE JOYS OF COLLABORATION

From my current vantage point, the theme underlying my professional career is the desire to understand the dynamic tension between self and other, between identity and difference, between the person and the relationships in which one participates. I am captivated by questions such as the following. How does one develop a coherent sense of self within a context of difference? What are the relational processes through which families manage difference? How do these processes work differently in adoptive families, in which there is no biological connection between parent and child and in which one's sense of self must be constructed in light of having two sets of parents, one of whom may be unknown? How do individuals and families construct narratives about their development? In what ways do these narratives regulate subsequent behavior?

Building on my dissertation, my early work was concerned with identity development from an Eriksonian/identity status perspective. I combined that interest with one in relationships by expanding interview (Grotevant, Thorbecke, & Meyer, 1982) and questionnaire measures (Grotevant & Adams, 1984) to include sections on interpersonal relationships. The identity work was conducted in tandem with research I conducted with Catherine Cooper exploring the interface between communication processes in families and identity outcomes, especially exploration of alternatives (Grotevant & Cooper, 1985).

Catherine and I had much in common, including our graduate training at Minnesota, and together we looked for opportunities to collaborate on research linking human development with family processes. In the bonding process of writing our first grant proposal together, we both experienced the joy of intense commitment to a project and to the collaborative relationship that created it. We both brought our "internal working models" of collaboration to our new effort–and in the process created our own collaborative process, which has subsequently involved many students. The content of our work and the process of our collaboration have mutually enriched each other and continue to do so.

Part of the joy of university life for me, then and today, is in the intensity of the intellectual experience and the interpersonal relationships that are built around it. I recall one Friday afternoon when Catherine and I were working on a grant proposal in the Cactus Café in the student union, against a rapidly approaching deadline. Both heavy coffee drinkers then, we had downed many cups in the process of talking through our ideas and capturing them on paper. Around 5:00 p.m. we looked up and, much to our surprise and amusement, discovered that we were the only ones working and that everyone else was celebrating the Friday happy hour. For both of us, it demonstrated how our work was also our play.

Of all my publications, the one with arguably the greatest impact has been Grotevant and Cooper (1986), which presented our theoretical model of the connection between individuation in family relationships and the development of identity and interpersonal skill in adolescents. This work challenged the wisdom of the time, arguing that the task of adolescence is not to sever relationships with one's parents, but rather that the transformation in parent-child relationships during adolescence involves the adolescent's ability to develop and advocate for a clear point of view while also remaining relationally connected to one's parents.

Catherine and I presented the first incarnation of the 1986 paper at the 1979 International Seminar on the Child and the Family at Gustavus Adolphus College in St. Peter, Minnesota. The well-known senior discussant for our paper blasted us for continuing in a line of work that he thought had been unproductive and inconclusive (using the Plan Something Together task to elicit family interaction.) Although I recall wishing the earth would open up and swallow me, I also remember a gentle Rueben Hill pulling us aside at the coffee break and telling us that the work we were planning had much merit and that we should persevere despite the critique. I'll never forget it.

That episode taught me several important lessons: (a) that unconstructive criticism doesn't help anyone (except perhaps the critic's ego), (b) that elders in the field have the responsibility to foster promising work of those more junior; and (c) that tenacity can pay off. The theoretical paper must have gone through at least five major revisions and must have been critiqued by at least a dozen reviewers before it was finally published in *Human Development*. The satisfaction of seeing it in print was immeasurable. Catherine and I have both continued an interest in this topic and recently wrote a new paper updating the model and expanding it to include our interests in ethnicity and adoption (Grotevant & Cooper, 1998).

The family therapy literature provided valuable insights for our emerging research program, but it required us to master this new literature and translate its highly abstract concepts into researchable terms. I attended workshops by Salvador Minuchin, James Framo, Carl Whitaker, and others; they inspired me to take preliminary steps toward training to become a family therapist. However, I soon realized that, despite my interest, there were not enough hours in the day to do it all well. I reluctantly decided to forego the possibility of clinical training in favor of conducting clinically relevant research. I don't regret that decision today, but I haven't ruled out the possibility that my future might yet hold some opportunities for clinical work of one kind or another.

Toward Understanding Adoptive Families

In 1980, I was contacted by Ruth McRoy, a graduate student in Social Work who was doing her dissertation on transracial adoption. She had heard that I had done similar work with Sandra and Richard. I served on Ruth's dissertation committee and enjoyed our interaction very much. After completing the PhD, Ruth was hired as an Assistant Professor in Social Work. We continued discussing our common interests. Over coffee one day, she mentioned that a colleague who worked in a residential treatment center commented that his unit had a large number of adopted children–why might this be? After reviewing the literature, we discovered repeated findings that adopted children were overrepresented in clinical populations. In collaboration with Ruth's mentor Louis Zurcher, we decided to pursue this question. We obtained funding from the Hogg Foundation for Mental Health to study adoptive and non-adoptive families who had adolescents in residential treatment. This project took about seven years from beginning to end, culminating in several articles and a book (McRoy, Grotevant, & Zurcher, 1988).

I have often told students that I enjoyed learning so much that I decided to do it as a profession. This project certainly stretched me professionally. It provided my first opportunity to be on the inside of treatment facilities, to talk with parents about the anguish their families had experienced, and to talk with kids whose behavior was unpredictable and whose constructions of the world were often skewed. This experience affirmed my interest in understanding adoptive family processes and the development of adopted adolescents. If my research and writing could help ameliorate the pain these families and kids described, I would have made a real contribution.

Midway through the residential treatment study, Ruth and I were contacted by the Vice President for Social Services of Lutheran Social Services in Texas, who told us that several of his agencies were beginning to advocate for adoptive placements in which the birthmother chose the adoptive family for her baby and actually met them at placement and continued to have contact with them. Although the agency heads were enthusiastic, he wanted to evaluate this practice before they went too far with it. Ruth and I agreed to do a small-scale evaluation if LSS would fund our interviews; in turn, we told LSS that we would apply for a grant to do a nationwide study of openness in adoption. The pilot study yielded several articles and another book (McRoy, Grotevant, & White, 1988), and the nationwide study has now become a four-site longitudinal project that has involved 190 adoptive families and 169 birthmothers (Grotevant & McRoy, 1997, 1998).

By the mid-1980s, I was teaching a full load, serving as director of the graduate program, and juggling four major research projects: the Family Process Project (with Catherine Cooper), the residential treatment study (with Ruth McRoy and Lou Zurcher); the openness in adoption study (with Ruth McRoy); and a review of family assessment techniques (with Cindy Carlson; Grotevant & Carlson, 1989). The pace was intense, but so was the satisfaction. My greatest satisfactions in teaching, administration, and research combined the intellectual and the interpersonal. In each venue, I had many opportunities to be a collaborator, a facilitator, a mentor. There was joy in discovery and joy in experiencing it with others.

The intensity of my career was matched by the intensity of Susan's. Her MBA had prepared her for work with several state agencies, including the Legislative Budget Board and the Sunset Advisory Commission. She and I wanted to have another child; however, as "older parents," the second took a bit longer to come along than did the first. Mark Ryan Grotevant was born in 1985. I was the only man in the auditorium full of prospective fathers who had gray hair.

Administrative Adventures

In 1989, having recently been promoted to full Professor, I saw an announcement for a position as Head of the Department of Family Social Science at the University of Minnesota. This was very appealing because it would allow me to continue administrative leadership at a higher (departmental) level. Moreover, it would put me in a well-established college in a well-established university, in which I hoped not to be continually fighting for existence. It would also put me in a department with well-known family scholars and would put us back in the Twin Cities, which held fond memories for us. (As with childbirth, the passing years mute the memory of Minnesota winters!) Susan and I were both restless, wondering what was next in our careers. Would we always be in Austin? We never thought so. But what would be next?

I approached the Minnesota position eagerly but with caution, constantly monitoring how it felt to project myself into the job. After extensive discussions with the faculty, staff, administrators, and students, and extensive discussions with Susan, I accepted the job. Paul was then a senior in high school, and Mark was completing preschool. I moved to Minnesota on January 1, 1990, and Susan and Mark followed at the end of June, after Paul's high school graduation.

I threw myself into the new position, attempting to strengthen an already-solid department and preserve our position against a series of annual university budgetary "reallocations." In my 5 1/2 years as head, we experienced budget cuts every year and were able to hire no new faculty. While heading the department, I also continued my research on openness in adoption. A proposal I wrote to NICHD while in Texas was funded once I arrived in Minnesota, and our work continued with new data collection from adoptive families and their children. Ruth continued research with the birthmothers in our project, and we had now become the Minnesota/Texas Adoption Research Project.

My enthusiasm for the job and my determination to keep my research program alive despite the administrative load led to many very long days and nights. I found that my waking moments were monopolized by administrative dilemmas and that the mental space necessary for the creative work of research was being choked out. I came to realize that my heart was in the world of ideas and action rather than in the politics of academic administration. After 5 1/2 years of working a day job (administration) and a night job (research), I decided to opt for sanity and return to the faculty role. I have never regretted this move, although it hurt financially and ran counter to notions of prestige in the academy.

During my time as department head, I was a member of the Family Story Collaborative Project, a small interdisciplinary team funded by the MacArthur Foundation to develop methods for assessing intergenerational continuities in families by way of narratives and to apply such methods to our own varied research populations. An SRCD monograph marked the successful conclusion of the first phase of our work together (Fiese, Sameroff, Grotevant, Wamboldt, Dickstein, & Fravel, 1999). It was an exciting stretch to explore the new world of narratives and to link this literature from diverse disciplines with more familiar work, such as that in the field of identity. I was also engaged in the collaborative production of an edited volume on identity and development with three wonderful Dutch colleagues (Bosma, Graafsma, Grotevant, & de Levita, 1994). Thus, the 1990s has been a time of great excitement in my research, because I have been able to connect my most passionate research interests within the context of the longitudinal follow-up of the participants in the openness in adoption research project. Those interests include adolescent development, identity, narratives, family relationships and communication processes, and adoption.

One of my greatest joys is mentoring graduate and undergraduate students in the context of my research team. As I construe it, my role is not unlike that of an orchestra conductor. One of the things that has always been rewarding to me as a musician is the opportunity to be a contributing part to a much greater whole. My job as research director is to orchestrate, to help individuals blend, to strengthen each individual so that they can most effectively contribute to the whole, to have a vision for where we might go but to draw on the strengths of the participants in getting there. Taking on this role gives me great satisfaction, especially when there's that magical synergy among the players that produces an amazingly beautiful sound.

My 51st birthday occurred when our adoption project research team was in Indiana participating in our annual multi-site project "summit meeting." Ruth's birthday is just one day later than mine, so it was a joy to celebrate together. At dinner on our last evening together, our students surprised us with limericks they had composed for the occasion. Many of them were clever (albeit too ribald for publication!), but this one particularly warmed my heart:

> There once was an old man named Hal
> whose colleague was also his pal.
> When students would tire,
> his mind would inspire,
> and lift up our sinking morale.

Adapting to an Open-Ended Career

I frequently tell my graduate students that one of the most exciting and potentially most stressful aspects of a career in academia is that it is completely open-ended. There are many more challenges than any one person could possibly take on. There will be many requests for your time and expertise, and no one but you will be able to say "no" when you have reached the limit.

Life as an Assistant Professor at Texas did indeed bring its stresses. Since we were a small program, faculty had relatively heavy teaching and administrative loads. The commitment to create and nurture an active research program involved a huge investment, because there was relatively little departmental infrastructure to assist. Assignments eagerly agreed to in the first years on the job were now piling up on each other, and the load was beginning to feel overwhelming. Having sprinted through undergraduate school, the Navy, graduate school, and the first years of Assistant Professorhood, it became clear that I needed to do some recentering. I became interested in Eastern philosophy and learned meditation. I studied the piano, picking up the instrument abandoned in childhood. Susan and I concluded our growing discontent with Catholicism by becoming Episcopalian. And I started singing in choirs in church and in the community. These years taught me the importance of personal, professional, and family balance, a goal easier to state than to achieve.

I continue singing today, now with the choir of the House of Hope Presbyterian Church in St. Paul. Choral singing is the ultimate embodiment of the systems theory dictum that the whole is greater than the sum of the parts. Singing is a physical act, a spiritual act, a relational act, and an intellectual act that demands one's full attention. Many of my most significant peak experiences have come while singing.

THE STORY . . . SO FAR

As Mark progressed through elementary school in the mid-1990s, it became increasingly clear that he had attention deficit hyperactivity disorder (ADHD), the dimensions of which were not then fully apparent. The next several years involved three changes of schools and many personal and family challenges. This journey has given me great empathy for parents and children who struggle with issues outside those considered normative. It has made me impatient with those who believe that every family and every child must fit a certain mold. It has connected my professional and personal life with an intensity I had not yet experienced. It has brought me face-to-face with institutions and professionals that "don't get it." It has also brought me into contact with caring adults who want to make a difference and with incredibly empathic parents known only to me via the Internet.

I feel incredibly fortunate to be a professor. I have more autonomy in my work than do most other people in the world. With privilege comes responsibility, and I hope that my work will make a difference for families and for children. At the same time, I am sure that many of the insights contributed by my work will be superseded by new research and theory, as they should be. Thus, an even more important contribution is how I relate to others day by day. Just as my mentors showed me the joy of research and collaboration, I hope that my actions as teacher, investigator, mentor, and friend touch the lives of others in positive ways. I know from my own experience that many of the most significant moments of connection occur at times when they are not planned, and that teachers may not be aware of the impact of the many individual interactions that involve them each day. I suspect that generativity in relationships has more staying power over time than do some of our cherished theories and results.

While completing this chapter in November 1999, I attended a conference on Ethics and Adoption. One of the speakers, Judge William Thorne of the Third Judicial District in Salt Lake City, included the following piece in his presentation. It serendipitously expresses the core idea I attempted to convey in the paragraph above:

The Little Things (Hillis)

> Springs are little things, but they are sources of large streams;
> Nails and pegs are little things, but they hold the parts of a large building together;
> A word, a smile, a frown are all little things, but powerful for good or evil.
> Think of this and mind the little things.

As I pause to look around me, I am thankful that both my sons are doing well. After graduating from the University of Texas at Austin with a major in history, Paul worked for a time as a computer network manager and then went west (San Francisco) to forge a new life. He now happily works at an independent bookstore in the city and is on the threshold of married life with his fiancée, Carolyn. They are fortunate to have found each other. Mark is completing his sophomore year in high school, is doing well academically, has a loyal band of friends, and is eager to drive.

I look forward to another 15 years of formal academic employment and to time beyond that writing and consulting. My goals include launching Mark into the world as a young adult with a good chance of success, advocating for children with special needs and supporting schools who educate such children well, understanding the complex issues facing adoptive families and attempting to improve their situation through research and education, balancing my professional work with music and spiritual growth, and deepening relationships with my wife and friends. The excitement of ideas and relationships I experienced in college continues to motivate me today. Both are touchstones that help me orchestrate my life.

AUTHOR NOTE

Harold D. Grotevant, PhD, is Professor of the Family Social Science Department, 1985 Buford Avenue, University of Minnesota, St. Paul, MN 55108.

REFERENCES

Bosma, H. A., deLevita, D. J., Graafsma, T. L., & Grotevant, H. D. (Eds.) (1994). *Identity and development: An interdisciplinary approach.* Newbury Park, CA: Sage.

Boxer, A.M. & Cohler, B.J. (1989). The life course of gay and lesbian youth: An immodest proposal for the study of lives. *Journal of Homosexuality, 17*, 3, 315-355.

Fiese, B.H., Sameroff, A.J., Grotevant, H.D., Wamboldt, F.S., Dickstein, S., & Fravel, D.L. (1999) The stories that families tell: Narrative coherence, narrative style, and relationship beliefs. *Monographs of the Society for Research in Child Development.* Vol *64*, 2, Serial No. 257, 1-162.

Grotevant, H. D. & Adams, G. R. (1984). Development of an objective measure to assess ego identity in adolescence: Validation and replication. *Journal of Youth and Adolescence, 13*, 5, 419-438.

Grotevant, H. D. & Carlson, C. I. (1989). *Family assessment: A guide to methods and measures.* New York: Guilford Press.

Grotevant, H. D. & Cooper, C. R. (1985). Patterns of interaction in family relationships and the development of identity exploration in adolescence. *Child Development, 56*, 2, 415-428.

Grotevant, H. D. & Cooper, C. R. (1986). Individuation in family relationships: A perspective on individual differences in the development of identity and role taking in adolescence. *Human Development, 29*, 2, 82-100.

Grotevant, H.D. & Cooper, C.R. (1998). Individuality and connectedness in adolescent development: Review and prospects for research on identity, relationships, and context. In E. Skoe & A. von der Lippe (Eds.), *Personality development in adolescence: A cross national and life span perspective.* (pp. 3-37), London: Routledge.

Grotevant, H.D. & McRoy, R.G. (1997). The Minnesota/Texas openness in adoption research project: Evolving policies and practices and their implications for development and relationships. *Applied Developmental Science, 1*, 4, 166-184.

Grotevant, H.D. & McRoy, R.G. (1998) *Openness in adoption: Connecting families of birth and adoption.* Newbury Park, CA: Sage.

Grotevant, H. D. Thorbecke, W. L., & Meyer, M. L. (1982). An extension of Marcia's identity status interview into the interpersonal domain. *Journal of Youth and Adolescence*, 11, 1, 33-47.

McRoy, R. G., Grotevant, H. D., & White, K. L. (1988). *Openness in adoption: New practices, new issues.* New York: Praeger.

McRoy, R. G., Grotevant, H. D., & Zurcher, L. A. (1988). *Emotional disturbance in adopted adolescents: Origins & development.* New York: Praeger.

Reflections of a Psychologist Turned Relationship/Family Scientist

Mark A. Fine

KEYWORDS. Autobiography, stepparents, divorce, remarriage, borderline personality

INTRODUCTION

In this article, I share some reflections on the path my career has taken–a path that has led me to view myself now as a social scientist, with a specialization in families and close relationships. My goal is to share some of my professional experiences and transitions in the hope that these may be helpful to other scholars whose career paths have not yet crystallized. I will share some non-professional experiences when they shed light on career choices and moves. First, through a description (in chronological order) of turning points in my academic career, I will describe why I became a psychologist and how my professional identity shifted from being a clinical psychologist to a psychologist/scholar to a family psychologist to a family scholar and to my present identity as a family and relationships scholar. Second, I will describe the transitions involved in my development from being disciplinary (i.e., psychologist), to multidisciplinary, to interdisciplinary, and, at rare moments, to transdisciplinary. Finally, I will share some of the changes that have occurred in my specific research and scholarly interests. Although I may present changes in my thinking and practices as if they reflect a desirable and/or preferable course, I do not mean to imply that they would be ideal for others.

CHRONOLOGY OF CAREER TURNING POINTS

Deciding to Be a Psychologist

Although I have always enjoyed reflecting on and talking about feelings, thoughts, experiences, and relationships, I made my decision to become a psychologist late in my undergraduate career. I was completing my major in Economics, with plans to go to law school, when I took a course in "The Helping Relationship" from Don Barr in the College of Human Ecology at Cornell University. In this course, I was exposed not only to basic elements of psychotherapy, but also to some of the social critiques of psychotherapy and the need to focus on community and social causes of individuals' problems. Not only was the content fascinating to me, but the manner in which Don taught the course, his eagerness and enthusiasm, and the commitment of other students made this experience a turning point in my life. From this point on, I took as many psychology courses as I could at Cornell and eventually graduated with majors in both economics and psychology. My experiences had convinced me that graduate school in community psychology was the best fit for my interests, but I found that community psychology programs were quite few in number and those that did exist tended to be combined with programs in clinical psychology. Therefore, I applied to clinical/community programs and found the going very rough; although I visited several programs, I only received one offer. I accepted and began my graduate training in clinical psychology at The Ohio State University under the mentorship of Andy Schwebel. I began my graduate training with a distinct bias against individual forms of clinical intervention (as they "blamed the victim") and with the goal of learning how to make changes at the community and societal levels. I was also skeptical of the value of empirical research, feeling that it had often been used "against" those who participated in it.

Becoming a Scholar

At The Ohio State University, I received a more "traditional" education than at Cornell and I became immersed in an academic culture that was strongly supportive of both research and clinical training. Consequently, my appreciation for empirical research grew and I concurrently became more interested in acquiring and enhancing my clinical skills. I still maintained my role as a "social critic" and retained my social consciousness, but came to believe that, under certain circumstances, individual forms of psychotherapy could be useful. It was during my third and fourth years in my graduate program that my roots as a scholar took hold. I had relatively little interest in publishing during my first two years (a remnant of my concerns with empirical research), but found that I greatly enjoyed the challenge and process of writing manuscripts that at least attempted to make a unique contribution to some field of study. By the time I graduated, I was strongly socialized into the role of a scholar and was committed to the principle that my work on a particular project or study was not completed until some contribution from the project had been published. I was taught that, although a master's thesis and a doctoral dissertation were important documents leading to important educational experiences and academic degrees, the projects were not completed until the results were published in a peer-reviewed journal. I also now realize that it was during this time that my love of collaboration began. I have very fond memories of long meetings with my advisor and other collaborators, editing a manuscript line by line, laughing and joking, and otherwise enjoying the process of trying to create a product that was greater than what any of us could produce alone. This love of collaboration has continued to be very strong in me and, when I am asked to write a piece or work on a particular project, my immediate reaction is to ask, "Who might I work with on this project?" I find scholarly collaboration to be a pleasurable social activity.

My interests in family issues actually began when I entered a research group under the leadership of my academic advisor, Andy Schwebel. This group was involved in studying divorce and its effects on family members. Thus, I inherited an interest in divorce and single-parent families, but I eventually internalized this interest and continued studying divorce and single parenthood throughout graduate school and into the beginning of my academic career. Another factor that cemented my decision to study families was a comment that my advisor made that I remember well to this day. He mentioned somewhat casually that he had made a shift in emphasis from the community to the family and I asked him why. He stated that he had come to the conclusion that he could effect more change by working with families than he could by working with communities as a whole. After thinking through his comments, I found some validity in them and this gave me further justification for focusing my academic interests in understanding and helping families more so than communities as a whole.

Progression Toward Becoming a Family Psychologist and Family Scholar

My first academic position was as an assistant professor in the psychology department at the University of Dayton. In this role, I functioned very much like a typical academic clinical psychologist, teaching clinical courses in personality assessment, psychopathology, ethics, and cognitive-behavior therapy; conducting research on clinical populations, particularly young women with eating disorders and/or personality disorders; and maintaining a small private practice outside of my academic position. I enjoyed engaging in these activities and took advantage of several opportunities in a community mental health center and area hospitals to improve my clinical skills.

Nevertheless, I retained my interest in families and decided to focus on remarriage and stepfamilies. An internship supervisor (Jan Kiecolt-Glaser) had given me the excellent advice to identify a programmatic area of research and build a reputation in that area, as opposed to publishing in a diffuse way across many different content areas. Because I increasingly saw divorce (and often single parenthood) as a step or stage along the way toward the formation of a stepfamily and because I concluded that there had not yet (in the mid-1980s) been an extensive amount of research on stepfamilies, I decided to focus the majority of my research efforts in that area. I still did some research on more traditional clinical topics (e.g., personality disorders, eating disorders), but my passion was directed toward furthering our understanding of stepfamilies.

Thus, there was a disconnect between my primary research activities (in families in general and stepfamilies in particular) and the remaining aspects of my professional functioning. For many years, I was quite comfortable being a fairly traditional clinical psychologist in teaching and clinical activities, while focusing on families in most of my scholarship. Into the early 1990s, I felt increasingly ill at ease regarding this disconnect and began to think of ways to try to forge a closer alliance between the different aspects of my professional academic identity.

By 1993, some aspects of my professional identity had crystallized. Although I enjoyed teaching and some clinical activities, my primary passion was in my role as researcher/scholar. For the first time, in some surveys of professional identity, I recorded my primary identities as "researcher" and/or "professor" instead of also adding clinician and other labels reflecting my various practitioner activities. In addition, at this point, I saw myself as a family psychologist, in the sense that I still felt like a psychologist, but one who focused more on family-related issues than clinical ones. Further, I stopped promoting my private practice and eventually stopped seeing clients. I have not seen a client in a psychotherapeutic capacity since 1993.

It is more than just a bit ironic that I now view my primary professional role as that of a scholar. As a child, I resisted my father's (and occasionally my siblings') attempts to correct my relatively frequent grammatical errors by invoking the following logic, "You know what I mean. What does it matter if I do not follow abstract and arbitrary grammatical rules?" Because of this populist attitude, no one in my family would have predicted that I would become a scholar who places a very great value on the quality of writing and who would later edit two scholarly journals. In part, this shift occurred because I found myself enjoying the process and challenge of writing clearly and received positive feedback on my writing skills. In addition, I have had the good fortune of working with some excellent writers, including Don Barr, Andy Schwebel, John Moreland, Carolyn Swift, Larry Kurdek, Katherine Allen, Dave Demo, Marilyn Coleman, and Larry Ganong, who not only write or wrote extremely well, but who also took the time to mentor me.

Movement Toward Becoming a Family and Relationships Scholar

In 1994, an opportunity arose to apply for the chair position in the department of human development and family studies at the University of Missouri-Columbia. This was a very attractive option at this point, because (I list academic and professional reasons below, although there were also a number of familial and personal issues that influenced my decision to apply for this position): (a) I was feeling less of an attachment to my disciplinary roots as a psychologist, and particularly a clinical psychologist; (b) I had felt for some time that an interdisciplinary department, such as human development and family studies, might be the most comfortable academic home for me; (c) I wanted to be in a department and university that placed the same very high priority on research and scholarship that I did; (d) The department at the University of Missouri had two scholars who also conducted research on remarriage and stepfamilies and the prospect of working collaboratively with them was very attractive; and (e) I was attracted to the challenge of assuming a leadership role in an academic department. After being interviewed and becoming even more enthusiastic about the position than I was before, I was offered the position and accepted it.

Since August 1994, when I assumed my new position at the University of Missouri, my primary identity as a researcher/scholar has only strengthened and I have increasingly thought of myself as a family scholar/researcher as opposed to a family *psychologist*. While I still have some attachment to psychology (particularly developmental and social psychology) and while my training in psychology still clearly influences my thinking (in both known and unknown ways), I now increasingly think of myself as a family researcher/scholar. In the last two years, in various surveys, I have identified my primary discipline as being HDFS or family studies, rather than psychology.

The change in my thinking has been subtle. For many years, when I thought of myself as primarily a psychologist, I was very open to publishing in multidisciplinary outlets, such as *Journal of Marriage and the Family, Journal of Family Issues, Family Relations,* and *Journal of Divorce & Remarriage,* and viewed these journals as appropriate places for psychologists to publish their work. Reflecting this multidisciplinary stance, I edited *Family Relations* from 1993 to 1996. Now, I still consider these journals as appropriate outlets for my work, but because I am a family and relationships scientist and not because I am also a psychologist. These multi- or interdisciplinary journals are now the most appropriate places for me to publish my work.

Relatively recently, my identity has been transformed yet again. I have become more active in the growing field of personal relationships and now think of myself as a family and relationships scholar. Reflecting this subtle change, I now serve as Editor of the *Journal of Social and Personal Relationships,* attend a wider range of conferences (such as Communication Studies, Head Start, and child development), and collaborate with an even broader array of scholars.

TRANSITIONS IN DISCIPLINARY-RELATED IDENTITY

Based on definitions proposed by Acitelli (1995) and others, my scholarly trajectory has moved from disciplinary (i.e., clinical psychologist), to multidisciplinary (i.e., working with scholars from other disciplines, but doing so in an independent manner), to interdisciplinary (i.e., truly collaborating with scholars from other disciplines), to, as often as I can, transdisciplinary (i.e., working with others in such a way that labor is assigned to collaborators on the basis of their skills, interests, and areas of expertise, rather than their discipline). In fact, the distinctions among these types of disciplinary collaborations are somewhat arbitrary and it is probably more useful to consider them as lying on a continuum from disciplinary to transdisciplinary. Although I review my development as if it followed a linear, continuous trajectory, these various "stages" overlapped considerably. A few examples from specific research projects may illustrate this personal transition.

Some of my earliest work was designed to investigate the effects of divorce on children and their relationships with their parents (e.g., Fine, Moreland, & Schwebel, 1983). This work was *disciplinary* in the sense that I viewed my task as taking a *psychological* approach to understanding how divorce affects children. The outcome variables of interest were primarily *psychological,* as opposed to socioeconomic or physiological. My collaborators were all clinical *psychologists* who had interests in using new knowledge in psychoeducational ways for the benefit of those experiencing divorce.

At the University of Dayton, in my first academic position, I engaged in a number of multidisciplinary research projects. The best example is work that I did with Randy Sansone, a psychiatrist specializing in the treatment of eating disorders. He and I conducted a number of studies on eating disorders and related phenomena (e.g., Sansone, Fine, Seuferer, & Bovenzi, 1989; Sansone & Fine, 1991). In most instances, my colleague identified the major research questions, wrote the introduction and much of the discussion, and was responsible for the management of data collection. My role was typically to help determine the research design, analyze the data, write the methods and results sections, and integrate the various sections together into the final version of the manuscript. Of course, I am exaggerating the specialization in the division of labor; for example, he was involved in aspects of data analysis and I was involved in writing some portions of the introductions to manuscripts. Nevertheless, my basic point is that our work was parallel in the sense that we, for the most part, did not work on our assigned tasks collaboratively. We somewhat independently completed our assignments and then put them together into an aggregate package (i.e., the manuscript). This approach has both virtues and limitations. It is efficient and brings together colleagues with skills and talents that can complement each other. At its best, such work can lead to the successful completion of projects that could not have taken to fruition had either investigator conducted the study alone. At its worst, there is the risk that the two investigators, because they may not have a thorough overview of the entire research project and all of the constituent parts, may contribute parts that do not fit together well. For example, if the individual conducting the data analyses misinterprets the meaning of some of the study hypotheses, analyses may be conducted that do not directly test the proposed hypotheses. If the individual writing the discussion section does not understand what some of the statistical results mean, inappropriate inferences may be drawn. Depending on the extent to which the colleagues can take on the tasks performed by the other, some of the risk can be lessened by having each colleague carefully review the work done by the other.

Most of my research collaborations have fallen somewhere between multidisciplinary and interdisciplinary. My work with Larry Kurdek (e.g., Fine & Kurdek, 1995; Kurdek & Fine, 1991), trained as a developmental psychologist, and also with Patricia Voydanoff and Brenda Donnelly (e.g., Fine, Voydanoff, & Donnelly, 1993; Voydanoff, Fine, & Donnelly, 1994), both sociologists, illustrates research collaborations that were primarily interdisciplinary in the sense that we: (a) did not divide up research tasks according to disciplinary affiliation, (b) most of the important tasks could be performed by any of the research partners, (c) and we were as likely to submit to multidisciplinary journals (e.g., *Journal of Marriage and the Family*) as we were to disciplinary ones (e.g., *Journal of Family Psychology*). Nevertheless, there were some tasks that were assigned on the basis of disciplinary training and/or expertise, such as when I, because of my clinical background and experience, would be more likely to write "implications for practitioners" sections of manuscripts, whereas my sociologist collaborators would be more likely to integrate a sociological theory into a manuscript.

Other collaborations that fall into the category of interdisciplinary would include my work on stepfamilies with Larry Ganong and Marilyn Coleman (e.g., Fine, Ganong, & Coleman, 1999) and recent work with Dave Demo and Katherine Allen (Demo, Allen, & Fine, 2000). For the most part, these research projects were conducted in a manner that was not greatly influenced by disciplinary roots, at least not explicitly. Perhaps because all of us (cited in this paragraph) professionally reside in departments of human development and family studies, I recall only minor attention devoted to how our work together might be influenced by our different disciplinary backgrounds. For the most part, tasks were assigned based on non-disciplinary related factors, such as skills, areas of expertise, the amount of time that an individual had to devote to an activity, research interests, enthusiasm for the task, and a host of others. Relatively infrequently would we explicitly mention a disciplinary-related factor as a meaningful consideration. Our work was certainly enriched by the fact that our differing backgrounds and training experiences led us to have varying and complementary competencies and exposure to certain literatures. Rather than our original disciplinary affiliation, however, it was these differing competencies and content knowledge that determined our division of labor.

As much as I aspire to function in a transdisciplinary manner, I have done so rarely, if ever. Perhaps the closest I come to functioning in this manner is in my editorial role. When I was editor of *Family Relations* (1993-1996) and now as editor of the *Journal of Social and Personal Relationships,* I try to make such editorial decisions as which scholars will be asked to review a particular manuscript or which Associate Editor to send a manuscript to with relatively little consideration of professional discipline. I attempt to make such decisions on the basis of the skills, interests, and competencies of the various individuals, although I acknowledge that there are rare instances when disciplinary training and identity are considered.

I struggle with the issue of whether it would be desirable for me and for others in the diverse relationship fields to think of ourselves as primarily *social scientists* and to *completely* abandon disciplinary boundaries–a transdisciplinary stance. I have a dream that at some point the current boundaries between and among disciplines will evaporate and we will all be part of one large group of social scientists. On the other hand, this abandonment of traditional disciplines would come with considerable costs. For example, we might have fewer scholars who have expertise in some unique methods that are tied to specific disciplines. No doctoral training program can possibly expose students to all research methods in the social sciences and, therefore, there may be a loss of some of the less commonly known, although useful, methods. In addition, given the academic tendency to compartmentalize, it is quite possible that academics and administrators would find other ways to subdivide the social sciences (e.g., by content area, by methodology), although, in my opinion, these other possible subdivisions might be less costly than are divisions on the basis of discipline alone.

CHANGES IN RESEARCH INTERESTS

A very common question asked of scholars is how they became interested in the content areas reflected in their research programs. Certainly, in many cases, such choices reflect the researcher's personal experiences and a desire to shed light on phenomena that have been personally impactful. For me, this was not the case and my original interest in divorce began in a relatively unexciting manner–my academic advisor at The Ohio State University was then interested in the effects of divorce on family members and, as an incoming graduate student in 1979, I joined his research team studying this topic.

Nevertheless, I found the topic of divorce to be an interesting one and found it easy to summon the enthusiasm and commitment necessary to study this topic. My early work examined the long-term effects of divorce on the quality of parent-child relationships (Fine et al., 1983). My dissertation research, reflecting my interest in race and culture, examined the effects of an afrocentric world view on how single mothers adapted to their circumstances (Fine, Schwebel, & Myers, 1985).

When I moved into my first academic position at the University of Dayton in 1984, research on divorce had become increasingly plentiful and it was becoming somewhat more difficult to make unique contributions to that area. At that time, I made a deliberate and reasoned decision to move into the area of stepfamilies and remarriage, for three reasons: (1) In contrast to divorce, relatively little empirical research on stepfamilies had been conducted by this point in time; (2) It became increasingly clear to me that divorce was a process and an event that typically led to remarriage and experiences in a stepfamily, suggesting that divorce was an intermediate step toward living in a stepfamily; and (3) I was intrigued by several aspects of stepfamily life, including the dynamics and possible consequences involved in adding a "new" adult, the stepparent, to an existing single-parent family unit. Key issues are concerned with the challenges of determining what role the stepparent "should" assume in the stepfamily. For these reasons, I began to study various aspects of life in stepfamilies, an interest and focus that I have maintained consistently through the present time.

In addition to my work on stepfamilies, I have forged new ways of thinking about my research program. For example, I began to think about my research agenda as one involving the study of how family members adjusted to the challenges of a wide array of transitions, ranging from marriage to divorce to remarriage. Further, most recently, I have been involved in national and local research into the Early Head Start program, which I consider to reflect a focus on how children and parents adjust to the challenging circumstances revolving around parenting young children within a context of poverty. This increased ability to find common underlying themes to my research interests and efforts has been very helpful to me in identifying new research directions. I recommend this to other scholars, because one will be more successful as a scholar to the extent that one has a clear sense of the overarching theme(s) that underlies one's research program.

Over time, I also developed research interests that truly were unrelated to my primary interest in families, including studies on fairly mainstream topics in clinical psychology, such as eating disorders and personality disorders. These topics were appropriate ones when I was functioning as an academic in a psychology department, but I discontinued my work in these areas when I moved to the University of Missouri. Somewhat more related to my work in families is an ongoing interest in ethics. In this broad area, I have published articles on a strategy for teaching a graduate course in clinical ethics, the ethics of managing clients with certain challenging forms of psychopathology, and, most recently, to the ethics of numerous aspects of the publication process, including authorship (Fine & Kurdek, 1993) and "piecemeal" publication issues (Fine & Kurdek, 1994). I view my work on ethics as related to my research program in families because ethics necessarily involve *relationships* among people, whether they be clinician and client, faculty mentor and graduate student, and/or scholar and journal editor. Thus, to me, ethical dilemmas are an integral part of human relationships.

Most recently, I have broadened my conceptualization of my research program to the general area of close relationships. In this broadened view, families are one type of close relationship. Reflecting this new view of my research program, I have engaged in some studies on factors related to the stability of premarital dating relationships and on social cognition.

OTHER TRANSITIONS AND CHANGES

Over the course of my professional career, there have been several other transitions that were not described earlier. First, from a philosophy of science standpoint, I have moved on the continuum from positivism to post-positivism. Although I always felt that it was overly simplistic and misleading to identify a "truth" through interpreting results from research studies, I functioned and wrote as if I believed that such an entity existed. Now, I believe that there are multiple "truths," and that the results of research studies are bound by the particulars of the context in which they were derived. I still believe that there is value in large-scale studies that attempt to generalize from a sample to a population of interest; I now, though, consider the generalizations with more qualifications and with a greater attention to context than I did at an earlier point in my career.

Methodologically, my original training, skill, and passion was in quantitative and statistical methods. I am a quantitative person by nature and have a natural excitement and enthusiasm for statistical methods. In fact, my peers in graduate school and faculty colleagues would tease me about the enjoyment I would experience reading statistics books as bedtime reading! Nevertheless, over time, I have become more comfortable and familiar with qualitative methodologies. Some of my current work in Early Head Start involves conducting in-depth interviews with young mothers in the program every four months and gathering additional qualitative data (e.g., focus group results, interview service providers). While I am gaining experience in the gathering of qualitative data, I still find the task of analyzing and deriving meaning from these data to be daunting and very challenging. By my nature, in my personal work, I still resonate more with quantitative and statistical approaches than with qualitative methods, but feel that using qualitative approaches allows one to answer a broader array of questions and that the quantitative and qualitative combination has the potential to make greater contributions than either could alone. For these and other reasons, I highly value qualitative work and attempt to promote and encourage it (e.g., in my editorial roles, in my role as advisor to graduate students) to the same extent that I do other types of research.

CONCLUSIONS

As I reflect on how my research interests have moved from divorce to remarriage/stepfamilies to families in transition to close relationships, there has been somewhat of a reversal in the extent to which my research interests and activities are focused vs. broad. The early part of my academic career was characterized by an increasing specialization and narrowing of research interests. I was (wisely) advised to develop a programmatic line of research around a relatively specific and narrow topic, so that I could establish a reputation in that area. Indeed, this strategy does serve to enhance one's reputation far more than if one were to publish a few articles on a wide array of topics. In addition, I tended to focus my reading of journals and books on topics related to divorce and later remarriage and stepfamilies, with less attention devoted to other topics that were relevant to my work as a clinical psychologist and to my growing general interest in families.

As my academic career has progressed (and I hope it is not yet in its final stages!), obtaining a broad view of the various fields of interest to me has become a greater priority. Perhaps this change has occurred because a journal editor, in my view, is responsible for being open and responsive to a broad array of topics within the purview of that particular journal. But, it is also possible that I sought to become a journal editor because of the increasing broad range of my scholarly interests and because editing a journal provides one with considerable opportunity to become more knowledgeable about a wide array of research areas. Regardless of the etiology of this shift, I find myself much more interested in publications that present a broad survey of a particular research area, an overview of a field as a whole, or that draw new and innovative connections between one or more areas of research.

At this point in my career, I generally operate in one of two ways. On the one hand, I still maintain my research programs in the area of divorce, single parenthood, and stepfamilies and have recently branched off into some new areas, such as the evaluation of early intervention programs. Even within these focused areas, however, I have assumed a broader role. For example, I have recently authored or co-authored some broad overviews of the divorce (Fine, 2000; Fine & Demo, in press) and stepfamilies/remarriage (Coleman, Ganong, & Fine, 2000) literatures, which take a more global view than do book chapters or articles that present research from a particular study. On the other hand, I read more widely, both in terms of content and discipline, than I once did, and am as likely to have my curiosity piqued by an article that attempts to present the "big picture" of a particular field as I am by one in my specific areas of interest and study. I do not know if this transition from being specialized to being more of a generalist characterizes the careers of other scholars in our field(s), but I suspect that this pattern is not an uncommon one.

AUTHOR NOTE

Address all correspondence to Mark A. Fine, PhD, Department of Human Development and Family Studies, University of Missouri-Columbia, 316 Gentry Hall, Columbia, MO 65221 (E-mail: finem@missouri.edu).

REFERENCES

Acitelli, L. K. (1995). Disciplines at parallel play. *Journal of Social and Personal Relationships*, *12*, 4, 589-595.

Coleman, M., Ganong, L., & Fine, M. (2000). Reinvestigating remarriage: Another decade of progress. *Journal of Marriage and the Family*, *62*, 4, 1288-1307.

Demo, D. H., Allen, K. A., & Fine, M. A. (Eds.), (2000). *Handbook of family diversity*. New York: Oxford University Press.

Fine, M. A. (2000). Divorce and single parenting. In C. Hendrick & S. S. Hendrick (Eds.), *Close relationships: A sourcebook* (pp. 139-152). Newbury Park, CA: Sage.

Fine, M. A., & Demo, D. H. (in press). Divorce: Societal ill or normative transition? In R. M. Milardo & S. W. Duck (Eds.), *Families as relationships*. Chichester, UK: Wiley.

Fine, M. A., Ganong, L. H., & Coleman, M. (1999). A social constructionist multi-method approach to understanding the stepparent role. In E. M. Hetherington (Ed.), *Coping with divorce, single-parenthood and remarriage: A risk and resiliency perspective* (pp. 273-294). Mahwah, NJ: Erlbaum.

Fine, M. A., & Kurdek, L. A. (1993). Reflections on determining authorship credit and authorship order on faculty-student collaborations. *American Psychologist, 48*, 11, 1141-1147.

Fine, M. A., & Kurdek, L. A. (1994). Publishing multiple journal articles from a single data set: Issues and recommendations. *Journal of Family Psychology, 8*, 4, 371-379.

Fine, M. A., & Kurdek, L. A. (1995). The relation between marital quality and (step)parent-child relationship quality for parents and stepparents in stepfamilies. *Journal of Family Psychology, 9*, 1, 216-223.

Fine, M. A., Moreland, J. R., & Schwebel, A. I. (1983). Long-term effects of divorce on parent-child relationships. *Developmental Psychology, 19*, 5, 703-713.

Fine, M. A., Schwebel, A. I., & Myers, L. J. (1985). The effects of world view on adaptation to single parenthood among middle-class adult women. *Journal of Family Issues, 6*, 4B, 107-127.

Fine, M. A., Voydanoff, P., & Donnelly, B. W. (1993). Relations between parental control and warmth and child well-being in stepfamilies. *Journal of Family Psychology, 7*, 2, 222-232.

Kurdek, L. A., & Fine, M. A. (1991). Cognitive correlates of adjustment for mothers and stepfathers in stepfather families. *Journal of Marriage and the Family, 53*, 3, 565-572.

Sansone, R. A., & Fine, M. A. (1991). Treatment impressions and termination experiences with borderline patients. *American Journal of Psychotherapy, 45*, 2, 173-180.

Sansone, R., Fine, M. A., Seuferer, S., & Bovenzi, J. (1989). The prevalence of borderline personality disorder among women with eating disorders. *Journal of Clinical Psychology, 45*, 4, 603-610.

Voydanoff, P., Fine, M. A., & Donnelly, B. W. (1994). Family structure, family organization, and quality of family life. *Journal of Family and Economic Issues, 15*, 3, 175-200.

Soft Ideas and Hard Methods: Family Sociologist or Social Psychologist?

Sheldon Stryker

KEYWORDS. Autobiography, identity, family sociology, social psychology

I have a second chance! The last (and first) time I was asked to tell a professionally relevant autobiographical story, I chose a bloodless title for the paper delivered and the ultimate publication (Stryker, 1994). I noted when delivering the paper and in the published piece that I should have chosen the first half of the title I have used for this paper (plus a different second half), one that described reasonably the content of the story to follow and yet had some life to it–one whose informal tone was in keeping with the purpose and the character of the piece. Given this second chance, I was determined not to blow it.

My title is descriptive of what I wish to say. The first half of it describes what is, for many, a contradiction entailed in the theoretical and empirical work that defines whatever contribution I have made to sociology in general, to family sociology or social psychology in particular. I, of course, do not see any contradiction–but that is a part of the story I have to tell.

The second half, it will be noted, is framed as a question, a question that appears to suggest an either/or alternative. Logically, of course, "social psychologist" and "family sociologist" are not mutually exclusive, but the identities one comes to hold and that serve to influence choices made among alternatives present in one's life experiences, the personal identifications with social categories that become central to one's sense of self and those that remain peripheral or even absent from self, are not necessarily governed by the criteria of logic. What underlies the way in which I have framed this matter in my title is the second part of my present story. So to the story itself.

THE ROAD TO SOCIOLOGY

I became a sociologist in part by accident. After a post-high school stint as a (pick and shovel) laborer building a defense plant, I entered the University of Minnesota in January 1942. Both my family and I assumed that I would become a "real doctor." A year-plus later, I had accumulated 15 quarter credits, tournament level bridge competency, a quite reasonable 3-cushion billiards game, and the advice from a psychologist-cum-career counselor–after taking the Strong Vocational Inventory on a whim while walking across campus to a favorite lunch spot–to "work with people."

At that time, having been drafted, I left the university for the military; I would have left earlier had I been allowed to enlist, but 20/800 eyes prevented that from happening and resulted in my service records being stamped "limited service" and "no overseas duty." Three years later, I was discharged from the army, having served as a company medic in a combat engineers outfit in France and Germany (winding up the last day of the war in Austria, south of Berchtesgaden). The hands-on experience of dealing with the consequences of shoe-mines, together with a personal hospital stay resulting from German mortar fire, persuaded me I was not cut out for medicine. A post-European war stint at the army-sponsored American University at Biarritz, where I tried my hand at "creative writing" and failed to impress my teachers, strongly suggested the same was true of that prospective career. I returned to Minnesota with no career plans at all. Nevertheless, I knew that I would re-enter the University.

To abbreviate a longer tale, the confluence of a friend discharged from the military who knew he wanted to be a social worker, memories of the "work with people" advice given me years before, and the fact that undergraduate social work was then a curricular sequence within the Department of Sociology led me to enroll as a undergraduate sociology major. I was, of course, eligible for GI bill support, but, as a disabled veteran, I was also eligible for support though a rehabilitation program. The program promised monthly payments of $120 rather than $90 and five rather than four years of support *if* a faculty member would attest that five years were necessary in order to achieve career objectives. To that point, I had given no thought to graduate school–indeed, did not yet know that I wanted to become a sociologist, much less what graduate school entailed. However, five years of free education was obviously better than four!

During the summertime absence of the then-chair of sociology, F. Stuart Chapin, I wound up asking Ray Sletto, later long-term chair at Ohio State, to sign the necessary papers. Ray spent about an hour telling me why I should not go to graduate school and should not become a sociologist, but finally signed. (Much later, I asked Ray why he had tried to discourage me. His response, paraphrased: If you could not be discouraged, that meant you really wanted to be a sociologist; and only if you really want it is it worth doing. Sage advice that, and advice I have given in modified form to others through the years. Incidentally, I have often offered others additional advice in the form of an iteration of a "law" enunciated by Karl Schuessler, my long-time colleague and friend at Indiana University. Schuessler's law is: Sociology must be fun! If it isn't fun, there are easier and more remunerative ways of making a living. Also incidentally, advised by Karl that if I wanted to be immortal, I too had to have a law to which my name was attached, I "discovered" my own sociological law, which is: "Good people don't have to be s.o.b.'s!")

BECOMING A PARTICULAR KIND OF SOCIOLOGIST

Enrollment as a sociology major, albeit in the social work sequence, led me into two courses, one in The Family and one in Social Psychology, both with Clifford Kirkpatrick. Kirk was eminent in both fields, perhaps especially in the sociology of the family. Through the next two years, he became much more than my classroom teacher; he became advisor, mentor, friend, role model, and the director of my undergraduate honors thesis. It was Kirk's encouragement that led me to enter graduate school at Minnesota, without really considering alternative possibilities. Later, just after Chapin–in the spring of 1950–put his arm around me in the hall outside his departmental office and told me it was time for me to get out into the world (I had been in graduate school for about one month more than two years at the time, and didn't take prelims until more than a year later), Kirk also invited me to come to Indiana University, where he had moved a year earlier to become chair. To create a position for me, Kirk put together two teaching assistantships, allowing a full-time salary of a munificent $2500 (in all honesty, $500 was added about two months after my arrival, fall 1950). I became a regular faculty member the following year, and I have been at Indiana ever since. My salary, I am pleased to say, has improved substantially in the intervening years.

Part of my duties during my early period at Indiana was to help Kirk with the preparation of his family textbook (Kirkpatrick, 1955). In particular, I undertook a revision, subsequently published as an appendix to the text, of Kirk's earlier "What Science Says About Marriage and the Family," on which I had worked at Minnesota, and sought to summarize extant quantitative work on dating, courtship, marriage, divorce, etc. The emphasis on quantitative methods in "What Science Says" mirrored the general ethos of the Minnesota department at the time. Reflecting Chapin's views, science was by definition quantitative, and the department was determined to be scientific. I understood there were limits to that aspiration, limits that in part reflected the historicity of human experience (and thus the unlikelihood of the existence of timeless laws describing that experience). Still, I accepted the wisdom of mimicking, to the degree possible, the logic and the procedures of science as we understood science at the time. And, in large degree–and with what I take as appropriate cautions, provisos, and caveats–I still do.

One caution, proviso, and/or caveat via the social psychology that I was first introduced to in Kirk's social psychology course, namely, the work of George Herbert Mead, needs to be noted. The brief discussion of Mead in that class was the stimulus for expanded readings of Mead then, later into and through graduate school, and subsequently as well. A number of themes of Mead's work resonated with me. In particular in this context, his argument that social life is characterized by a principled indeterminacy hit home, probably because it was consonant with how I came into sociology in the first place. Also, related themes in Mead's work reinforced this argument. The significance of self and of subjective experience more generally, the self control made possible by mind and the internal manipulation of symbols–these and other themes permitted one to accord a dignity to humans that alternative social psychologies did not and could not warrant. In short, Mead's themes left room for both chance and choice in accounts of human personal and social experience. Yet, while implying the limited utility of deterministic models of natural science for sociology, at least as I read him, Mead's arguments implied the appropriateness of applying the logic of experimental science to social behavior. And, while chance and choice argued the inevitably probabilistic character of fit between theory and empirical findings, properly formulated theory could indeed be rigorously tested.

As any hard-nosed scientist will tell you, Mead's are indeed "soft ideas." Nevertheless, they are to me and to others attractive and powerful ideas. Neither attractiveness nor power, however, testifies to the validity of ideas. As I have just suggested, a question that early intrigued me and motivated my own work was whether or not these and related ideas could be stated in the form of a theory. By theory, in turn, I refer to a set of propositions developed logically from definitions and explicit assumptions. Theories include propositions with interrelated concepts, having empirical indicators that permit their empirical test.

I was convinced by my reading of the literature that many who expounded Mead's ideas in sociology took them as givens, as true beyond any doubt and beyond any need for empirical verification; I did not–and do not–think that this attitude pays Mead the respect he deserves. Further, many others who applied Mead's ideas to social phenomena accepted Herbert Blumer's (1969) claims that his presentation of symbolic interactionism replicated Mead's views and implied a methodological position denying the possibility of general sociological (or social psychological) theories, predictive social science, the utility of structural concepts for social analyses, and the applicability of numerical (mathematical or statistical) methods in social research. I did not–and do not–believe any of these claims. Certainly, there are sociological problems worthy of interest and research that are not amenable to numerical methods; and certainly there are limits to the useful application of any of the methods available to sociologists for their research. Surely, also, a quest for universal empirical generalization and predictive explanatory theory is likely to have its limits. Nevertheless, there are empirical regularities, even if not universals, in social life; we can and ought to formulate testable theories to explain such regularities as exist; and we can and ought to test those theories in as rigorous a manner as is possible. To do otherwise is to resign ourselves to power as the decisive regulator of what is deemed to be true about social life. As I have often said about possible epistemologies underlying what one does as a sociologist, since none can be argued unequivocally to be more valid than another, we pay our nickels and take our chances.

In any event, my Minnesota training would not permit me to accept a state of affairs in which the implied nihilism of an anti-science stance ruled; and in my dissertation, initiated (in 1952) and completed (in 1955) while working as a full time faculty member, I set out to draw together some (not all) of Mead's ideas, systematizing conceptions and theoretical propositions, in order to test them as rigorously as possible.

This "program" has undergirded much of the work I have done as a sociologist and social psychologist.

ENTER FAMILY

Obviously, my introduction to sociological work on the family came early in my nascent career as a sociologist. As an undergraduate, I had the benefit of Kirk's courses as well as continuous *informal* contact with him. As a graduate student, I participated in a seminar group which conducted an experimental study of attitudes toward male sex behavior, a study replicated when members of the group were reunited at Indiana (Kirkpatrick, Stryker, & Buell, 1952). And, at both Minnesota and Indiana during my first year there, I joined Kirk in working on his family text and on the revision of "What Science Says."

Given that background of focus on the family in my undergraduate and graduate training as a sociologist, there can be little wonder why I chose a family setting for my dissertation work—though it was not automatic. That is, it was my interest in the ideas of Mead, and my determination to "do right" by Mead by subjecting his ideas to as rigorous an empirical test as I could manage, that took precedence in my thinking. More specifically, at that time, I saw the concept of role-taking as pivotal in his discussion of the development of self, of personhood. I believed that I could justify, on the basis of Mead's discussions, a set of hypotheses concerning circumstances permitting accurate role-taking as well as the consequences of accuracy in role-taking. Further, I believed, I could develop operationalizations of key concepts entailed in these hypotheses that would enable a reasonable test of the hypotheses and therefore of the ideas underlying them.

But, given those ideas themselves, the operationalizations required specifying an institutional context for the research. Central to Mead's thought is the concept of meaning. And I, as a researcher, had to know a good deal about the meanings entailed in the role relationships in which role-taking accuracy was to be assessed before I could find, or build, an adequate index of role-taking accuracy or of the expected outcomes of that accuracy. Moreover, because the hypotheses spoke to specified sources of differential role-taking accuracy and differential consequences of accuracy, there was methodological advantage to be gained by finding some setting in which multiple persons' role-taking accuracy could be assessed in relation to multiple others. Thinking about such necessities and/or desiderata, as well as the practical limitations on what I as an individual researcher with very limited sources could manage (the kinds of support now routinely available or possible for dissertation research then are not what they are now; an analogy of desktop computers, now versus counter-sorters, then, comes to mind) led me to choose family units composed of a married pair and the parents of one of that pair as the arena in which I could carry out my study.

That choice was based on another consideration. My prime dissertation problem was high risk–it could well have produced negative results; and then, as now, research producing negative results holds little interest for sociological audiences (including dissertation committees!). Consequently, I built into my research a hedge study. My reading in the family literature circa late 1940s, early 1950s, led me to doubt Talcott Parson's then popular and generally accepted thesis that argued the demise of the extended family and its replacement by the nuclear family of mother, father, and their immature children. My hedge had to do with cross-generational interaction, in particular patterns of helping, between adult children and their parents. I never fully analyzed the resulting data, since my risky research problem did not fail me, but I did examine them enough to know they cast serious doubt on Parson's argument. (I think the data are still somewhere in my files; just a bit later, Marvin Sussman nicely exploited his own research findings that made the same point.)

There is, I think, a general lesson in the story being told that is worth brief elaboration before going on. If, as for Mead, symbolic interaction is the defining characteristic of human social experience; if, as they are, meanings are at the heart of symbolic interaction; and if meanings, as they do, vary across institutional settings, abstract social processes (for example, role-taking) must be located with some concrete institutional setting (for example, family) before they can be effectively researched. It is this lesson that, importantly, has led symbolic interactionists away from experimental settings in their research. But, even for experimental researchers, the lesson holds. If experimental social psychologists do not locate their procedures in some explicit institutional setting, their subjects will find one to give their participation meaning. (And, if their subjects either provide a singular but unknown setting or variable settings, there exists uncontrolled alternative accounts of the experimental findings.)

A QUESTION OF IDENTITY: FAMILY SOCIOLOGISTS OR SOCIAL PSYCHOLOGIST?

In my own mind, the theoretical issues emanating from my reading of Mead took precedence in my dissertation over its substantive concerns with family relationships. Yet, clearly and perhaps inevitably, the early publications (Stryker, 1955; 1956; 1957) flowing from the dissertation research served to identify me to the external sociological world as a sociologist of the family. That identification, reinforced I am sure by Kirk's sponsorship, led to a number of opportunities that had the effect of further reinforcing that identification while at the same time allowing me to think about what was of greater interest to me, namely, the theoretical ideas of symbolic interactionism. An early opportunity came in the form of a Groves Conference invitation to present a paper, later published (Stryker, 1959) on symbolic interaction as an approach to family research. A subsequent opportunity to expand the thinking presented in the Groves Conference paper was an invitation from Harold Christensen to write a chapter on the interactional and situational approaches for his *Handbook of Marriage and the Family* (1964). Perhaps the most significant of these opportunities, significant both in terms of the way in which my work has developed ever since and with respect to my own sociological identity, was an invitation to address a 1966 plenary session of ASA's Section on the Family. For that session, I wrote the paper "Identity Salience and Role Performance," subsequently published (Stryker, 1968), which contained the initial statement of what has come to be known as Identity Theory, a theory of role-choice behavior. Two observations should be added to this recital: (1) the impetus for much of the effort to infuse family sociology with sociological theory of one sort or another came from family sociologists like Reuben Hill who were reacting to the subfield's reputation in the broader discipline as being singularly a-theoretical; (2) that the ideas entering Identity Theory were hardly mine alone is indicated by the fact that after my 1966 address, a man I had never seen before came up to me and said: "You've just delivered our book!" The man was George McCall, and the book was *Identities and Interactions* (McCall & Simmons, 1966).

However, I never felt myself to be a family sociologist. This is my own view, despite my external identification as a family sociologist and the public manifestations of that identification in the form of published papers in which family figured prominently. This is also evident to me, despite the fact that family relationships have entered, albeit less centrally, into most of my subsequent research and writing efforts. Indeed, I was vaguely uncomfortable with being so identified and have tried to think about why this was so.

One reason has only become clear in retrospect: Only once in my life have I taught a course in the family, and that was not at Indiana University. Kirk, God love him, had a Depression mentality with regard to the courses he taught. That is, as an academic in the 1930s he not unrealistically had come to worry about the loss of enrollment as a threat to employment–and not even the very plush post-World War II enrollment days persuaded him that this worry was out of date. Consequently, the courses he taught were "his" courses, and he could not accept the idea of sharing them. By the time of Kirk's retirement, I was no longer interested in teaching in the family area.

Partly my vague discomfort at being labeled a family sociologist stemmed from other sources, not excluding the snobbishness of youth. I shared the view of family sociology as being largely a-theoretical, despite the work of people like Reuben Hill and William Goode, and too much devoted to doing good rather than doing science; and my early participation in the Grove Conference had not dissuaded me of that judgment. (I must add, in all fairness, that same youthful snobbishness led me to see all but a very few of the "famous" sociological theorists I listened to through my early ASA meetings as having very large feet of clay.) However, the decisive turn with respect to my identification as social psychologist rather than family sociologist came in the mid-1960s, when I was offered a position in the Department of Family Relations at Cornell University. Despite the attractiveness of joining a vigorous department containing people like Urie Bronfenbrenner, John Harding, and Ed Devereaux, and despite the heady compliment (to a young sociologist) of being offered a position in that department, I ultimately decided that I could not accept the offer, that doing so would confirm and likely fix an exclusive identity as a family sociologist; and I was just unwilling to accept that possibility. Surely, we learn who we are through the eyes of others; just as surely, we also learn who we are by reflecting on what we do.

But having chosen an alternative identity did not mean that I lost contact with family sociology. For one thing, much of my theoretical and research efforts in social psychology continued (and still continues) to incorporate in one way or another family-based relationships. For another, I have watched developments in family sociology, often with considerable concern over what I seemed to be seeing. In short, then, the evidence is that I did indeed carry a salient identity as family sociologist, despite my failure to recognize that fact. And, I'm feeling chagrined by my belated recognition that this is so. Let me explain by reference to what I think I've seen.

In my earlier years, interpersonal relationships and interaction–what were then called dating and courtship, marital interaction, parent-child relationships and their consequences–were the focal sociological concerns with the family, and interest in such provided a natural, powerful and attractive entry point for neophyte sociologists and a bridge to more general sociological and differentiated sociological concerns. Too, in my earlier years, family sociologists writing about interpersonal relations and interaction were highly visible in the general sociological journals. In more recent years, those earlier focal concerns seem to have dissipated or at least in important degree gone underground–i.e., become less visible in our general journals. I don't doubt that the total amount of sociological writings about family matters is very large, perhaps larger than it has ever been, but more of it seems to be sociological history of the family, comparative institutional analysis of the family, demographic analysis of family size and structure, or the byproduct of interest in other topics–delinquency and crime, feminist theory and research, sexuality, etc.–and it is such work on the family that comes to wider sociological attention through publication in the general journals. Please do not misunderstand: I am not contending that work related to family on other than family relationships and interaction is of lesser import, only asserting that lesser attention and import attached to relationships and interaction–assuming such is real and not the product of my overwrought imagination–is disturbing. Admittedly, cause and effect may be confounded in my analysis. Still, for one thing, the field's ability to recruit major talent is mitigated. For another, work that once was central to the sociology of the family has flowed from sociologists to persons trained in "family studies," health and recreation, social work, human development, psychology; and less of it is done by sociologists–a prime example is the study of love, of intimate relationships. It does not denigrate the contributions of non-sociologists to the study of family relationships and interactions to say that family relationships and interaction are too important in a variety of sense to forego in any degree the potential contributions of sociology.

Herein my chagrin. I am not sufficiently the egomaniac to believe that I could have significantly changed the scenario just sketched. But, had I explicitly recognized my identity as family sociologist, altered my own research and publication agenda to accommodate that recognition, and participated over more recent years in the professional life of family sociology, perhaps in concert with like-thinking sociological brethren I could have made some difference. At least I could have tried, rather than only engaging in posthoc commentary. And I would now feel less guilty!

AUTHOR NOTE

Sheldon Stryker, PhD, is Distinguished Professor of Sociology, Indiana University, Bloomington, IN 47405.

The reading of a draft of this essay by my colleague, Brian Powell, made the essay more clear and more cogent than it otherwise would have been. I appreciate that reading.

REFERENCES

Blumer, H. (1969). *Symbolic interactionism: Perspective and method.* Englewood Cliffs, NJ: Prentice-Hall.

Christensen, H. (Ed.) (1964). *Handbook of marriage and the family.* Chicago: Rand-McNally.

Kirkpatrick, C. (1955). *The family as process and institution.* New York: Ronald.

Kirkpatrick, C., Stryker, S. & Buell, P. (1952). An experimental study of attitudes toward male sex behavior with reference to Kinsey findings. *American Sociological Review, 17*, 5, 580-586.

McCall, G. J. & Simmons, J.T. (1966). *Identities and interactions.* New York: The Free Press.

Stryker, S. (1955). The adjustment of married offspring to their parents. *American Sociological Review 20*, 2, 149-154.

Stryker, S. (1956). Relationships of married offspring and their parents: A test of Mead's theory. *American Journal of Sociology, 62*, 3, 308-319.

Stryker, S. (1957). Role-taking accuracy and adjustment. *Sociometry, 20*, 4, 286-296.

Stryker, S. (1959). Symbolic interaction as an approach to family research. *Marriage and Family Living 21*, 2,111-119.

Stryker, S. (1968). Identity salience and role performance. *Journal of Marriage and the Family, 30*, 4, 558-564.

Stryker, S. (1994). Identity theory: Its development, research base and prospects. In N. Denzin (Ed.) *Studies in symbolic interaction, Vol. 16* (pp. 9-20). Greenwich, CT: JAI Press.

The Admiral's Son with an Independent Spirit

Walter R. Schumm

KEYWORDS. Autobiography, research, career, military, childhood

INTRODUCTION

My Father's Family

Most of my family's oral tradition was associated with my father's stories that framed much of my childhood and my values. My earliest forebear was orphaned as a child in Germany around the age of ten or so and departed Germany in 1841 to avoid the draft, becoming a cabinet-maker in Switzerland. In 1849 Christian Schumm went to California via Panama to find gold. He didn't find enough, but I still have a piece of a watch chain made from the gold he panned. He moved to Wisconsin to take up farming, which he also failed at, and eventually died in 1881 or so as a saloon keeper in Sauk City, where he and his wife are buried (albeit in different cemeteries). His son Walter, one of several children, earned a degree in architecture from Columbia University, I think, and had a hand in designing the old Grand Central Station in New York City. It is reported that he also designed a building specifically to warehouse/sell china. Once a Catholic bishop offered him all the contracts on Long Island if he would convert and he told him "No way!" At any rate, Walter and his wife Alberta Brooke didn't get along well and they separated about 1911 when my father Brooke Schumm was five or six years old. They tried to persuade my father at that age to choose living in an orphanage rather than living with one of them, but my father refused and ended up living with his mother. My father's family was so poor that as a teenager he cried in thankfulness one Christmas when his mother got him, as his only Christmas present, a bar of soap designed to help reduce acne. He was so happy just to receive anything. One time he thought his mother would be upset with him because he came home from school with bullet holes in his new jacket (gang warfare, he was an innocent bystander) but she was happier he had escaped harm.

Because his mother highly valued education, he entered the private Ethical Culture School (they gave scholarships to one third of their students to allow their better off students to rub elbows with a wide variety of students) and did well enough that he was able to pass the admissions test for the Naval Academy in the middle of his junior year (so he never finished high school). The military became his ticket to the middle class. He was five feet ten inches tall, weighed only 116 pounds, and had to eat a full meal to make the weight limit for getting into the Academy. He was known as the "walking death" because of his thinness. He had to beg his father to loan him the admissions fee and was disappointed that his father was so reluctant to help him out. Later his father would visit him at the Academy and state that his primary reason for coming was to see the buildings. It was a family secret for a long time but his father committed suicide in the early years of the Depression when his business was failing.

At the Academy, he roomed with Charles Tooke, who had a photographic memory. Charlie's father would ask my father if Charlie was studying hard and my dad would lie about it. My father was really proud the one time that he bested Charlie by a couple of points after studying for an exam for days, even though Charlie hadn't bothered to study at all. Another time my father caught someone cheating and this led to a boxing match that my father lost, allowing the cheater to avoid being turned in. But my father was pleased that the cheater had to miss class the next day, being in the hospital for a broken thumb from the damage he had received in his win.

Although some people have a lack of respect for the military, I was raised with the ideals associated with being an officer. These ideals consisted of being a gentleman, scholar, thinker, and someone with integrity, whose word was his bond. Someone who would try to minimize killing on all sides as well as take care of one's own people, enemy prisoners and civilians, with particular assistance rendered to defenseless women and children. Some of my better assignments later in the Army Reserve would be as commander of two prisoner of war units (Schumm, 1998). While I have spent twenty-seven years in the family field, I have lived my whole life under the assumption I would be an 'officer and a gentleman' when I grew up. That is not to say the professor image didn't occur fairly early–as early as the second grade, my teachers were suggesting that I might be a professor when I grew up.

My Mother's Family

On my mother's side, I know less. My ancestors there go back to the Mayflower, though one of the seven from that ship was reportedly hanged as a horse thief. They remained in the New England area, moving back and forth from Boston to Newbury, Vermont, with my mother's father running antique shops. I wasn't told as many stories about this side of the family. There was some degree of alcohol abuse by the males in the family, which may have had something to do with the family secrecy that resulted.

STORYTELLING AND MORAL TEACHING

It seemed that my childhood was beset with stories with morals. My Dad loved the *The Count of Monte Cristo,* a book about a hero who got even with all his enemies after overcoming many difficulties. One story revolves around Jig Jig Brown. He was a harsh sea captain of a U.S. destroyer who was not liked by his crew, but who cried when they presented him with a model of his ship when he left the ship for another job in the Navy. The moral: Everyone has a soft side, which a thoughtful gift revealed, even though it had been made in celebration of his leaving rather than in honor of it.

Another story is about supporting your boss. My father had been doing off duty work on the ship's engines and their capabilities. My father's immediate boss came into the wardroom very depressed one day because the ship's captain had ordered him to produce some engineering analyses that very day and he knew they would take several days. My father told him that he had already been working on those problems and had them figured out, so it was not a problem. My father's boss said that my father could do no wrong in his eyes after that. The moral: If you save your boss's situation, you save your own; going beyond basic requirements, surpassing expectations, can pay off in unexpected ways.

Once my father was told there was some delicious lobster for lunch (he loved lobster but hated crabmeat). So he chowed down and was wondering why everyone was standing around laughing at him. It was actually crab. The moral: Be careful about being too picky with your food.

The Military Influence

Several stories are based on my father's military experiences. During World War II, they saw a parachuting Japanese aviator floating by. My father was in charge of the guns on the U.S.S. San Diego, an anti-aircraft ship, and was afraid someone might fire on the helpless man. He ordered the crews to hold their fire and let the man go, though some wanted to avenge the deaths of their friends. Later, a U.S. destroyer picked the man up, who turned out to be a sunburned American pilot (who had been terrified when this ship passed by with most of its heavy guns aimed at him). The moral: Never forget the all important "milk of human kindness" as my father called it.

Another time, his ship was ordered to bombard a Japanese-held island in order to silence an enemy radio station somewhere on the land. They raked the island with shells and got the radio but my father always worried that they might have killed innocent civilians in the process, though no one really ever knew what had happened. The moral: If you have to be hard on an issue, be careful–don't shoot everyone to get rid of one troublemaker, if you can help it.

When the war started, it was a Sunday in Boston and they could not open the safe with the war plans. So they had to get a thief out of the Boston jail to help them, which he did, successfully. The moral: In a crisis, it's the expertise you need, more than the source.

A corollary of this was his story of how the Navy had to get rid of many of its high ranking officers who were good diplomats but lousy fighters at the start of the war. Of course, after the war, the Navy brought back more of the diplomat-types, those who knew, in my father's words, how to "hold the handle of the teacup properly in their pinky finger." The moral was that what really counts is knowing your job but that much of the time those with political skills will get more credit (and higher promotions), until the bullets start flying.

Many of the stories involved family members. In 1940, when my brother was nine years old, he climbed a 300 foot radio tower outside Boston Navy yard, diverting the attention of both an outgoing and an incoming work force shift, costing thousands of man-hours and dollars. The Captain in charge of the Navy yard was trying to see Admiral Tarrant to complain and demand the head of the child's father. My father got there first, however, because he was the admiral's aide, and talked to him about my brother climbing the radio tower. The Captain then came in and ranted and raved about the cost of this fiasco and the damage to the war effort. However, he had nothing to say and stomped out angrily when the admiral responded simply that he liked a boy with spirit. The moral: Sometimes there are personal things more important than what seems urgent at the moment.

The same admiral demonstrated the value of truthfulness over tact (a family theme)–when riding with the Secretary of the Navy, President Roosevelt, and my father, the Secretary asked the admiral what he thought about tearing down the blue collar housing in the area to make more room for the base. Contrary to the politically correct answer, the admiral said "I think it stinks!" and along with my father was promptly dismissed, to walk back to the headquarters. I used to think this value of truth over authority was a personal virtue until I read that all INTJ (introverted, intuitive, thinking, judgmental) personality types like myself tend to see the world that way. In our family, the idea of "kissing up" to an authority figure has always been an anathema. It is rather amazing that I have survived over 29 years in the military reserves with such an attitude.

There was the story about the mentally challenged sailor who wasn't competent enough for any regular job (nobody wanted him assigned to their section) but wanted to feel significant, with an important job. The Captain and my father thought and thought about the issue, finally coming up with the idea of assigning him the responsibility of keeping the hallway into the Captain's cabin absolutely spotless, scouring every inch of it with a toothbrush, daily. This gave the man a job he could do, and he felt so proud to be keeping the Captain's area clean. The moral: Everyone has an important role if you use his or her talents creatively.

In September 1942, a Japanese submarine sent a fan of torpedoes towards a series of U.S. ships and sank or damaged several of them. My father's ship, the U.S.S. San Diego, was hit by the torpedo, which failed to detonate. Men inside the ship heard the thud and saw the dent in the hull, but those topside (including my father) saw the torpedo reach the ship and assumed it had passed underneath the ship. My father thought it was human error, setting the torpedo depth too low, thinking that the ship was a larger cruiser than it was. Instead, the actual reason was probably simple mechanical error. The moral was that sometimes it takes luck or God watching out for you (leaving open the question of what happened to the other ships that were sunk!).

One story was one I may have witnessed, even though I was so young that I might have missed the meaning at the moment. My father was waiting to get a haircut at Cameron Station, an installation (since dismantled) in Alexandria, Virginia, our hometown. An Army general sauntered in and demanded to be served first, in front of a line of about a dozen or so people waiting along with my father. My father waited until the general was seated and then he slowly walked up to the barber, handed him his identification card, with the rank of Rear Admiral (technically one rank higher than the brigadier general, though my father was retired at the time–but no one dared ask about that) and said "I always thought that two stars were higher than one." The meaning was that if the general had the right to jump the line because of his rank, my Dad had the right to get in front of the general. This angered the general so much that he stomped out, much to the tittering and amusement of the others in line. The moral: Lack of consideration for others, pride, and arrogance can lead to extremely humiliating personal embarrassment.

Self as an Influence

My own birth has a story. I was born two months premature at a time when 25% of such babies went blind. The cause of this birth defect was the pure oxygen given to these infants so they could breathe, which caused blood vessels to grow into the center of the eye. The pediatrician, an optimistic fellow, told my mother there was a 100% chance that I would die. This was complicated because my father's mother, who was living with us, resented my arrival and had told my mother she wanted me to die. Fortunately for me, I ate like crazy, gained weight rapidly, didn't go blind, and became a rather chubby baby by age one. The fact that I looked like my grandmother turned her guilt into doting and she had the honor, among other things, of teaching me how to tie my shoelaces for the first time. The moral: The will to survive is important!

It seems that my father and I always talked, sometimes for hours at a time, more like college roommates do. In contrast, my mother was a woman of few words, though they were terribly significant when she did say something. But I think my father was deliberately trying to reverse what he had experienced from his own father. Thus, talking a lot and spending time together was his prime solution. The moral: Children need their parents' time more than anything else. Although I enjoy talking with my children as much as almost anything in life, I have not achieved (consistently) the same amount of time with each of them that my father did with me.

The most memorable issue we debated was the Vietnam War. My Dad would take the Viet Cong side and make me argue the U.S. side. He was really good–the V.C. should have hired him as their spokesperson, except he didn't totally believe his own arguments. One of the more early debates, when I was about 15 (with my father present), was between myself and my cousin Phil Dodd, who was a reporter for the *Chicago Tribune* and used to appear on *Meet the Press*. I had worked up a good argument on why Vietnam was wrong, because it was sending well educated, highly trained American boys like myself (except older) to their deaths, which was a tragic waste of human potential. To finish the argument I added that it was especially bad because they were being killed by uneducated, ignorant Viet Cong (who would probably never amount to anything anyway) who were, for the most part, using cheap 50-cent bullets. My cousin jumped all over that idea by reminding me, correctly, that the life of a Viet Cong was worth every bit as much as mine, no matter the relative level of education. I had thought my argument invincible and here it had been revealed as so terribly flawed.

EARLY HOME LIFE

I grew up in the "classic" fifties home. My father worked full-time while my mother ran the household. I have thought about challenging feminist theorists as to whether my parents' situation was all that bad. My mother always had a car and a checkbook at her disposal. My father was driven to work each day by a chauffeur (and he was only a Captain in the Navy). When he came home, he had at least an hour to unwind, get a drink, and just relax. Yes, my mother was busy preparing dinner but she got to have a nap of 1-2 hours each afternoon and we had a maid who did most of the chores, most notably cleaning of the kitchen and bathrooms. I did some of the chores (garbage, dishes, cleaning up after the cat) while my Dad did most of the outdoor work, gardening, mowing, repairs. I also trimmed the ivy along the sidewalks and curbs, raked leaves, weeded, and swept the sidewalks and walkways. My mother did wash and dry our clothes.

I think our chores were divided fairly equitably, but having the maid was critical to the balance. Nor was my mother "stuck" at home. She did an extensive amount of volunteer work for the community, especially the League of Women Voters. After she died, the League dedicated a small garden to her, in Alexandria, Virginia. I never had the impression from my mother that she considered herself "oppressed." She had worked in canning factories during World War II and seemed to be glad to not have to be doing that sort of work for a living. When Betty Friedan's *The Feminine Mystique* was published it was a source of discussion. However, from the tone of the discussions, it seemed to capture only part of the experience of my mother and her friends, and made a woman's life seem more negative than they experienced it.

Another impression of mine was that the rules were pretty straightforward. My parents would do all they could to give me a good upbringing, spending time with me, setting a good example for me, paying for my education. In return, I was expected to be the highest quality person I could be, which would eventually reflect well upon them. It was never stated out loud, but it seemed a reasonable quid pro quo to me; in fact, I thought that I was getting the better end of the deal. The idea of rebelling against my parents or bringing shame on them, in my mind, was totally illogical–why bite the hand that is feeding you so well? This logic extended to others in society. My parents often picked up people needing a ride around town, often poor, black women, and asked only that they help someone else in return.

This is not to say we had a perfect family. My father was, I suspect, by today's standards, some degree of an alcoholic. By the standards of the 1950s Navy, he was a routine social drinker. I felt badly about it because he occasionally fell asleep in his chair before going to bed, to which alcohol seemed to contribute, and I missed talking more with him. One evening, he had a bit too much and forgot to serve me my dinner at the table–it was potatoes and chipped beef. Actually, I had taken the potatoes and mashed them, with butter, but he forgot to serve me the beef and cream, which was one of his favorite toppings. Somehow my mother could keep silent no longer and made a mildly sarcastic comment on the situation and they both ended up speaking sharp words to each other. This was such a shock to me that I turned pale white and stopped their comments dead in their tracks. They both realized how much out of norm the situation must have gotten. It was the only time in twenty years that I heard them exchange such critical comments.

The only other problem was that, in my mind, they were not nearly affectionate enough. My Dad would hug Mom and make comments about how nice it would be for me to grow up and have a woman to hug. I thought that his approach was a bit demeaning to Mother. Somehow I picked up the notion that, at that time, sex wasn't all that great for women and that it was more of a sport for men. Once I said that, when I was about eight, and the audience of adults and my parents thought my views were terribly humorous. However, it wasn't clear if the humor was about to my being correct or my being wrong, or just my precociousness in having views about sexuality at all.

Another time, I was asked, about the same time, to say grace at Thanksgiving when we were having dinner at the Dodds, my cousins (Marty, my cousin Phil's wife, died only this past January, 1999). I resented the superficiality of only offering thanks once or twice a year, so I protested by taking them literally and saying "Grace, Amen." I don't know if they got the point but they muttered something to themselves like, "Well, what can we say, he did just what we asked!"

This theme of superficiality versus authentic depth was an undercurrent of a war led by myself. I would come down for breakfast and Dad would say, "Here comes the dour monk! Don't you know that (starting to sing) life is just a bowl of cherries, la la la la la la!" I would say something about taking life more seriously, but smile, and then we would move on. I don't know where that idea of seriousness being virtuous came from, perhaps from my mother's stoic New England roots, but it seemed as if wired into me from my earliest recollections. The down side of this is that I have never been a "fun-seeker" and have been rejected by quite a few people for not being "fun enough."

This has occasionally led to some unusual conversations. In high school, a private Episcopal school at which my father taught when he retired from the Navy, I studied each night from the time I got home until nine or ten, each night, sometimes forsaking dinner. College was the same routine, more or less. When I came home from college, a neighbor friend challenged me by asking if I had ever laid any women, gotten drunk, or smoked pot. When I said no, he responded "Man, you've never lived!" My thought was that such a life wasn't really living at all.

I was born in 1951 when my mother was 43 and my Dad was 46, so it was sort of like being raised by grandparents. My brother, my only sibling, was 20 years older and he was my idolized role model. If he did it, then I was going to do it. That desire to imitate him led to me to get a PhD, be an Army Reserve officer, attain the rank of colonel, command a unit as a full colonel, have four children, and be a research scientist, all of which I accomplished–except I've had more children. I am not sure if this seemed like imitation or competition to my brother!

The Neighborhood

Society wasn't perfect either. My Dad had tried to register to vote in 1954 in Virginia and they said he had to print his name, last name first, middle initial, address, date of birth, and perhaps a couple of other things. He tried to do this but put his age instead of his date of birth. They said since he was white, they'd overlook it–the implication being that the whole reason for giving such rambling, long, verbal only instructions was to disenfranchise blacks. Our own home was purchased in 1954 for about $18,000 but my parents got it because the owners didn't want to sell it to the highest bidders, who happened to be Jewish. According to the previous owners and the realtor, there was already one Jewish family in the neighborhood and two would be too many. My Dad loved to point out the hypocrisy of our local congressman, who was named Broyhill. Once he challenged him in a town meeting because Broyhill had voted for a bill but not its funding–he was trying to take credit for both sides of the issue. Mr. Broyhill didn't take to my Dad's approach, from what my Dad said.

My Dad told stories about his going to the back of a bus in Norfolk, Virginia, in about 1928, and being inspected by the driver who then told him to move up front where the whites belonged. He was proud that his (white) Aunt Beatrice Fetz was a life member of the NAACP. Today, this general tenor would seem improper, less activist than it should have been. The stories clearly decried racism, anti-Semitism, and political hypocrisy, but the theme seemed to be that changing things would be up to my generation, more than theirs. I think the idea was that, if you raised your children right, they would make more progress with such issues than if you took on the system by yourself.

Religion versus Spirituality

Another major issue was religion. Spirituality was seen as intrinsically important but religion was the realm of hypocrites. The classic family story on this was the Long Island church contract story, mentioned previously. When my Dad had been about eight, he had skipped one Methodist Sunday school lesson to attend a Catholic service with a close friend, which cost him his perfect attendance pin for the year. This struck him as grossly unfair, for the rest of his life. My parents generally refused to attend church, though my mother liked to go to the Thursday services before Easter. Nevertheless, they sent me to a local Episcopal church when I was only five, by myself, which led to much emotional pain, sitting in church week after week, like an orphan, with everyone afraid to interact with me. But I loved to hear the Bible stories and sing the songs, for they were good by themselves and also relieved my loneliness and isolation. I prayed for years that my parents would go to church with me and finally my Dad did one Sunday. Sadly, the priest, who was otherwise a very honorable man, could not resist pointing out the hypocrisy of parents who sent their children to church alone for years but wouldn't come themselves. This stinging criticism, accompanied by what seemed to be the eyes of all in the church scowling at us, ensured that my Dad never went to either that church or any other ever again. It would be easy to judge, but I erred myself because years later my Dad came into my room while I was praying and I basically gave him the cold shoulder.

My brother tried to visit the same church once, but the church members also gave him the cold shoulder. Those two visits pretty much killed any prospects of my family ever going to church as a family. My Dad always said that parents should teach children nothing about religion and let them make up their own minds when they turned eighteen. However, I ran into some Protestant evangelicals at my Episcopal high school who said that God wanted everyone to have a personal relationship with Him. At first this seemed like heresy to me, for God was too almighty or at least too busy to permit such a thing. At the Youth for Christ and Young Life meetings, however, the people seemed to be about the only ones I ever met who genuinely accepted people for themselves, without looking for what they could get out of them. I was stunned one time when a girl–a really nice-looking girl–actually said hello to me, someone for whom most girls wouldn't give the time of day (I wasn't exactly known as Mr. Fun). Later, in twelfth grade, after reading a Billy Graham book, I made a bedside commitment to Christ. The inner change wrought by this spiritual quest seemed to be a new, deep sense of meaning and joy that, on the positive side, has persisted through various difficulties. On the negative side, however, this change has often been obscured by either my melancholy temperament or my preoccupation with professional or family responsibilities. My Army Reserve obligations also have limited my formal church attendance to an average of one or two Sundays a month, which appears to be the height of spiritual unreliability to many regular church attenders.

Actually, the story is more confusing because, when I was six years old, I had the strongest intuitive sense that God wanted me to be a church pastor. This seemed to me to be the most absurd idea because I was so clearly unprepared for the task. In addition, I have always been an "idea" person, the classic "INTJ" researcher personality. I believe that pastors should be warm, fuzzy, people persons whose effusive personalities naturally draw people to them. They must be individuals about whom people would say "Pastor Smith is just so warm and loving"–not that his ideas are so incisive and meaningful. Nevertheless, this feeling has led to some frustration because I have many ideas on how churches could operate more effectively, but my ideas appear to have no credibility to anyone within institutional Christianity. If there was any rule based on tradition per se, I would try to break it, deliberately so people would learn to depend on God rather than more superficial things. I would focus on what Jesus taught rather than the many things usually preached about other issues. You wouldn't believe the weird looks I get from priests and pastors when I fail to restrain myself and mention ideas like these. I should say, as an aside, that my Dad was very proud of having raised two religious sons, himself not being religious other than burying the dead at sea during World War II. He used to nag the Episcopal priests at my high school mercilessly because his sons were religious without any training while their sons were often anti-religious following much religious training.

Another early event occurred when I was walking home from school when I was about seven, looking down at the asphalt pavement and wondering what I was going to do. I was feeling discouraged, probably for not being as popular at school as I wanted and possibly because, at that moment, I wasn't feeling like my parents loved me very much. I took inventory of my assets and figured I'd never make much of a mark with my athletic talent or looks. I might do well, however, in having a caring heart (as much as anyone else could) and intelligence, the latter being my best approach to earning people's respect. I believe I asked God to help me by giving me wisdom (remembering Solomon had been given credit for asking that). As a strategic life decision, that was partly good (discounting looks, favoring wisdom over materialism) and partly bad–I should have given more emphasis to loving people as opposed to more or less outsmarting them.

Early Aspirations Nipped in the Bud

When I was eight, my Dad and I had a discussion about what I wanted to do when I grew up. At any rate, I told my Dad that I was thinking of getting a PhD in psychology. To that he said, "Any jerk can get a PhD in psychology." His comment ended those aspirations on the spot, and I decided instead to pursue a PhD in astronomy or oceanography, that being "real science." Ultimately, this goal led me to attend William and Mary College because of its good physics and oceanography programs. However, I learned that I became seasick easily and I nearly flunked out of physics. One of my physics professors remarked how "If you work really, really hard, you might get a bachelor's degree," which was not exactly encouraging. When I was a senior, I tried to build an electrostatic cooling machine, based on ideas of an engineer who worked down the hall from my brother at Union Carbide's Cleveland office. It was a lesson by itself because none of my esteemed professors thought it would ever work; some of them expected that I would flunk out of college for failing my senior project. But I believed in my brother's descriptions of what his friend had accomplished and, to the amazement of students and professors, the device I built eventually cooled a red hot wire coil very effectively. Upon seeing it work, it took my professors only about five minutes to figure out how it worked. In other words, they had to believe in order to understand or comprehend–their faith had to precede their understanding in this totally non-religious situation.

This "handwriting on the wall" problem in physics led me to finally take courses in psychology, anthropology, and political science. While I was struggling to get average grades–not to mention respect–in physics, I found myself at the top of the class in the other areas, without trying nearly as hard. I concluded it would go better to be an "A" sociologist rather than a "C" physicist. This discrepancy led me to consider a career change even though it was too late to change majors. The net result was that while physics got me into the Signal Corps for two years at the end of the Vietnam era (even though I volunteered for infantry and artillery first), I had decided to pursue graduate education in an area outside of physics.

I have mentioned the family secrets of the hanged horse thief and my grandfather's suicide. Another secret is that one of my ancestors may have been black, something my nephew has failed to confirm or deny (he is our family's history researcher). When I first learned of this, it was interesting to speculate on how my life would change or would have been different had I been known to be of African-American descent! My family had joked about the possibility of a relative having been touched by the "tar brush." Actually, I had more important ties. The maid who worked with my family for 15 or more years became a virtual relative. She probably spent as much time with me as my mother when I was young. When I had to leave to join the Army, she walked up to our house that morning, early, with roast chicken and a cake to send me off. I was very touched that our maid was treating this like an important occasion, while my own parents were treating it like any other day. They probably felt differently but didn't want to say so.

When my mother lay dying a few years later, she could not recognize my own brother but she recognized our maid Sarah and made a major effort (given her dying condition) to introduce her to a visitor. After my mother died, her wedding ring disappeared. It was only recovered through Sarah's efforts (upon my Dad's request); she visited the nursing home and scolded and shamed the staff into surrendering the ring that they had stolen. The net result was that my mother was buried without her ring and one of my nieces was given it later on.

I have kept up correspondence with Sarah and visited her a couple of years ago in Ashland, Virginia. She put all of her daughters through college and has her own home where she takes care of her invalid husband to whom she has been married for 40-plus years.

My Parents' Death

My mother died in 1973 and my father in 1985. Both deaths provided a hard lesson for me, in terms of trusting intuition versus logic. My mother was diagnosed with polyarteritis nodosa, but when I asked the doctor what that meant, he said it meant she would be cured and perfectly well in six months. I asked him twice because my intuition and my mother's actions (having my Dad buy a nice suit, a new car, and other things he might not do by himself without her help) suggested she had something more serious. I prayed about it but still had a sense this was a terminal condition, incurable. But I figured the doctor knew more than I did and I pretended all through her last Christmas that all was well. By the time the truth came out, she was too dysfunctional to engage in communication with very effectively.

My father died quickly of a heart attack on April 15th but did and said things that last day that suggested he knew something was not right and he had to get his affairs in order as best he could. I was driving to Iowa for a meeting [I believe that Pauline Boss was at the same meeting and was very consoling] and en route had a strong intuitive feeling I should call home if I wished to talk to my father. But I dismissed it as not being logical to stop in the middle of nowhere to call, when there was no indication of any problems at home. If I had, I would have reached him; by the time I arrived at the meeting, it was too late to call. Ken Kennedy drove with my family to Lawrence, Kansas, so we could trade cars out and we drove as fast as we could to Maryland, reaching the funeral home just as they were closing. Thus, my son Jonathan got to see his grandfather one last time. I explained the meaning of each ribbon on his uniform, that included fifteen battle stars from World War II, and a bronze star medal. I told the story often to my three-year-old son but he cannot be sure today, at 20 years of age, if he remembers the event or just the telling of it.

BACK TO SOCIAL SCIENCE

While I enjoyed the Army as a lieutenant, it was not something I enjoyed day after day. The challenge and frustration of it was mostly that, no matter how well you did yourself, only one person below you or above you in the military hierarchy could screw up the works and ruin much of what you had done. Later in life I came to view this as more of a challenge–how do you design redundant structures that overcome this flaw–but at the time it seemed to make my life a great waste of effort.

I met some college girls who really liked the Family and Child Development Department at Kansas State University and I applied there for a graduate degree and to VISTA, the domestic peace corps. When VISTA failed to come through, I went to graduate school. This started off well but I soon ran into roadblocks. In one class, I failed the midterm so badly the instructor pointed out that I was the worst in the class, with a score of less than 20 out of 120 maximum points. I recovered because he didn't weight the midterm very much in the final grade, but at the moment I was very worried that I had erred in leaving my steady, well-paying job as an active duty lieutenant.

Then, my money ran out and only the offer of a research assistantship by Dr. Steve Bollman saved my bacon at the last possible moment. If I recall correctly, at least three times my car broke down and Dr. Bollman showed up out of nowhere to help me get it towed/fixed. It seemed as if he was either my guardian angel or else he was tracking me. Steve is one of those rare silent caretakers, who does tremendous amounts of good for people but doesn't ask for any fanfare. Hence, much of what he does goes unnoticed by those not close to him. As one can tell from the references, Steve and Tony Jurich have formed a very long-term publishing team with me. One of the nice things about my graduate education at K-State was the freedom to think about unconventional approaches to issues.

One time I tackled a paper by Tony Jurich and developed a new interpretation of his data, which he handled very well (Schumm & Rekers, 1984). Ken Kennedy also allowed us wide latitude in what we did for our papers and considered spiritual issues to be legitimate topics in his human development classes.

Going for the PhD

In 1978, I had decided to pursue a PhD and the only question was where. K-State offered me a lucrative assistantship but I knew if I took it, I could never take a job there. Purdue University offered me the least money for an assistantship, which given my theoretical predilection against things material, sealed the deal. Purdue was a great experience because I was able to study methodology in depth and to engage in learning with my professors as colleagues. Purdue expected its graduate students to be fully qualified to assume the professional role of assistant professor upon graduation and expected them to gain proficiency at teaching, research, and publication. Professor Figley's goal was for his best students to publish up to six articles before graduation, which was quite a challenge (I did three). One of the more interesting events was when I reviewed an article in press in *Family Relations* by Dr. Figley, I determined that its analysis had been flawed. In an attempt to reanalyze the data I contacted the graduate student who had collected the data. She had, in fact, just tossed the computer cards into her trash can that very day, frustrated over her academic research for reasons I have forgotten. She was able to retrieve half of the data so I could analyze it. In the end, the *Family Relations* article was withdrawn, but three other articles were published from the same data (Schumm, Figley, & Jurich, 1979; Schumm, Figley, & Fuhs, 1980; Schumm, Figley, & Fuhs, 1981). At my prelim defense jokes were made about why I should be or would be failed because of my daring to force a professor's paper to be withdrawn after it had been accepted for publication. Dr. Figley, to his credit, took all this in stride like a statesman. I also had a great time working with Dr. Wallace Denton in the area of premarital counseling, which has led to a research track for me in that area, largely shared with Ben Silliman (Schumm & Denton, 1979; Schumm & Denton, 1980; Silliman & Schumm, 2000; Silliman & Schumm, 1999).

What Was Really Important

I graduated in August 1979, just six days after marrying my wife, Kimberly Ring Schumm. We had first met at an Intervarsity Christian Fellowship retreat at Rock Springs ranch south of Junction City, Kansas, in the fall of 1974. She had sparked my interest because she was thinking of becoming a marriage counselor at the time we first met. We corresponded for years, somewhat to my parents' disapproval because they disliked her lower social class background and her relative lack of tact.

They actually offered me $1,000 cash if I would send her away at one point. However, the fact was that I happened across very few women who would entertain the idea of having at least four children, who were theologically conservative, but politically moderate, and who loved cats, and didn't despise "godless social science." Not to mention having to deal with my relative lack of social skills, my being in the military, and my unusual approach to religious issues. As for loving cats, when I was a baby, I had a cat that followed me around almost like a babysitter and would bring me presents, such as dead rats and mice (my parents loved the babysitting part but not the dead stuff part). My cat was my hero and friend when I thought no one else was.

In 1978 my future wife moved into an apartment above mine, so we spent most of our meals together, though sleeping separately. We were engaged on Valentine's Day 1979. After we were married, we were en route to Kansas when I found a folded note inside the gas cap of our car which said something like "Please help! This man is kidnaping me. Call the police and have him arrested!" The note was left by another family scholar who is now a professor of long standing at a major university. We have seven children now, ages 4 to 19: four boys (Jonathan, Joshua, Phillip, and Daniel) and three girls (Miriam, Deborah, and Martha). The older ones have been our greatest critics on occasion but they all are our greatest source of joy. We are proud of each of them, even though they are uniquely different from each other. To write about them in more detail would take another paper!

RETURN TO KANSAS STATE UNIVERSITY

To the dismay of Texas Tech and Indiana University, I turned down positions there to accept a temporary job at Kansas State. Eventually, I got the job at K-State on a permanent basis. At that time, getting a job at K-State in our department was a genuine ordeal by fire. One job applicant was so badly raked over the coals during her research presentation that she was found weeping in the restroom afterwards. Knowing what I was in for, I knew I had to change tactics to spare myself the same grilling. I took the approach of criticizing others' research, so my prospective antagonists would have to defend that research in order to attack me. Since the research was so poor it couldn't possibly be defended, this would silence them. And it did, with the attack switching from me to the issue of the quality of research in the field in general. I got the job!

However, my approach to undergraduate teaching was deficient in several aspects and it nearly cost me my job until I was switched into mostly graduate teaching. Fortunately, I worked as a teacher for the Army Reserve for eight summers in a row and learned much of what I know about teaching from that experience. I learned that you have to start teaching with the assumption that the students love you and then use eye contact, body language, and directed discussion to reach out (as if with the tentacles of a friendly octopus) and touch each of them emotionally and intellectually.

I briefly worked with Gary Bauer, one of the Republican presidential candidates in 2000, when he was deputy secretary of Health and Human Services under President Reagan. He wanted me to review grant proposals or make a presentation on family strengths, my memory is foggy on which now. But, the trip was going to cost nearly a thousand dollars, a tremendous sum of money for me at the time; I was delivering pizzas to supplement my income as an assistant professor. He graciously loaned me the money but was disappointed (I think) that I couldn't pay it back until the government reimbursed me, which took several weeks. I have always thought the Christian Right would at least show an interest in some of my research, but my independent spirit has probably gotten the better of that aspiration. So, I have never been invited to Focus on the Family (Dr. James Dobson) or the American Family Radio Network (or any other religious talk show for that matter!), unlike some of my more famous students (e.g., Dr. Ken Canfield, President of the National Center on Fathering in Kansas City), who even have their own daily radio shows now.

Mobilization for Desert Storm

In my early years at K-State, I helped develop some of their methodology courses and the beginning graduate level theory course. I had a personal goal of putting K-State on the map in terms of publications and largely succeeded though that criterion was later given lower priority by higher administration than grants and numbers of students taught. Then on December 9, 1990 I was informed that, as of December 11th, I would be on duty in San Antonio, Texas, in support of Desert Shield. That led to the busiest day of my life, as I had to close out my classes, do a will, say goodbye to my family, and pack for an undetermined stay in Texas or possibly the Mideast. For a year, I worked 16 hour days, seven days a week, lost hair, gained weight, and developed hypothyroidism, possibly as a result of that stress.

My career was seriously disrupted, with my publication rate being reduced to just five articles for the next two years (1991-1992) after having published 103 articles over the previous 12 years. But it was fun to work for an organization with focus (support the war effort at all costs!), clear guidance, and unlimited resources, at least compared to most universities. I was also helped because my creditors reduced my interest rates, which helped me pay off many of my debts (I had to go to Consumer Credit Counseling Service to avert bankruptcy earlier in 1990; their help was just fabulous!).

I evaluated the impact of my Desert Storm service, my active duty days, and my extra drill days on the number of publications I've had each year between 1980 and 2000 in a regression analysis. The results suggest that my Desert Storm service cost me 11 publications ($p < .001$). Every 27 days of active duty (i.e., duty away from home) added one publication (because I can work on my writing in the evenings when I am off duty ($p < .07$). However, every 13 days of extra drills (i.e., every 8 hours spent near home doing reserve work) cost a publication ($p < .10$). The adjusted R-squared for the regression analysis was 30.6% ($p < .03$). And who says you can't use statistics to analyze your own personal life!

Since then, I've gotten back on track slowly, with most of my research concerning military families–since the military has probably paid a third or more of my income each year since 1991 for reserve duty or consulting on family issues. In terms of teaching, I have become known for playing dead family theorists in my class on family theory, an approach that introduces humor and helps stimulate creative thinking in a class that might otherwise be much more dull. Even in my research classes, a lot of humor is derived from my poking fun at myself for all of the mistakes I've made or seen over the years in family research. I am busy trying to publish research on the health and family outcomes of Desert Storm (Schumm, Reppert, Jurich, Bollman, Castelo, Sanders, & Webb, 2001).

About two years ago, I was selected to command the Sixth Brigade of the 95th Division, which means I supervise nearly 200 military instructors. At the same time, my family and I are working a small farm, with sheep, guinea hens, a llama, chickens, ducks, cats, dogs, and goats. Many days it seems there just aren't enough hours in the day. But, it's basically my own fault, so I shouldn't complain! More seriously, I must admit that many of the most important things I have learned about marriage and parenting have come more from experience than from books. In the end, I have probably focused more on military family research than I might have expected and somewhat less on general family research or on the religious aspects of family life (Schumm & Rotz, 2001) than I might have intended.

Research Themes

My most consistent lines of research have been with respect to premarital counseling (Schumm, Silliman, & Bell, 2000; Schumm, Resnick, Silliman, & Bell, 1998) and with respect to methodology (Schumm, Southerly, & Figley, 1980; Schumm, 1982; Schumm, Barnes, Bollman, Jurich, & Milliken, 1985; Acock & Schumm, 1993; Schumm, 1990, 1993). Somewhat in the middle I have done work on marital satisfaction, in terms of measurement (Schumm, Paff-Bergen, Hatch, Obiorah, Copeland, Meens, & Bugaighis, 1986; Schumm & Hemesath, 1999), family life cycle factors (Schumm & Bugaighis, 1986), mate selection (Grover, Russell, Schumm, & Paff-Bergen, 1985), and gender effects (Schumm, Jurich, Bollman, & Bugaighis, 1985; Schumm, Webb, Farrel, & Bollman, 1998), even polygamy (Gwanfogbe, Schumm, Smith, & Furrow, 1997).

I have lately published more in the military family research area. Here, one of my recent articles is one in which we found a 21.5% divorce rate over two years after a six month overseas peacekeeping deployment (Schumm, Bell, & Gade, 2000). Some other areas include marital communication (Schumm, 1983; Schumm, Anderson, & Griffin, 1983; Schumm, Barnes, Bollman, Jurich, & Bugaighis, 1986), home schooling (Schumm, 1998), family violence (Schumm, Martin, Jurich, & Bollman, 1982; Martin, Schumm, Bugaighis, Jurich, & Bollman, 1987; Schumm & Bagarozzi, 1989), spanking (Larzelere, Klein, Schumm, & Alibrando, 1989), religiosity (Olson, Schumm, Bollman, & Jurich, 1985; Schumm, Hatch, Hevelone, & Schumm, 1989; Schumm, Jeong, & Silliman, 1990), and program evaluation (Eggeman, Smith-Eggeman, Moxley, & Schumm, 1986; James, Kennedy, & Schumm, 1986; Christian, Dwyer, Schumm, & Coulson, 1988; Moxley, Eggeman, & Schumm, 1986).

Some might expect me to mention my editorship of the *Sourcebook* (Boss, Doherty, LaRossa, Schumm, & Steinmetz, 1993) as a major source of accomplishment, but I credit it mostly to my fellow editors. Some may think I would be proud of my measurement research, for which I was awarded the Moran Award in 1990, but some things, like the Kansas Marital Satisfaction Scale, were created more by accident and with the brainstorms of colleagues than by some genius on my part. One of the small things of which I am most proud is a note in *Journal of Marriage and the Family* in which I predicted how an analysis would turn out if done differently (Schumm, 1984) and, fortunately, it did when the authors redid it.

In the near term, I plan to continue to assess the impact of Desert Storm and more recent deployments on service members and their families (Bell & Schumm, 2000; Schumm, Bell, & Gade, 2000; Schumm, Jurich, Stever, Sanders, Castelo, & Bollman, 1998). This research is a challenge because it confronts the traditional military assumptions that deployments affect neither family stability nor retention. Even today, I engaged in a discussion in which a general officer took the traditional position (no harm done) while a senior warrant officer argued the other side (spouses get fed up with soldiers being gone too much). Of course, some people believe that Desert Storm veterans aren't really sick, either.

As far as long-term goals, I would like to do more to develop models of family strengths (Schumm, 1985b) and satisfaction (Schumm, 1999), including the impact of positive and negative aspects of religiosity on family variables, particularly if it could be tied into John Gottman's extensive patterns of research findings (Eggeman, Moxley, & Schumm, 1985). I expect I will continue to try to publish on controversial issues from a conservative viewpoint (Schumm & Rekers, 1984; Schumm, 1985a, 1987, 2000). One such controversial idea is my new theory about Pearl Harbor, based on my statistical analysis of the events prior to December 7, 1941–as a way of showing my methodology students how simple statistics can change even the way history might be interpreted. That idea was developed after I had much success in class with showing students how a proper statistical analysis could have prevented the Challenger disaster, which killed seven astronauts in 1986.

I also plan to develop my typological view of religion, in which there are five "types" of moral operations. Types I (total evil) and V (total good) are benchmarks for Type II (love only yourself), Type III (love your friends, hate your enemies), and Type IV (love your friends and your enemies). The moral law, in this model, has much to do with the boundary between Types II and III, while much of what Jesus seemed to teach appears to be on the boundary between Types III and IV. Thus, his teachings surpassed but did not supercede the moral law, in this model. My LDS friends have commented that they see a reflection of Mormon afterlife theology in the three types, II, III, and IV. However, my view is that God's hope is for more people to pursue a Type IV lifestyle no matter what their stage in the life cycle. The catch is that such a lifestyle may not be sustainable without an experiential relationship with a God who loves you like crazy, which takes me back to remembering how Jesus lived and died (and lived!). At any rate, the model has made for good discussions as "prescientific theory" in my family theory class.

AUTHOR NOTE

Walter R. Schumm, PhD, is Professor of Family Studies, School of Family Studies and Human Services, Justin Hall 343K, Kansas State University, 1700 Anderson Avenue, Manhattan, KS 66506-1403.

REFERENCES

Acock, A. C., & Schumm, W. R. (1993). Analysis of covariance structures applied to family research and theory. In P. B. Boss, W. Doherty, R. LaRossa, W. R. Schumm, & S. K. Steinmetz (Eds.), *Sourcebook of family theories and methods: A contextual approach* (pp. 451-468). New York: Plenum.

Bell, D. B., & Schumm, W. R. (2000). Providing family support during military deployments. In J. A. Martin, L. N. Rosen, & L. R. Sparacino (Eds.), *The military family* (pp. 139-152) Westport, CT: Greenwood Publishing Company.

Boss, P. B., Doherty, W., LaRossa, R., Schumm, W. R., & Steinmetz, S. K. (Eds.). (1993). *Sourcebook of family theories and methods: A contextual approach.* New York: Plenum.

Christian, R., Dwyer, S., Schumm, W. R., & Coulson, L. A. (1988). Prevention of sexual abuse for preschoolers: Evaluation of a pilot program. *Psychological Reports*, *62*, 2, 387-396.

Eggeman, K. W., Smith-Eggeman, B., Moxley, V., & Schumm, W. R. (1986). A marriage enrichment program for newlywed couples. *Wellness Perspectives*, *3*, 2, 32-36.

Eggeman, K. W., Moxley, V., & Schumm, W. R. (1985). Assessing spouses' perceptions of Gottman's temporal form in marital conflict. *Psychological Reports*, *57*, 1, 171-181.

Grover, K. J., Russell, C. S., Schumm, W. R., & Paff-Bergen, L. A. (1985). Mate selection processes and marital satisfaction. *Family Relations*, *34*, 3, 383-386.

Gwanfogbe, P. N., Schumm, W. R., Smith, M., & Furrow, J. L. (1997). Polygyny and marital/life satisfaction: An exploratory study from rural Cameroon. *Journal of Comparative Family Studies*, *28*, 1, 55-71.

James, D., Kennedy, C. E., & Schumm, W. R. (1986). Changes in parental attitudes and practices following a religiously oriented parent education program. *Family Perspective*, *20*, 1, 45-59.

Larzelere, R. E., Klein, M., Schumm, W. R., & Alibrando, S. A. (1989). Relations of spanking and other parental characteristics to self-esteem and perceived fairness of parental discipline. *Psychological Reports*, *64*, 3 pt. 2, 1140-1142.

Martin, M. J., Schumm, W. R., Bugaighis, M. A., Jurich, A. P., & Bollman, S. R. (1987). Family violence and adolescents' perceptions of outcomes of family conflict. *Journal of Marriage and the Family*, *49*, 1, 165-171.

Moxley, V., Eggeman, K., & Schumm, W. R. (1986). An evaluation of the "Recovery of Hope" program. *Journal of Divorce*, *10*, 1-2, 241-261.

Olson, L., Schumm, W. R., Bollman, S. R., & Jurich, A. P. (1985). Anomia and religiosity in the Midwest. *Journal of Social Psychology, 125*, 1, 131-132.

Schumm, W.R. (1982). Integrating theory, measurement, and statistical analysis in family studies survey research. *Journal of Marriage and the Family, 44*, 4, 983-998

Schumm, W. R. (1983). Theory and measurement in marital communication training programs. *Family Relations, 32*, 1, 3-11.

Schumm, W. R. (1984). Comments on "Age at marriage, role enactment, role consensus, and marital satisfaction." *Journal of Marriage and the Family, 46*, 4, 985-986.

Schumm, W. R. (1985a). Marriage and parenthood are necessary for a happy life for both men and women. In H. Feldman & M. Feldman (Eds.), *Current controversies in marriage and family* (pp. 91-99). Beverly Hills, CA: Sage.

Schumm, W. R. (1985b). Beyond relationship characteristics of strong families: Constructing a model of family strengths. *Family Perspective, 19*, 1, 1-9.

Schumm, W. R. (1987). Feminism and family studies: Another viewpoint. *Journal of Family Issues, 8*, 2, 253-256.

Schumm, W. R. (1990). Evolution of the family field: Measurements principles and techniques. In J. Touliatos, B. F. Perlmutter, & M. A. Straus (Eds.), *Handbook of family measurement techniques* (pp. 23-26). Newbury Park, CA: Sage.

Schumm, W. R. (1993). On publishing family research using "sophisticated" quantitative methodologies. *Marriage & Family Review, 18*, 1-2, 171-175.

Schumm, W. R. (1995). Non-marital sexual behavior. In G. A. Rekers (Ed.), *Handbook of child and adolescent sexual problems* (pp. 381-423). Lexington, MA: Lexington Books.

Schumm, W. R. (1998). Trends in homeschooling in a Midwestern community. *Psychological Reports, 82*, 2, 364-366.

Schumm, W. R. (1999). Satisfaction. In D. Levinson, J. J. Ponzetti, Jr., & P. F. Jorgensen (Eds.), *Encyclopedia of human emotions* (Volume 2) (pp. 583-590). New York: MacMillan.

Schumm, W. R. (2000). Psychology of the scientist: LXXXIII–An assessment of Herek's critique of the Cameron group's survey studies. *Psychological Reports, 87*, 3 Pt. 2, 1123-1132.

Schumm, W. R., Anderson, S. A., & Griffin, C. L. (1983). The Marital Communication Inventory. In E. E. Filsinger (Ed.), *Sourcebook for marriage and family assessment* (pp. 191-208). Beverly Hills, CA: Sage.

Schumm, W. R., & Bagarozzi, D. A. (1989). The Conflict Tactics Scales. *American Journal of Family Therapy, 17*, 2, 165-168.

Schumm, W. R., Barnes, H. L., Bollman, S. R., Jurich, A. P., & Bugaighis, M. A. (1986). Self-disclosure and marital satisfaction revisited. *Family Relations, 35*, 2, 241-247.

Schumm, W. R., Barnes, H. L., Bollman, S. R., Jurich, A. P., & Milliken, G. A. (1985). Approaches to the statistical analysis of family data. *Home Economics Research Journal, 14*, 1, 112-122.

Schumm, W. R., Bell, D. B., & Gade, P. A. (2000). Effects of a military overseas peacekeeping deployment on marital quality, satisfaction, and stability. *Psychological Reports, 87*, 3 Pt 1, 815-821.

Schumm, W. R., & Bugaighis, M. A. (1986). Marital quality over the marital career: Alternative explanations. *Journal of Marriage and the Family*, *48*, 1, 165-168.
Schumm, W. R., & Denton, W. (1979). Trends in premarital counseling. *Journal of Marital and Family Therapy*, *5*, 4, 23-32.
Schumm, W. R., & Denton, W. (1980). Premarital counseling: Approaches, objectives, content, and evaluation–a bibliography. *Pastoral Psychology Journal*, *28*, 3, 181-187.
Schumm, W. R., Figley, C. R., & Fuhs, N. N. (1980). Similarity in self-esteem as a function of duration of marriage among student couples. *Psychological Reports*, *47*, 2, 365-366.
Schumm, W. R., Figley, C. R., & Fuhs, N. N. (1981). Predicting self-disclosure anxiety in the marital relationship. *Journal of Psychology*, *107*, 2, 273-279.
Schumm, W. R., Figley, C. R., & Jurich, A. P. (1979). The dimensionality of the Marital Communication Inventory: A preliminary factor analytic study. *Psychological Reports*, *45*, 1, 123-128.
Schumm, W. R., Hatch, R. C., Hevelone, J., & Schumm, K. R. (1989). Attrition and retention among Christian Church (Disciples of Christ) congregations in three metropolitan regions: A mail survey of 1,149 active and inactive members. In D. N. Williams (Ed.), *A case study of mainstream Protestantism: The Disciples' relation to American culture 1880-1989* (pp. 521-553). Grand Rapids, MI: Eerdmans.
Schumm, W. R., & Hemesath, K. K. (1999). Measurement in family studies. In M. Sussman, S. K. Steinmetz, & G. Peterson (Eds.), *Handbook of marriage and the family* (pp. 291-305). New York: Plenum.
Schumm, W. R., Jeong, G. J., & Silliman, B. (1990). Protestant fundamentalism and marital success revisited. *Psychological Reports*, *66*, 3 pt. 1, 905-906.
Schumm, W. R., Jurich, A. P., Bollman, S. R., & Bugaighis, M. A. (1985). His and her marriage revisited. *Journal of Family Issues*, *6*, 2, 221-227.
Schumm, W. R., Jurich, A. P., Stever, J. A., Sanders, D., Castelo, C., & Bollman, S. R. (1998). Attitudes of Reserve Component service members regarding the consequences of frequent overseas deployments. *Psychological Reports*, *83*, 3 pt 1, 983-989.
Schumm, W. R., Martin, M. J., Jurich, A. P., & Bollman, S. R. (1982). Classifying family violence. *Journal of Family Issues*, *3*, X, 319-340.
Schumm, W. R., Paff-Bergen, L. A., Hatch, R. C., Obiorah, F. C., Copeland, J. M., Meens, L. F., & Bugaighis, M. A. (1986). Concurrent and discriminant validity of the Kansas Marital Satisfaction Scale. *Journal of Marriage and the Family*, *48*, 2, 381-387.
Schumm, W. R., Polk, B. B., Bryan, J., Fornataro, F., & Curry, J. (1998). Treat prisoners humanely. *Military Review*, *78*, 1, 83-93.
Schumm, W. R., & Rekers, G. A. (1984). Sexual intercourse should not occur prior to marriage. In H. Feldman & A. Parrot (Eds.), *Current issues in human sexuality* (pp. 105-124). Beverly Hills, CA: Sage.
Schumm, W. R., Reppert, E. J., Jurich, A. P., Bollman, S. R., Castelo, C. S., Sanders, D., & Webb, F. J. (2001). Pyridostigmine bromide and the long-term subjective health status of a sample of female Reserve Component Gulf War veterans: A brief report. *Psychological Reports*, *88*, 1, 306-308.

Schumm, W. R., Resnick, G., Silliman, B., & Bell, D. B. (1998). Premarital counseling and marital satisfaction among civilian wives of military service members. *Journal of Sex and Marital Therapy*, *24*, 1, 23-30.
Schumm, W. R., & Rotz, P. L. (2001). A brief measure of intrinsic religiosity used with a sample of military veterans. *Psychological Reports*, *88*, X, 351-352.
Schumm, W. R., Silliman, B., & Bell, D. B. (2000). Perceived premarital counseling outcomes among recently married Army personnel. *Journal of Sex and Marital Therapy*, *26*, 2, 177-186.
Schumm, W. R., Southerly, W. T., & Figley, C. R. (1980). Stumbling block or stepping stone: Path analysis in family studies. *Journal of Marriage and the Family*, *42*, 2, 251-262.
Schumm, W. R., Webb, F. J., Farrel, J., & Bollman, S. R. (1998). Gender and marital satisfaction: Data from the National Survey of Families and Households. *Psychological Reports*, *83*, 1, 319-327.
Silliman, B, & Schumm, W. R. (1999). Improving practice in marriage preparation. *Journal of Sex and Marital Therapy*, *5*, 1, 23-43.
Silliman, B., & Schumm, W. R. (2000). Marriage preparation programs: A literature review. *The Family Journal*, *8*, 2, 133-142.

Trying to Make Sense of Self: A Work in Progress

Gary W. Peterson

KEYWORDS. Autobiography, parental behavior, parental influence, adolescent social competence, parent-child relationships, parent-adolescent relationships

INTRODUCTION

Looking back, it amazes me that I'm doing what I do today! I don't intend to sound overly self-satisfied–I'm not. Compared to what my life might have been like, however, things have gone pretty well! Whatever I ultimately do accomplish in life and career, however, I would still like to think that I remain a "work in progress," rather than simply contemplating my later years. Frankly, I have struggled a lot about whether to include my own autobiography in this collection of essays by some truly stellar scholars. Sue Steinmetz, a great friend, to whom I owe much for saving my career from post-midlife doldrums, has been relentlessly after me to do this. She once stated that my pathetic protests about writing this essay (e.g., claiming writer's block, among other silly excuses) were nothing but "bullshit" and that I should just "start writing." She was right–and because my roots are blue-collar, I found this direct approach very compelling–so I agreed to give it a shot and started constructing my tale as best I can!

Although I have (in streaks) enjoyed constructing theories about things "out there," actually constructing a theory about the "self" is hard to do and elicits conflicting emotions, difficult to describe. So, I will focus on those happenings that I believe may have influenced me to study families and to focus on parent-child relations. A couple of cautions first–I'm not really too sure why I became what I am, so some of this is, at best, a rough guess or seems like a series of haphazard events, rather than a result of careful planning. One thing I'm convinced about, however, is that who I am is, in part, a product of several people with whom I have been privileged to know and share everyday experiences. I hope I've done them justice in describing how much they have helped and influenced me.

FAMILY MEMBERS WHO MADE A DIFFERENCE

I know it may sound like pandering to my ancestors, but I may have chosen to study families because, although my own early family experience wasn't perfect, overall, it was very good. I was born in St. Cloud, Minnesota, the oldest child of Warren Omer Peterson and Netti Mae Peterson (Alexander). When I was six months old my parents loaded up our Model A Ford and moved from Minnesota and the Peterson (father's) side of the family to Grand Island, Nebraska, to live near the Alexander (mother's) side of the family. Later, in 1951, my twin brother and sister (Allen and Annette) were born to round out our family. The Petersons (paternal side) were second generation immigrants from Sweden, whereas my mother's side (the Alexanders) were a compelling mixture of Scotch-Irish, German, English, and "who knows what" (as Grandma Alexander used to say). Although I seem to have inherited some of the Petersons' temperamental qualities, my social self is much more a product of the Alexanders.

The Alexanders are a difficult group to describe, but I guess the best way would be tough, practical, down-to-earth, folks who commonly populated midwestern railroad and farm towns in the '30s, '40s and '50s. None of them, except strangely myself, ever pursued a university degree of any kind, but their lack of formal education was no real impairment that I could ever see. They were simply the best damn people that I have ever known–and I was so very privileged to have them (warts and all) start me off in life. What a great childhood they provided me, and if given enough space (and the acute eye of the fiction writer), I might take a crack at writing a novel about them!

None of them had much money, but it didn't seem to matter much. Two great things about the Alexanders were that many of them lived near me when I was young and, above all, they were inclined to be very loud and rowdy. My good fortune was to be raised within a large extended family, centered around my grandparents, Warren and Netti Alexander. Moreover, besides my grandparents, there were many aunts, uncles, and cousins in the Alexander clan, which meant that our family picnics and gatherings were often huge affairs (ranging from 200-300 people) and absolutely joyous occasions full of raucous laughter, chaotic banter, a profusion of dirty jokes, and impressive beer drinking.

The Alexanders had one claim to fame–Grover Cleveland Alexander (my grandfather's brother and my great uncle), a very famous major league baseball pitcher (played from 1911-1931) who was enshrined in Baseball's Hall of Fame and still holds the National League record for the most life-time wins by a pitcher (373, tied with Christy Matthewson). He (variously referred to as "Alex the Great," "Ole Pete," or "Uncle Dode"–his family nickname) won 30 games per season three times during his career, pitched 16 shutouts in one season, and almost single-handedly beat the powerful New York Yankees in the 1926 World Series (with Babe Ruth). A modestly successful actor, Ronald Reagan, portrayed him in a biographical Hollywood movie entitled *The Winning Team*, with his wife, Amy, being played by Doris Day! When I was a very young child, I vaguely remember "Uncle Dode" as a kindly old man, quietly sitting in the corner of my grandparents' house, fighting a losing battle against cancer, with diminished resources from too many nights on the town. He remains the focus of great family pride, though baseball aficionados are well aware of his well-publicized shortcomings, but he was an amazing athlete! The good parts of his legend have always been a great inspiration for me.

Some of my best childhood memories are those of going to Florence's Tavern (Saturday afternoons) with my grandfather, a railroad engineer for the Union Pacific R.R. for 50 years. For Grandpa, the tavern was his place to hang out with railroad buddies, play cards and shuffle board, generally whoop it up (without ever causing any harm), and buy me all the Nehi chocolate pop and corned beef sandwiches that I could possibly consume. To this day, whenever I think of happy places, I think of a warm Nebraska tavern on a frigid winter's day, the rowdy but lovable railroad guys, and Polka music pulsating from the jukebox in the background. Today, when I ever hear Polka music, I immediately conjure up my grandfather's beaming, alcohol-flushed face (he liked to hum the song "Irene Goodnight") and the smell of freshly drawn draft beer from the tap. Although not very "cultured," these outings were good old-fashioned excuses for male bonding–and wonderful times for me!

My grandmother, Netti Alexander (Boufinch), had one of the most gentle but powerful personalities I have ever known. She was the unquestioned center of the Alexander clan and received deference (without asking for it) from everyone in the family. Although my grandfather (a very fine man in his own right) thought he was "in charge," he was clueless of the fact that everyone viewed grandma as the cement holding the family together and the one who provided us with our collective meaning. She often let Grandpa believe he was in charge, but, in reality, she was the real source of most of "his" brilliant ideas. The ironic thing, however, was that grandma, who was such a powerful authority figure, accomplished all this while being very frail in a physical sense. She was victimized by a terrible form of rheumatoid arthritis and spent the last 20 years of her life in a wheelchair, being ravaged by this cruel disease. Despite her handicap and the constant pain, she rarely let her agony show through and get her down. She was the personification of determination, endurance, and courage–a real inspiration for others. I wish I could look her in the eyes today and tell her how much her memory has been an inspiration for me.

When you look back at your parents and firmly believe that they have done a great job, it's very difficult not to make saints of them. To me, however, it seems like pointless nitpicking to dwell on their human weaknesses and moments of failure–especially since the overall story is so good. My father, Warren Peterson, was born in Litchfield, Minnesota, in 1922, the youngest son of Frank and Minnie Peterson. Frank, his father (my grandfather), died of a sudden heart attack while driving my Dad (age 5) and his two brothers from town to a friend's farm. My grandmother, Minnie Peterson, was suddenly a widow and faced the challenge of raising 3 boys during the '20s and Depression years as a single mom. Both of my parents, in fact, were raised during hard times and acquired the attributes commonly associated with this experience–obsessions with getting and keeping a good job, an emphasis on saving money, a strong belief in hard work, and considerable preoccupation with how things might again become difficult in the future (saving for a rainy day–never be extravagant, etc.).

My father was unfortunate to graduate from high school as part of a generation of young men who confronted World War II. However, he didn't seem to see it that way because, as a wide-eyed, innocent 19-year-old in 1942, he enthusiastically enlisted in the Navy. He received training as a combat medical corpsman and (because the Marines did not have their own medical corps) was assigned to the 2nd Marine Division in the Pacific theatre of the war. Eventually, he participated in desperate amphibious assaults against heavily defended Japanese-held islands in the Pacific, first on Tarawa and then Saipan, where he received serious wounds. He has only begun to talk about these experiences in old age, perhaps to understand if there was any human meaning to the horror he experienced. As a child, I remember that he would occasionally awaken at night in complete terror, haunted by memories, and have to be consoled by my mother. These were deeply disturbing events for him, some in which he now has begun to take pride, but other aspects of which remain very troubling for him.

During my early years of childhood I remember my father working most of the time, either holding down two jobs (e.g., an appliance repairman for Sears & Roebuck and a night clerk in a liquor store) to make ends meet or repairing something around the house. We did not have much money, but I did not become aware of being deprived until I was a teenager. Some would probably characterize Dad as a classic "inexpressive male" because he had difficulty communicating affection. He loved to talk, laugh, and had many friends, but he had difficulty dealing with deeply personal issues. Despite this reticence, I never felt that he failed to communicate love. He did so by being absolutely reliable, honest to the point of obsession, fixing things for us, providing us with food and shelter, and by always being there for us when anything went wrong. Somehow he communicated through his actions that he would walk through fire for us if need be. You could see it in his eyes. I have never doubted his love, and with age, he has become better at communicating his feelings, though still somewhat awkwardly.

Dad is not someone who reads much, except perhaps newspapers. Highly educated people would probably describe him as inarticulate because, though he talks a lot, he often struggles to find elaborate words to describe what he means. Despite some shortcomings in verbal polish, however, he has a great gift for understanding mechanical things (something he did not pass along to me!!). He can fix just about anything he puts his mind to, a talent that never ceases to amaze me when I've watched him in action. He sees mechanical things abstractly in terms of multiple dimensions and begins at any point in a mechanical problem to solve it, whereas I struggle to think in two dimensions and must follow written directions step by step. He is also a perfectionist in solving mechanical problems and doing repair work. This genuine mechanical talent (and incredible hard work) allowed my father to overcome a lack of higher education and ascend the occupational ladder from that of an appliance repairmen, to working in one of the first nuclear power plants in the country (something that we are now somewhat ambivalent about), to being a supervisor of a large regional power station. He was a model of making the most of one's talent and of working very hard on our behalf.

Finding adequate words to describe one's mother is probably difficult for most, and my mom is certainly no exception. She was simply the person who influenced who I am more than anyone, and I have missed her so very much since her death in 1995. She was one of 8 children and had both natural intelligence and incredible common sense that showed through immediately in any conversation. She could be incredibly gentle, listen to you patiently about problems, provide innovative solutions, but there was a point when she would lose her patience and say "Oh cut the crap, Gary . . . it's time to get off your fanny and get to it!" In short, she had a variety of natural therapeutic skills ranging from those used by Carl Rogers to those of Albert Ellis that somehow seemed to work together (she knew nothing about these men). She taught me to combine the attributes of humility with the ability to "stick up for yourself and those who matter when you need to."

My mother was a gifted athlete and may have inherited some of her ability from "Uncle Dode," whom she worshiped and conveyed to me his legendary accomplishments. She was extremely thin, only slightly over 5 feet tall, and could run like the wind. She could pitch a baseball like a rocket with pinpoint control and taught me how to play this wondrous game. She was a baseball fanatic and I grew up immersed in deep emotions about this sport, probably best captured in Hollywood movies like *Field of Dreams* and *The Natural*. She was a "dyed in the wool" St. Louis Cardinal fan (my uncle had pitched for them), and though she expressed dislike for the New York Yankees, she had a deep and abiding respect for their great talents (especially Yogi Berra). To this day, I share all of these cherished beliefs with her–though sometimes I find it amusing that I have persisted with such things.

My mom also was very tough (probably a better word is "feisty") and she taught me how to a box. During several of my years in Grand Island, we lived in low-income housing (government surplus housing created for veterans' families after World War II) next to some pretty tough kids, so pugilistic skills occasionally came in pretty handy. She taught me never to be the aggressor, but to be capable of defending myself if need be. Her training worked and I eventually acquired a fairly notable reputation as someone not to mess with, so I was rarely challenged and seldom needed to use these skills (after a couple of impressive boundary-setting displays of my abilities).

Mom was an interesting combination of great adventurer and victim of certain phobias like fear of heights. She only liked mountains from a distance and was a devoted "flatlander" from Nebaska. Later in life, she would only grudgingly board an airplane to visit me, and sit there in white-knuckled terror during the flight. At the age of 19, she and her older sister Amy had moved to Seattle, Washington, where she worked in a wartime airplane factory riveting together airplane sections in a role many women performed, now immortalized as "Rosie the Riveter." Later she moved to Waukeegan, Illinois, where she met my father in a local night spot towards the end of the war. My father had been assigned there after recovering from his war injuries–and attracted my mom's attention at the local nightclub because he would frequently be asked to join the band on stage to sing "Fuzzy Wuzzy Was a Bear"! She never really explained to me why she found this to be so attractive.

My mother worked hard inside the home raising my brother, sister, and me until I was in junior high (8th grade) and we moved to Lincoln, Nebraska. A very unselfish person, she was satisfied with what she got in life and had a sense of contentment with things. Subsequently, she worked in my school's cafeteria and later as a secretary in a school supplies business in Lincoln. I remember the terrible year in her early 50s when she experienced the sudden onset of rheumatoid arthritis that ravaged her body, in even more devastating ways than it had for my grandmother. The first year of this affliction was psychologically catastrophic for her. By the second year, however, I witnessed a remarkable transition as she began to cope with this terrible affliction by demonstrating the same great courage that I had previously seen in my grandmother. Like her own amazing mother, she became the heart of our family, the one everyone listened to, and the cement that gave us our meaning. It makes me very happy today when I hear my daughters speak of my beloved mother (their Grandma) with the same reverence that I use to describe my own grandmother. She would be so very pleased by that.

CHILDHOOD AND ADOLESCENCE

My childhood was greatly shaped by the people I have just described. Early childhood was spent in the midst of the Alexanders, playing, being in school (which I almost always enjoyed), and listening to radio programs. Television didn't come to Grand Island until I was about 7 years old, so my early childhood memories are those of listening to radio programs. Later, during my elementary school years, I spent most of my time playing baseball, collecting baseball cards, tending to my paper route, and reading countless books. I'm not sure how I developed an interest in reading so much, though my aunt Amy (my mother's older sister) was an avid reader, and perhaps my close relationship with her influenced me to love reading. I particularly remember being enthralled by Laura Ingalls Wilder's books about her frontier childhood, Mark Twain's (Samuel Clemens') novels, and the historical fiction of Kenneth Roberts. Early in grade school, I also developed an intense interest in history, and especially in Abraham Lincoln and the American Civil War period–endeavors in which I continue to dabble to this day. I have never been content to limit my intellectual pursuits to a narrow area of academic specialization, without at least some reprieve. Given the expectations of academia today, this has not been a very adaptive quality for establishing a single-minded academic record on a highly focused theme. However, this is a price worth paying for the sake of pursuing broader intellectual interests and questions that I truly find interesting.

I was a very good student during my grade school years and won local writing contests for my grade. Essays I wrote on Abraham Lincoln and the Battle of Gettysburg were published in the local town paper. This was a great source of pride for me and, I believe, encouraged me to pursue scholarly endeavors in the future. My parents were approached by my second grade teacher and the school principal about the possibility of moving me up a grade, but Mom and Dad had the good sense (in my opinion) not to take them up on this. In terms of social and physical development, this decision not to move me up a grade was a wise one for me. I was a pretty capable athlete and really enjoyed participating in sports. Moving me up a grade might have made me less capable compared to more mature peers and could have diminished some of the positive times I had later in childhood and adolescence.

We moved to Lincoln, Nebraska, when I was in the 8th grade. Except for a transitional period of 2 or 3 months following our move, I remember my adolescence as a happy time. In fact, during my later academic career, this might explain why I have studied adolescent social competence, rather than following the huge mob of social scientists who have focused on the social and emotional problems of teenagers. Perhaps, because my own adolescence was so much fun, I long ago rejected the view that adolescence is inherently a period of storm and stress. Instead, I have always been an advocate of what has now become the mainstream view–that most young people make it through adolescence without experiencing deep-seated psychological disturbances. In fact, my own experience has led me to the conclusion that adulthood is substantially more crisis-prone than I ever recall about my teen years.

If I were asked to give a general characterization of my adolescence, I would have to say "watch the movie *American Graffitti,*" which absolutely fascinated me when I first saw it years after my own adolescence was only a memory. Cruising with Beach Boys songs on the radio, hanging out at the local drive-in, drinking booze underage, dating, mooning, greasers, jocks, and preppies all were part of my teen years. My grades declined from the 8th through the 10th grade, primarily because I was spending a lot of my time on sports, girls, and having fun. I was a bit of a jock, with varsity letters in football, gymnastics, and track. Individual athletic competition was enjoyable for me, particularly in sports like gymnastics, or track and field, but football, a team sport, was barely tolerable. I persisted with football (as a halfback) primarily because it provided peer status and the fact that weekly games weren't nearly as painful as the practices (I guess because my adrenaline was up and I didn't notice the pain so much). Football practice, however, was a truly miserable experience for me (I only weighed 145 lbs. in a sport composed of behemoths). And, to this day, I can only watch football in small doses.

Although I often lived for the moment during adolescence, there was always a practical, self-monitoring side to me that began to reassert itself, especially during the latter part of high school. This duality in my temperament, the risk-taker (adventurer) who likes change combined with the pragmatist who charts a judicious course, seems to be a continuing theme in my life. During high school, my academic interests gradually began to reassert themselves and to temper some of the fun subculture in which I had immersed myself. During my senior year, my grades had again improved and I was making the honor roll, though I never remember spending much time studying during junior or senior high.

An important influence on my reemerging academic success was a particular friendship that continues to this day. I had a great diversity of friends including jocks, preppies, greasers, and brains (the teenage slang of the day for these groups). Depending on the particular day, I would have a somewhat different subcultural identity shaped, in part, by the friends I was hanging out with at the moment. A relationship of particular importance for me was my friendship with John DeFrain, who probably would have classified himself as a member of the "brain" subgroup and is now a Professor of Family Studies at the University of Nebraska. It was my friendship with John that renewed my interest in scholarly activities and got me thinking about going to college. Although my parents instilled the work ethic, discussions with John stimulated interest in literature, philosophy, and social issues. John was extremely well-read and was constantly provoking me to think about novel and unconventional ideas. I owe him much for helping me to become excited again about ideas and for introducing me to many of the provocative ideas that were emerging in the 1960s. In exchange for intellectual stimulation, I once paid John back by rescuing him from an irate teenage thug who, at a local hangout, was intent on "ringing his bell." Later I watched with great amusement as John got "blitzed" for the first time on orange-flavored vodka (John hated the taste of alcohol). When I see him today at conferences, I truly enjoy reminding John of our youthful escapades. (He enjoys doing the same to me!) For a sense of life continuity, it's been great over the years to have a boyhood friend, working in the same profession, who is a constant reminder of how things were long before academe.

UNDERGRADUATE YEARS

Besides my friendship with John, another reason I attended the University of Nebraska in the fall of 1965 was the low cost involved, primarily because I lived in Lincoln where the university was located. My decision to attend a university after graduating from high school (spring 1965) was initially a somewhat tenuous commitment. I had a vague notion that I might want to be a teacher and, since I had always liked history, I chose this discipline as my academic major. Throughout my subsequent undergraduate and master's work, I continued to pursue an integrated program of history and education. I loved the history component of my program of study (especially 19th century American history), but just put up with uninspiring education courses to prepare for some kind of employment. Ironically, the worst examples of teaching were provided by faculty in the College of Education, where real course content seemed somewhere between elementary and nonexistent. The history courses, however, were truly inspiring and remain among the best examples of college teaching that I have experienced. During my undergraduate years, however, becoming a university professor did not yet seem very realistic (the prospect of completing 3 degrees seemed formidable), so I was vaguely oriented toward becoming some kind of high school teacher–though my career aspirations were quite hazy.

When I entered the university, I made a commitment to myself that I was going to get serious about my studies, and give this higher ed. thing a decent chance. Frankly, attending a university was very intimidating because I truly believed that many people who attended such hallowed places were far smarter than me. Nonetheless, I made a pledge to myself that, instead of just reading and studying what interested me (something I'd done since childhood), I was going to discipline myself and devote study time to what the instructors actually assigned (i.e., in junior and senior high school I had never done this very consistently). Consequently, my goal was to get Cs (and occasional Bs), the best that I thought was possible, given that many people who attended universities were so smart! Well, I really surprised the hell out of myself–instead of Cs, I got straight As in my coursework and, after my first semester, I received the first of a series of scholarships that covered all my tuition throughout my subsequent undergraduate and graduate work. The fall of 1965 (my first semester) was the last time that I hit-up my parents for college money. From then on, my tuition was covered by scholarships and, by working part-time, I paid for all my living expenses. Mom and Dad were really proud of my achievement, but also quite stunned by the suddenness of my success–and no one was more surprised than me!

During my undergraduate years, another transition was my inclination to pal around with very academically capable students, and live what I thought was the lifestyle of an intellectual. I dressed in nerdish clothes, grew long hair, and hung out with people who discussed historical ideas, literature, philosophy, politics, and the revolutionary ideas of the time. I know, Lincoln, Nebraska, seems like a strange place for a bohemian period; There were probably only about 35 or so bohemian intellectuals in the whole town, but somehow I found them all. I spent hours studying, often well beyond what was needed, and sometimes went to a local tavern called Casey's for long discussions with bookish friends. In the 1960s, there were so many interesting social and political developments providing fodder for our discourses. Occasionally, when I now think back to my "bohemian" undergraduate days, I sometimes become amused at all the hot air we expended, yet I also remember that we were really excited about knowledge. During our discussions, we'd bounce ideas off each other and have a lot of fun along the way. It was probably an unusual way to spend one's undergraduate years, but I thoroughly enjoyed it.

Certain aspects of my life seem contradictory, difficult to reconcile, and have to do with my previously mentioned dualism involving both a pragmatic and adventurous self. Somehow, I have often been able to reconcile what some people would define as contradictory aspects of my life. So, by the time my undergraduate years were waning, I was becoming increasingly concerned about the prospects of impending military service with the Vietnam War raging. My selective service number made prospects for getting drafted after graduation virtually a foregone conclusion. So, as my "bohemian period" faded somewhat, I cleaned myself up a bit and grudgingly signed-up for Army ROTC, a decision made with great moral reservation–my pragmatic side had kicked in again. Despite believing that the Vietnam War was terribly wrong, I was not inclined to live in Canada and alienate myself from my family members over this issue. My pragmatic side decided that it might be better to serve my impending time in the military as an officer rather than an enlisted man.

Once this difficult decision was made, I continued to work diligently to finish a bachelor's degree in 1970 and then a master's in 1971. I remember, with some amusement, the dumbfounded reactions of my parents and friends when I completed the bachelor's degree with highest distinction. Most of these responses were evoked by a picture and accompanying article about me that appeared in the local newspaper alongside a couple of truly legendary scholars from whom such things were expected. Because my scholarly renaissance had been largely unnoticed by those who had known me since high school, I was frequently asked if some mistake was made. I was never offended by these comments because I had, if you remember, originally hoped only to "get by" in college. All this extra stuff was just gravy. My parents were again very proud, but also completely stunned that a kid of theirs could do this well in college (a very foreign world for them)–and no one was more surprised about it than me!

TRANSITIONAL YEARS

My adult years immediately following master's degree work were spent first as an officer in the U.S. Army, followed by a brief stint as a junior high school teacher. In 1971, I was commissioned a 2nd Lieutenant and embarked on what I thought then was an awful experience working for two very long years. Initially, I received orders assigning me to Vietnam–which were subsequently cancelled with reassignment at Aberdeen Proving Ground, Maryland. I was assigned to supervise the post Officer's Club and related recreational facilities–something for which I had no training and about which I was completely clueless. Nonetheless, for two long years, I managed the post nightclubs, formal dining facilities, swimming pools, golf courses, and the post liquor stores. My duties ranged from dealing with generals and their wives, entertaining many domestic and foreign dignitaries, hiring chefs and bartenders, scheduling big name entertainment, to hiring go-go girls (not a very politically correct task by today's standards, though I found them far more pleasant to deal with than generals and their wives). Only much later have I realized that I was acquiring a great variety of organizational and personnel management skills that were helpful for my later duties as an administrator in academe. Academics, most of whom have never experienced the military, are surprised when I assert that very little difference exists between managing a bunch of university professors and managing personnel in the Army.

During my military experience, I also met and eventually married Sharon Meyers, who worked as a secretary at Aberdeen Proving Grounds. Just before getting out of the military, I applied for and received a teaching position at a junior high school in the Washington, D.C. area. I enjoyed this job much more than the military, and spent my time teaching social studies, English, physical science, and coaching gymnastics. More than anything, my time as a junior high teacher fueled my interest in adolescence and convinced me that families remained powerful influences on the lives of young people during these years. I began to talk to Sharon about the possibilities of doing something different.

GRADUATE SCHOOL

During all these years, I had maintained a long-distance friendship with John DeFrain, who was pursuing doctoral work at the University of Wisconsin-Madison in the Department of Child and Family Studies. I was completely undecided about my future, though during my military stint, I started to think about becoming a college professor (though exactly what kind was still a mystery). Teaching at junior high level was OK, but I was beginning to develop bigger plans, and John kept prodding me to apply for admission to doctoral studies at Wisconsin. I considered further graduate work in history, my first love, but job prospects were dismal at best and my practical side warned me that I should probably choose another field. I figured that I could continue reading history as a hobby, which I have done to this day.

My initial reservation about following John's advice was rather fundamental. My entire repository of knowledge about children and families was limited to what I had learned from once being a kid, from being raised by good parents, from growing up amidst the Alexanders, and from daily experiences with teenagers as a junior high teacher. Hardly a firm basis upon which to build an illustrious academic career, I felt the need to learn more about families and children so I selected (I think, based on John Defrain's advice) and read Bert Adam's brand new textbook *The Family* (1973), John Flavell's book *The Developmental Psychology of Jean Piaget* (1963), and Erik Erikson's book *Identity, Youth and Crisis* (1968). Well, I found this stuff to be pretty interesting and understandable, though perhaps a little less intriguing than history. Anyway, I applied to enter the doctoral program in Child and Family Studies (CFS) at Wisconsin, and despite having never graced a child and family studies classroom during my previous education, I was admitted and given a graduate assistantship. Sharon was very enthusiastic about living anywhere but Maryland, so we boxed up our stuff and drove a U-Haul to Madison.

My first and last year at Madison, Wisconsin was both an interesting and a peculiar introduction to the serious world of academia. I was a research assistant for a major longitudinal study on the development of Piagetian concepts headed by a brilliant, engaging developmental psychologist who unfortunately was also suffering from severe drinking problems. I spent my first year administering Piagetian tasks to youngsters and running statistical analyses for his project, the results of which I would carry dutifully to the local tavern so that he could peruse them over several beers. I remember sitting with him in the tavern trying to figure out the analyses with him (as he progressively became more plastered), while he would watch Mr. Rogers on the television above the bar and laugh hysterically. Apparently, for him, having several beers under his belt turned Fred Rogers into a remarkable stand-up comedian!

The rest of the CFS department was experiencing great political struggles to an extent that threatened the department's very existence. Moreover, though I was primarily interested in family studies, and especially parent-child relations; few if any opportunities existed in these areas, through either specific courses or faculty expertise. The discontent among many graduate students and my growing friendship with another student, Randy Day, eventually led me on what might seem a bizarre transition into the doctoral program at Brigham Young University. But why on earth would a secular guy who is politically liberal decide to pursue doctoral work at Brigham Young University, a bastion of religious faith and political conservatism? Frankly, some of this decision still puzzles me today, but perhaps one quote by the great worldly philosopher, Yogi Berra, best sums things up: "When you come to a fork in the road, take it!" Frankly, at this primordial time in my career development, I was pretty naïve about the politics of academia, the relative reputations of academic institutions, and where this might lead me. I had always thought about higher education primarily as a means to experience ideas and become an intellectual, but had remained pretty ignorant of the political/academic pecking order of things.

But actually, when I think about it, there were several sound reasons for my decision. First, the situation in CFS at Wisconsin was continuing its downhill trajectory. Second, my friendship with Randy (the only Mormon I knew personally) gave me some assurance that members of the Latter Day Saint (LDS) religion weren't some strange religious cult of which I should be wary. Third, I had met Reuben Hill, a legendary LDS scholar, when he came for a seminar in our department at Wisconsin. Reuben was to become for me the personification of what being a scholar was all about–the range of his intellect was truly amazing. Getting to know him early in my graduate education was very important in solidifying my professional identity and what it meant to be a family scholar. A fourth reason for considering BYU was the concerted effort by the BYU family studies and sociology faculties to recruit "non-LDS students," a somewhat offensive designation to which I eventually adjusted (the assumption here being that the "non" indicated that those who were not LDS *lacked* an important quality). Today, I would certainly not choose BYU (though I greatly value the training I received at the time) because the openness to student diversity that existed during my doctoral years has not continued, nor have any "non-LDS" faculty ever been hired there in family sociology, family science, or family therapy (i.e., at least of which I am aware).

Returning back to 1975, Randy also put me in contact with both Wesley Burr and a student then at Brigham Young, Geoffrey Leigh, who later became a major collaborator of mine on several projects. These conversations and helpful discussions with Bert Adams in the sociology department at Wisconsin were key elements in solidifying my decision to move to Provo, Utah. Consequently, my overall feelings about my decision to attend BYU remain reasonably positive to this day. It was excellent graduate training in the 1970s, surprisingly free of religious bias, and provided opportunities to work with excellent scholars who were shaping the fields of family studies and family sociology. Most notably among these were Wesley Burr, Darwin Thomas, Reuben Hill (who was at BYU as a Visiting Professor), and of particular importance for me, Boyd Rollins. It was a very exciting time to be in Provo, with Wes Burr providing leadership for the huge *Contemporary Theories About the Family* project (Vols. 1 and 2) (Burr, Hill, Nye, and Reiss, 1979) that greatly expanded our knowledge about families and child development. We were exposed to a constant stream of symposia involving nationally known scholars such as Carlfred Broderick, Ivan Nye,

Jetse Sprey, William J. Goode, Diana Baumrind, and Lawrence Kohlberg.

The other major reason why BYU was a good choice involved my position as Research Assistant to Boyd Rollins and Darwin Thomas for the NIMH funded research project entitled "Parental Influences on Child Compliance." This experience provided me with valuable introductions both to survey assessments of parents and adolescents (Peterson, Rollins, and Thomas, 1985) as well as the assessment of parent-adolescent relations through simulation game and behavioral observation strategies (Peterson, Rollins, Thomas, & Heaps, 1982). The primary objective was to examine how a variety of parental behaviors predicted the development of various adolescent outcomes such as conformity to parents, academic achievement, and self-concept development. An important outgrowth of working on the Rollins and Thomas project was how it got me interested in a research topic that continues in modified form to the present day. Another outcome was the theoretical model I developed for my dissertation and tested with data from this project.

My dissertation topic was deeply rooted in the social psychology of parent-adolescent relationships, an application of social power theory. The particular focus of my study sought to determine whether two forms of conformity to parents, external compliance versus internalized conformity to parents' expectations, were fostered by different parental behaviors and dimensions of parental power. Results from my study indicated that, most notably, parental support and coercion distinguished between these two forms of adolescent conformity. External compliance by adolescents (i.e., complying with parents while under their direct surveillance) was fostered by contingencies of reinforcement provided by parental support and by parents who used coercive parental approaches. Internalized conformity to parents' expectations (i.e., complying when not observed based on personal commitment) was encouraged by parental reasoning (induction), was not responsive to supportiveness, and was diminished by coercive behavior used by parents (Peterson, 1978).

When I think back to those I learned from during my graduate school days, I remember Darwin Thomas, Wesley Burr, Reuben Hill and, most importantly, Boyd Rollins. Darwin encouraged my inclination to read outside the family and sociological literatures in philosophy, literature, philosophy of science, history, and theory. He exposed me to truly intellectual dimensions of family studies and family sociology and taught me to think in novel ways about issues. Wes provided me with the most useful intellectual skill of my graduate education–how to take abstract theoretical ideas and large unsynthesized bodies of knowledge and shape them into precise theoretical propositions about how things operate in families. Although middle range theory has unfortunately fallen out of fashion (often due to critiques by scholars who never developed anything better), it continues to provide me with the best thought process I have ever acquired for getting to the point (or essential meaning) in a large body of information. From Reuben Hill, during his brief stint at BYU, I got to observe a truly great mind at work during discussions in his office. I would go to see Reuben only occasionally, because each time I went with only a brief purpose in mind, the discussion would last two or three hours, which I then affectionately called "billowing cloud" sessions (i.e., ideas kind of billowed forth from Reuben, almost endlessly, one from the other). Reuben was absolutely full of ideas and loved lengthy discourse through which he would wander from idea to idea. I learned much from him–but If I had gone to him regularly, I would never have had enough time to complete my dissertation and probably would yet be a student at BYU!! Reuben had the most impressive range of intellect that I have ever witnessed and it was fascinating to watch him analyze an issue. I wish that we had more true scholars like him today and I feel very privileged to have known him as well as I did.

The person I owe the most for helping me during my BYU days was Boyd Rollins, the Chair of my dissertation committee. Boyd taught me methodology, how to cope with mainframe computers requiring punch cards, and to appreciate the value of multivariate statistics. Although he provided guidance, he treated me as an equal, and allowed me tremendous freedom to initiate papers from the project data. He also became a close friend and I have great memories of climbing Mount Timpanogas (just east of Provo) and helping to assemble a stable for his horses with him. Boyd was a very good mentor, a man of great wisdom, and a person of noble humility whom I respect immensely.

None of these wise mentors did any of my work for me, but simply created great opportunities that, fortunately, I had the foresight to pursue and use somewhat. I went to NCFR in late October 1978 and in the hallway literally ran into Barbara Armstrong, then the Chair of the Department of Human Ecology at the University of Akron. After almost knocking her flat, I chatted with her for a while and it came up during our brief conversation that she had an open faculty position that fit me perfectly. I was hungry to start my career and be on my own so I told her I was very interested, was subsequently invited to interview, and accepted the position. I made this decision against everyone's advice (Rollins, Thomas, and Burr), all of whom thought I should hold out for a better position. However, "when you get to a fork in the road, take it"–I again followed Yogi's advice. The only problem was while I now had a job, I had not even begun my dissertation. So with great resolve and the benefit of the Rollins and Thomas data set, I lived and worked like a medieval monk for three months, laboring to finish my dissertation (I remember being up at 12 o'clock New Year's Eve plugging away at my dissertation, watching Dick Clark on television greet the 1978 New Year). By March 1978 I was a new Assistant Professor at the University of Akron–my professional life had begun.

ROCKY TOP YEARS

I have been fortunate to be able to move to different positions during my career and work in varied settings. I only remained at the University of Akron for a year and a half, having been lured away to the Department of Child and Family Studies at The University of Tennessee, Knoxville (August 1979). During my time at Akron and the early years at Tennessee I continued to work long distance with Boyd Rollins and Darwin Thomas and began a long distance collaboration with Geoffrey Leigh who was then a faculty member at the University of Iowa. Early in my career, I established a lasting pattern of teaching undergraduate and graduate courses in parent-child relations, parent-adolescent relations, adolescence, and family theory. At Knoxville, I competed for and received a 12-month Agriculture Experiment Station appointment that included about $20,000 per year in research funding, including a Research Assistantship to offer a graduate student each year. I kept this appointment for the 8 years I was on the faculty at UTK and it was a wonderful means of starting my career. Probably the only downside to having this funding was the reduced incentive to seek other forms of external funding–but I certainly had enough resources to keep me busy and engaged.

During the Tennessee years, my family life also experienced dramatic changes. Sharon and I became the parents of two beautiful daughters, Erin (1982) and Aimee (1983). We privately arranged to adopt our first child, Erin, when she was 3 days old. What a sudden transition to parenthood it was to receive a phone call at the office and be told to drive immediately to the hospital in Sevierville, Tennessee, to pick up our daughter! I remember being both completely overwhelmed with joy and quite anxious about the new responsibilities of fatherhood. We had decided to adopt a child because, up to that point, medical reasons had prevented the biological birth of a child for us. Well, about 2-3 weeks after Erin arrived, Sharon totally stunned me with the announcement that she was pregnant. Eight months and 2 days after Erin was born, my second daughter, Aimee, came into the world. So, at 36 years old, I suddenly found myself not only teaching parent-child relations, but also living this reality every day as the father of two beautiful daughters–the most demanding but also the best thing we ever do in our lives! And there was still more to come!

I continued to publish from the BYU project (Peterson, Rollins, & Thomas, 1985; Peterson, Rollins, Thomas, & Heaps, 1982), but also gathered new data in suburban Knoxville high schools that both replicated and opened up new avenues of inquiry raised by the Rollins and Thomas project. Basically, the major focus of my research became how parental behaviors (or influence attempts) and perceived parental authority dimensions (or power) predicted such aspects of adolescent social competence as conformity to parents' expectations, autonomy from parents, and self-esteem (see Peterson & Rollins, 1987). This resulted in studies that I (and several collaborators) have continued to build upon and elaborate both empirically and theoretically to the present day. Generally, this work has indicated that such variables as support, reasoning, monitoring, and punitiveness, as well as expert, legitimate, coercive, and reward influence, either foster or hinder the development of social competence in adolescents (see Peterson & Hann, 1999; Peterson & Leigh, 1990).

This work also began to reveal that seemingly contradictory dimensions of social competence, such as adolescent autonomy and conformity in reference to parents, are not at odds with each other, but instead, are complementary qualities for the young (at least in moderation). Although specific parental attributes (e.g., coercive influence) did predict these outcomes differently (Henry, Peterson, & Wilson, 1989), many of these behaviors predict adolescent autonomy and conformity in a similar manner (Peterson, 1986a; Peterson, Bush & Supple, 1999; Peterson & Leigh, 1990; Peterson & Rollins, 1987), suggesting that competent parents seek to encourage a balance between these two important attributes in their young. Other closely related articles reversed the typical socialization model (i.e., parental influence models) and assumed a "child effects" perspective by examining how adolescent social competence and aspects of the parent-adolescent relationship affected the well-being of parents (i.e., parental satisfaction) (Henry & Peterson, 1995; Henry, Peterson, & Wilson, 1997).

A second focus of scholarship, the family circumstances and life attainment obstacles faced by low-income rural youth, related to the rural mission of my Agriculture Experiment Station appointment. I (and graduate student collaborators) helped to collect longitudinal data for a large regional project and used the data for several studies on the family circumstances of low-income, Appalachian youth from southern rural areas of the U.S. Several of our publications explored the implications of familism, Appalachian culture, low-income status, and class-based socialization values on the life-attainment and well-being of rural youth from these isolated mountain areas (Peters & Peterson, 1988a, 1988b; Peters, Wilson, & Peterson, 1986; Peterson & Peters, 1985; Peterson, Southworth, & Peters, 1983; Peterson & Stivers, 1986; Peterson, Stivers, & Peters, 1986; Wilson, Henry, & Peterson, 1997; Wilson & Peterson, 1988; Wilson & Peterson, 2000; Wilson, Peterson, & Wilson, 1993).

During my years at Tennessee, I also began to pursue a major interest in writing theoretically based review articles that sought to integrate large bodies of literature on a variety of parent-child/parent-adolescent relationship topics. I have agreed to do this fairly frequently because I am probably better at doing this than any other form of scholarship. Because I frequently get bored focusing exclusively on a narrow research topic (I also like to read outside our field a lot), I often look forward to doing review pieces, both for intellectual variety and to see if I can think about topics in new ways. My most demanding early attempt to integrate and interpret a large body of material was a collaborative chapter with Boyd Rollins that examined the huge literature on parent-child relationships (Peterson & Rollins, 1987) for the *Handbook of Marriage and the Family* (Sussman & Steinmetz, 1987). When I began writing this chapter, I had to come to grips with the harsh reality that I was eminently unqualified to do this!! I was a young Assistant Professor who had read little about parenting children younger than adolescents, with my primary expertise being the parent-adolescent literature relating specifically to my own research. Meanwhile, the literature on younger children, especially infancy and early childhood, was massive, even by the early to mid-1980s. I remember how disconcerting it was for me to suddenly realize how limited my knowledge was–especially after I had promised to produce a chapter of major consequence for a field I had only recently joined! Writing this chapter was initially a very humbling and anxious time for me, but it was also the period when I learned the most about my chosen area of expertise.

Other theoretical papers that I either wrote myself or in collaboration sought to apply family (mostly sociological) conceptual frameworks to aspects of the parent-adolescent relationship and the impact of divorce on children (Peterson, 1986b; Peterson, 1987a; Peterson & Cleminshaw, 1980; Peterson, Leigh, & Day, 1984; Peterson & Peters, 1983). Related activities involved a collaborative effort with Ron Cromwell (then a faculty member at Tennessee) on the application of systems concepts to conceptualize a methodology for assessing aspects of the family system (Cromwell & Peterson, 1982, 1983; Peterson & Cromwell, 1983). Another scholarly endeavor was that of being a guest editor for special issues of journals on "Theories of Adolescence" (Peterson, 1987b) and "Ethnic and Cultural Perspectives on the Family" (Peterson & Ellis, 1986a, 1986b). My collaboration with Geoffrey Leigh also resulted in our co-edited book *Adolescents in Families* (Leigh & Peterson, 1986), a collection of original articles used in courses on families and adolescents around the country. Chapter authors included such nationally prominent scholars as Patricia Bell-Scott, Greer Litton Fox, Hamilton McCubbin, Patrick McKenry, Raymond Montemayor, Ann Petersen, Thomas Ewin Smith, Darwin Thomas, and Hershel Thornburg.

I mostly remember my years at Tennessee in terms of the great personal relationships that helped me to get my career on track and survive "running the tenure gauntlet." My long-term professional collaboration and friendship with Geoffrey Leigh was extremely valuable and was a major influence on my career and personal life. I was also very fortunate to work with (mostly as a doctoral committee chair) a great bunch of graduate students who truly made possible whatever I accomplished during those early years. Several of these individuals are now life-long collaborators and friends (Carolyn Henry, David Peters, Mary Elizabeth Stivers, and Stephan Wilson). During my 8 years at Tennessee, I chaired 13 doctoral students to the completion of a dissertation and served on the committees of numerous other graduate students. When I have ever given serious thought to the real meaning of my career, working with these wonderful people has certainly been one of the best parts!

SUN DEVIL COUNTRY

Yogi started whispering in my ear again in 1987, so I said good-bye to Knoxville and moved to Tempe, Arizona, as Chair of the Department of Family Resources and Human Development (FRHD), a program in deep trouble at Arizona State University (ASU). FRHD had a very uneven history, and when I was hired as Chair (much to my surprise and probably many others'), productivity among the faculty was extremely low. Recent political wars among key department faculty members had greatly harmed faculty morale and endangered the department's continued existence. A further issue was the complicated nature of the department, with programs in child development and family studies, both of which I was familiar with, and those in which I had no background, such as home economics education, clothing and textiles, and foods and nutrition. I soon found myself having to learn about such things as scientific research laboratories for the biological sciences and to accommodate the expectations of faculty members whose scholarly endeavors were very different from social scientists'.

I was recruited for the position by ASU faculty members and eventually accepted the offer, partly because the financial incentives were good. Sharon and I also liked the idea of living in Arizona. Our decision was made against the advice of several colleagues, who suggested that becoming chair of this troubled department might be something akin to walking a greased tightrope with no net! This was further complicated by the fact that I knew very little about administering an academic department and no one in the department was likely to give me some initial pointers. Upon my arrival, I was confronted with a demoralized faculty and a brand new office staff, none of whom had previous experience in academe. Consequently, my initiation into Department Chair duties was one of learning by trial and error, or on bad days we began to use the term "foxhole management" to characterize it.

To top things off, three months after arriving in Arizona, my marriage broke up and I soon found myself in a little apartment with half-time joint custody of my 4- and 5-year-old daughters. This was initially the low point in my adult personal life and reinforced my view that adulthood is a far more turbulent time period than adolescence. Thanks to friends like Rick Fabes and Woodrow Monte (a member of our foods and nutrition faculty), plus personal determination of my own part, I got through this period and focused for awhile on just being a good half-time single parent and an effective administrator.

Somehow it worked. During the years that I was Chair, FRHD experienced a major renaissance and became one of the truly successful child and family programs in the country. Although FRHD was in bad shape when I began my stint as Chair, its major advantage was the nucleus of young talented faculty members in the department who were just launching their careers and had great potential to improve the department (e.g., Scott Christopher, Richard Fabes, Mark Roosa). The other advantage was a supportive Dean whom I repeatedly convinced to provide several new positions for recruiting additional faculty of considerable talent (e.g., Carol Martin and Hector Balcazar). During these years, we greatly improved our graduate programs in both child/family development as well as in foods and nutrition. Key developments in the department's progress were the establishment of a Marriage and Family Therapy graduate program and a PhD program in Family Science. The publication rates of department faculty members soared and great progress occurred in the acquisition of external funding.

I learned to be an effective administrator in FRHD and gradually came to the opinion that building a department with talented faculty and innovative programs can be as rewarding as maintaining a productive line of scholarship–though I have tried to do both in my career. I maintain this view about chairing departments, despite the widespread belief that managing a group of academics is often analogous to "herding cats"!

Over the 11 years I have been a Chair, I have also become increasingly theoretical about leading departments and have conceptualized this challenge in terms of several principles of departmental administration that I try to follow: (1) Respect faculty governance–or the best way to make long-term progress is to gain the support of your faculty, through democratic processes, for a particular departmental vision; (2) Listen carefully to faculty opinions about preferred departmental directions and structure a precise strategy about how to effectively articulate that collective vision; (3) Don't be an autocrat, but know when it is crucial to exercise strong leadership to make departmental decisions that are absolutely necessary (and where indecisiveness will be costly); (4) Lead a department to focus increasingly on its strengths rather than scattering resources and talent over too many areas; (5) Understand that the best strategy for leadership is to be a good opinion leader (i.e., gain faculty support because your ideas are sound); (6) Realize that a Chair's primary job is to foster the careers of others rather than one's own self-interest; (7) Recognize that it takes a variety of talents (or diverse faculty roles) to make a great department (i.e., faculty members will differentially emphasize research, teaching, and service); (8) Identify how each faculty member can best make a contribution to the departmental vision and reward them as best you can for doing this; (9) Articulate the department's vision clearly in written documents (mission statements, strategic planning documents), marketing tools, and by being the department's primary representative; and (10) Implement this vision through appropriate curriculum changes and long-term plans for hiring faculty. I have tried to follow these principles as Chair of three different departments–and, as I write this essay, I will soon be returning to The University of Tennessee as Head of the Department of Child and Family Studies, my fourth department in this capacity. After leaving FRHD, I have chaired in succession the Sociology Department at ASU and the Department of Human Development at Washington State University. Major achievements for both departments included successful strategic planning in which focus areas and clear visions of departmental directions were articulated.

During my later years at ASU and my time at WSU, my research and scholarship has continued on several fronts. Besides the continuation of work on parental influences on adolescent social competence, I also collaborated with Hector Balcazar on interdisciplinary research that crossed the boundaries of several fields such as public health, family studies and family sociology. Specifically, our papers examined how immigrant status, the acculturation process, and Hispanic family values were influential in predicting health outcomes and risk-taking behavior among Mexican and Mexican-American youth (Balcazar, Krull, & Peterson, in press; Balcazar, Peterson, & Krull, 1997; Balcazar, Peterson, & Cobas, 1996; Peterson, Cobas, Balcazar; & Amling, 1999; Peterson, Balcazar, & Castro, 1995). This work also encouraged me to attend and present papers at international meetings in Mexico City, Puebla, Mexico, and London, England, the result of which caused me to be increasingly interested in comparative work across cultures.

This growing interest in cross-cultural research has also led me to apply this focus to earlier work I had pursued on the influence of parental behavior and parental authority on aspects of adolescent social competence. Consequently, I am currently providing leadership for a group of scholars including Kevin Bush, Jose Cobas, Andrew Supple, and Stephan Wilson to gather data using the parent-adolescent questionnaire I developed at The University of Tennessee based on the work of Rollins and Thomas. As of today, we have gathered data from publicly funded schools (adolescent respondents) located in large urban areas of Chile, China, India, Kenya, Mexico, Russia, and the U.S. We have only begun to analyze some of this data and have several papers in progress (Bush, Peterson, Cobas, & Supple, in press; Peterson, Cobas, Bush, Czaplewski, under review). Increasingly, we are conceptualizing parent-adolescent relationships across these cultures in terms of two general cultural orientations, individualism and collectivism (Peterson, 1995a). Specifically, we are interested in how parents foster these general cultural values differentially across cultures in the form of autonomy and connectedness (i.e., the parent-adolescent relationship indicators of individualism and collectivism). Our research supports the view (i.e., a working hypothesis) that both autonomy and connectedness in reference to mothers and fathers are encouraged by parents of adolescents in most, if not all these cultures. However, the exact balance encouraged between these two values and the precise parenting mechanisms used to encourage autonomy and connectedness may vary across cultures (Bush, Peterson, Cobas, & Supple, in press; Peterson, Cobas, Bush, Czaplewski, under review; Peterson, Madden-Derdich, & Leonard, 2000; Peterson & Steinmetz, 1999). Moreover, it appears that autonomy and connectedness coexist, develop together, and are partially reconciled as connectedness with parents becomes the secure base from which competent youthful autonomy arises. The result is that variable amounts of autonomy and connectedness become components of the concept *interdependence*–or the idea that parent-child relationships involve the development of individuality as well as the continuation of relationship ties with parents (Peterson, 1995a).

I have also continued my interest in theoretical and integrative scholarship by collaborating with co-authors to write several major review chapters. Some of these writing efforts include surveys of the parent-child/adolescent research (Bodman & Peterson, 1995; Peterson, 1999b; Peterson & Bush, in press; Peterson & Rose, in press; Peterson, Madden-Derdich, & Leonard, 2000), a theoretical conceptualization of the existing literature on parental stress using family stress theory (Peterson & Mathieson, 2000), an analysis, across a variety of social science literatures, of the relationship issues autonomy and connectedness within families (Peterson, 1995a), an analysis of the limits of family systems theory (Peterson, 1990), an identification of common principles for prevention programs (Peterson, 1995b), and an examination of how gender plays a vital role in defining the nature of parent-child relations (Peterson, Bodman, Madden-Derdich, & Leonard, 2000). I also continued to collaborate with others on topics relating to parent-child relations (Day, Peterson & McCracken, 1999).

My most demanding writing project in recent times was again the update (with Della Hann) of the massive literature on parent-child relations for the revised version of the *Handbook of Marriage and the Family* (Sussman, Steinmetz, & Peterson, 1999). Much to my chagrin, I found that the literature had expanded almost exponentially since the 1987 *Handbook* (Sussman & Steinmetz, 1987) and I again faced the grim reality of doing an extended crash course to bring myself up to date in this immense literature. In the end, we kept much of the same conceptualization as the 1987 chapter, but massively updated the content of the literature review sections (Peterson & Hann, 1999).

One of these alternative lines of scholarship was that of editor for a variety of projects, one of which was a special issue of the journal *Sociological Inquiry* on parent-adolescent relationships (Peterson, 1999a). The most demanding editorial project, however, was that of co-editor for the revised *Handbook of Marriage and the Family* (Sussman, Steinmetz, & Peterson, 1999) at the request of Suzanne Steinmetz and Marvin Sussman. This was a great project and I am very thankful to Sue and Marvin for this opportunity. Coordinating such an undertaking, however, is an immense task, difficult to describe. Many times during the "progress" of this tome, I began to believe it would never end. In fact, I used to joke that "a likely definition of Hell" for me would be that "when I die, I would suddenly be revived only to find myself in Hell with the eternally assigned task of editing the same handbook for infinity!" The major plus of this project, however, was how it compelled me to reconnect with the larger domains of family research and the many talented scholars who were creating it. I felt like I was, once again, learning a huge range of material, much like I had once accomplished for doctoral comprehensives. A principle that became crystal clear to me during this process was that extensive handbook projects are held hostage largely by their slowest author. Much to my eventual surprise (and relief), however, the book was eventually published and forged perhaps the most productive academic relationship of my career–with Suzanne Steinmetz, my "e-mail collaborator" on both the *Handbook* and the journal *Marriage & Family Review*.

About the time that the *Handbook* project was winding up, Sue and I were asked by Marvin Sussman and The Haworth Press to become editors of *Marriage & Family Review*. This has been another rewarding experience, the key goals of which were to improve the quality of this journal and arrange for worthy thematic projects proposed by Guest Editors. An offshoot of our role as editors of *Marriage & Family Review* has been the enlargement of several thematic projects for the journal into recently published edited books on fatherhood (Peters, Peterson, Steinmetz, & Day, 2000; Peterson & Steinmetz, 2000) and new theoretical conceptions of the family (Settles, Steinmetz, Peterson, & Sussman, 1999). Sue and I have made plans for a large number of special issues (and books) on a variety of innovative themes that will be guest edited by some of today's foremost family scholars.

Overall, I would classify myself philosophically as somewhere between a positivist and social constructionist in the way I think about parent-child relations. This affirms the belief that scientific methodologies are capable of revealing useful family patterns, but that these patterns become known to us at least partially through meanings we have constructed in our everyday lives. Although the quality of parent-child research continues to improve, I am not sure that we are making as much progress as I once thought possible when my career began. Frankly, I don't think that I would advise parents much differently about effective ways to raise their children than I would have years ago during my graduate work. We seem to be using more sophisticated statistics, better methodologies, and researching new populations, but I wonder if we aren't too enamored with style rather than substance. I am somewhat reluctantly suspicious that the best insights into the lives of families have been achieved by perceptive novelists, insightful social commentators, and great theoreticians.

AND NOW FOR SOMETHING COMPLETELY DIFFERENT

During my ASU years, I married Polly Anderson, who got me into family life on an everyday basis, even more so than before. Polly is a talented social worker with extensive experience as a supervisor for Child Protective Services. She keeps me focused on things that are important in life and is a great source of daily strength for me. I owe her much for tempering the heady abstractions that I often spout with her reasoned pragmatism that is deeply rooted in her daily experiences with families. Together, we raised my two daughters, Erin and Aimee, as part of a joint custody arrangement with Sharon, my former spouse. It worked pretty well and today my daughters are either attending a university or headed there next year. They are well on their way to adulthood and they are the real legacy and meaning of my life thus far.

A few years after our marriage, Polly and I decided to have another child. So in 1996, when I was 49 years old, Luke was born, a beautiful little boy who ensures that I will not only be studying, but also living parent-child relationships for my remaining years. He is a constant source of joy for us and is busily disconfirming many expectations that we had about young children from our experience of raising two daughters. Though I remain devoted to the "nurture side" of the nature-nurture controversy, I am getting somewhat suspicious that boys may really be different in ways that many social scientists (including me) are reluctant to acknowledge. I have also become a grandfather with a beautiful granddaughter, Myka Mae, daughter of my oldest child Erin, who has become a wonderful young mother. In short, my family life is a great source of joy and contentment for me, a constantly evolving source of challenges and wonder. For me, being a parent does not end–it just changes and evolves into something completely different.

As I write this, Polly and I are packing our things to move to a new position at the University of Tennessee, this time not as an Assistant Professor, but as Head of the same department where I spent my early career. I loved living in Knoxville and being at UTK better than any career or living situation I have experienced since. I am happy, excited, and challenged by the new opportunities there. I really believe that Yogi is right about this one! "If the game ain't over, you can make it home again."

AUTHOR NOTE

Gary W. Peterson, PhD, is Professor and Head, Department of Child and Family Studies, the University of Tennessee, Knoxville, TN 37996-1900.

REFERENCES

Adams, B.N. (1973). *The American family: A sociological interpretation.* Chicago: Rand McNally.

Balcazar, H., Krull, J., & Peterson, G.W. (in press). Acculturation and family cohesiveness: Exploring their relationships to psychosocial and health-related risk behaviors among Mexican American pregnant women. *Behavioral Medicine.*

Balcazar, H., Peterson, G. W., & Cobas, J. (1996). Acculturation and health-related risk behaviors among Mexican American pregnant youth. *American Journal of Health Behavior, 20,* 6, 425-433.

Balcazar, H., Peterson, G.W., & Krull, J. (1997). Acculturation and family cohesiveness in Mexican American pregnant women: Social and health implications. *Family and Community Health Journal, 20,* 3, 16-31.

Bodman, D. & Peterson, G.W. (1995). The parent-child relationship from a family science perspective. In R.D. Day and W.R. Burr (Eds.) *Advanced Family Science* (pp. 205-225). New York: Brooks-Cole.

Burr, W.R., Hill, R., Nye, F.I., & Reiss, I. L. (Eds.) (1979). *Contemporary theories about the family vols 1 & 2.* New York: Free Press.

Bush, K.R., Peterson, G.W., Cobas, J. A., & Supple, A.J. (in press). Adolescents' perceptions of parental behaviors as predictors of adolescent self-esteem in Mainland China. *Sociological Inquiry.*

Cromwell, R. E. & Peterson, G. W. (1982). A framework for multisystem-multimethod assessment. In E. Filsinger and R. Lewis (Eds.) *Marital observation and behavioral assessment: Recent developments and techniques* (pp. 45-63). Beverly Hills, CA: Sage Publications.

Cromwell, R. E. & Peterson, G. W. (1983). Multisystem-multimethod family assessment in clinical contexts. *Family Process, 22*, 2, 147-177.

Day, R., Peterson, G., & McCracken, C. (1998). Predicting spanking of younger and older children. *Journal of Marriage and the Family, 60*, 1, 79-94.

Erikson, E.H. (1968). *Identity: Youth and crisis.* New York: Norton.

Flavell, J.H. (1963). *The developmental psychology of Jean Piaget.* New York: Van Nostrand.

Henry, C. & Peterson, G.W. (1995). Adolescent social competence, parental behavior and parental satisfaction. *American Journal of Orthopsychiatry. 65*, 2, 249-262.

Henry, C., Peterson, G. W., & Wilson, S. M. (1989). Parental power bases and processes as predictors of adolescent conformity. *Journal of Adolescent Research, 4*, 1, 15-32.

Henry, C., Peterson, G. W., & Wilson, S. W. (1997). Adolescent social competence and parental satisfaction. *Journal of Adolescent Research, 12*, 4, 389-409.

Leigh, G. K. & Peterson, G. W. (Eds.) (1986) *Adolescents in families.* Cincinnati, OH: Southwestern Publishing Co.

Peters, D. F. & Peterson, G. W. (1988a). The socialization values of low-income Appalachian mothers: Implications for mental health intervention. In S. E. Keefe (Ed.) *Appalachian mental health* (21-39). Lexington, KY: University of Kentucky Press.

Peters, D. F. & Peterson, G. W. (1988b). Mental health services and the persons who influence the career decisions of rural Appalachian youth. In S. E. Keefe (Eds.) *Appalachian mental health* (pp. 75-92). Lexington, KY: University of Kentucky Press.

Peters, D. F., Wilson, S. M., & Peterson, G. W. (1986). Adolescents and rural Appalachian families. In G. K. Leigh and G. W. Peterson (Eds.), *Adolescents in families* (pp. 456-471). Cincinnati, OH: Southwestern Publishing Co.

Peters, H. E., Peterson, G. W., Steinmetz, S. K., & Day, R. D. (Eds.) (2000). *Fatherhood: Research, interventions, and policies.* Binghamton, NY: The Haworth Press, Inc.

Peterson, G.W. (1978). The nature and antecedents of adolescent conformity. Doctoral Dissertation, Provo, Utah: Brigham Young University.

Peterson, G. W. (1986a). Parent-youth power dimensions and the behavioral autonomy of adolescents. *The Journal of Adolescent Research, 1*, 2, 231-249.

Peterson, G. W. (1986b). Family conceptual frameworks and adolescent development. In G. K. Leigh and G. W. Peterson (Eds.) *Adolescents in families* (pp. 12-35). Cincinnati, OH: Southwestern Publishing Co.

Peterson, G. W. (1987a). Role transitions and role identities during adolescence: A symbolic interactionist view. *The Journal of Adolescent Research, 2*, 3, 237-254.

Peterson, G. W. (1987b). Theories of adolescence. Guest editor, Special issue of the *Journal of Adolescent Research, 2*, 3.

Peterson, G. W. (1990). Recognizing the limits of systems concepts: Paradigm warfare versus integration. *Family Science Review, 3*, 1, 5-10.

Peterson, G. W. (1995a). Autonomy and connectedness in families. R. D. Day and W. R. Burr (Eds.) *Advanced family science* (pp. 20-41). New York: Brooks-Cole.

Peterson, G.W. (1995b). The need for common principles in prevention programs for children, adolescents, and families. *Journal of Adolescent Research. 10*, 4, 470-485.

Peterson, G. W. (1999a). The parent-adolescent relationship. Guest editor, Special issue of *Sociological Inquiry, 69*, 3.

Peterson, G. W. (1999b). The renewed importance of studying parent-adolescent relations. *Sociological Inquiry, 69*, 3, 426-430.

Peterson, G.W., Balcazar, H., & Castro, F. (1995). Hispanic-American adolescents at risk. In P.C. McKenry and S.M. Gavazzi (Eds.) *Visions 2010: Families and adolescents* (pp. 36-37). Minneapolis, MN: National Council on Family Relations.

Peterson, G. W., Bodman, D., Bush K., & Madden-Derdich, D. (2000). Gender and the parent-child relationship. In Demo, D., Allen K., & Fine, M. (Eds.) *Handbook of family diversity* (pp. 82-104). New York: Oxford University Press.

Peterson, G. W. & Bush K. R. (in press). Promoting healthy development with adolescents living in nuclear families. *Encyclopedia of primary prevention.* New York: Kluwer Academic/Plenum.

Peterson, G.W., Bush, K. & Supple, A. (1999). Predicting adolescent autonomy from parents: Relationship connectedness and restrictiveness. *Sociological Inquiry, 69*, 3, 431-457.

Peterson, G. W. & Cleminshaw, H. K. (1980). The strength of single-parent families during the divorce crisis: An integrative review with clinical applications. In N. Stinnett, B. Chesser, J. DeFrain, and P. Knaub (Eds.) *Family strengths: Positive models for family life* (pp. 431-443). Lincoln, NE: University of Nebraska Press.

Peterson, G. W., Cobas, J.A., Balcazar, H., & Amling, J.W. (1998). Acculturation and risk behavior among pregnant Mexican American females: A structural equation model. *Sociological Inquiry, 68*, 4, 536-556.

Peterson, G.W., Cobas, J.A., & Bush, K.A., & Czaplewski, A. (under review). Parent-youth relationships and the self-esteem of Chinese adolescents: Collectivism versus individualism. *Journal of Marriage and the Family.*

Peterson, G. W. & Cromwell, R. E. (1983). A clarification of multisystem-multimethod family assessment. *Family Process, 22*, 2, 173-177.

Peterson, G. W. & Ellis, G. E. (1986a). Ethnic and cultural perspectives on the family. Guest editor, Special issue of *Family Perspective, 20*, 4, 1-7.

Peterson, G. W. & Ellis, G. J. (1986b). Countering ethnic and cultural myopia in the study of families. *Family Perspective, 20*, 4, 307-322.

Peterson, G. W. & Hann, D. (1999). Socializing parents and children in families. In S. Steinmetz, M. Sussman & G. Peterson (Eds.), *Handbook of marriage and the family* (pp. 327-370). New York: Plenum Publishing Co.

Peterson, G. W. & Leigh, G. K. (1990). The family and social competence in adolescence. T. Gullota, G Adams & R. Montemayor (Eds.), *Advances in adolescent development, vol. 3* (pp. 97-138). Newbury Park, CA: Sage Publications.

Peterson, G. W., Leigh, G. K., & Day, R. D. (1984). Family stress theory and the impact of divorce on children. *Journal of Divorce, 7*, 3, 1-20.

Peterson, G. W., Madden-Derdich, D., & Leonard, S. (2000). Parent-child relationships: A life-course perspective. In S. J. Price, P.C. McKenry, & M.J. Murphy (Eds.) *Families across time* (pp. 187-203). Los Angeles, CA: Roxbury Publishing Co.

Peterson, G. W. & Mathieson, K. (2000). Understanding parental stress: A family perspective. In P.C. McKenry & S. J. Price (Eds.) *Families and change: Coping with stressful events* (revised edition) (pp. 71-93). Thousand Oaks, CA: Sage Publications.

Peterson, G. W. & Peters, D. F. (1983). Adolescents' social construction of reality: The impact of television and peers. *Youth and Society, 15*, 1, 67-85.

Peterson, G. W. & Peters, D. F. (1985). The socialization values of low-income Appalachian white and rural black mothers: A comparative study. *Journal of Comparative Family Studies, 16*, 1, 75-91.

Peterson, G. W. & Rollins, B. C. (1987). Parent-child socialization. In M. Sussman & S. K. Steinmetz (Eds.). *Handbook of marriage and the family* (pp. 471-538). New York: Plenum Press.

Peterson, G. W., Rollins, B. C., & Thomas, D. L. (1985). Parental influence and adolescent conformity: Compliance and internalization. *Youth and Society, 16*, 4, 397-420.

Peterson, G. W., Rollins, B. C., Thomas, D. L, & Heaps, K. (1982). Social placement of adolescents: Sex-role influences on family decisions regarding the careers of youth. *Journal of Marriage and the Family, 44*, 3, 647-658.

Peterson, G. W. & Rose, H. (in press). Promoting healthy development with children living in nuclear families. *Encyclopedia of primary prevention.* New York: Kluwer Academic/Plenum.

Peterson, G. W., Southworth, L. E., & Peters, D. F. (1983). Children's self-esteem and maternal behavior in three low-income samples. *Psychological Reports, 52*, 1, 79-86.

Peterson, G.W. & Steinmetz, S. K. (1999). Perspectives on families as we approach the twenty-first century–Challenges for future handbook authors. In M.B. Sussman, S.K. Steinmetz, & G.W. Peterson (Eds.), *Handbook of marriage and the family* (pp. 1-10). New York: Plenum.

Peterson, G. W. & Steinmetz, S. K. (2000). The diversity of fatherhood: Change, constancy, and contradiction. In H. E. Peters, G. W. Peterson, S. K. Steinmetz, & R. D. Day (Eds.), *Fatherhood research, interventions and policies* (pp. 315-322). New York: The Haworth Press, Inc.

Peterson, G. W. & Stivers, M. E. (1986). Adolescent autonomy and family connectedness in rural Appalachia. *Family Perspective, 20*, 4, 227-239.

Peterson, G. W., Stivers, M. E., & Peters, D. F. (1986). Family versus nonfamily significant others of low income youth: A longitudinal study with intervention implications. *Family Relations, 35*, 3, 417-424.

Settles, B., Steinmetz, S., Peterson, G.W., & Sussman, M.A. (Eds.). (1999). *Conceptualizing families: International perspectives*, Binghamton, NY: The Haworth Press, Inc.

Sussman, M., Steinmetz, S., & Peterson, G.W. (Eds.) (1999). *Handbook of marriage and the family* (revised edition). New York, NY: Plenum Publishing Co.

Sussman, M. & Steinmetz, S.K. (Eds.). (1987). *Handbook of marriage and the family* (pp. 471-538). New York: Plenum Press.

Wilson, S.W., Henry, S.W., & Peterson, G.W. (1997). Life satisfaction among low-income, rural youth from Appalachia. *Journal of Adolescence, 20*, 4, 443-459.

Wilson, S. M. & Peterson, G. W. (1988). Life satisfaction among young adults from rural families. *Family Relations*, *37*, 1, 84-91.

Wilson, S. & Peterson, G. W. (2000). Growing up in Appalachia: Ecological influences on adolescent development. In R. Montemayer, G.R. Adams, & T. Gulotta (Eds.) *Advances in adolescent development*: *Ethnicity and adolescence* (pp. 75-109). Thousand Oaks, CA: Sage Publications.

Wilson, S. M., Peterson, G. W., & Wilson, P. (1993). The process of educational and occupational attainment of adolescent females from low-income, rural families. *Journal of Marriage and the Family*, *55*, 1, 158-175.

PART V: INDEPENDENT SPIRITS

In Memoriam
Evelyn Millis Duvall
(1906-1998)

The flow of life blurs the shadow of death as we glimpse the sublime in many an early moment. Life is good and we feel blessed to be part of it.

Independent Spirits

Suzanne K. Steinmetz
Gary W. Peterson

This section is dedicated to Evelyn Duvall, a truly independent spirit, who had extensive impact on how we think about families. She is best known for her family development concept through such descriptions as that of the "family life cycle," which brought into our awareness such constructs as "launching stage" and "empty nest stage." Duvall's accomplishments range from developing a pure culture for mushroom growers to publishing over 20 books on most aspects of childhood, parenting, and marital interaction. Many of these books were published in other countries and went through multiple editions. In her essay, "Evelyn Duvall's Life," she notes that she began her first grade of formal schooling by walking three miles to a one-room schoolhouse; the following year she boarded in a nearby town during the week and walked four miles home for the weekend. Because she was quarantined with measles when she was scheduled to take the New York State Regents examination in Geometry, her teacher monitored the exam at her bedside–she received a grade of 99. Her life was characterized by beliefs in family and her abilities to identify important needs and to marshal resources (often by doing it herself) that respond to these issues.

In many ways, Duvall's life and career and those of the other authors in this final section of our autobiography project are similar to the essays in other sections. Many were first generation members of their families to attend college, while others were carrying on a rich tradition of following their parents, and in some instances, grandparents in obtaining a college education. Similar to essays in previous sections, the age, gender, and stages in one's career of the authors were quite diverse.

Despite these similarities with previous essays, however, the authors of these autobiographies are somewhat different. Many of these authors experienced their early childhood and adolescent years in rural settings. Not only did Duvall, Day, Lee, Miller, Settles, and Boss live in small, rural towns, they specifically noted the influence of these contexts on their subsequent lives and careers. Unlike earlier sections where most authors came from the east coast, the majority of these contributors are from the Midwest or west coast. Only Furstenberg can claim an east coast background, whereas McAdoo's childhood is rooted in the deep south and Midwest. The influence of rural life and the prominence of state universities with cooperative extension programs are aspects of the culture of the Midwest, inter-mountain west, and the northwest environments that may have played a role in these authors' decisions to study families. Three authors are members of the Church of Latter-Day Saints, with family being a critical component of their religious, social, and educational life. Only Furstenberg, with his east coast roots, describes his background as being imbued with social activism. The other authors write at length about their early desires to help people, often in a direct manner, and not, as Burr notes, indirectly by becoming a geologist who explores for oil. Ultimately, these authors did provide service to society, mostly in terms of teaching students and conducting research, which like the geological aspirations of Burr, are primarily indirect influences.

Yet, in many different ways, like Evelyn Duvall, these authors demonstrated independent spirits, or to apply an overly used phrase, they "pushed the envelope." Simply stated they did not settle for the roles that had been expected of them. As Miller states in his essay, "Among professional colleagues I'm viewed as a conservative, but among family, friends, and religious leaders, I'm suspiciously liberal." Although an undergraduate education might have been the most expected of most of these authors, they all went the extra mile and obtained a doctorate and pursued academic careers. Moreover, both in direct as well as indirect ways, they questioned and challenged stereotypes relating to sexism, ageism, and racism. Many completed their educations on "their" time, which was interspersed between missions, work, child-bearing, adoption, and parenthood. Others, specifically Settles and Furstenberg, completed their theses in a shorter time than their advisors anticipated in order to meet their own deadlines.

Randal Day notes that, like several authors in previous sections, he is a product of the baby boom era. In his essay "Migration into Middle Class: Social Capital at Work," Day notes that he began life in a lower-income family living in Dufur, Oregon, located in a small farming and cattle area in the rural northwest, that claimed a one-party phone line. Day suggests that there were four factors that influenced his development: (1) being an outsider with no contacts with universities, (2) knowing few peers with academic aspirations, (3) wanting to serve in the military as a pilot, and (4) being a member of the Mormon church. Membership in the Mormon Church, for example, made his family an outsider, but provided Day with individual relationships (social capital) that imbued him with aspirations for higher education. A later move to Pullman, Washington, associations with schoolmates that were university bound, and service on a Mormon mission to England provided the support from friends and family that changed his life. He describes the personal struggles he experienced making the transition from a marginal student to a solid academic. Day's path to becoming a family scholar illustrates the identity change required in moving from a nonacademic definition of self to the abstract world of academe.

In "How a Kid from the North Woods Got Lucky," Gary Lee notes that his story is one of serendipity, opportunism, and sheer dumb luck. His parents were faculty at a small northwestern Minnesota college, Moorhead State, who taught at both the college and the high school that the college sponsored on its campus. Upon learning that he could take classes at the campus high school that also counted for college credit, Lee became inspired to get things done through "double credit" in a very pragmatic way. He was halfway through his sophomore year of college by the time he graduated from high school. Lee, a free spirit, got bored with accounting, toyed briefly with becoming a lawyer, and rejected the overtures of Harvard because they wouldn't transfer credits he'd earned at Moorhead State! Later, he held a faculty position at St. Cloud State and became serious about studying families only when he stumbled accidentally into the country's most prestigious family sociology program at the University of Minnesota. His primary reason for choosing this program was, again, a pragmatic, goal-oriented one–he discovered, much to his surprise, that Minnesota would actually pay him (through a traineeship) to go to graduate school! He became aware of Minnesota's prestige and the advantage of studying families only after he had entered the program and looked around a bit. Lee's essay illustrates how his individuality and creativity became channeled by the array of high quality family scholarship that was then prevalent at the University of Minnesota.

Another Minnesota graduate, Brent Miller, entitles his autobiography, "Mountains, Mormonism, Marriage, and Family: Life and Career Reflections." In doing so, he underscores the importance of his religion, family life, and his desire to remain close to the mountains and open spaces that were formative elements of his youth. Raised in the mountains of Logan, Utah, he notes that the Rocky Mountains and his Mormon religion are major anchors for his life. Combined with this need for stability, however, Miller describes himself as a curious youth, always exploring and attempting to find new approaches to old problems such as "tying a chicken down inside a crate to get it to hatch another chicken's eggs." His Mormon mission turned his keen interest for investigating things into a desire to achieve greater scientific understanding of family life.

"The Way Things Were and Still Are," by Harriette P. McAdoo, explores the tremendous educational progress made by her ancestors that are only four generation removed from slavery. However, despite the fact that McAdoo's mother completed a master's degree and taught on the college level for three years, she was forced to do housework for whites in Ann Arbor, Michigan. Simply stated, no other jobs were available for African Americans and the contradictions of American society were very prevalent, even for highly educated Blacks. After marriage and parenthood, McAdoo and her husband, John McAdoo, decided to attend the University of Michigan during the 1960s. Her venture into the feminist movement at Michigan was short lived because white women were attempting "to reassure themselves that it was OK to go to work." Instead of being a novel issue for her, she came to the realization that Black women faced the challenge of working outside the home as an everyday necessity of life. As McAdoo states "I was already working, going to school, and still having time for my three children." Her essay illustrates how involvement in the politics of the family field can be a time-consuming and valuable experience. Her scholarly career also illustrates the importance of a long-term collaborative relationship with John, her husband and colleague.

In "Observing Families: Their Contexts and Consequences," Rand Conger suggests that important influences on his life were his mother's spirit, her value of education, and the importance she placed on showing children that they were loved. His father's search for knowledge, his work ethic, and his heavy workload in taking second jobs to support his family also influenced Conger. These early family influences provided him with the importance of the hard work and an interest in children and families that motivated him to pursue higher education and to rise to the middle class from a lower income status. Several high school teachers and notable university mentors inspired him to look beyond his own experiences and try new pathways. His initial career was marked by considerable creative potential, though somewhat unfocused by early administrative roles that he eventually decided not to pursue. Conger describes how individual initiative, repeated connections with the best scholars in the field, and important collaborative relationships transformed his research career into one he initially did not imagine would be possible.

"An Interest in Lost Persons," the title of Pauline Boss's essay, can be traced to her childhood interest in a favorite radio program called, "Mr. Keen, Tracer of Lost Persons." Her initial research was on MIAs, which led her to conceptualize the construct "boundary ambiguity." Boss was born into a Swiss immigrant family on a Wisconsin farm at the end of the Great Depression. She followed her older sister to a one-room schoolhouse and, although only four years of age, the teacher allowed her to stay. When her family later moved to a larger town, she became marginalized as a "farm girl," and thus spent her time studying. Married during the semester break of her sophomore year of college, she moved back to the rural village and became a married, commuter student. This again marginalized her and she faced losing a much-needed scholarship since married women were considered bad investments. Boss subsequently describes how her own tenacity and experiences within the university propelled her to expand her roles beyond housewife and mother to that of prominent family scholar.

"Threads in My Professional Career," by Wesley Burr, traces his interest in families to a desire, developed during childhood, to help others. However, from his perspective, the ambiguity complexity, and controversy in the study of law and his dislike for the sight of blood (i.e., a physician), left some type of work in the teaching profession as the only reasonable option. A scholarship to study in the new department, Human Development and Family Relationships, with an interventionist perspective, caused him to change his goal of teaching biology and to transfer from the Zoology Department. His graduate experience in the Sociology Department at the University of Minnesota again illustrates the considerable role that this program has played in developing original thought about families.

Furstenberg, in his autobiography "Life Course Reflections," notes that he came from a family committed to social activism (i.e., an activist physician father and an activist mother employed as social worker) that valued education highly and supported his decision to obtain a Ph.D. in Sociology. He notes that, during his undergraduate education, sociologists still wrote for the general public and this inspired his desire to do meaningful research that would help people. Perhaps one of his most famous studies, The Baltimore Study–a 30-year longitudinal investigation of adolescent pregnancy–resulted from his mother's request to prepare questions that were needed "on Monday" for an evaluation study. He notes that, being a good son, he wrote a set of questions with a disclaimer because he had not had the opportunity to investigate the program's goals and services. The rest, as you might say, is history, with the result being a project that has become a model of longitudinal research in the social sciences. Furstenberg's essay illustrates how frustrating the early career of a scholar can be as well as the rewards of reaching maturity in one's profession.

Barbara Settles, in her autobiography "Everyday Life in Family Scholarship and Family Life: Sketches and Interpretations," notes that her family has its roots in rural Appalachia. Perhaps unusual for such ancestry, the thirst for knowledge and success was evident in her forbears because each generation obtained increasingly higher levels of formal education. Her maternal grandmother was a midwife and was proud to note that all of her own children taught school. Since her public grade school was double grades through eighth grade, her father ran for school board to ensure there would be a junior high school and a new high school complex. Settles credits her fifth and sixth grade teacher, a history buff, for inspiring her and providing her an opportunity to tutor other students. Her career is illustrative of a scholar who has worked systematically to improve the position of women within her university and to approach the study of family both from the perspective of theorist and practitioner. Her career is also a model for those who wish to engage is successful collaborations with others and become involved extensively in organizations that foster the study and welfare of families.

These authors, like those in the previous sections, have contributed in many ways to family scholarship, but perhaps, even more importantly, to how families might be strengthened in the future.

Evelyn Duvall's Life

Evelyn Millis Duvall

KEYWORDS. Autobiography, family life development, marriage and family, research

EARLY LIFE AND EDUCATION

Evelyn learned early to stand on her own two feet. Just as she had started in first grade in Oswego, New York, her parents decided to go into farming. They bought an abandoned farm four miles from town, building a cottage on the shore of Lake Ontario, a mile from the highway. There they lived through the summer months, moving into town after the crops were in and returning in time for spring planting.

Evelyn walked three miles to the one-room rural school by a young woman engaged to marry a local man. The teacher dozed at her desk after late night dates, while those in the higher grades taught the younger students. Evelyn, born left-handed, was made to use her right hand by her conscientious classmates. She began to stutter, so her parents transferred her to school in town where she lived with nearby friends. She walked four miles home every Friday afternoon, returning to school on Monday morning. Her neighbors provided room and board but otherwise left Evelyn to her own devices–an early lesson in independence.

By the time she entered high school, her younger sister Esther and she lived spring and fall in the family home in town. Esther resisted Evelyn's guidance with "You can't tell me what to do; you're not my mother." These clashes left wounds in both sisters that took years to fully heal.

University Education

When Evelyn was scheduled to take the New York State Regents examination in Geometry, she was quarantined with measles. Her Geometry teacher personally monitored the exam at Evelyn's bedside and was rewarded with Evelyn's regents grade of 99. Grades were important. Ten state scholarships based on grades allotted to each country had been awarded, with Evelyn in eleventh place. Then a classmate with a special grant from Cornell released the tenth award to Evelyn. Her church gave Evelyn their four-year scholarship in recognition of her establishing and leading their junior church. Since Syracuse University had a policy of only one scholarship per entering student, Evelyn appealed to the Vice-Chancellor who permitted both scholarships and referred her to remunerative work to help with her other costs ordering supplies for Home Economics laboratories. When her work with a local doctor's family became too demanding, her dean got her a job waiting tables in a dormitory. Soon she was tutoring failing fellow students at university rates. Her financial situation now was secure, and she gave herself to her studies and graduated in three and one-half years Summa Cum Laude.

Research on Mushrooms

The summer between her Junior and Senior years she sold farm books in the Hudson River Valley. A thriving mushroom grower there was losing millions because of a fungal infection that ran through his crop. As she closed the deal on his farm books, she convinced him that his problem could be solved. He immediately set her up in a laboratory in the cellar of his home. She finished her degree at the university while he built a five-room fully equipped laboratory. She started her research there upon graduation in January 1927 and by November she had solved the problem by developing pure culture spawn free of the disease and finding a way to fumigate the houses and sterilize the compost on which the mushrooms grew.

Vera Charles of the United States Department of Agriculture invited Evelyn to join her staff in Washington to extend her methods to other fungal infections. But by then Sylvanus Duvall asked Evelyn to come as his bride to Nashville, Tennessee, where he had his first job on the faculty of Scarritt College.

Three options lay open for Evelyn: (1) to marry and go to Tennessee as Sylvanus' bride, (2) to take the position in Washington that USDA offered, or (3) to return to West Camp, New York, laboratory that awaited her direction in producing pure culture mushroom spawn on a commercial basis. She decided to see the mushroom project well underway and then to marry Sylvanus and go as his bride to Nashville. He, patient man that he was and is, agreed to wait as long as it took. They were married in December 1927 in her home church in Oswego and proceeded south after a brief honeymoon.

MARRIAGE, MOTHERHOOD, AND GRADUATE WORK

Evelyn was thrilled to find Vanderbilt University nearby and, with her husband's blessing, applied for admission as a medical student. But she had three strikes against her–she was a woman, she was married, and she had not taken the pre-med courses at Vanderbilt. There was no appeal, so she took graduate work in biology and received her Master's degree the same month her first child, Jean, was born in 1929.

The Great Depression meant the dismissal of recently hired faculty, so Sylvanus was out of work with a wife, a daughter, and a second child on the way. The little family did what many another did at that time–they went to their parents. Mother Duvall found it hard to crowd a grown son, his pregnant wife, and two-year-old daughter into her three-bedroom house already occupied by her sister Cora, her husband and herself, but all three generations made do.

That fall Sylvanus found a pastorate in rural Vermont and moved into the parsonage with Aunt Cora to keep house until Evelyn was able to join him. Her doctor forbade her to travel in order to avoid a threatened miscarriage. This meant that Evelyn and her firstborn, Jean, stayed on with the Duvalls until baby Joy arrived.

January 1932 found Evelyn with two young daughters joining Sylvanus in a draughty Vermont parsonage, where everyone was ill, and a practical nurse was in charge. By spring, all were well and the young family found its place in the little rural community. Evelyn started a youth fellowship, Sylvanus had a reading group underway, and their daughters enjoyed going with their parents on pastoral calls around the far-flung parish.

When the First Congregational Church of Marietta, Ohio, called Sylvanus as its pastor the following year, the little family left for this better position with mixed feelings. By fall 1934, the Duvalls were living in the university area of Chicago where Sylvanus was a professor at George Williams College.

Evelyn soon found work with the Chicago Association of Child Study and Parent Education leading groups of mothers throughout the area (Duvall, 1939). This meant traveling by streetcar from "back of the yards" where first generation immigrants lived to the North Shore where wealthy families maintained an upper class way of life.

It soon became clear that the parents in the inner city slums had quite different perceptions of their parental roles than did those of the affluent suburbs. Graduate courses toward her Ph.D. at the University of Chicago had taught Evelyn about differences between the social classes, so it was with a feeling of *AH-HA* that Evelyn recognized that the ways parents disciplined their children and the ways they viewed themselves were related to their social class position (Duvall, 1937, 1944).

Using two simple questions: "Who is a good mother?" and "Who is a good child?" enabled Evelyn to find the conceptions of parenthood held by mothers at various social class levels. Selecting from among parents' groups Evelyn was leading at the time, four at the lower class level, six at higher social class levels, and fifteen in between, Evelyn had twenty-five groups of parents further classified as black or white. At regular meetings of each of these mothers' groups, Evelyn asked each mother to jot down on one side of a blank 3 × 5 index card "five things a good mother does" and on the other side, "five things a good child does."

This yielded a stack of 433 cards (one from each parent) with ten items on each to be categorized. The only surface large enough for such a cumbersome process was the Duvall's dining room table; so the family ate in the kitchen during the weeks of classifying the verbatim responses.

Early in the process of sorting these parental responses, Evelyn recognized that members of the lower social class levels tended to see their roles as "make the child mind," while parents of high social class viewed their parental functions largely in terms of furthering the child's development. This developmentalism of higher status mothers in contrast to the more traditional stance of mothers at lower social class levels was consistent for both black and white parents.

Digests of her Ph.D. research *Conceptions of Parenthood* were published in the *American Journal of Sociology* (Duvall, 1946a), and in the *Human Development Bulletin* (Duvall, 1950a). This research inspired Elder's study "Traditional and Developmental Conceptions of Fatherhood" Iowa State University thesis 1947, and Robert Blood's dissertation at Merrill Palmer in 1952, and has been widely quoted over the years.

While teaching the family course in the Sociology Department of the University of Chicago, the first White House Conference on the Family in Washington, D.C., invited her participation and displayed materials prepared for it by her students in The Family (Duvall, 1949).

Meanwhile, Evelyn had been elected secretary of the newly established National Council on the Family Relations. Soon she became its first Executive Secretary with an office on the University of Chicago campus. From this home base, she set up state and regional councils across the country as she lectured and conducted workshops for professionals with central interests in family life "carrying the National Council on Family Relations with her in her briefcase," said her mentor, Professor Ernest W. Burgess of the University of Chicago.

The Duvalls lost a stillborn son in 1942 leaving Evelyn with a year's maternity leave to fill. About that time, the University of Chicago opened its interdivisional program in Human Development under Robert J. Havighurst. Its appeal for Evelyn lay in its covering the major fields of how humans are conceived, born, develop, and mature through the years with courses open to its students in departments of Anthropology, Biology, Psychology, and Sociology.

Evelyn was one of the first three graduate students in what was to be an exciting educational experience for which she is still grateful. Upon her graduation her 14-year-old daughter, Joy, congratulated her with the question, "Fine, that's done; now what will we do?" The meaning was clear–it was the whole Duvall family that had worked with Evelyn in earning the degree. Both daughters had enrolled in French courses while their mother struggled to pass the language examinations at the new higher level required. The girls told their mother it was to share the many French workbooks, dictionaries, and supplemental readers she found helpful. But they told their father they might help Evelyn get through if they worked with her. After three tries, she finally found her name on the list of those passed at the new higher required level. The Duvalls all celebrated when Evelyn cleared the last hurdle and got her Ph.D. in Human Development in June 1946.

ACADEMIC PUBLISHING

Meanwhile, Evelyn's writing skills had developed through the years of preparing materials for *The Christian Home* and *The National Parent-Teacher*. Her immediate motivation had been the modest remuneration. Five dollars meant meat on the table augmenting the macaroni and cheese and other frugal fare dictated by Sylvanus' modest teacher's salary. But the long-term rewards were becoming established as a published writer.

Along about then, the United States Armed Forces Institute asked Evelyn to help prepare materials for Marriage and the Family credit courses to be available for military personnel around the world awaiting active duty (Duvall, 1942, 1945a; 1945b). This led to D.C. Heath's request for "a civilian edition" of the course for college students. Professor Reuben Hill and Evelyn wrote the text published as *When You Marry* (Duvall & Hill 1945). It went through a number of editions under that title and finally as *Being Married* (Duvall & Hill, 1960; 1962; 1965; 1967).

Macmillan asked Evelyn to write a high school text for courses on the family at the secondary level, and her *Family Living* (Duvall, 1950b) was followed by a number of other editions including one in Japanese for that country's post-war effort to introduce democratic principles through their emphases in family life.

Over the years as she spoke to conferences, convocations, and a great many varied groups of young people, she had them write their questions on blank 3×5 index cards anonymously except for age and gender identification. Soon there were 25,000 questions that Evelyn analyzed by sex and age of the young person and categorized into the several areas of interest expressed.

Evelyn's response to these many questions was published as *Facts of Life and Love for Teenagers* (1950c; 1956) and later as the emphases in youth's questions shifted, *Love and the Facts of Life* (1963, 1965, 1967). There were paperback editions of these titles that sold in the millions. Association Press celebrated this their best seller by producing a gold embossed leather-bound special edition. Arco Publications, London, published a British edition of *Facts of Life for Teenagers* (1957) with further impressions in 1960, 1962, and 1969.

Sylvanus and Evelyn Duvall's *Sense and Nonsense About Sex*, clarifying myths and fictions about inter-relationships between the two sexes with facts emerging from the various fields of study, first appeared in 1962 in a series of paperbacks (Duvall & Duvall, 1962). Lutterworth Press, London, put out its first British Edition of *Sense and Nonsense About Sex* in 1967.

When her daughters married, Evelyn was impressed anew with the prevalence of the mother-in-law joke and wondered why it was considered funny. Deciding to try to find what was behind the stereotype, she conducted group interviews with mothers with whom she was meeting in her parents' classes. Spring Byington, playing the mother-in-law in

CBS *December Bride* network radio show, offered Evelyn their contestants' responses swelling the numbers to 5,020 individuals with mother-in-law experiences to share. It was an exciting chore to make sense of what all these persons were saying about their in-laws. In addition to a journal article (Duvall, 1954a), Association Press convinced Evelyn that her *In-Laws: Pro and Con* was worth the effort and presented the statistics and anecdotal materials well enough to see the book through several editions (Duvall, 1954b).

Among the reader responses, we cherish a handwritten note from Dr. Mirra Komarovsky of Columbia University, saying in part:

> *I am reading with great interest your book* In-Laws: Pro and Con. *You are to be congratulated for having tackled this neglected subject in such a stimulating way.*

Evelyn's daughter, Joy, found dating questions she heard from young people with whom she was meeting professionally paralleled those Evelyn had been getting for years: How do you get a date? What do you do with a date when you get it? How does one break off a dating relationship?, and so on and on. If there was that much interest, why not do a book on dating? *The Art of Dating* (Duvall, Johnson, & Duvall, 1958; 1967) by Evelyn and Sylvanus Duvall and their daughter Joy Duvall Johnson was the happy result.

Sylvanus and Evelyn enjoyed working as a team never more than when they led the North American Conference on Church and Family for the Councils of Churches of the United States and Canada on controversial issues where church and family meet: abortion, illegitimacy, infidelity, mixed marriage, and family planning (Duvall, 1961). As co-chairmen, the Duvalls chose eminent authorities in each area to share their expertise in conference presentations and in the conference workbook published as *Sex Ways, in Fact and Faith: Bases for Christian Family Policy* (Duvall & Duvall, 1961). This volume served the conference well and became a benchmark thereafter.

Family Development arose out of postwar disruption in the mid-1940s when Reuben Hill and Evelyn Duvall were appointed to prepare working papers for the First National Conference on the Family to be held in 1948. The co-chairmen enlisted twenty-three family specialists from many disciplines nationwide each to prepare a four-section report on what could be expected at each stage of the family life cycle: (1) developmental tasks of children, (2) developmental tasks of parents, (3) challenges, crises, and problems to be expected at each stage, and (4) implications for needed services. The combined report "Dynamics of Family Interaction" (Duvall & Hill, 1948), 199 pages of mimeographed materials were the working papers for the conference and the basic framework for the six editions of *Family Development* (Hill & Duvall, 1957, 1962, 1967, 1971, 1977; Duvall & Miller, 1985).

The thesis of *Family Development* is that families grow through predictable stages of development through the family life cycle: Beginning families (Married couple without children); Childbearing families (Oldest child birth-30 months); Families with preschool children (Oldest child 30 months-6 years); Families with school children (Oldest child 6-13 years); Families with teenagers (Oldest child 13-20 years); Families as launching centers (First child gone to last child leaving home); Families in the Middle years (Empty nest to retirement); Aging families (Retirement to death of both spouses) (see chart in Duvall, 1957: 13).

Many families do not pass neatly through the model eight-stage family life cycle. Girls have babies before they marry, many while still in their teens. There are single parents at all stages of the family life cycle. Thousands of couples live together before they are married or while still married to others. Marriages end in divorce sooner than in death, while remarriage brings his children, her children, and their children into the family system. Gay couples of either gender rear children. Abortion, adoption, abandoned, abused, and neglected children as well as runaway parents are headlined challenges for whom family theory and policies have no comfortable solution.

Nevertheless, *Family Development* has influenced family theorists, inspired creative family research, and brought about innovative family practice and teaching. It has helped such professionals as counselors, social workers, teachers, and therapists know what to look for within an individual's stage of personal and family development.

For instance, if you know three things about a person: (1) stage of his family life cycle, (2) ethnic, racial, and national background, and (3) socio-economic class level, before you meet face to face, you can have a general idea of where that individual is, what challenges he faces, what crises he may be coping with, and what may be helpful at this stage of his development.

The family development conceptual framework has provided a foundation for teaching, research, and counseling by combining the dynamic flow of the family life cycle with that of the developmental tasks of each family member and of the family as a whole at each stage of its development.

Why Wait Til Marriage (1965a) was written to young people who still have a choice to consider reasons for delaying full sexual expression until marriage: (1) avoiding sexually transmitted disease, (2) abstinence is the only completely sure contraceptive, (3) unwanted pregnancy can cut short plans for education and future choices for both the boy and the girl, (4) family, friends, and those who matter most usually expect young people to behave in sexually responsible ways, (5) overstepping the bounds of one's culture can pose real problems for both members of the pair, their families, and their future, (6) "being in love" is a poor guide for marriage readiness since most young people are in and out of love a number of times through their teens. Evelyn also wrote a number of articles discussing the dilemmas that families with teenagers face (Duvall, 1962; 1964a; 1964b; 1965b, 1969).

Evelyn tried not to be "preachy." She avoided the words "should" or "ought to." She was gratified by the Introduction to the Special Catholic Edition (1965) written by Father Francis L. Filas, S.J. Chairman of the Theology Department of Loyala University, in which he concludes:

> *The author does not base her conclusions on Catholic moral theology but rather on statistical, psychological, and sociological considerations. These conclusions are, however, quite in accord with sound Catholic moral teaching.*

A paperback edition of *Why Wait Til Marriage* came out in (Duvall, 1966s), a first British Edition appeared in 1969, and editions in other countries appeared in Dutch, French, German, Portuguese, and Swedish.

Face-to-face contact with thousands of teenagers over the years helped Evelyn understand the issues they face: dropping out of school or continuing on, cheating or trying to create a climate of honor, going steady or dating widely, marrying at the first opportunity or pursuing one's goals until really ready to settle down, using an automobile responsibly, dealing with smoking, drinking, and drugs in line with one's own long-term values.

Although *Today's Teenagers* (1966b) is about teenagers, it actually addresses the adults who live and work with them in home, school, and community. This book is a bridge between teenagers and their significant adults. As such it is widely read and may have filled some of the gaps between young people and the adults who care about them.

Faith in Families (1970) is Evelyn's attempt to restore faith in the family as the basic unit of society so essential for survival. Criticism of

American families is often unwarranted and tends to undermine confidence in what families are doing: bearing and rearing children, guiding adolescents, living with difference, learning to communicate fully, solving family problems, and becoming at home in the larger community.

January 1968 found Evelyn and Sylvanus Duvall in New Zealand with an assignment from its government to find out why divorce and venereal disease rates were so high there. They were taken to every city in both North and South islands where they met with parents, teachers, ministers, and young people each day and conducted town meetings every evening when the day's questions (especially from youth) were reviewed and discussed. It soon became clear that in this recreation-oriented culture where no community is more than sixty miles from a beach, young people generally were more interested in fun than in work or further education. Even though all college costs were government-funded, few teenagers were interested in further education. They tended to gather in their beach cabins for mutual enjoyment of one another with little adult supervision. It was not surprising that sexual activity began early and resulted in sexually transmitted disease, and hurried-up marriage so often ending in divorce. Sex education and family life education were but sporadic efforts eliciting little interest. There may have been changes in this scenario since 1968.

At the December 1971 White House Conference Evelyn presented the keynote address in the Family Life Section. Upon her return to Sarasota, she organized and led a Conference on Creative Retirement for which she enlisted Dr. Arthur Fleming, Chairman of the national conference and Special Consultant to the President on Aging as keynoter, and Dr. Lawrence Carlson, Associate Dean of the Institute of Lifetime Learning with headquarters in Washington, D.C., to climax the Sarasota conference with a challenge to form a local institute. This was immediately underway, and by early spring 1972, the Sarasota Institute of Lifetime Learning had programs going throughout the County.

As Program Director, Evelyn set up six-week seminars on such topics as Ecology, Money Management, Maintaining Vigor in the Later Years, Religious Movements in America, Gerontology for Professionals, and International Relations. Enrollees received "Certificates of Completion" dated and signed by the Dean of the Sarasota Institute of Lifetime Learning.

The Sarasota Institute of Lifetime Learning continues to be a vigorous community enterprise, enrolling more than 13,000 retirees in its programs during the current season.

Kenneth J. Waite, State Director of AARP for Southwest Florida, credits Evelyn when he said, "We wouldn't have a Sarasota Institute without Evelyn Duvall. It's amazing the number of outstanding people she knows well. The Sarasota Institute is uniquely successful because of the people involved in it." What was true in 1972 is equally true now as the Institute draws outstanding leaders from far and wide who volunteer their time and talents in return for hearty response from their audiences. As one popular professor put it, "The questions your retirees ask are more penetrating and challenging than I get from my brightest graduate students."

In May 1972, Evelyn was given a ten-pound block of cheese by a friend returning from a cruise, so she invited representatives of the field of aging in the area to a punch and cheese party at her home in Plymouth Harbor. As hostess, she guided the discussion that afternoon toward the possibility of a clearinghouse on aging in which common concerns might be considered, and the Sarasota Council on Aging was launched that afternoon. It was sufficiently funded to maintain an office in downtown Sarasota for several years. Unfortunately, political changes in personnel saw its termination.

POLITICAL INVOLVEMENT

Evelyn had her fingers in several political pies at that time. She has a Certificate of Appreciation from Reuben Askew, Governor of the state of Florida, for "Your help, support, and assistance in the 1974 Gubernatorial Campaign." Another cherished certificate of thanks is from Lawton Chiles for Evelyn's help in his 1976 Senatorial Campaign; he now is Governor of Florida. Cherished, too, is an engraved invitation to participate in the inauguration of Jimmy Carter as President of the United States on January 20, 1977, given in appreciation for her work in his support. In 1979, Ted Sperling ran for Sarasota's mayoralty with Evelyn as his campaign manager. He didn't win, but their work in his campaign cemented a cherished Sperling-Duvall family friendship. Then, in 1991, Evelyn was named one of the "thousand points of light" in President Bush's recognition of volunteers in American life.

NATIONAL AND INTERNATIONAL CONFERENCES

A report, *Emanating from the National and International Conference for Family Living*, prepared in 1948, covers content from the Conference on Housing for Family Living at Rye, New York, November 1946, for which Evelyn was one of seven committee chairmen. Use of the family life cycle was evident in the four stages around which the conference and this volume were organized: (1) Early years (1-3); (2) Crowded Years (2-15); (3) Peak Years (12-27); and (4) Later Years (25-40); dealing with the ways in which a family's housing needs change as it moves through the family life cycle.

Christian Family in Changing East Asia (1954c) reports on the Manila Conference (November 2-16, 1954) in which delegates from Korea, Japan, Okinawa, Formosa, Hong Kong, Burma, Thailand, Malaya, and the Philippines participated. David Mace, Evelyn and Sylvanus Duvall were the three Western leaders of the two-phase meetings: the first, a leaders' seminar for the 120 East Asia family life leaders, and the second, a general conference open to church leaders from across the Philippines. The Duvalls contributed nine chapters for this volume using content from their plenary session presentations at both the seminar and the general conference.

Foundations for Christian Family Policy (1961) covers what happened at the North American Conference on Church and Family, held April 30 through May 5, 1961, under the auspices of the Canadian Council of Churches and the National Churches of Christ in the USA. Evelyn and Sylvanus Duvall, co-chairmen of the conference, determined the issues (abortion, divorce, mixed marriage, etc.) and chose outstanding experts in each area to lecture and present their materials in the workbook *Sex Ways, in Fact and Faith* (1961). The Duvalls wrote the first and final sections of the proceedings.

The Church Looks at Family Life (1964) contains the content of the 1963 Family Life Conference in Nashville, Tennessee, in which Evelyn's four addresses appear as the first four chapters, David Mace's lectures as the second four chapters, and Paul Popenoe's the final four chapters. As a whole, it presented the factual bases of what was happening in American family life at the time and proposed approaches churches might make to strengthen families struggling with such questions as working mothers, mixed marriage, broken homes, family crises, etc.

International Conference on the Family (1966) reports that conference theme "Changing Family Patterns in Asia." Evelyn's plenary lecture at this conference in New Delhi, India, appears as Chapter 5 "Preparation of the New Generation for Responsible Living: Childhood, Adolescence, Adulthood." Evelyn spoke as President of the International Liaison Committee, National Council on Family Relations at the invitation of the Family Planning Association of India, the Association for Moral and Social Hygiene, and the Tata Institute of Social Sciences, all of India.

Scandinavian Seminars for teachers, social workers, and family leaders were led by Evelyn through Norway, Sweden, Denmark, and Finland. They met with the secretaries of Education, of Health, and of Welfare in each country and then toured sites of special interest throughout the summer of 1954. Evelyn and her sister, Esther Millis Coon, in 1978 retraced the earlier Scandinavian visit and added the Norwegian Mail Boat Vesteralen trip up the West Coast of Norway from Bergen to Kirkenes, cruising in and out of the fords delivering mail and passengers along the way.

In January 1979, Evelyn and her sister, Esther, flew to Mexico City where they stayed in the same hotel where the Duvalls had been before. Highlights of the trip were the National Folk Ballet in the Palace de Belles Artes and the Museo de Anthropologia in Chapultepec Park. They went on to Taxco and Acapulco where the Shah of Iran had just bought a huge estate built by a Hollywood personality. By the time he had refurbished it to his liking, he had invested some five million American dollars in it, a tidy sum even in those days.

PROFESSIONAL RECOGNITION

At various times over the years, Evelyn's biography has appeared in *American Men of Sciences*, *Dictionary of International Biography*, *The International Review of Sociology*, *National Registry of Prominent Americans*, *Who's Who*, *Who's Who of American Women*, *The Who's Who in the World*, *World Book Encyclopedia*, and *Writers' Directory*.

The George Arents Pioneer Award was presented to Evelyn by Syracuse University in 1952. The American Academy of General Practice honored her with their Certificate of Appreciation at the 1954 Scientific Assembly of Family Physicians in America. The Cooperative Extension Service gave her their National Citation in 1969. Hood College presented their honorary degree "Doctor of Humane Letters" to Evelyn in 1970. Reuben Askew appointed Evelyn to the Florida Division of Aging Council in 1973. She was named "A Valuable Human Resource of the United States of America" in 1973. The E. W. Burgess Award of the National Council on Family Relations came to Evelyn in 1981 in "recognition of continuous and meritorious contributions to theory and research in the family field."

A gracious letter from Major General Gerhardt W. Hyatt, Chief of Chaplains of the Department of the Army, thanked Evelyn for her leadership of the Command Chaplains Conference in Washington, D.C., July 24-27, 1972. The American Bicentennial Research Institute (1776-1976) put Evelyn's name in their Library of Human Resources. In 1981, Evelyn was given the key to the City of Sarasota in recognition of her community work.

The Psychiatric Out Patient Centers of the Americas (POCA) gave its 1987 "Award for Outstanding Contributions to Mental Health" to Evelyn in a plaque that reads, "Presented to Evelyn Millis Duvall, Ph.D., as college professor and author of thirty books, she has demonstrated a lifelong commitment to teaching, advocating and exemplifying healthy family and personal relationships."

The Evelyn Millis Duvall Endowed Chair in Family Development was established at the University of South Florida at Sarasota in 1986 with matching funds from the State of Florida providing one million dollars for ongoing research and teaching in family development, in perpetuity. Whereupon, USF President John Lott Brown presented her with a certificate of Life Membership in the President's Council "in recognition of outstanding leadership in providing support to higher education" on July 17, 1986.

The University of South Florida Student Ambassadors gave Evelyn a plaque, "In appreciation of your outstanding support and service to the University of South Florida at Sarasota, May 2, 1989."

The Sarasota Institute of Lifetime Learning founded by Evelyn in January 1972 began with discussion groups on a wide variety of topics across Sarasota County and since has grown to attract thousands who now fill two large movie theaters on topics that range from "The Best in Art" to "International Challenges." In recognition of her role in its birth and development, she has been given life membership and is listed as "Founder and Consultant" in each season's programs.

Twelve Ph.D. candidates in Family Development at the University of Minnesota brought Evelyn to their campus in June 1990 to discuss with them "Family Development: A Personal Perspective." While there, she addressed convocations of students and faculty on both the Minneapolis and the St. Paul campuses under the direction of Dr. David Olson who wrote in appreciation of her presentations,

> We have received rave reports of your presentations and I'm so pleased that we have copies of the video here to enjoy and share with others. It was wonderful to see you again and I am so pleased you agreed to visit us. Hope you enjoy the tape! Warmest regards, David.

Memberships in such professional associations as the American Association of Marriage and Family Therapists (Fellow), the American Sociological Association (Fellow), the International Union of Family Organizations (Member of the General Council), and the National Council on Family Relations (Founder and Life Member) continued on over the years.

FAMILY AND FRIENDS CHERISHED

Evelyn notes, "My greatest blessing has been my husband with whom I have lived throughout my entire adult life. We have seen our marriage flower and fruit and continue to grow through more than six decades of personal and marital development."

Good friends from childhood on through the years mean more and more as time passes and many dear ones are no longer among us. Each of these losses is mourned and adds a comfortable acceptance of death as an intrinsic part of life.

As older relatives leave and the generations overlap, there comes heightened enjoyment and appreciation of youngsters growing up in the family. Nieces and nephews, grandnieces and grandnephews, grandchildren and now great-grandchildren give promise of welcoming great, great, grandchildren before we, too, pass beyond life's curtain. The flow of life blurs the shadow of death as we glimpse the sublime in many an early moment. Life is good and we feel blessed to be part of it.

AUTHOR NOTE

Evelyn Duvall prepared a draft of her autobiography when invited by Marvin Sussman in the early 1990s. Unfortunately, she died before it could be revised. Her essay was written in the third person, and did not include references. Dr. Steinmetz gratefully acknowledges her husband, Tom Pickett, for considerable work locating references to include in this essay. Duvall's essay was left in the third person as she had written it.

Address correspondence to Evelyn Duvall's daughter: Joyce Duvall Johnson, 526 Saint Andrew Court, Lady Lake, FL 32159.

REFERENCES

Christian Family in Changing East Asia (1954c) report on the Manila Conference (November 2-16, 1954). E. M. & S. M. Duvall contributed 9 chapters to this report.

The Church Looks at Family Life (1964) contains the content of the 1963 Family Life Conference in Nashville, Tennessee.

Duvall, E. M. (1937). Child-parent social distance. *Sociology and Social-Research*, 21, 458-463.

Duvall, E. M. (1939). The Association for Family Living. *Marriage and Family Living*, *1*, 4, 75+.

Duvall, E. M. (1942). Marriage in war time. *Marriage and Family Living*, *4*, 4, 73-76.

Duvall, E. M. (1944). Growing edges in family life education. *Marriage and Family Living*, *6*, 2, 21-24.

Duvall, E. M. (1945a). Loneliness and the serviceman's wife. *Marriage and Family Living*, *7*, x, 77-81.

Duvall, E. M. (1945b). Soldier come home; a listing of current books, pamphlets, reprints and articles pertaining to readjustment of returning servicemen. *Marriage and Family Living*, *7*, 3, 61-63+72.

Duvall, E. M. (1946a). Different conceptions of parenthood. *American Journal of Sociology*, *52*, 193-203.

Duvall, E. M. (1946b). *Building your marriage*. New York, Public affairs committee.

Duvall, E. M. (1949). *Family life materials*. Syracuse, NY: Syracuse University Press.

Duvall, E. M. (January, 1950). *Human Development Bulletin* (pp.18-20).

Duvall, E. M. (1950). *Family Living* New York: MacMillan.

Duvall, E. M. (1953). *When you marry*. Boston: Heath.

Duvall, E. M. (1954a). In-laws in your life. *Pastoral Psychology*, *5*, 49,39-46.

Duvall, E. M. (1954b). *In-Laws: Pro and Con*; An original study of inter-personal relations. New York: Association Press.

Duvall, E. M. (1950c, 1956). *Facts of life and love for teenagers*. NY: Association Press.

Duvall, E. M. (1957; 1962; 1967; 1971). *Family development*. Chicago/Philadelphia: Lippincott.

Duvall, E. M. (1957, 1960, 1962, 1969). *Facts of Life for Teenagers*. London: Arco Publications, (British edition).

Duvall, E. M. (1963, 1965, 1967). *Love and the Facts of Life*. New York: Association Press.

Duvall, E. M. (1968). About sex and growing up. (Illustrated by Simon Frankel) New York: Association Press.

Duvall, E. M. (1961). International conference on the family. *Marriage and Family Living*, 23, 12-14.

Duvall, E. M. (1961). Foundations for North American Conference on Church and Family. *Marriage and Family Living*, 23, 270-272.
Duvall, E. M. (1962). Where do they get their ideas of love and marriage? PTA-Magazine, 56, 8,10-14.
Duvall, E. M. (1964a). Adolescent love as a reflection of teenagers' search for identity. *Journal of Marriage and the Family*, 26, 2, 226-229.
Duvall, E. M. (1964b). Identifying potential conflicts areas in high school dating. *Journal of Marriage and the Family*, 16, 1,103-106.
Duvall, E. M. (1965a). *Why Wait Til Marriage*. New York: Associated Press (Paper 1966a).
Duvall, E. M. (1965b). Family dilemmas with teen-agers. *Family Coordinator*, *14*, 2, 35-38.
Duvall, E. M. (1966b). *Today's Teenagers*. New York, Association Press.
Duvall, E. M. (1969). Teen Agers and the generation gap. *Family Coordinator*; *18*, 3, 284-286.
Duvall, E. M. (1970). *Faith in Families*. Chicago, Rand McNally.
Duvall, E. M. (1974). *Handbook for parents*. Nashville: Broadman Press.
Duvall, E. M. (1976). *Parent and teenager: living & loving*. Nashville : Broadman Press.
Duvall, E. M. (1977). *Marriage and family development*. Philadelphia: Lippincott.
Duvall, E. M. & S. M. (1946). *Leading parents groups*. New York: Abingdon-Cokesbury Press.
Duvall, E. M. & Duvall, S. M. (Eds.) (1961a). *Sex ways, in fact and faith: bases for Christian family policy*. New York: Association Press.
Duvall E. M. & Duvall, S. M. (Eds.) (1961b). *Foundations for Christian Family Policy*. Proceeding of the North American Conference on Church and Family, April 30-May 5, 1961. Sponsored by the Canadian Council of Churches and the National Churches of Christ in the USA.
Duvall, S. & Duvall, E. M. (1962). *Sense and Nonsense About Sex*. New York: Association Press.
Duvall, S. & Duvall, E. M. (1967). *Sense and Nonsense About Sex*. London: Lutterworth Press (British Edition).
Duvall, E. M. & Hill, R. (1945). *When you marry*. Boston, D. C. Heath and Company.
Duvall, E. M. & Hill, R. (1948). Report of the committee on the dynamics of family interaction. Washington, DC: Mimeographed.
Duvall, E. M. & Hill, R. (with chapters in collaboration with S. M. Duvall) (1953; 1960; 1962; 1965; 1967). *When you marry*. New York: Associated Press.
Duvall, E. M. & Johnson, J. Duvall (1958, 1967). *The Art of Dating*. New York: Association Press.
Duvall, E. M., Mace, D., & Popenoe, P. (1964). The church looks at family life. Nashville, TN: Broadman Press.
Duvall, E. M. & Miller, B. C. (1985). *Marriage and family development*. New York: Harper & Row.

Migration into Middle Class: Social Capital at Work

Randal D. Day

KEYWORDS. Autobiography, social capital, fatherhood, family science

EARLY YEARS

This article is a narrative about a boy from lower socio-economic class making the transition into "polite" middle society within the gates of the academy. As the featured character in this drama, I try to demonstrate how my life is an example of how social capital (e.g., family and community relations that benefit children's cognitive and social development (Amato, 1998; Coleman, 1988, 1990; Hagan, MacMillan, & Wheaton, 1996) operated in my life.

I was born in Vancouver, Washington and grew up in the Northwest in the middle of the last century. I am a "baby boomer" who was heavily influenced by Roy Rogers, Howdy Doody, Sky King, Twinkies, Duncan Yo-Yos, and Topp's baseball cards. I was sure I would meet Annette Funicello and she and I would be friends. I was crushed to find out, following the release of the movie *The Parent Trap*, that there was only one Hayley Mills which, I reasoned, seriously decreased my chances of meeting her (them).

Most of my pre-high school years were spent in and around a small farming/cattle community of The Dalles, Oregon, that is perched on the Columbia River. For many years we lived in a small town near there called Dufur. Dufur had a ten-party line telephone system with no dial phones . . . just the crank on the side of the box. The absence of a dial phone symbolizes the idea that I lived in the transitional time between rural isolated America and the technology age of the latter 20th century. Dufur was very rural and isolated, few people owned TVs, our phone number had no prefix, there were no zip codes, no computers, no foreign cars to speak of, no people of color (except our local Native American neighbors who were completely shunned by the our community), and a grade school with fewer than 60 children. Technology for me, until after high school, consisted of a small brown Toshiba transistor radio that (at night) would pick up a radio station in Portland that played rock and roll music and during school hours in October would broadcast the World Series that I would secretly listen to through the tiny ear piece.

Dufur's Impact

From a social capital point of view, spending my youth in Dufur had at least four effects on my later life as a university professor. Social capital can be found in the school systems in varying amounts and densities.

Insider vs. Outsider. The level of social capital in the Dufur elementary school was high if you were connected within the local wheat farmer community, low if you were an outsider and a "town kid."

After the sixth grade, I experienced an academic decline that culminated in last minute heroic measures to actually graduate from high school. I had two very poor teachers in my seventh and eighth grade years that nearly squashed any desire to participate in educational pursuits. Their attention was clearly directed at children to whose parents they were socially connected. A small disenfranchised sub-group of us who were unconnected and socially dislocated from mainstream social interaction were actively shunned and dismissed as irrelevant.

In addition, the actual quality of instruction was so poor that when we moved to a larger town during my high school years, I found myself seriously behind my peers in foundational instruction. In the early '60s there was a severe teacher shortage. The only 7th grade teacher the Dufur Elementary School could attract was a fellow who had just finished four years in the Navy and had three semesters of general undergraduate training. He was given an exemption and allowed to teach.

No Contact with Universities. Second, few people in Dufur, including none of my immediate family members (except one distant uncle) had ever seen a university up close. We were a "Rooseveltian" Democratic, blue collar, working class family still recovering from World War II and the Great Depression. My father worked in print shops and my mother was the office staff for the local Forest Service Station of the Mt. Hood National Forest. There was a general notion in our family that universities were good things; however, few had any idea what that actually meant. Again, through social connection, modeling, and leveraging of social capital, one finds a place in his/her social locations. By my estimation, I was tagged early as someone who had limited potential and on whom resources (e.g., time, special attention, and mentoring) should not be wasted.

Our family members voted for John Kennedy and were very awed by his majestic presence. We adopted the local twist on Kennedy's inaugural speech, "Ask not what Dufur can do for you, instead ask what you can do for Dufur."

In Dufur, few of the men (nor their children with whom I played) had educational aspirations. Some of the men in the Forest Service had been to a university, but most had not. Therefore, my personal expectations for job and career were limited. I spent most of my youth in a semi-illiterate daze: While I could read (barely), I only chose to do so if I found an interesting short action novel about World War II. I had no idea of what I wanted to do as an adult, except I was pretty sure I wanted to be like either Mickey Mantle, Johnny Unitas, or a fighter pilot on an aircraft carrier. The only consistent activities I participated in as a youth were going to church activities (at my parents' insistence), working on local farms, and playing sports (at which I was very average). When I did go to church activities willingly it was when they involved scouting, which was very closely tied to my military fantasies.

Serving in the Military. Third, most of the men I knew in Dufur and most of the men in my family had served in the military and there was an expectation that my four brothers and I would do something similar. Several of my friends and I would spend endless summer hours playing a very real form of war with BB guns in hand on "patrol" in "hostile enemy territory."

Joining the Mormon Church. While living in Dufur, my mother joined the Church of Jesus Christ of Latter-Day Saints (Mormon), which caused a major loyalty split among the other family members on both sides and led to several years of marital conflict. It also further alienated our family from friends and acquaintances in the Dufur social scene. However, in the long run, this proved to be the most important change our family made. It was through my experiences at church and social connections with those men and women that eventually led me toward upward social mobility and a chance at university life. My ability to tap into a different reserve of social and community capital dramatically changed.

As a younger teen, I loved to listen to Buddy Holly and other early rock-n-roll stars. Later, I became especially fond of The Beach Boys and the heavy rhythm-and-blues beat of The Animals and Kinks. These songs created a fantasy world for me and I dreamed of participating in the endless summer of fast cars and beach parties, but never really did. I did learn how to play the guitar and have played in bands of many types for more than 40 years. My country roots have recently led me back to playing bluegrass music which I find strangely comforting even though it can be corny and annoying to many listeners (I am thinking of family members who tease me constantly).

During my high school years, our family moved to Washington. The first two years of high school were completed in Ephrata, another small rural farming community. I was very involved in three activities: working in the hay fields in the summer, sports, and trying to keep from getting kicked out of school. I was a bit of a behavior problem child. I rarely did anything that was really bad, but was a class clown who cared little about the educational process.

Pullman, Washington. During my senior year of high school, our family moved to Pullman, Washington. Wow! What a contrast. My friends and peers in Ephrata had work aspirations that had virtually nothing to do with university; my new schoolmates were suddenly talking about going to Stanford and the University of Washington rather than joining the Navy or working for Boeing. By the end of my senior year in 1966, I started doubting my long-held desire to join the military. My friends at high school began to suggest that war was bad thing: a thought that had never really occurred to me. Again, through modeling and connection with those who had a different idea about life, my life's goals, dreams, aspirations, and directions were forever changed.

The effects of community connection have been dramatic in my life. Those connections substituted for important lessons my parents and family members could teach. Instead, key lessons about upward mobility came from a new school that was sitting a few blocks from a major university, and a three-month high-school relationship with my first girlfriend. I somehow connected with a young woman whose father was a dean at the university. In a very few months, she educated me about the value of education and our frequent walks on campus began to break the barriers as I learned what higher education could do for me.

Additionally, I had a respected teacher at Pullman High tell me that my thoughts and ideas were unique, interesting, and worthy of exploration. Although I was close to failing her class, she read some of my poetry and listened patiently to me in class as I provided rambling explanations of Dylan Thomas poems. Mrs. Hegland let me know that I had potential and that I should not waste it. I will be forever grateful.

That summer I worked for the U.S. Forest Service as a first-response attack firefighter in a national forest in Montana. One hot summer night on a steep unforgiving mountainside fighting a monstrous forest fire, I realized that there are many jobs in life that are very physically demanding. I began to wonder if I really wanted to spend my life in those types of jobs.

That fall I enrolled in a small college in Havre, Montana (Northern Montana College), and spent nine miserable months not playing sports (one of the reasons I had enrolled) and freezing to death. By spring quarter, my grades were so miserable they asked me not to return.

I was now in the adult world and had a problem. It was clear that I was not going to play sports for a living, nor was being a warrior for one's country as glamorous as I had originally envisioned. Most of my friends were safely tucked away in university life preparing to become attorneys, doctors, and captains of industry, whereas I could not even compete in the lowest form of university environment. In addition, the Pullman draft board began to remind me on a regular basis that I would soon reach the magical age of 19. My mother provided the solution.

Missionary Experience

She knew I was seriously thinking about joining the military rather than waiting to be drafted, and she was fundamentally opposed to the war in Vietnam, long before it was popular to be against it. She counseled instead that my personality and temperament were much more suited to helping people than shooting at them. She pushed hard for me become a Mormon missionary. After many long weeks of agonizing about that decision, I decided she was right. I also felt, for the first time, a strong spiritual confirmation of another potential my life could have.

Finances were always difficult for our family and I knew sending me to be a missionary would be a real sacrifice for them to support me for two years. It was a crossroads moment and my family and friends from church rallied around to encourage me to make this commitment. Once again, the investment from those around me made the difference.

From 1967 through 1969 I served as a full-time missionary for the LDS church in England. My time in Great Britain was a watershed experience. So much of who I am today can be traced back to the experiences of those 24 months. First, I actually read several books and learned how to study and retain information. I discovered that I could persist at difficult tasks, such as learning that I could teach and be successful at this. More importantly, I gained a broader eternal perspective of my worth as an individual and that my contribution to others could be significant. The connections made during my missionary experience were classic examples of how social capital works in one's life. Many of the young men I met came from families who had higher educational aspirations and experiences. The showed a different kind of life that was clearly within my grasp. They also frequently commented about my teaching style and my ability to think abstractly. These were messages that I had never heard before.

MARRIAGE AND COLLEGE

I came home from that experience with a new lifelong goal. I was determined to gain an education and focus my life on activities that make a difference in the lives of those with whom I come in contact. In the fall of 1969, I enrolled in Southwestern Oregon Community College in Coos Bay. I met my wife Larri-Lea and we committed early on to make our family and our service to God the focus of our lives.

Our first son was born in the fall of 1970. To pay for school, I worked full time at a local sawmill on the afternoon and midnight shifts. Going to school full time and working full time were very difficult but provided movement toward my goal of securing a fulfilling job.

As a result of contacts made during my missionary experience, we moved to Provo, Utah, in January of 1971. Once there I began attending Brigham Young University. I originally wanted to become a high school English teacher with an emphasis in drama. I had been in several plays and loved the theatre. A former missionary companion's mother worked at Utah State Mental Hospital. Through that connection I secured a job in Provo to pay for school and continued to work full time there for two years. For the last two years of my bachelor's degree, I worked full time (usually on the midnight shift), maintained full time student status (including summers), attempted to remain connected to family as husband and father, and did the best I could at participating in church duties.

By 1973 we had two children and I managed to graduate with a degree in speech therapy and audiology. However, during my last very stressful semester, I offended a temporary faculty member. She made sure that I would not continue on to graduate school in audiology. Her decision to scuttle my academic boat also prevented me from securing a teaching certificate and could not, therefore, work in that field. I explored options with Air Force and found that I could still become a pilot.

However, as I thought about my responsibilities to my two young children, I decided that the necessary time away from them required of pilots was not for me.

Child Development and Family Relations

The idea of social connection and taking advantage of social capital continued to play an important aspect of my life. Our church leader of the student church group we attended was Dr. Alvin Price, who was a professor in Child Development and Family Relations. For two years he had been a part of our spiritual life and I had worked closely with him as he worked with the 100 student families of our group. He also believed in me. In my hour of desperation, Al came to our house one evening and offered to personally take me on as a graduate student in CDFR, complete with a teaching assistantship. He was sure I could do it. I agreed to try and will be forever grateful to him for this support.

My love for the study of the family and children was born in the CDFR department at BYU. Prior to my work with Al Price, I had taken no classes about children or families and generally regarded such courses as being suited for women who were bent on being mothers or were looking for ways to find a marriage partner. I had no idea that a legitimate field of study existed that focused on families.

I loved it and plunged in with all my heart. I completed my Master's degree in one year. For my thesis, I focused on moral development and cheating among students at BYU (Day, 1973). I found out that there were a substantial number of students who cheated even though they held high moral standards. Even in the face of expulsion, when the stakes were high and they were not doing well, many resorted to cheating.

University of Wisconsin. While working on my thesis, I became interested in the area of cognition and learning. This area crossed over into my work on cheating and moral development, with Piaget's work taking a central role in my thinking. As I finished my thesis, another serendipitous event occurred. One of my committee members attended a conference at the University of Wisconsin-Madison on cognition and learning. He had been a strong supporter of me during my program and spoke to a conference speaker about me as a potential doctoral student Dr. Wilder replied that indeed he was looking for another doctoral candidate and had assistantship money. Within a few days, contact was made, I was accepted, and was committed to entering the program at Wisconsin.

Our third child had just arrived, and my supportive, loving wife nearly came apart at the seams when I began exploring this opportunity with her. I announced that it would take three more years in school. It was a major test of our relationship.

From the first day at the University of Wisconsin, I knew there was trouble. My mentor/employer was being considered for tenure and apparently did not have the support necessary to stay. The department was in turmoil and there were many conflictual faculty confrontations on a variety of topics. The graduate students huddled together for survival and tried to steer clear of the open hostility. In the huddle were future family science professionals like John DeFrain, Pauline Boss, Gary Peterson, and several others. About mid-year, Gary and I decided that the prospects of long-term survival at Wisconsin were dimming and we began to formulate other plans. Both of us decided we would rather study issues focusing on family life and adolescents. I contacted Wesley Burr at Brigham Young University and began making inquires about a new Ph.D. program in family studies offered at BYU. He was very clear, however, that they would not admit me if I did not have a degree from another school. Having all of one's degrees from the same institution is generally frowned upon. It became clear that I needed to secure a master's degree from the University of Wisconsin as part of my return to BYU.

By spring of 1975, the climate between Dr. Wilder and me had seriously deteriorated as his general disengagement from the department became more pronounced. I would have to finish a thesis on my own. The acting department head, Dr. Jane Pillivian, saw the situation and intervened. She spent the remaining months we lived in Madison working with the system requirements so that I could leave with a degree and completed thesis without help from a chair and essentially without a committee. I have never forgotten this act of kindness and assistance. Her intervention was a Godsend.

Brigham Young University. Our move back to the Utah increased our family stress to an all time high. As both my wife and I reflect back on those times, both of us have difficulty to this day talking about what happened or even remembering the details of the events.

For the next two years, I immersed myself in the family literature. I was very fortunate to be at BYU during the years Wesley Burr was assembling *Contemporary Theories about the Family* (Burr, Hill, Nye, & Reiss, 1979). I took a class from him in the first year of my program in which he invited three class members (including me) to assist him in writing the chapter on symbolic interaction and the family. The excitement and energy present in the department during those years was unlike anything I had experienced. I began teaching undergraduate courses in family and had an abundance of excellent educational opportunities.

Among my most cherished experiences are the marriage and family therapy clinical courses I was permitted to take which introduced me to the family systems approach. I began to believe that through my teaching and research efforts I could make a difference in people's family life, and I began studying the literature on divorce. At that time, most of what had been researched on divorce could be collected into a modest-size file drawer. I decided to do my dissertation on the effects of divorce on economic well-being in families. For my data source, I chose the relatively new National Longitudinal Survey of Youth (NLS).

In the early years of the NLS, the codebooks were on microfiche and could only be read in two places on campus; it was very inconvenient and difficult to use. During my last year Wes took a sabbatical to Arizona State University and I changed chairs to Dr. Stephen Bahr. We worked together to create a statistical model that neither one of us had tried. The idea was to collapse the information of a longitudinal group into time periods rather than the year an event occurred and then estimate the effects of divorce on economic trends one, two, and three years following the divorce (Day & Bahr, 1986).

For younger readers, there was a time when this type of statistical analysis was very new, frustrating, and difficult. We used an early version of SPSS that resided only on the university's mainframe computer. The NLS data were purchased and came packaged on large data tapes that one left archived in the computer center. There were hundreds of computer cards that had to be punched by machine that gave the commands to the computer. The university only allowed grad students to run our data between 12:00 midnight and 5:00 a.m. Therefore, batches of cards were submitted in the afternoon and results retrieved the next morning. The computer would cease working on a program if it encountered any kind of error. Consequently, each and every error cost at least one day. Most who remember running data in those days (back when we had to walk to school everyday and it was uphill both ways) would experience weeks or even months of depression, high stress, and even rage at the slowness of the turnaround time. What took me several months to generate then can now be done with my desktop today in a few hours (or less).

I felt fortunate to participate in three publications while in graduate school. The first was being a part of the chapter on symbolic interaction and family life in *Contemporary Theories about the Family* with Wes

Burr (Burr et al., 1979). This was an exciting experience and has had lasting impact on how I think about theories and human interaction. I also worked with Richard Galbraith at BYU. We produced a paper that was accepted by *Child Development* (Galbraith & Day, 1978). This paper followed up on my interest in cognition and learning. Additionally, my dissertation findings were published in the *Journal of Divorce* (Day & Bahr, 1986). My graduate program had instilled in me a lifelong commitment to the research process.

SOUTH DAKOTA STATE UNIVERSITY

In the early spring of 1977, I finished my coursework and had most of the work done on my thesis. Additionally, we were pregnant with our fourth child. Larri-Lea indicated in very strong tones that it was time for us to seek gainful employment. I knew it would be difficult to complete my degree by summer but I began the job search process. As luck would have it, there were very few openings that year. During the search process a student in our office suite pointed out that there was a position open at South Dakota State University: I shivered but applied.

My interview at SDSU came during a severe ice storm, and it was their spring break. The one thing I remember most about that interview was that the weather was terrible but the faculty were warm, accepting, and eager for me to come. I remember being flabbergasted that someone would actually hire me.

Another reason I took the job was that the dean in the College of Home Economics made it very clear that, if a candidate agreed to come for an interview, was offered the job, and then turned it down, he/she would not be reimbursed for expenses. If the faculty did not want the candidate, then she would reimburse him/her for the interview. Once they offered me the job, it would have been a minor financial disaster for us to absorb the expense. We decided to take the job, despite its limitations.

Our years in South Dakota were some were "the best of times and worst of times." Larri-Lea loved Brookings, especially our association in our church, and still frequently comments on the high quality of life we found there. We both agree that it was a first-rate town in which to raise our five children.

My struggles in the university system were somewhat difficult from the first day. The teaching loads were extreme (4 and 5 courses per semester), the committee workload was equally difficult, and the pay was low. I had no prior experience with the Home Economics aspect of our profession and had never heard the phrase "Land Grant School." Our dean was the President of the American Home Economics Association (AHEA) and very persistent in suggesting that all in the college (Home Economics) should accept that movement and their definition of how family issues should be taught. I made a tactical error by suggesting that most of what she was promoting would retard and even kill the study of family issues. She insisted on pushing through the South Dakota legislature a bill that provided money to build a home management house in which our students (all in the college) would be forced to live in residence for at least one semester. The rent they would pay would then be used to retire the building cost. It was an idea that had many flaws. As I kid I learned many important rules: Never try to take the mask off the Lone Ranger; never step on Superman's cape; and never make fun of Howdy Doody's freckles. No one told about stepping on dean's toes. It was not a good idea for a new assistant professor to challenge the plans of a dean in his first year out of graduate school; in fact, it was a very bad idea.

I was able to survive my own impetuous confrontation with the dean by receiving excellent teaching evaluations and by publishing a few articles in peer-reviewed journals. Among them were two articles written with a very talented undergraduate student named Daniel Hooks. Our first study was an examination of how spontaneous abortion affects women's sense of family crisis (Day & Hooks, 1987a). The second came about as a result of a term paper written by Daniel Hooks (Day & Hooks, 1987b). The two of us did an exhaustive search of what was available about the history of divorce in western civilization. I mention this because it signaled a turn in the way I taught. It was at this time I began to find a deep and abiding love for teaching and working with students. That deep love for students remains to this day.

Research activities came, however, at very high cost. Our department had few resources and only one secretary who provided support for ten-plus faculty and a very large pre-school program. Photocopying was very limited and class material was produced on a ditto machine purchased in the 1950s. No typewriters were available in the department, and there was very limited graduate student assistance. Most of the manuscripts I produced were written at night by hand and then given to a paid typist. It was not until four years into the job that I was given access to one of the typewriters in the college. The computer at SDSU consisted of an antiquated mainframe that was setup in a basement hallway of the administration building. Eventually, the school purchased six primitive terminal monitors onto which some code could be submitted. For most data runs, however, one had to hand-punch cards. The turnaround time often was measured in days before a faculty member's data would be run.

In addition to teaching four and sometimes five different preparations each semester, the advising load was very high. The committee work was difficult, filled with politics, and the long winter months generally were oppressive.

Each year I would hopefully apply for positions in other parts of the country, but to no avail. My peer group competing for the same positions had the advantage of departmental situations in which strong mentoring systems were in place, more resources for research were available, and department cultures were prevalent that fostered professional productivity.

In 1978-79, Wade Mackey came to SDSU as a visiting assistant professor in the Department of Sociology. We connected and I became fascinated with his research. He suggested that we should pay closer attention to Michael Lamb's notion that fathers were the forgotten parent. Wade had been trained as an anthropologist and brought a very unique perspective to the study of fathers. He had garnered a small grant from the Guggenheim foundation to observe fathers in public places. Based on a fundamental anthropological approach he suggested that fathers' involvement with their children (as an observational measure in public places) should vary depending on underlying cultural mandates. Cultures in which high compliance is necessary for survival (agricultural societies) should produce father-child relationships that would be very different from cultures which were much more egalitarian. He traveled to 20 different cultures in Africa, Near and Far East, Europe, and in the U.S. and collected thousands of hours of observational data of men in public places with children. I collaborated with him on several papers resulting from this effort, one of which was published in the *Journal of Marriage and the Family* in 1979 (Mackey & Day, 1979; Day & Mackey, 1986a; Day & Mackey, 1986b; Day & Mackey, 1989). More importantly, my association with Wade began a twenty-plus-year interest in studying fathers in families.

It was during this time that our family finances were at a low point. I decided to develop and design a summer study-abroad program for SDSU that would provide added summer money. For more than ten summers, I took students to Europe for three to six weeks for a travel/educational experience. Much of the time, the trips were centered in England, my second home. I recruited the travelers, designed the trips, hired guides, found the hotels, invented the educational experience, and made all arrangements. While the experiences were unforgettable and the extra pay useful, it did not assist me in my efforts to find a another job where I could do the research and writing I felt I needed to.

In 1985, after eight years at SDSU, I attempted to leave South Dakota one last time: Washington State University was looking for an assistant professor. I had tenure by this time (despite my relationship with the dean) and was an associate professor. I made it very clear in my application letter that I was willing to come to WSU, even if it involved a drop in rank and meant the uncertainty of competing for tenure again. I was successful and excited at the thought of returning to the Northwest.

My initial year at WSU was exhilarating. I began to revive research interests, teach only two courses a semester, and found the university climate much more supportive. Lurking under the surface, however, were some significant and dramatic changes in our department and my career. By the second and third year at WSU, it was clear that our department head was very unhappy at WSU and he eventually left. His leaving coincided with other major changes impacting the College of Agriculture and Home Economics. Enrollments were decreasing and several faculty members and department heads began to challenge the ideas of the new dean. It became clear that by 1990 that our department was being considered for a potential program cut. It was also clear to us that unless we merged with the failing Department of Adult and Youth Education, we would be dissolved or at least forcibly reorganized. During a very stressful three-year period, with an interim chair, we set out to reshape the department. Again, my personal research agenda was put on the back burner for more immediate needs.

During this time, I was elected to represent the Family Discipline section in the National Council on Family Relations. Several of us proposed that it was time to establish the study of the family as a separate discipline rather than have that endeavor be a stepchild to several other disciplines. In concert with Wes Burr, Geoffery Leigh, Kathleen Gilbert and many others, we established the Family Discipline section, started the journal called *Family Science Review*, initiated the Teaching Family Science Conference, and began writing a text that reflected this shift in our thinking about our field.

Additionally, Wes Burr, Kathleen Bahr, and I spent several years writing, testing, and rewriting a text called *Family Science* in an effort to capture the study of the family, as it is unique from a sociological, historical, psychological, or anthropological approach. Over the course of several years, the book had modest sales but was adopted by more than 40 family science programs. I think our book and the other efforts also resulted in the increased use of the term *family science* (Burr, Day, & Bahr, 1993). I am currently rewriting this text and trying to recast it as a book about family processes, which I believe is one element in the study of the family we call *family sciences.*

During this time, I continued my research about fathering issues (Day & Mackey. 1989; Mackey, White, & Day. 1992). However, the work on the text, department turmoil, a heavy church commitment to work with 15 teenage boys in a struggling scout program, and very difficult family struggles with my own teenagers seriously reduced the time spent on creative activities.

The years of departmental disorder resulted in a significant rebuilding of our unit into one that had more than twice the number of faculty. This also involved a move to a new location a complete recreation of our curriculum, the hiring of a new chair, and establishing ourselves as a viable and integral part of the college. We were very fortunate to hire Dr. Jay Teachman as our chair.

Jay had been a colleague and friend before he joined us at WSU. From the first, it was clear that Jay would bring to the department a unique direction and emphasis. First, Jay was a member of the prestigious newly formed Child and Family Well-Being Network and had an established, nationally recognized research record. As a result of the large federal grant that accompanied his membership in the Network, he was able to use accrual grant money to build our program and provide incentives for faculty members to do research and teaching projects that brought a much higher level of visibility and viability the department. Within a five-year period, we were able to add more than ten new faculty members to our department, and our productivity levels increased significantly.

With the pressing duties of the chair position, Jay called upon me to assist him with his duties within the Network. Over this period, I began a career-changing association with some of the more visible and productive scholars in our field. From the onset, the Network sensed that there would be a revival in researchers' and policymakers' interest in father involvement issues. The network called on me to assist them in building a research and policy response to the events happening at the national level. They reasoned that as changes in the government welfare programs shifted, there would significant efforts afoot to include men in the calculus.

As a member of the network, I helped create a series of five seminal meetings in Washington, D.C., about fatherhood and related topics. This series of workshops and forums involved researchers, law and policymakers, and intervention providers. For the first time, I was rubbing shoulders with researchers and public figures that I had only been distantly associated with previously. One result of our efforts was that Vice President Al Gore recognized the Network with the National Performance Review award for our efforts at bringing the topic of father involvement to the forefront.

Additionally, the Network charged me with building an association between them and the National Center on Fathers and Families (NCOFF). For the last seven years, I have been very actively involved in NCOFF's efforts to build a research/intervention program that brings scholars and practitioners together in a united effort to change the well-being of families by increasing effective father involvement.

From my association with the Network and NCOFF, I have been able to participate in several publications, national level programs, and high impact conferences about father involvement and children's well-being (Day, 1992; Day, 1998; Day, Peterson, & McCracken, 1998; Teachman, Carver, & Day, 1995; Teachman, Day, & Carver, 1995; Teachman, Paasch, Day, & Carver, 1997; Day, 1998; Teachman, Day, Carver, Call, & Paasch, 1998; Marsiglio, Day, Lamb, 2000; and Marsiglio, Amato, Day, & Lamb, 2000). I also pushed hard in the Network for much greater attention to be paid to family processes. I suggested that father involvement and many other family dynamics would be understood much better if we understood them from the view of the multiple people within a family. As a result of that initiative, I was asked to present a major paper at an invited conference sponsored by the Network in the fall of 1997 at the Arlie Center in Washington, D.C. At this conference, the Network brought together the best researchers and scholars possible to spend several days in a think-tank setting and discuss the direction that the study of children and families should/could go for the next several years. I assembled a team (Alan Acock and Steve Gavazzi) to help write this paper and it appears in *The Well-Being of Children and Families: Research and Data Needs* (Day, Gavazzi, & Acock, 2001).

In the midst of these research activities, Jay and college level administrators called upon me to develop a distance education degree for our department. It was becoming very clear to us (at the department, college, and university levels) that WSU needed to compete for student credit hours via distance education venues. I led the effort in our department to write a competitive grant to initiate our effort. We were selected by the university to proceed with our distance education degree initiative.

Over the course of two and one-half years, I directed and helped develop 17 courses that formed the core upper-division distance education degree in Human Development at WSU. This degree was officially approved in 1997 and we launched the program that fall. The delivery system was high production video with some Web applications. Department faculty created and filmed course materials and our program became a prototype for a campus-wide initiative to introduce distance education. Additionally, I wrote several articles about distance education and the changing nature of classroom instruction (cf., Bailey, & Day, 1999; Day, & Baugher, 1999).

In the summer of 1998, my life took another serendipitous turn. Dr. Teachman unexpectedly resigned as chair of the Department of Human Development and the task fell to me to be the interim head while a search was conducted. It was somewhat stormy year that included very difficult staff and faculty problems. The search for a new department head did not go well and, additionally, I decided to not apply for the position. In the midst of the turmoil, I was approached by BYU about an opening in the newly formed College of Family Life that was to be advertised at Professor rank. After many long months of indecision, upheaval, and negotiations between BYU, WSU, and me, we painfully decided to leave the Northwest and embark on a new adventure. All but one of my children had completed high school and was out of the nest. Our youngest boy put up a valiant fight to stay in Pullman, but in the end, we decided that a move to BYU would be best for all concerned.

While at BYU, I have reinvested my energy in my research program. I am currently developing a research agenda centering on the use of the newly collected National Survey of Youth 1997 and the National Survey of Adolescent Health (ADD Health). These projects will focus on changes in family processes that influence important life-changing decisions by adolescents. Of course, my interest in how fathers play a part in those family processes will be featured.

As I finish this piece, there are several themes that are clear to me. First, very few events of my professional life were preplanned. Most of the time, I trekked onward and the adventure has unfolded before me. My pre-college tests predicted an almost zero chance of my even attending university, let alone graduating. My participation in university life has been an unanticipated blessing that far exceeds my expectations that were formed in Dufur. The difference has been my contact with those who were willing to invest in my future. The principle of social capital has been a significant one in my life. Of course, I had to be teachable, willing to listen, and work. But without the social connection of others, I shudder to think where my life would taken me. My parents were unable to provide the leverage that others could. Girlfriends, scout leaders, church ministers, authentic friends, and loving family have all contributed in significant and dramatic ways.

In particular, I would not have the wonderful job I do if it were not for the love and support of my sweetheart of 31 years. Her contribution to our survival in this enterprise is inestimable. She never gave up (but wanted to), she rarely complained (even when she had every right to), and she believed in me (when I did not believe in myself).

It has been a long and difficult apprenticeship for me. After nearly three decades of trying to make the journey into a different social and the academic world, I am beginning to discover a place where I can make a difference. As I prepare for the next 15 years of my career, I am sure there will be more surprises–and that is one of the things that keeps me coming to work each day.

I am convinced that university life is changing. I recently wrote a piece for *Family Science Review* (Day & Baugher, 1999) about the changing nature of university life. In this piece we suggest that how we approach teaching and research will dramatically shift in the next few years. We will be required in the near future to find ways of assisting students as *they* sort through mountains of information, sift out the relevant elements, and synthesize those informational bits into a useful whole that will solve a problem. We will also have to do that task when the student is not in our physical presence. Our ability as university professors will necessarily transcend our abilities to perform in class (usually a strategy designed to entertain instead of one that creates real learning), to act as surrogate parents to students (a common and destructive form of teaching), or to pretend that we are the all-knowing high priests and of knowledge, authoritatively bringing the tablets down from the mountain to the eager peasants below. This meaningful shift in university life will, I predict, be a dramatic change for many.

I remain hopeful and enthusiastic about my calling to serve in education as we work in the academy. The future success of that endeavor will necessarily be tied to my ability to adapt and constantly rethink how I do education. It will also hinge upon our collective abilities to support one another and join together to bring the best from one another as we continue to unravel the intricacies of inner family life.

REFERENCES

Amato, P. (1998). More than money?: Men's contributions to their children's lives. In A. Booth & N. Couter (Eds.), *Men in families: When do they get involved? What difference does it make?* (p. 241-278). Mahwah, NJ: Lawrence Erlbaum Associates.

Bahr, S., & Day, R. D. (1978). Females employment, role performance and role consensus. *Journal of Comparative Family Studies, 2*, 53-68.

Bailey, S. J. & Day, R. D. (1999). Beyond traditional classroom walls: The development and effectiveness of a human development extended degree program. *Family Science Review, 12*, 204-215.

Burr, W.R., Leigh, G. K., Day, R. D., & Constantine, J. (1979). Symbolic interaction and the family. In W. R. Burr, R. H. Hill, F. I. Nye, & Reiss, I. (Eds.), *Contemporary Theories about the Family: Volume II*. New York: Free Press.

Burr, W. R., Hill, R., Nye, F. I., & Reiss, I. (Eds.) (1979). *Contemporary Theories about the Family: Volume II*. New York: Free Press.

Coleman, J. (1988). Social capital in the creation of human capital. *American Journal of Sociology, 94*, 95-120.

Coleman, J. (1990). *Foundations of social theory.* Cambridge, MA: Harvard University.

Day, R.D. (1973). Moral Development and Moral Behavior. Unpublished Master's Thesis, Brigham Young University, Provo, UT.

Day, R. D. (1992). The transition to first intercourse among racially and culturally diverse youth. *Journal of Marriage and the Family, 54*, 4,749-762.

Day, R. D. (1998). *Social fatherhood: conceptualizations compelling research, and future direction.* National Center on Fathers and Families. University of Pennsylvania.

Day, R.D. & Bahr, S. J. (1986). Income changes following divorce and remarriage. *Journal of Divorce, 9*, 75-88.

Day, R.D. & Baugher, S. (1999). Distance education and the changing nature of university life. *Family Science Review, 12*, 154-160.

Day, R.D., Gavazzi, S. & Acock, A. (2001). Compelling family processes. In A. Thornton (Ed.) *The Well-Being of Children and Families: Research and Data Needs.* University of Michigan Press: Ann Arbor, MI.

Day, R.D. & Hooks, D. (1987). Miscarriage: A special type of family crisis. *Family Relations, 36*, 305-310.

Day, R.D. & Hooks, D. (1987). A short history of divorce: Jumping the broom and back again. *Journal of Divorce, 10*, 57-73.

Day, R.D. & Mackey, W.C. (1986a). The role image of the American father: Examination of the media myth. *Journal of Comparative Family Studies, 17*, 371-388.

Day, R.D. & Mackey, W.C. (1986b). Children as resources: A cultural analysis. *Family Perspective, 20*, 251-264.

Day, R. D. & Mackey, W.C. (1989). An alternative benchmark to evaluate the American father. *Journal of Family Issues, 10*, 401-408.

Day, R.D., Peterson, G. W. & McCracken, C. (1998). Predicting spanking of younger and older children by mothers and fathers. *Journal of Marriage and the Family, 60*, 79-94.

Gallbraith, R. & Day, R.D. (1978). Child developmental changed in clustering criteria. *Child Development, 49*, 889-891.

Hagan, J., MacMillan. R., & Wheaton, B. (1996). New kid in town: Social capital and the life course effects of family migration on children. *American Sociological Review, 61*, 368-38.

Mackey, W.C. & Day, R.D. (1979). Some indicators of fathering behaviors in the United States: A cross-cultural examination of adult male-child interaction. *Journal of Marriage and the Family, 40*, 287-299.

Mackey, W. C. & White, U., & Day, R.D. (1992). Rationales for entering into the U.S. fathering role: Men's divulgences, women's perceptions. *Journal of Genetic Psychology, 53*, 4, 435-446.

Marsiglio, W., Amato, P., Day, R.D., & Lamb, M. (2000). Fatherhood in a social context. *Journal of Marriage and the Family, 62*, 439-460.

Marsiglio, W., Day, R.D., & Lamb, M. (2000). Exploring fatherhood diversity: Implications for Conceptualizing Father Involvement. *Marriage & Family Review, 29*, 269-294.

Teachman, J.D., Paasch, K.M., Day, R.D. & Carver, K.P. (1997). Poverty during adolescence and subsequent educational attainment. In G. J. Duncan & J. Brooks-Gunn (Eds.) *Consequences of Growing Up Poor*, Russell Sage, New York.

Teachman, J., Day, R.D., Carver, K., Call, V. & Paasch, K. (1998). Sibling resemblance in behavioral and cognitive outcomes: The role of father presence. *Journal of Marriage and the Family, 60*, 835-848.

Teachman, J., Carver, K. & Day, R.D. (1995). A model for analyzing paired data. *Journal of Marriage and the Family, 57*, 995-1024.

Teachman, J. D., Day, R.D. & Carver, K.P. (1995). The impact of family environment on educational attainment: Do families make a difference? In B.C. Ryan et al. (Eds.) *The Family-School Connection*, Vol. 2: Issues in Children's Lives. Sage, Thousand Oaks, CA.

How a Kid from the North Woods Got Lucky

Gary R. Lee

KEYWORDS. Autobiography, cross national research, gerontology, caregiving

Most of the autobiographies in this collection, if I can judge from the examples I've read, are stories of inspiration, deep intellectual curiosity, and heroic struggles to advance the cause of knowledge. Mine is a story of serendipity, opportunism, and sheer dumb luck.

EARLY SOCIALIZATION AND EDUCATION

I grew up in an academic family, although not of the type I'm familiar with now. My parents worked at a small state college in northwestern Minnesota, where they bounced back and forth between appointments in the college itself and in the high school that the college operated on its campus (known, not surprisingly, as the "Campus School" by the locals). The Campus School was disbanded in 1969, two years after I graduated as a member of a class of nineteen. By this time my parents were both employed full-time at the college level, my father as a professor in the business department (well, actually assistant professor; he never finished his doctorate) and my mother as a librarian.

I had no designs on an academic career, but instead had planned on being a lawyer since about third grade. I have no idea why. Perhaps it's because I loved to argue, and thought as a lawyer I could get paid for it. In any event, this was my goal, and I was in a serious hurry to get there. Again, I have no idea why. Perhaps this trait came from my mother's side of the family. She's now an 84-year-old widow, in marginal health, who can't stand to watch television because it's a waste of time. What, I ask quite reasonably, is she saving the time for? She doesn't know, beyond the general principle that time is not a thing to be wasted, particularly on anything that might be construed as enjoyable. She is, after all, Swedish. I was also Swedish once, but have gotten over it; I am now the envy of all for my time-wasting abilities.

But as an adolescent and young adult I was still in a serious hurry. And I got what turned out to be a great opportunity to hurry even faster. My father, for some reason, related to me one day a story of some previous student at our Campus School who had been allowed to take a class at the college, and had received dual (both high school and college) credit for it. I thought this was a fine idea, and inquired into what the rules were for doing this sort of thing. Turned out there really weren't any. The college would allow me to take a class if I paid the tuition. So, the summer after my sophomore year in high school, I signed up for Introductory Sociology at the college. I think I took it because it met at 7:30 a.m. and wouldn't interfere with my afternoon paper route.

I earned an "A" in the class, thus learning I could compete on that level. I also learned that I could substitute that college class for a social studies requirement at my high school. This sort of double dipping was too much for an opportunist such as myself to resist, so I inquired into the rules about how many times I could do this. Again, there weren't any. So I proceeded to sign up for all the college classes I could fit into my schedule, which wasn't too hard since my high school principal thought I could be gotten along pretty well without (we'd had a few disagreements) and was happy to facilitate my absence. By the time I graduated from high school I was a second-quarter college sophomore.

I had taken a year of introductory accounting because my father (who, coincidentally, taught introductory accounting, but not to me) had a plan. I was to get a degree in accounting, practice for a couple of years until I was qualified to become a CPA, then go to law school. Then somehow we'd all be rich. I'm a little hazy on the details of how this would work, but it may have involved the enormous salary I could earn. Alas, I was bored to death by accounting, and also didn't see the connection to my ultimate dream of becoming a lawyer–what did Perry Mason know about debits and credits? I decided to major in pre-law.

About this time a recruiter from Harvard came through town. I was interested in Harvard Law School after college, so even though I hadn't yet graduated from high school I responded affirmatively to the invitation to a meeting. The recruiter, of course, was interested in potential undergraduates, not law students. He explained to me that they took a certain number of scholarship students from each state and that they had no one from North Dakota in the class of '71. So if I'd take out a post office box in Fargo (adjacent to my hometown) I'd have a good shot at a scholarship to Harvard.

I asked if Harvard would accept transfer credits from Moorhead State College. In hindsight, this might have been a dumb question. But if you don't ask, they don't tell you. The recruiter was a nice man, so he didn't laugh in my face, but he nearly grinned himself to death. He's probably put this story in his memoirs too. The answer, of course, was no, and I allowed as to how I wasn't going to let several years of hard work go to waste, so thanks, but I'd just stay here. Some opportunist I turned out to be.

The recruiter, however, happened to have a degree from Harvard Law School, and told me that they and other law schools really preferred that their students not major in pre-law as undergrads; learn law in law school, he said. He suggested either some sort of business major or a social science, depending on what kind of lawyer I wanted to be. At this point I didn't know lawyers came in kinds, but since I'd already tried a business major with unhappy consequences the social science part sounded good. I remembered fondly my first college class in sociology, and thought maybe that was where I belonged.

Shortly after high school graduation my high school sweetheart Naomi and I decided to get married, and to make a break from home and move up the academic ladder. So I transferred to St. Cloud State College, about 170 miles down the road from home. It's not Harvard, but they did accept transfer credits from Moorhead. For those of you familiar with *Prairie Home Companion*, when the kids from Lake Wobegon go to college they go to St. Cloud State. Since they're all above average, the competition was a little stiffer than at Moorhead. Plus St. Cloud had a larger and better sociology department, with a chair, Herb Goodrich, who took me under his wing, found me a work-study job in the department, and taught me a lot about academic life as well as sociology.

Naomi and I, soon joined by our daughter Laura, lived in an 8'-by-33' trailer on the outskirts of St. Cloud while I took a full load of classes and worked in the department and as the weekend manager of the student union on campus. I was on schedule for graduation after fall quarter of 1969, and of course planned to head directly to law school. But I was enjoying my sociology classes, and ran across one particularly terrific professor, Virgil Kroeger, whose classes really excited my intellectual curiosity. He was an older man who had never published a word, who had held a number of academic jobs usually for short times, and who many students found to be too difficult, too acerbic, too empirical, or too theoretical. I thought he was wonderful.

One night I was relating something he'd said in class to Naomi. She said I was so excited by all this that maybe I didn't want to be a lawyer after all; maybe I wanted to be a sociology professor. I thought maybe she was right. So, virtually the next day, I sent off applications to two graduate schools: Minnesota, because it was only 75 miles away and we could move our trailer down there; and Duke, because . . . I have no idea–maybe I liked the name. Obviously a lot of deep thought and research went into this process.

Duke admitted me, but wouldn't take me until the fall of 1970; they didn't take mid-year admissions. I was graduating in December of 1969, and had nothing to do with myself until the following fall if I wasn't in school. Then I received a letter from Joan Aldous, telling me that I'd been awarded an NIMH-sponsored traineeship at Minnesota beginning in January of 1970, and mentioning money. I hadn't known that anyone would pay me to go to grad school. I was so thrilled by this that I hopped in my old Rambler and drove down to the university to accept in person. I'm sure Joan had no idea what to do with me when I got there, but she was very gracious and answered all my silly questions. I was thrilled.

The only problem was that my traineeship was in family sociology. To that point it had not been revealed to me that there was such a thing. I vaguely recalled a couple of courses in marital and family relations on the curriculum at St. Cloud State, but I had never thought of taking them. I hurried to change my registration for my last quarter. As I recall, one course was good and the other was awful, but I can't remember which was which. I certainly didn't suspect that within a couple of years I'd be teaching these courses.

GRADUATE SCHOOL

When I arrived at Minnesota in January of 1970, I discovered several interesting things. One was that I had a desk in a large office, shared by other family sociology trainees; they were to become a terrific source of my professional socialization. Another was that I really didn't have to commit my life to family sociology just because I was on a family traineeship. However, I also realized rapidly that I had stumbled into a truly powerful program, with the best faculty in the country in this particular specialty–Reuben Hill, Ira Reiss, Joan Aldous, and Irving

Tallman–and that developing a specialty in family under their tutelage wouldn't be a bad thing. Further, I discovered that the subject matter was much more interesting than I had expected it to be, and that the family was an excellent arena for the study of all kinds of social processes and human relations. I decided pretty early on that I'd stick with it.

I also discovered, at about this point in my fledgling career, that sociologists did research. As an undergrad I had, of course, taken methods and statistics courses, but I thought these were sort of like the foreign language requirement–needed for a liberal education, but not related to anything I might really need to know. I thought that "doing research" and "going to the library," meant essentially the same thing. Not so, I found. It became evident to me, through my classes and the more informal sessions in the trainee "bullpen," that sociologists are indeed scientists who can discover new knowledge, test hypotheses, formulate explanatory theory, and write things other than textbooks. In my classes with Hill, Reiss, and others, I learned that ideas are wonderful things and necessary for the advancement of knowledge, but that the ability to assess the credibility of one's ideas against the evidence is equally essential. I am still a committed positivist, and expect to remain so throughout my declining years. I blame this on good training.

My advisor was Ira Reiss. I was moving through the graduate program with my usual speed until I hit the point of having to do a master's thesis. I had an idea, borrowed in some part from Durkheim's anomie theory, and I had a data set, borrowed in its entirety from the Social Science Research Center at neighboring Augsburg College, where I did some occasional part-time research work. Ira was terrific about turning around rapidly on drafts of the thesis, but his response was always the same: "This is good, but you need to do a little more." He told me I was raising more questions than I was answering, and that one more chapter would make the thesis really good. When I did that chapter, he thought another one would be nice.

I was, for the first time in my academic life, late. By winter quarter of 1972, I had been in graduate school for over two years and didn't have a master's degree, although I was within a quarter of having all the course work done for the doctorate. This was something of a problem for the Graduate School, but also a problem for my alma mater, St. Cloud State, where I had started teaching part-time in the fall of 1971. We had all assumed I'd have my master's degree by that time, but I didn't. When it looked like I wouldn't have it done by spring quarter, the new chair there spoke sternly to me about my lack of progress. This was a new experience for me.

When Ira used the words "one more chapter" in our next meeting about my thesis, I summoned every ounce of courage I had and squeaked out a protest. It was something along the lines of the thesis already being about 250 pages, and I knew plenty of people who'd done a lot less for Ph.D. dissertations. Ira's response, and I remember it verbatim, was, "OK, let's call it a dissertation." My response, which I also recall verbatim, was, "Huh?"

Ira explained that Minnesota was inaugurating a new graduate program, which encouraged non-thesis master's degrees. If I converted to the new program, I could take four exams and turn in two seminar papers, which I'd already done, in place of the thesis. If these were judged adequate I'd get the master's, and my thesis could become my dissertation. The only problem was that the exams were scheduled for Wednesday; this was Monday.

I thought about it for maybe thirty seconds, switched to the new program, and took and passed the exams. I was awarded the master's degree in the spring of 1972, and my chair at St. Cloud was so happy he offered me a full-time, tenure-track position for the next year. I took it, and spent part of the year working on that last chapter of the dissertation. Ira finally said it was enough already–I think he was as sick of the thing as I was; he mentioned something about having it bound on all six sides–and I got the degree in the spring of 1973.

RESEARCH

Although I had a good tenure-track job at St. Cloud, I'd been bitten by the research bug. Washington State took a chance on me even though I didn't have a publication to my name at that point, and I accepted. We moved west in the summer of 1973, and stayed at Washington State for fourteen years. This position gave me a chance to pursue my research interests; the teaching load was reasonable, and there was an excellent crop of graduate students. Because Washington State was also known for its family program and many students came there specifically to study family, I got to work with some of the best. I learned a lot from them.

My research agenda was directed by interests that were, by and large, purely intellectual. I had read William Goode's (1963) *World Revolution and Family Patterns* in graduate school and become very excited about comparative research and the interrelations of properties of societies and properties of family systems. When I discovered the existence of cross-cultural surveys and data sets, such as the Ethnographic Atlas, that were largely untapped by sociologists, I realized that many of my ideas were testable. In a year-long seminar entitled "Practicum in Family Research" that I taught in 1976-77, we coded about fifteen variables from the Human Relations Area Files for 122 societies and added these variables to the Standard Cross-Cultural Sample. They dealt with everything from the socialization of children to the status and treatment of the elderly. At last count over twenty articles had been published from the work of this seminar, on topics ranging from parental socialization values (Ellis, Lee, & Peterson, 1978; Peterson, Lee, & Ellis, 1982) through mate selection (Lee & Stone, 1980; Atkinson & Lee, 1984), marital structure (Lee, 1979; Cassidy & Lee, 1989; Lee & Whitbeck, 1990), divorce (Seccombe & Lee, 1986), and conjugal power (Lee & Peterson, 1983; Warner, Lee, & Lee, 1986) to the status of the elderly (Lee & Kezis, 1979, 1981; Lee, 1984; Ishii-Kuntz & Lee, 1987).

My continuing interest in comparative research resulted in my first book (*Family Structure and Interaction: A Comparative Analysis*, 1977; 1982), which turned out to be something of a cross between a text and a monograph. I remain fascinated by comparative research and, increasingly, its fellow traveler historical research, because these are the only means we have of apprehending relations among the properties of social systems. Although I've done less actual research in the comparative arena in recent years, I've written several chapters on comparative methods (Lee & Haas, 1993) and on substantive issues such as variations and changes in extended-family households (Lee, 1999). A discussant at a meeting once dismissed one of my papers as irrelevant because it had nothing to do with contemporary concerns or people, consisting as it did of an analysis of the characteristics of small, nonindustrial societies. My defense was that the paper tested hypotheses that were based on a theory that also had many contemporary applications. Thus, we learned something about the utility of the theory, which I thought was important. The discussant didn't. You don't win them all.

In recent years I've been much less involved in comparative simply because I've been pulled in other directions, although the International Section of the National Council on Family Relations was nice enough to give me the Jan Trost Award for comparative research in 2000. Some of these directions involve gerontology and, particularly, the family lives of older people. Again my interest in these things doesn't stem from any particular personal experiences, but rather because I became fascinated with gerontological analyses in graduate school. I took a seminar from Don McTavish, which he began by introducing us to the difficulties of distinguishing age, period, and cohort effects. The intellectual challenge of understanding this issue got me interested in the sociology of aging in general, and I've pursued it in my teaching and research ever since.

One of the things I find fascinating about gerontology is the great number and variety of myths in our culture about older people. Some of these myths are shared, and even perpetrated, by social scientists. Correcting them is great fun.

In 1975, I received a small grant from NIMH to do a study of psychological well-being among older persons. One of the concerns my research team had involved the role of adult children. We had read repeatedly, in textbooks and elsewhere, that children play a critical role. Older persons who see their children regularly, who are involved in their children's lives, and whose children care for them and see to their needs were alleged to be happy, content, well-adjusted old folks. Those who rarely see their children, due to distance, alienation, or apathy, were unhappy and maladjusted. At the time, everyone knew this.

Our interest was simply in estimating the magnitude of the effect of interaction with children on older parents' psychological well-being. We had no doubt that the correlation was positive, but we hadn't found any reports of actual data on the issue. Many authors who asserted the existence of this positive correlation seemed to take it as self-evident; no documentation was necessary. Others cited other authorities, and when we tracked down the citations we expected to find, eventually, the evidence. We didn't. Instead we discovered an instance of the hallowed academic tradition of the circular citation: he said it because she said it because he said it. There *was* no evidence.

So we did a survey. We measured interaction frequency in several different ways, and had several measures of psychological well-being. No matter where we looked or how we looked for it, we found no correlation whatsoever between these measures (Lee, 1979). Our first thought, which anticipated many subsequent critics, was that frequency of interaction was too simplistic a measure, and that interaction might be an occasion for arguments as well as the exchange of positive strokes. But we had measured frequency of interaction with friends in exactly the same way, and it correlated positively and rather strongly with our well-being measures.

Others suggested that intergenerational interaction might not be satisfying to older folks because of the "generation gap." Fortunately we had identical measures for frequency of interaction with siblings; these measures were also perfectly uncorrelated with well-being (Lee &

Ihinger-Tallman, 1980). It appeared that interaction with friends was associated positively with several dimensions of well-being, while interaction with family members wasn't. Our argument was (and is) that it is psychologically gratifying to be chosen as a friend, by someone who has an infinite set of possible choices (Lee & Ishii-Kuntz, 1987). Family interaction may be harmonious or rancorous, a source of delight or irritation, but is known to be motivated in some part by sentiments of obligation. And our choices are constrained: if we're supposed to visit our mothers, we can't pick the best one.

Home was once described by Robert Frost as the place where "when you have to go there, they have to take you in." He didn't say they have to be glad to see you. Mostly, of course, they are. But sometimes they're not, and sometimes they really don't care.

A large part of the message I've attempted to convey in my research on intergenerational relations is that families are not the source of all things good. For older people, in fact, their benefits may be more instrumental than psychological. We're all aware of the huge amount and proportion of care for infirm elders provided by families. Some authors, in fact, have argued that the family caregiving system works so well that the government should keep its great big hands off to avoid interfering with it. This ignores the tremendous costs sustained by family caregivers, for one thing. But it also assumes that older people who need care want to get it from their loved ones.

I've argued in several ways that this is not necessarily the case (Lee, 1985). I've included an item in three different surveys of older persons that asks where the respondent would live if he/she were unable to live independently due to declining health. In one of these surveys, 13 percent of the parents said they'd live with a child, while nearly 54 percent chose a nursing home. The differences in the other two surveys weren't this extreme, but were definitely in the same direction. I don't think this indicates any surge in the popularity of nursing homes, but rather an aversion to being a burden on one's children. We spend most of our lives struggling to maintain and achieve independence, particularly from our families of orientation. When we can no longer be independent, dependence on our children is a less attractive option to most people than dependence on others who are being paid for their services. I think we assume that most older people want to be cared for by their children in large part because we haven't asked them.

Another indicator of this, I think, is the study I did with colleagues (Jeff Dwyer and Ray Coward) at the University of Florida. I wrote a chapter for a book Jeff and Ray edited on gender differences in family caregiving (Lee, 1992). My job was to review theory in the area, which didn't leave me a lot of reading; there wasn't much. The conclusion of my chapter was that we really didn't know why women provide so much more care to infirm elders than do men, except that this was an example of family division of labor, which is highly gendered in virtually all of its manifestations.

That was unsatisfying. To "explain" something as a special case of something else that is largely unexplained doesn't advance the cause of knowledge very much, as I continually remind my grad students. In discussing this frustration with my colleagues, it became clear that we knew pretty much why wives provide more care for husbands than vice versa: husbands tend to be older than their wives and have shorter life expectancies. Wives care for husbands during the husbands' last years, and by the time the wife needs care she's a widow. So the real unanswered question involves the "second line" of defense: why do daughters provide more care for infirm parents than do sons?

It struck me one day that perhaps the answer to the second question was embedded in the answer to the first. In other words, maybe daughters provide more care to parents than do sons for the same reason that wives provide more spousal care than husbands. If one accepts the premise that spouses provide most care to infirm elders when they are available and able (and one should; it's richly documented), then most of the parents for whom children are the primary caregivers are widowed or otherwise without spouses. And most of *these* people are women. Perhaps, with the exception of spouses, there's a strain toward gender consistency in the caregiving dyad: women care for women, and men care for men.

We found (Lee, Dwyer, & Coward, 1993) that the first part of this is definitely true. The vast majority of child caregivers for elderly women are daughters; most of the exceptions to this consist of sons who have no sisters. When the care recipient is a father, however, child's gender is a very poor predictor of caregiving; there's no clear tendency for either sons or daughters to predominate.

From this we learn three things. First, adult daughters are more likely to be caregivers than adult sons in large part because mothers are more likely than fathers to require the care of a child, and women are overwhelmingly more likely to care for women than are men. Second, it's the strain toward gender consistency in the caregiving networks of females that we need to explain: why is it that older women are cared for by their daughters, while older men are cared for by whoever is most available? Third, maybe we should ask this question of older people themselves, which we virtually never do. It strikes me that almost all of our efforts to explain gender differences in caregiving behavior have concentrated on the properties of the children who might (or might not) provide care. When daughters provide care and sons don't, we look for explanations among the circumstances and characteristics of the children. But maybe older women don't *want* their sons to give them baths or help them to the bathroom. Men may be more accepting of such help from daughters because the caregiving role is indeed more institutionalized for women (OK, that's pretty weak; we're still working on it). And, most importantly, perhaps adult children of both genders are doing pretty much what their parents want them to do.

The same principle applies to the resolution of a dilemma in the study of intergenerational coresidence. While the gerontological literature is quite unequivocal about the important role of children in providing a home for aging parents who are widowed, infirm, and incapable of independent residence, several studies done from the perspective of family sociology have argued that intergenerational coresidence occurs primarily, if not exclusively, for the benefit of the junior generation. The latter makes sense in light of our finding that elderly parents neither want nor intend to live with their children when they become infirm. But it really isn't consistent with the evidence. The conclusion that coresidence benefits the adult child generation resulted from a failure to separate the relatively small number of older people who might actually need to live with children (the very old, the ill, the impoverished, the widowed) from the much larger number of younger, healthier, wealthier, married older persons who often provide homes for their adult children because of either delayed launching or returns to the nest. Lumping these two types of parents together (and using linear estimators of the effects of variables such as age, when the underlying relation is nonlinear) makes it appear as if the former group doesn't exist, when the reality is that they are simply numerically overwhelmed by the latter (Lee & Dwyer, 1996). They are very real, and they're out there living with their kids.

But the evidence is overwhelming that living with children is not the first choice of older Americans. It's not that they don't like their kids; they do. In the same study where we found a 4-to-1 preference for nursing homes over children, we were unable to use Bengtson's scale of affection for children because it produced no variance–everyone clustered at the top of the scale. Perhaps it's because they *do* like their kids that they don't want to live with them. They don't want to sour the relationship with unrelenting togetherness and the conflict it may produce, and they don't want to interfere with their children's lives or consume their resources. When older people go to live with their adult children, they go not by choice but by necessity. "Home is where, when you have to go there . . ."

Recently I've been engaged in a study of the psychological consequences of widowhood, focusing particularly on the fact that, at least in cross-sectional data, the loss of a spouse seems to be a more difficult experience for men than for women (Lee, Willetts, & Seccombe, 1998; Lee, DeMaris, Bavin, & Sullivan, 2001). However, we're now starting to look at some longitudinal data that appear to lead to the opposite conclusion. This paradox will prove to be either really interesting or really irritating, depending on whether we can resolve it.

At the moment I find it irritating, but that's because I haven't had much chance to try to resolve it yet. I'm ending my fifth year as department chair. This is our program review year, I have three positions to fill, two tenure/promotion cases, three applications for faculty improvement leaves, a lab full of new computers that haven't been housebroken yet, and my granddaughter started playing soccer last Sunday. Plus I'm writing this autobiography. Those widows will have to wait a bit.

REFLECTIONS ON MOBILITY

I am now working at my fifth institution of higher education, counting St. Cloud State, where I taught prior to receiving the doctorate. We left Washington State for the University of Florida in 1987, went from there to the University of Nevada-Reno in 1995, and departed hastily for Bowling Green State in 1996. (The Reno story is too long for this chapter; maybe someday it'll be a book.) Each time we moved we did so because we expected an improvement in our situations. At this point I'd say we're two-for-four. The last move was certainly an improvement, and we think we're hunkered down in Bowling Green for the long haul. This is partly because we like it here, and partly because our daughter and granddaughter moved here last year, so we're gradually colonizing the place.

All this moving around has generated two thoughts. First, academics are great ones for thinking that the grass is greener in someone else's pasture. When we've been around a university for a while we get to know its shortcomings intimately. Colleagues at other institutions who might want to recruit us tell us all the good stuff about their schools, but of course they're in the "courtship" mode at the time. When we get there the "marriage" mode takes over pretty quickly, and we discover that our new university has its own set of shortcomings, sometimes more noxious than the ones we left. Mobility is risky.

Second, somebody ought to do a study. Academics must be among the most mobile people in the world in the sense of being generally unable to work in their hometowns. For most of us, if our local college or university has a position available for which we're suited, we have to compete with applicants from all over the country, and being a local is no advantage whatsoever. When we need jobs, we're virtually always on the national market. In each of the three major sociology departments in which I've been employed, there's been precisely one faculty member who was born in the state in which the university is located. Sometimes, if we stay long enough, we adopt our institution's location as our home. And sometimes our children stay in these adoptive homes, or, as in our case, move there. But for most of us in academe, our families of orientation are elsewhere. And the places we grew up are rarely the places we live now. This should have some pretty serious implications for the kinship relations of academics. Some day I'll do a study.

My primary thought on mobility, though, is that we've left a lot of good people when we've moved. We've had some great friends everywhere we've lived, and we miss them. Fortunately, we also have great friends here in Bowling Green, and some terrific hobbies (golf, cross-country motorcycling) we share with them. I've also been lucky to have had some of the best graduate students in the history of graduate students–I won't mention particular names, but you guys know who you are. I've been married to the same marvelous lady for around 33 years now, and she only gets better with age.

Meanwhile, I still think of myself as a Minnesota kid, and hope to return there eventually, at least for retirement. It is, as we say, only cold in the winter. But that's probably fifteen years away, and I'm mostly enjoying being a department chair. More time for research would be nice, but it'll keep; nothing I'm doing is an emergency. And my granddaughter has another soccer game this Sunday.

AUTHOR NOTE

Gary R. Lee is affiliated with the Department of Sociology, Bowling Green State University, Bowling Green, OH 43403.

REFERENCES

Atkinson, M. P., & Lee, G. R. (1984). Structural correlates of marriage payments: Antecedents of the bride price. *International Journal of Sociology of the Family*, *14*, 1, 67-79.

Cassidy, M. L., & Lee, G. R. (1989). The study of polyandry: A critique and synthesis. *Journal of Comparative Family Studies*, *20*, 1, 1-11.

Ellis, G. J., Lee, G. R., & Peterson, L. R. (1978). Supervision and conformity: A cross-cultural analysis of parental socialization values. *American Journal of Sociology, 84*, 2, 386-403.

Goode, W. J. (1963). *World revolution and family patterns*. New York: The Free Press.

Ishii-Kuntz, M., & Lee, G. R. (1987). Status of the elderly: An extension of the theory. *Journal of Marriage and the Family, 49*, 2, 413-420.

Lee, G. R. (1977). *Family structure and interaction: A comparative analysis*. Philadelphia: J. B. Lippincott.

Lee, G. R. (1979). Marital structure and economic systems. *Journal of Marriage and the Family, 41*, 3, 701-713.

Lee, G. R. (1982). *Family structure and interaction: A comparative analysis* (second edition, revised). Minneapolis: University of Minnesota Press.

Lee, G. R. (1984). Status of the elderly: Economic and familial antecedents. *Journal of Marriage and the Family, 46*, 2, 267-275.

Lee, G. R. (1985). Kinship and social support of the elderly: The case of the United States. *Ageing and Society, 5*, 1, 19-38.

Lee, G.R. (1992). Gender differences in family caregiving: A fact in search of theory. In J.W. Dwyer & R.T. Coward (Eds.) *Gender and family care of the elderly* (pp. 120-131). Newbury Park, CA: Sage.

Lee, G. R. (1999). Comparative perspectives. In M. B. Sussman, S. Steinmetz, & G. W. Peterson (Eds.), *Handbook of marriage and the family*, 2nd ed (pp. 93-110). New York: Plenum.

Lee, G. R., DeMaris, A., Bavin, S., & Sullivan, R. (2001). Gender differences in the depressive effect of widowhood in later life. *Journal of Gerontology: Social Sciences, 56B*, 1, S56-S61.

Lee, G. R., &. Dwyer, J.W. (1996). Aging parent-adult child coresidence: Further evidence on the role of parental characteristics. *Journal of Family Issues*, 17, 1, 46-59.

Lee, G. R., Dwyer, J.W., & Coward, R.T. (1993). Gender differences in parent care: Demographic factors and same-gender preferences. *Journal of Gerontology: Social Sciences, 48*, 1, S9-S16.

Lee, G. R., & Haas, L. (1993). Comparative methods in family research. In P. Boss, W. Doherty, R. LaRossa, W. Schumm, & S. Steinmetz (Eds.), *Sourcebook of family theories and methods: A contextual approach* (pp. 117-131). New York: Plenum.

Lee, G. R., & Ihinger-Tallman, M. (1980). Sibling interaction and morale: The effects of family relations on older people. *Research on Aging, 2*, 3, 367-391.

Lee, G. R., & Ishii-Kuntz, M. (1987). Social interaction, loneliness, and emotional well-being among the elderly. *Research on Aging*, 9, 4, 459-482.

Lee, G. R., & Kezis, M. (1979). Family structure and the status of the elderly: A preliminary empirical study. *Journal of Comparative Family Studies, 10*, 3, 429-443.

Lee, G. R., & Kezis, M. (1981). Societal literacy and the status of the aged. *International Journal of Aging and Human Development, 12*, 3, 221-234.

Lee, G. R., & Peterson, L. R. (1983). Conjugal power and spousal resources in patriarchal cultures. *Journal of Comparative Family Studies, 14*, 1, 23-38.

Lee, G. R., & Stone, L. H. (1980). Mate-selection systems and criteria: Variation according to family structure. *Journal of Marriage and the Family, 42*, 2, 319-326.

Lee, G. R., & Whitbeck, L. B. (1990). Economic systems and rates of polygyny. *Journal of Comparative Family Studies, 21*, 1, 13-24.

Lee, G. R., Willetts, M. C. & Seccombe, K. (1998). Widowhood and depression: Gender differences. *Research on Aging, 20*, 5, 611-630.

Peterson, L. R., Lee, G. R., & Ellis, G. J. (1982). Social structure, socialization values, and disciplinary techniques: A cross-cultural analysis. *Journal of Marriage and the Family, 44*, 1, 131-142.

Seccombe, K., & Lee, G. R. (1986). Female status, wives' autonomy, and divorce: A cross-cultural study. *Family Perspectives, 10*, 3, 241-249.

Warner, R. L., Lee, G. R., & Lee, J. (1986). Social organization, spousal resources, and marital power: A cross-cultural study. *Journal of Marriage and the Family, 48*, 1, 121-128.

Mountains, Mormonism, Marriage, and Family: Life and Career Reflections

Brent C. Miller

KEYWORDS. Autobiography, adolescent sexuality, adolescent pregnancy, adolescent parenthood, transition to parenthood

ORIGINS

Childhood

I was the second child and oldest son of four children born to my parents in Logan, Utah. Logan is located in Cache Valley, which is ringed by mountains that are capped with snow seven to eight months of the year. Cache Valley was named by fur trappers in the 1820s and 1830s as the place where they sometimes "cached" (stored or hid) their furs through the winter. In the 1850s and 1860s my ancestors from Prussia, Norway, and England all immigrated to America and to Utah because of their religion.

In the mid-nineteenth century members of the Church of Jesus Christ of Latter-Day Saints (Mormons) gathered in Utah from all over the world, seeking freedom in general, and religious freedom in particular. They were seeking to establish their "Zion," a promised land in the great American West that was then an unsettled territory. I mention the Rocky Mountains and the LDS religion at the outset because these are important anchors in my life. The mountains are home to me, and I enjoy hiking, camping, fishing, and just being in the mountains all seasons of the year. My religious beliefs and activity also greatly influence the ways I work, play, and understand the world.

I had a happy childhood in Logan during the 1950s. In the summers our group of same-age friends explored the open fields west of town, and at night we played games in the neighborhood until our parents called us home. During the school year I walked about half a mile to the Ellis Elementary School. My natural curiosity sometimes led to mischief and trouble. For example, as a toddler my hand got caught running graham crackers through the rollers of the old washing machine, and in middle childhood I tied a neighbor's chicken down inside a crate to get it to hatch another neighbor's eggs. Outdoor activities were a fun part of my life, and in the summers I rode my bike to fish for trout in the clear, cold streams that ran out of the canyons, and in some of the irrigation canals that ran through town. I especially liked to fish and explore the mountains with my dad.

Adolescence

When I was 12 (in the summer of 1959) my family moved about 40 miles south to Ogden, which was at that time Utah's second largest city. My father was a commercial roofing contractor and we moved so that he could locate his business in a larger population area. I remember the move being hard for me at first; the kids wore different style clothes and it took several months for me to fit in. But the foothills of North Ogden, where we lived, was another place of openness and freedom where I enjoyed my teenage years. We built our own house in a peach orchard on the brow of a hill; quail, pheasants, and rabbits lived in the brushy hollows nearby, and deer were plentiful in the mountains within a mile of our home.

Because we lived in the outlying county school district, I rode the bus for quite a distance to attend junior high school. The bus driver kept the radio turned up loud so that we could listen to it (and maybe so that he didn't have to listen to us) on the way to school. At the same time every morning the radio station would broadcast the names of infants born the previous day at the Ogden City hospitals. I still remember the jingle that preceded the birth announcements, which reflected the pronatalist and profamily messages of the era and the area: "Across the street and a few houses down, a tiny little baby has come to town. To brighten up the household and make two hearts so glad, the sweetest little baby . . . just for mom and dad."

My adolescence was pretty typical for kids in that culture. I participated in school, scouts, and church activities in addition to family outings and reunions with our extended families. I also did manual work to earn money–picking fruit when I was young, and roofing and other construction work after my mid-teens. Beginning in my mid-teens I usually had a girlfriend until one of us got bored, and then we would drift apart and pair up with someone else. I had fun in high school, especially the social and sports dimensions. I was elected to student offices and lettered in track (throwing the javelin) and football (defensive cornerback). I liked to write and I was intellectually curious, so I enjoyed science, but I wasn't very good at the tedious detail required to do well in math and chemistry.

One of the most significant experiences of my late adolescence was serving a two-year mission for the LDS Church. Soon after high school graduation (from March 1966 to 1968) I was a representative of the Church in what was then called the Northern States Mission, headquartered in Chicago. This was truly a life changing experience. Being a missionary required self-discipline to live with an assigned companion, to get up early in the morning, to study scriptures daily, and to go out every day to discuss religious principles with anyone who would listen. We taught investigators in the evenings, and were in our apartment by 10 p.m. at night. My mission experience was also life altering in the sense that I grew close to many individuals and families whose lives were dramatically changed for the better by their acceptance of the principles we taught. It also helped me get a clearer picture of who I was, what I believed, and what I wanted to do in my life.

YOUNG ADULTHOOD

I was unsure what my future career would be. I had thought sometimes about becoming a medical doctor or an attorney, but I didn't know anyone to model those careers. After returning from my mission I decided to major in psychology and minor in family studies at Weber State College in Ogden. I think this educational turning point, after my mission, came about because I wanted to understand more about human relationships. The more that I studied the social and behavioral sciences, the more interested I became in understanding human behavior, and especially close (marriage and family) relationships.

Marriage and Post Graduate Education

The older I got the more seriously I dated. When I left on my mission at age 19, I thought that I would marry the girl I was dating then. We exchanged letters regularly at first, but she was still in high school, and during my two-year mission we both changed a lot. Her family moved away from Utah, and when I came home in 1968 it was several months before I went to see her in California. We still had romantic feelings, but getting married wasn't as simple or sure as before. It seems strange, but I began to feel that I should marry someone I had never dated. I had known Kevon Costley for almost 10 years, since our family moved to North Ogden. On double dates and with groups of friends we had gone lots of places together. After returning from my mission I had a peaceful, calm feeling whenever I was around her or thought about her, and I had a growing impression that we should get married. We respected and liked each other as friends but, because we never had dated, it was more than a little awkward to become engaged. I knew in a spiritual way that we were right for each other; this deep conviction and our commitment to each other has helped us to make it through difficult times. We married as college students when I was 22 and Kevon was almost 21.

At first we lived in Ogden, near Weber State College, where I was going to school and Kevon was student teaching. Because I had done well academically and I continued to be interested in higher education, I applied to Utah State University to begin the master's program in Family and Child Development in the fall of 1971. Jay Schvaneveldt became my major professor and eventually a respected friend who later served as department head at USU for nearly 20 years. For my thesis research I compared the fertility-related attitudes of three generations of Mormon women within family lineages. During my master's program I got a clearer understanding that it would be possible to make a career out of teaching and research in this field, so I applied to and was accepted at several of the leading doctoral programs. The University of Minnesota seemed to have the most to offer and gave me the "best deal," a $5,000 per year graduate traineeship sponsored by the National Institutes of Mental Health.

Doctoral Studies in Minnesota

In the fall of 1972 I entered the program in family sociology at Minnesota because Reuben Hill, Ira Reiss, Murray Straus, Joan Aldous, and Irv Tallman had built such a great reputation there in family scholarship. The Minnesota Family Study Center and the NIMH traineeship provided a rich learning environment. I also soon discovered that there were other strong complementary programs at Minnesota in Family Social Science and the Institute of Child Development.

In my first year I had the good fortune to work closely with Reuben Hill and others on the Family Problem Solving project. Reuben and

Marion Hill were wonderful in helping us feel personally and professionally welcome. I developed a friendship and worked with David Klein, who was Reuben's senior graduate assistant, and Steve Jorgensen who was in my graduate student cohort (Klein, Schvaneveldt, & Miller, 1977; Klein, Jorgensen, & Miller, 1978; Miller & Klein, 1981; Miller & Jorgensen, 1988). Joan Aldous was my first-year advisor, and after she moved from Minnesota, Ira Reiss became my major professor. I benefited greatly from the personal qualities and professional abilities of all these professors and graduate student colleagues at Minnesota.

Some of my most memorable graduate school experiences reflect how naive I was about academia. When I began the family sociology graduate program at Minnesota it didn't occur to me that family was only one of several emphases. Somewhat to my chagrin, I had to take foundation courses in social theory, complex organizations, population, deviance, and so on. Soon after my arrival I was enrolled in a basic history of social thought course, taught by a senior professor who had written the textbook. He still lectured by turning yellowed pages of handwritten notes that he had delivered to thousands and thousands of students before. Entering the Social Science Tower elevator one day, I found myself standing alongside this distinguished older professor with mutton chop whiskers. When I called him by his first name his face reddened with obvious displeasure. It was uncomfortable being confined with him in the elevator, and I learned that not all professors like to be on a first-name basis with students. That first fall quarter I also remember barging through Reuben Hill's closed office door one day without knocking, to find him meeting with one of his colleagues. Reuben was among the most patient of people; he just turned in his chair and regarded me quizzically. Although he didn't say anything, I could tell that even he wondered how long it would be before I learned more professional manners. Nowadays, when a graduate student enters my office with little or no regard for what I am doing, it helps to remember that I was once similarly naive.

Another memorable experience at Minnesota came about because I did something out of order in my graduate program. The Director of Graduate Studies for the department was by temperament rather formal in his interactions with students, and he was displeased that I had not followed the proper order. I wanted to find a way to move ahead with my program, and he suggested that he could resign and be replaced on my supervisory committee. With diplomatic intercession from Reuben Hill and Ira Reiss, he agreed at least to discuss the matter. When he came to the meeting I could see from his facial tics and coloration that he was highly agitated. Before even sitting down, he announced that he wanted to read a prepared statement, which went like this: "In recent weeks, and especially in the past several days, I have been the victim of repeated prank calls in the middle of the night. Because of the difficulty we have been having with this committee, and its temporal proximity with these phone calls, I am resigning from Brent Miller's committee." It was quite a shock to have the Director of Graduate Studies indirectly accuse me of harassing him and resign from my doctoral committee. Of course I was not responsible for the prank calls, but eventually we all agreed that it would be best to replace the offended faculty member on my committee, and my doctoral program moved ahead.

I always had been interested in human development as well as in marriage and the family. So, as part of my doctoral program in family sociology, I decided to take a supporting area through the Institute of Child Development at Minnesota. These developmental courses, and the professors who taught them, were truly excellent. Willard Hartup was a member of my doctoral supervisory committee, and in one oral exam he asked: "What is development?" His simple, direct question caught me off guard, and I remember stammering around about stages and sequences, after which he reduced development to its essential meaning–change over time. My thinking has been influenced by the seminars I took in social development (Andy Collins and Willard Hartup), cognitive development (John Flavell) and genetics and development (Sandra Scarr). I also met many strong doctoral students in developmental psychology, including Hal Grotevant with whom I am now collaborating 25 years later.

In the sociology doctoral program our training in research methods was first rate, and I took the opportunity to become an RA with David Olson in Family Social Science on the St. Paul Campus. That was the beginning of a constructive collaboration and friendship. My dissertation was a cluster analysis of types of young married couple interaction, based on data collected by David and others in the Intramural Research program at NIMH (Miller and Olson, 1990). Many nights I carried boxes of punched computer cards in to the mainframe computer center (there were no PCs!) between midnight and 4 a.m. so that I could do dissertation analyses without being interrupted during high-demand times.

Social theory was also an important part of our training at Minnesota. A graduate seminar taught by Paul Reynolds was especially infamous; all students received incomplete grades; because the papers we were expected to write could not be finished in one quarter. My paper for the course (which ran 100+ pages) was a reformulation of Ira Reiss' theory of premarital sexual permissiveness, which I presented at the NCFR Theory Construction preconference, and which later became the basis for a handbook chapter that Ira and I coauthored (Reiss & Miller, 1979).

There weren't any mountains to explore in Minnesota, but Kevon and I took a memorable canoe trip into the Boundary Waters Canoe area. It was an enjoyable wilderness experience of a different kind, paddling through mosquitoes and portaging between lakes in Southern Canada. In about 1973 I grew a full beard. Kevon and I were both very involved in the LDS University Branch that met on University Avenue in a huge old cavernous protestant church with massive stained glass windows. That branch was a great religious and social group, where we formed many friendships.

In the spring of 1975, anticipating graduation that summer, I interviewed for several jobs and decided to take a faculty position in the Department of Child and Family Studies at the University of Tennessee in Knoxville (UTK). After I defended my dissertation in August, Kevon and I prepared to make the move to Tennessee, but first we had to fly to Salt Lake to attend NCFR and to gather belongings in Utah. We were waiting for a ride to the airport when the phone rang, and the caller said "We have a baby for you." We were stunned. Hoping to have children for nearly six years, we had been through infertility testing and applied two years earlier to become adoptive parents. This call caught us completely by surprise because we had been told that we would be waiting longer. We spent the night in a frenzy of physical and emotional preparation for becoming parents the next day. We changed our plane reservations to fly to Chicago where we finally became parents of a beautiful, good-natured six-week-old baby boy who we named Clay.

ACADEMIC CAREER

First Faculty Position: The Tennessee Years

The Child and Family Studies faculty at UTK were mostly young and energetic, and we shared an unusually positive esprit de corps. It was an enjoyable position, teaching introductory marriage and family courses and graduate research methods. Developing and teaching that graduate research methods course (with Jo Lynn Cunningham) solidified a framework and structure that I later conveyed in journal articles (Miller, Rollins, & Thomas, 1982) and a textbook (Miller, 1986).

In Knoxville I conducted a short-term longitudinal study of the transition to parenthood, based on a literature review I had completed for my written prelims at Minnesota. We studied 120 expectant couples for about a year, and found that the transition to parenthood was associated with increases in individual and marital stress (Miller & Sollie, 1980) but that most couples also mentioned many positive aspects about having their first baby (Sollie & Miller, 1980).

In Tennessee, I enjoyed some hiking and trout fishing in the Great Smoky Mountains, but I still longed for the Rockies. Kevon and I were very involved with the LDS Church in Tennessee; she taught weekly religion classes for youth, and I was a bishop (lay minister) and counselor in the Knoxville stake presidency. Our years in Knoxville were wonderful, both personally and professionally, and we developed some of our closest lifetime friendships there. While there, we also adopted our second son, Micah, who was a bundle of energy and a funny little character when he joined our family at 6 months of age. We left Tennessee as a family with two young boys, Clay (age 4) and Micah (age 2).

Back to Utah State

We loved many things about Tennessee, but when a position came open at USU in the fall of 1979 we moved back to Logan. Having little children, we wanted to be closer to our families (especially their grandparents), and I had a longing for the Rocky Mountains. Changing university positions, I decided to develop a research program to address an applied, social problems type of marriage or family issue. Soon after my arrival at USU, the Utah State Office of Education issued a request for proposals to study what differentiated teens who began having sexual intercourse from those who remained sexually abstinent during their school years. I submitted a proposal that was funded in 1981, and that small sponsored project began two decades of research from which I have published many papers about adolescent sexual behavior and pregnancy.

In the early 1980s I became the evaluation researcher for a pregnancy prevention demonstration project Terry Olson had funded by the federal Office of Adolescent Pregnancy Programs (OAPP) in the Department of HHS. The sexual abstinence demonstration programs sponsored by OAPP had little chance of making (or of showing) a major difference in teen pregnancy, partly because the interventions themselves were relatively weak, and also because, by legislation, only a small amount of the budget (5%) could be used for research. However, using the data we collected to evaluate the program, I published a number of correlational studies linking adolescents' individual and family characteristics to their sexual intercourse experience (Miller, McCoy, & Olson, 1986; Miller, McCoy, Olson, & Wallace, 1986; Miller, Christensen, & Olson, 1987; Miller & Sneesby, 1988).

Our personal family life changed again in November 1983 when our third child, a cute little dark-haired girl, was adopted through friends who knew about her unstable situation. Erin's early years often had been chaotic and traumatic, and she was two years and 9 months old when she came to our family. We naively believed that our normal and mostly average family life would eventually (maybe even quickly?) smooth things out for her. The mid-1980s were mostly fun and enjoyable for our little family, and I carried a significant religious role as bishop of the North Logan 2nd Ward.

My studies about adolescent sexual behavior, and my involvement with OAPP, led to many opportunities to become acquainted with researchers and agency officials, and to participate in national grant review panels usually focused on adolescent pregnancy issues. In the late 1980s I conducted an evaluation study of the Kennedy Foundation's Community of Caring program, designed to help pregnant and parenting teens (Miller & Dyk, 1991). I also submitted a demonstration project, which was funded by OAPP, called FACTS and *feelings*, designed to help families talk about sexuality so that teens would avoid adolescent pregnancy by remaining sexually abstinent. The program itself was based on a series of videotapes and newsletters our team developed, intended for parents and children to view and discuss at home. Unusual for projects of this kind, our evaluation study was a true pre-test, post-test control group design with random assignment of families. Program families talked more about sexual issues, but there were not significant differences in teens' sexual attitudes and behaviors (Miller, Norton, Jenson, Lee, Christopherson, & King, 1993).

Sabbatical Experiences

Research on teen sexual behavior and pregnancy placed me in contact with people from whom I wanted to learn more, so I planned a sabbatical that took our family from coast to coast during the 1987-88 academic year. It began with me spending the summer of 1987 at the University of Michigan, taking quantitative methods courses and becoming better acquainted with Arland Thorton. I returned to Utah by bus (that was an education!), and our family packed up the barest essentials to move to Seattle, Washington.

We rented a two-bedroom apartment in Kirtland, across the Lake from Seattle, and Kevon worked on getting the kids settled in schools while I began commuting to Battelle Human Affairs Research Centers near the University of Washington. My commute around or over Lake Washington was a frustrating 30 to 40 minutes each way, and getting the children settled in unfamiliar schools also was challenging. I was a visiting scientist at Battelle, located in an idyllic wooded park around a pond (with ducks). Battelle's professional environment was similarly impressive. Steve McLaughlin and John Billy were my primary colleagues, from whom I learned how full-time social science researchers work, and especially how they craft winning contracts and grants. Our family enjoyed the Seattle area; the environment was beautiful, and we took opportunities to travel up and down the Pacific Northwest coast. After public schools were out in December we drove back to Utah for a week of Christmas holidays with our extended families.

The final leg of our family sabbatical journey was across the country to the Washington, D.C., area. We drove our station wagon, pulling a small 4 × 6 trailer with only our clothes and essential belongings. Starting school in an unfamiliar environment was more difficult for the children in January (mid-year) than it had been in the fall, but they did all right.

Wendy Baldwin was then Chief of the Demographic and Behavioral Sciences Branch (DBSB) at the National Institutes of Child Health and Human Development (NICHD). I sought an opportunity to work at DBSB because they had funded much of the early research about adolescent pregnancy and childbearing, and Wendy was an important leader in that area. We worked out a role for me to help around DBSB, and in the process, I became acquainted with how the Branch, the Institute, and the federal Government fosters research. It was a valuable experience to participate in meetings with the DBSB staff (Wendy Baldwin, Sandy Hofferth, Jeff Evans) and some of the leading social scientists in the country. DBSB was located in the old Landow Building in Bethesda, but in the spring of 1988 the Branch moved to a new location on Executive Boulevard in Rockville. Dawn Upchurch was an intern at the same time, and Susan Newcomer joined DBSB as I was leaving. Our family enjoyed seeing the amazing sights in the Washington, D.C., area. Being there in the winter and early spring gave us time before the crowds of tourists arrived, and we took advantage of the weekends to see as much as we could in six months. We also took some extended weekend trips up and down the East Coast.

Back to Utah Again

It has been said that you can never go home again (because it doesn't stay the same), but returning to Utah in the summer of 1988 truly felt like coming home. The sabbatic leave was a tremendously valuable learning experience, but we were tired of being temporary and moving. It had been a hassle commuting to and from work in Seattle, Bethesda, and Rockville, going into and out of the District, and traveling a lot on the weekends. When we returned to Cache Valley in the early summer of 1988 it was quite a contrast. Driving into the valley was like entering a peaceful, pastoral painting. Everyone and everything seemed to be moving in slow motion. The mountains were waiting too.

Returning to USU I resumed my research about adolescent sex and pregnancy. Kris Moore and I collaborated on a state of the science article about adolescent sex, pregnancy, and childbearing for the 1990 Decade Review issue of the *Journal of Marriage and the Family* (Miller & Moore, 1990). Soon thereafter we were funded by OAPP to analyze the antecedents of adolescent sexual behavior, using longitudinal data from the National Survey of Children. Analyses were done by several of the graduate students at USU who wrote articles about forced sexual intercourse (Miller, Monson, & Norton, 1995) and education (Schvaneveldt, Miller, Lee, & Berry, in press) and religiosity as correlates of adolescent sexual intercourse.

In 1991 I agreed to be Acting Head of the Department at USU while Jay Schvaneveldt was a Fulbright Scholar in Thailand. When he returned I was glad to give the administrative chores and headaches back to him. My memories of administrivia gradually faded, however, and by 1995, when Jay took another exotic leave to the Arab Gulf States, I became head of FHD on a permanent basis. Over the years I have reflected that Reuben Hill, Ira Reiss, and David Olson were never department heads, and I believe they avoided it deliberately. Being a full professor with external funding is a great career; one has the time and freedom to set one's own research agenda, and the financial resources to reduce day-to-day departmental obligations. Being a department head is a difficult balancing act, trying to maintain a scholarly research program while responding to the daily and sometimes competing needs of students, faculty, and staff.

During the childhood years our family had fun activities virtually every week, took many family vacations, and planned special "dates" where the children took turns going out with mom and dad. We held family home evenings regularly, and were quite religious as a family. As our children entered their teens, there was a different texture than we had expected, and it seemed to stem from our teens' trying to come to grips with their adoptive identities. Gradually we began to realize that some (many or most?) adopted children have issues that neither they nor their adoptive families understand very well when the children are young (Brodzinsky & Schecter, 1990). This realization started me on a new line of research to better understand adopted children's feelings and behavior (Miller, Fan, Christensen, Grotevant & van Dulmen, 2000), why adopted children are so much more likely to receive mental health counseling (Miller et al., 2000), and to test possible mediating mechanisms that would explain why some adopted children do well, while others have more problems (work in progress).

REFLECTIONS

The baby boom, the pro-family era of the 1950s, and the defiant Sixties are among the larger events and movements that shaped my life and outlook, in addition to being born in the Rocky Mountains and being raised as a member of the Church of Jesus Christ of Latter-Day Saints. I was born at the beginning of the baby boom, and was indoctrinated during the conservative, traditional, profamily 1950s. Although I was a teenager during the rebellious 1960s, I was also a Mormon missionary at the height of this tumultuous decade, and while protests and riots were going on around the country, I lived in a faith community that wasn't really of the "world." Among professional colleagues I'm viewed as a conservative, but among family, friends, and religious leaders, I'm suspiciously liberal. "Families, Science, and Values" was the theme of my NCFR presidential address (Miller, 1993).

I have had especially close ties with the National Council on Family Relations over the years, starting with the Preconference and Theory workshop, the Research and Theory Section, and then becoming Vice President for Publications, Program Vice President, and NCFR President in 1991. I also have participated actively in the American Sociological Association, the Population Association of America, Society for Research on Adolescence, and the National Campaign to Prevent Teen Pregnancy (Miller, 1998).

Early in my professional career I studied marriage quality (Miller, 1975, 1976) and the transition to parenthood (Belsky & Miller, 1986; Miller & Meyers-Walls, 1983). One of the shifts in my professional focus has been away from studying such normal developmental patterns in marriage and family life to an emphasis on social problems (teen pregnancy), and finally to issues with which our family has had personal experiences (adoption). By far I have written the most about teen sexual behavior and pregnancy, especially linking these topics to family contexts and patterns (Miller, 1995; Miller & Fox, 1987; Miller & Heaton, 1991; Miller, Norton, Curtis, Hill, Schvaneveldt, & Young, 1997; Miller, Benson, & Galbraith, 2001). This is one area where my work will probably have a lasting impact. I also have had some influence on students and colleagues in my teaching and writing about family research methods.

The adoption research that I am just beginning also has the potential to influence the field, partly because our family's experiences have given me personal insights that complement my professional training. My collaboration with Hal Grotevant and other colleagues to analyze the National Longitudinal Study of Adolescent Health (AD Health) is beginning to produce some important insight about the adjustment of adopted adolescents (Miller, Fan, Christensen, Coyl, & Grotevant, 2000; Miller, Fan, Christensen, Grotevant, & van Dulman, 2000). It has been interesting (and refreshingly honest) to observe how the social scientific approach has shifted from denying the values and biases of investigators to recognizing that values are inherent in all of our work. I don't think it is wise to overreact, however, by discarding a century of research methods. In current research I consciously combine a constructionist perspective (Miller, 1993) with positivist methods of conducting research. This seems to be an appropriate reconciliation for me and perhaps for other researchers who seek to understand human behavior and family relationships. Most of all, I've appreciated working with graduate students, trying to figure out marriage and family issues, and enjoying the ride.

REFERENCES

Belsky, J. & Miller, B.C. (1986). Adolescent fatherhood in the context of the transition to parenthood. In A. Elster and M. Lamb (Eds.), *Adolescent fathers* (pp. 517-522). Hillsdale, NJ: Erlbaum.

Brodzinsky, D.M. & Schechter, M.D. (Eds.). (1990). *The psychology of adoption*. New York: Oxford University Press.

Klein, D.M., Jorgensen, S.J. & Miller, B.C. (1978). Research methods and developmental reciprocity in families. In R.M. Lerner and G.B. Spanier (Eds.), *Child influences on marital and family interaction: A life span perspective* (pp. 107-135). New York: Academic Press.

Klein, D.M., Schvaneveldt, J.D. & Miller, B.C. (1977). The attitudes and activities of contemporary family theorists. *Journal of Comparative Family Studies*, *8*, 1, 5-27.

Miller, B.C. (1975). Child density, marital satisfaction, and conventionalization: A research note. *Journal of Marriage and the Family*, *37*, 2, 345-347.

Miller, B.C. (1976). A multivariate developmental model of marital satisfaction. *Journal of Marriage and the Family*, *38*, 4, 643-657.

Miller, B.C. (1986). *Family research methods*. Beverly Hills: Sage.

Miller, B.C. (1993). Families, science, values: Alternative views of parenting effects and adolescent pregnancy. *Journal of Marriage and the Family*, *55*, 1, 7-21.

Miller, B.C. (1995). Risk factors for adolescent nonmarital childbearing. In *Report to Congress on out-of-wedlock childbearing*, (pp. 217-227). Washington, DC: Dept. of HHS. (DHHS Pub. No. (PHS) 95-1257).

Miller, B.C. (1998). *Families matter: A research synthesis of family influences on teen pregnancy*. Washington, D.C.: National Campaign to Prevent Teen Pregnancy.

Miller, B.C., Benson, B., & Galbraith, K.A. (2001). Family relationships and adolescent pregnancy risk: A research synthesis. *Developmental Review*, *21*, 1, 1-38.

Miller, B.C., Christensen, R. & Olson, T.D. (1987). Adolescent self-esteem in relation to sexual attitudes and behavior. *Youth and Society*, *19*, 1, 93-111.

Miller, B.C. & Coyl, D.D. (2000). Adolescent pregnancy in relation to infant adoption in the United States. *Adoption Quarterly*, *4*, 1, 3-25.

Miller, B.C. & Dyk, P.H. (1991). Community of Caring effects on adolescent mothers: A program evaluation case study. *Family Relations*, *40*, 3, 386-395.

Miller, B.C., Fan, X., Christensen, C., Coyl, D., Grotevant, H. R., & van Dulmen, M. (2000). Why adopted adolescents are more likely to receive psychological counseling: Adoptees' problems or parents' lower threshold for referral? *Journal of the American Academy of Child and Adolescent Psychiatry*, *39*, 12, 1504-1511.

Miller, B.C., Fan, X., Christensen, M., Grotevant, H. & van Dulmen, M. (2000). Comparisons of adopted and non adopted adolescents in a large nationally representative sample. *Child Development*, *71*, 5, 1458-1473.

Miller, B.C. & Fox, G.L. (1987). Theories of adolescent heterosexual behavior. *Journal of Adolescent Research*, *2*, 3, 269-282.

Miller, B.C., & Heaton, T.B. (1991). Age of first sexual intercourse and the timing of marriage and childbearing. *Journal of Marriage and the Family*, *53*, 3, 719-732.

Miller, B.C. & Jorgensen, S.J. (1988). Adolescent fertility-related behavior and its family linkages. In D. Klein and J. Aldous (Eds.), *Social stress and family development* (pp. 210-233). New York: Guilford Press.

Miller, B.C. & Klein, D.M. (1981). A survey of recent marriage and family texts. *Contemporary Sociology*, *10*, 1, 8-21.

Miller, B.C., McCoy, J.K., & Olson, T.D. (1986). Dating age and stage as correlates of adolescent sexual attitudes and behavior. *Journal of Adolescent Research*, *1*, 3, 361-371.

Miller, B.C., McCoy, J.K., Olson, T.D. & Wallace, C.M. (1986). Parental discipline and control attempts in relation to adolescent sexual attitudes and behavior. *Journal of Marriage and the Family*, *48*, 3, 503-512.

Miller, B.C., Monson, B.H., & Norton, M.C. (1995). The effects of forced sexual intercourse on white female adolescents. *Child Abuse and Neglect, 19*, 10, 1289-1301.

Miller, B.C. & Moore, K.A. (1990). Adolescent sexual behavior, pregnancy, and parenting: Research through the 1980s. *Journal of Marriage and the Family, 52*, 4, 1025-1044.

Miller, B.C. & Myers-Walls, J.A. (1983). Parenthood: Stresses and coping strategies. In C. Figley and H. McCubbin (Eds.), *Stress and the family* (pp. 54-73). New York: Bruner-Mazel.

Miller, B.C., Norton, M.C., Curtis, T., Hill, E.J., Schvaneveldt, P., Young, M.H. (1997). The timing of sexual intercourse among adolescents: Family, peer, and other antecedents. *Youth and Society, 29*, 3, 54-83.

Miller, B.C., Norton, M.C., Jenson, G.O., Lee, T.R., Christopherson, C.R., & King, P.K. (1993). Impact evaluation of FACTS & *feelings*: A home-based video sex education curriculum. *Family Relations, 42*, 4, 392-400.

Miller, B.C. & Olson, D.H. (1990). Types of marital interaction: Using cluster analysis. In T.W. Draper & A.C. Marcos (Eds.) *Family variables: Conceptualization, measurement and use* (pp. 67-89). Newbury Park, CA: Sage.

Miller, B.C., Rollins, B.C. & Thomas, D.L. (1982). On methods of studying marriages and families. *Journal of Marriage and the Family, 44*, 4, 851-873.

Miller, B.C. & Sneesby, K. (1988). Educational correlates of adolescents' sexual attitudes and behavior. *Journal of Youth and Adolescence, 17*, 6, 521-530.

Miller, B.C. & Sollie, D.L. (1980). Normal stresses during the transition to parenthood. *Family Relations, 29*, 4, 459-465.

Reiss, I.L. & Miller, B.C. (1979). Heterosexual permissiveness: A theoretical analysis. In W. Burr, R. Hill, I. Nye, and I.L. Reiss (Eds.), *Contemporary theories about the family* (pp. 57-100). New York: Free Press.

Schvaneveldt, P.L., Miller, B.C., Lee T.R., & Berry, E.H. (in press). Academic goals, achievement, and age at first sexual intercourse: Longitudinal, bidirectional influences. *Adolescence.*

Sollie, D.L. & Miller, B.C. (1980). The transition to parenthood as a critical time for building family strengths. In N. Stinnett, B. Chesser, H. DeFrain, and P. Knaub (Eds.), *Family strengths: Positive models for family life* (pp. 149-169). Lincoln, Nebraska: University of Nebraska Press.

The Way Things Were and Still Are

Harriette P. McAdoo

KEYWORDS. Autobiography, family, African American, self-concept, racial identity

INTRODUCTION

The educational and social achievements of my family are one of the family events of which I am most proud. For an African American family that is only four generations from the enslavement of Africans, these achievements are significant. As a family researcher of a certain age, I am in the position of knowing persons, for instance, my maternal grandfather, who grew up on a plantation and whose parents and older brothers were enslaved. I was raised in the segregated south, with all of the rampant injustices, but tempered by the securities provided to us by our families at that time. I lived through the civil rights movement. I missed being part of the Little Rock Nine only because, during that time, my father took a sabbatical in Detroit and we then went to Michigan State. Later my high school in Detroit, Central, was the campground for military tanks during the riots after Martin Luther King's death. So my impressions of events will naturally be at odds with many of those who did not have these experiences.

While I am on an integrated life projectory, I still am caught when persons not of color say or do things that I know are sexist and racist. Being Black is something that I am never able to forget. This double consciousness noted by DuBois (1903) is an element that does not go away. It is a way of seeing the world through White eyes and at the same time seeing it through Black eyes as a reality check. All together my family denies the expectations that many family researchers often believe about Black families: that they were born in poverty or are only one generation from poverty at the most. I feel that the grounding that I experienced within my own family contributed to my interest in conducting research and writing about children and families, particularly those of color.

GENEALOGY

My father was the first to finish elementary school in his family and he went on to obtain a Ph.D. from The University of Michigan in Speech and to be President of the first land-grant college for Negroes, Alcorn State University. My mother's family had been middle class for five generations, even in the last generation of enslavement. Every person, male and female, for the past four generations has obtained at least a Master's degree.

Paternal Family

I am the daughter of Anne Howard Russell Pipes and William Harrison Pipes. My father grew up in the Delta region of Mississippi, in an all-Black town by the Mississippi River, that had been all Black since the period of enslavement. My father's people were sharecroppers. Under the sharecropping system you didn't own the land, you had a little plot, you worked the land, and you turned over everything on that plot to the owner, and then he subtracted the food and the cost of living. Of course, you never made enough to get ahead so it ended up being a means of perpetuating enslavement. The schools for Negroes only went to the sixth grade, and to go higher, a person had to leave the state of Mississippi and go to Tuskegee Institute in Alabama. My father came back the first Christmas and the money he had saved for his bus back to school was spent by his mother. That scared him so much that he never came back until he finished high school. In Alabama, he went all the way through high school and college (BA English), and taught there for a year. He received his master's from Atlanta University in Atlanta, Georgia, and there he met my mother.

My paternal grandmother, Ada L. Bankhead Pipes, was from Alabama from the area in which the Bankheads originated. Senator Bankhead was one member, and Tallulah Bankhead was another, and all of them were related, Black and White. My grandmother was Black, White, and Native American. My paternal grandfather, Hezikiah Pipes, was from Mississippi and he was mostly Black and very poor. He died when my mother was in her seventh month of pregnancy with me, so I did not know him.

My father was one of two children. He had a sister, Hattie, who was two years older. My grandmother saved them both from a fire and in the process lost a third child. She never had any other children, a result that probably enabled my father to obtain a good education. This was a factor that contributed to my father's ability to leave Mississippi, one of Billingsley's (1968) "screen of opportunities."

Maternal Family

My mother's side was different because Anna Howard Russell was born to a professional family and they were the fourth generation of middle-class families. During the enslavement period, my maternal great-grandparents were slaves on a plantation in Kentucky. Her mother was a seamstress, and her father was a regular slave. My maternal grandfather was the youngest of the 16 boys, the only Russell son who was born after enslavement. The period of slavery is very real to me because people in my lifetime lived around people who had been slaves or whose parents were enslaved.

My mother's father was Harvey C. Russell. He went to Kentucky State for undergraduate work and received master's degrees from the University of Cincinnati in Business and Education. He worked both as a teacher and in real estate, and was considered "well off." He married Harriett Tucker Russell, who graduated from Fisk University. Her parents were Annie C. Vance Tucker and Rev. William Tucker, who had met as students at Berea College in Kentucky *before* it was segregated under the Jim Crow laws. She went on to become Lady Principal of Livingstone College. The Music department was named after her, as was a dormitory in the 1980s. Her mother, Harriett Vance, had a huge brick home that had been built by her white owner. The money from that house paid for my wedding in 1962, four generations later, along with other major expenses of the family expenses over the years.

When my mother was twelve years old, her mother died. My grandfather married again, to Julia Jones Russell, the daughter of a physician. Dr. Jones had been enslaved and his family had been hidden in the attic of a Quaker family for two years, where he was taught to read. He escaped and joined the Union army. He put himself through elementary and high school as well as college. He went to Howard University and received a medical degree.

My step-grandmother, Julia Jones Russell, was the grandmother I knew. She was my grandmother for 50 years. She died in December 1991 at the age of 96. I was very fortunate that I had grandparents until I was age 52, and parents up to age 53 years. So I was able to get a feeling of the family going back for generations because people were actually living. My mother was 76 when she died in 1991, whereas my father was 74 when he died in 1981.

My mother, the oldest of four, went to Kentucky State, where she completed her undergraduate work in three years because there were four other kids coming up right behind her and she wanted to go to graduate school. She received her master's degree from Atlanta University in English Literature. My parents worked for a while in the Black southern colleges, and then went to the University of Michigan for my father's doctorate.

Early Years

I was born in the student infirmary at Fort Valley State College in Georgia. We stayed there for three months and then returned to Ann Arbor. In 1943, my father finished his degree when I was three years old. Even though my mother had a master's degree and had taught on the college level for three years, she was forced to do housework for whites in Ann Arbor, for there were no other jobs for Negroes.

We moved from Ann Arbor to Southern University in Baton Rouge for two years, where my father was the head of the English Department. My mother also taught there. When I was five, we went to Alcorn State University, the first land-grant school for Negroes, where my father was president for four years and my mother taught in the English and Literature Department. When I was eight years old, we went to Little Rock, Arkansas, to Philander Smith College, where my father was the academic vice president and my mother was a member of the English faculty. We remained there for eight years and then my parents, my two siblings, and I moved to Wayne State for my father's sabbatical. Philander's President cut off my father's pay after three months because they suspected that he was not coming back. He then refused to go back. We cashed in all of our insurance and stayed in the Midwest. He went to Michigan State and was a member of the faculty for about twenty-five years. He retired as professor and lived about eight years after his retirement.

Thus, my family consists of traditional (multi-generations) middle class on my mother's side, and newly entered middle class on my father's side. My father helped his sister and niece go to Alcorn University. I find I'm very close to both of them. I am the oldest, and my sister, Willetta, is ten years younger. My mother and father had lost three children because of the RH-negative factor. Since Blacks usually don't have the RH-negative factor problem, my mother didn't get the medical diagnosis and care she needed, so the babies died. I was ten years old when my sister, Willetta Ada Pipes, was born, and this was something to which I looked forward. Even now, I do not recall ever being jealous, because it was something that we all wanted since my mom lost so many babies. When my sister was two months old my mother got pregnant again, a real surprise. This time they had a son, named William Howard Pipes.

Marriage and Family

I met John McAdoo when I was at Michigan State as a first-year graduate student. He was taking courses at Michigan State even though he was going to get his Master's of Social Work at the University of Michigan.

We married in December of 1962 and lived in East Lansing, Michigan, the year I finished my master's degree. John was doing social work in Flint on his state-sponsored award. We then moved to Ann Arbor, where John finished his last year of the MSW. I established the first classroom for special education at Milan High School and taught there for several years. At that point, I decided that I did not want to be teaching 20 years from then, so we decided to pursue our Ph.D.s together at Michigan.

John had two children by a previous marriage; his first wife had died after the second child was born prematurely. Thus, we have four children: a son, Michael, who was born in 1958; a son, John III, who was born in 1961; a daughter, Julia, who was born in 1964; and a son David, who was born eight years later in 1972, after we finished Michigan.

Doctoral Work

The period of our doctoral work in Ann Arbor in the '60s was very significant and was a very special time for us. We made friends who have remained dear to us throughout our lives. We were older than most and we had three children by that time, so our house was often where parties were held. This was the period of Viet Nam protest movements, which we participated in, with Julia in a stroller as we marched. The women's movement flourished and I participated in one of the main groups, composed of mothers of young children who stayed at home while their husbands were faculty members or graduate students. Then I realized that what we as Black women had all along, White women were just beginning to assert their rights to do. They were trying to reassure themselves that it was OK to go to work. Like my mother and grandmothers, I was already working, going to school, and still making time for my three children. I dropped out of the group because I did not have time to waste.

The Black Panther Party was active in Ann Arbor and all of our children were active in their Saturday morning schools. The Black movements were growing across the country. The growing demands for more Black enrollment resulted in our leadership in closing down the University of Michigan down under the BAM Strike. John and I had almost completed our dissertations and had more to lose than the other students, if the university had cracked down on us. But Michigan listened to us. John was even put on the faculty admission committee for the College of Education and the Psychology Department. Many Blacks were able to enter doctoral programs because of these actions.

I went to the University of Michigan at a time when there was a child development program major within the school of education. It was an excellent program because they had an experimental school doing creative research and scholarship. My three children were stimulus, the main emphasis for my area of work. My degree was in educational psychology, and my major professor was from the developmental psychology department. Dr. Lorraine Nadelman, a gifted developmental psychologist, was a significant factor in my professional development.

Although there was an undergraduate Introduction to the Family course in the sociology department, there were no graduate courses in family when I was there. I became interested and did a lot of reading and ended up emphasizing the study of families more than children in my educational program.

I became involved in research even though I had no initial interest in such endeavors. Initially, I believed that research was something you suffered through, but eventually I found that I really liked it. I ended up taking the three basic research courses required in education and psychology as well as sociology research courses in the Detroit Area Study for my fieldwork. I became adept in instrument and questionnaire development and also worked as a statistical consultant for about a year and a half. This training matured into helping faculty and students identify research problems, the design of studies, and methods of implementation. I found that I could do this consulting very well and the experience taught me the desire to do research on my own.

ACADEMIC TEACHING AND RESEARCH

Howard University

With all of the activism and the growing emphasis on the Black Consciousness Movements, we decided that we would not go to a White university, but to Howard University instead. After graduation, we went to Howard University in 1970, where they wanted me to teach human development and not primarily to do research. I chaired the Human Growth and Development Sequence and John chaired the Research Sequence. In the 1970s, social work schools employed graduates from different disciplines. We joined the faculty with three psychologists, an economist, and someone in African History. This occurred mainly in the 1970s, when there were few persons with Doctorates in Social Work (DSW). Consequently, social work graduate schools had to rely on psychology, sociology, and education departments to obtain faculty to teach their classes at the graduate level. As a result, it was a very exciting time.

I wanted to keep my research skills, but I had to teach the two courses in Human Development. I always kept a separate research course. I was teaching a 50% overload, but had a lot of energy and didn't even think anything of it. I was able to use my research skills and at the same time, remained current in human development. John taught at Howard for five years and then joined the University of Maryland faculty. Howard was a very interesting place to be for twenty years because it was winding down from the pinnacle where Howard was considered the capstone. It had experienced the student riots in 1969. The majority of white teachers were driven away from Howard. Howard needed to get away from an almost anti-Black attitude than many of the professors had. Many of these faculty were good but held antiquated attitudes about Blacks. The ones who stayed on ended up being very good because they were the ones who had gone through all the questioning and had decided to stay and those are the ones who greeted us upon our arrival.

We came when Andrew Billingsley was the Academic Vice President and, at that point, he was hiring young Black Ph.D.s from all over the country to replace the white teachers who left. We had a very interesting period, because there were older, well-trained people, and then younger people who had the degrees not only from Black schools, but also from White universities that were not Ivy League. Many of the older ones had gone to the Ivy League schools, Harvard, Yale, and

Princeton, and many had an MSW, but not a PhD. There was a real mix, and it was a real challenge. Many of those new people thirty years later stayed at Howard and assumed leadership positions. It is very interesting that the group that arrived during the 1970s ended up taking over the University in the 1990s. The Academic Vice President, the Research Vice President, deans, and many other professors were people who came from that particular group of young Ph.D.s in the 1970s.

We worked strenuously and did a lot of fighting at faculty meetings. I have strong memories of what happened and it was basically the old group fighting against all the new people. We had many scars from it, but I think we did very well. All those coming to Howard were young people in their 30s, and the people who were over 50 were quite threatened and they did everything they could to stop us. We ended up prevailing.

I enjoyed teaching and did a good job. Eventually, I started going into my classes without any preparation. It went well for a couple of years, then it began to get boring. At that point, I was very active in getting my proposal funded and I began taking visiting professorships. I went to Smith College School for Social Work for three summers, because they do didactic teaching during the summers, and the students have placements in the year. I could stay at Howard and still do something different. I was a visiting professor at the George Brown School of Social Work in St. Louis and at Michigan State University and the University of Minnesota. I had opportunities to teach policy and about ethnic minority families because of a pattern in which all of the White schools brought Blacks to teach the ethnic courses. And one of the things we know is that ethnicity is something that can be tacked on. It's not really worth hiring somebody full-time, but it's something you could bring people in to do. So, although I did that at Smith, I was also doing policy on both the master's and doctorate levels, and supervising research.

Research Grants

In my dissertation at Michigan, I had examined the variables of racial attitude and self-concept. I used two samples, one involving children from Mound Bayou, Mississippi, where my father grew up, and a second involving children from Dearborn Heights, Michigan. What I wanted to do was examine whether growing up in an integrated environment had an impact on children that was different from growing up in an all-Black community. I found that, in both cases, self-concept was positive. I didn't find any support for the idea that Black children had deficits in self-concept. Instead, their self-concepts were very normal with the same standard deviation found in White children. I did find, though, that children who live within an all-Black area are significantly higher in self-esteem. This was explained by the fact that children who grew up in an all-Black area did not have to deal with racism in subtle ways that children in the North faced. Although the racial attitudes of the children were very similar, they preferred White over Black, probably because they were watching TV everyday. That is, they were getting the same messages as children living in integrated areas–it is better to be White than it is to be Black.

I received a small faculty grant at Howard University and went back five years later to talk to the parents and retest the children. Although their self-concepts were still high, the same racial attitude persisted in a very pro-Black area. I became interested in families because I realized you can't look at children and ignore families.

With a grant from the Office of Education, I was able to bring in faculty from public school systems all over the country and give them a solid grounding in research methodology. They would return home, collect their data, and then, during the second summer session, write their result. This was a large grant and the first major grant that our school had ever received, which meant that the university had to make rules left and right. I guess that if I had been any older, I would have given up, but it really was very good.

A research project from the Office of Child Development replicated one of my dissertation topics, the racial attitudes and self concept of Black children. Using children in the Washington, D.C., area, I selected 100 children who were Black. These children represented both the American population and children from Africa attached to the various embassies (both children of embassy staff, and children whose parents were workers). So we had a very marked class difference, as well as income difference, between working class and middle class Black children.

I found that the children from Africa (and they represented many different countries) had a much stronger sense of self-concept and racial identity. This was probably because African children were not forced to deal with non-Black people at a very early age like children from the D. C. area, Michigan, and Mississippi areas in the U.S.

Then I received a faculty grant to go to Nairobi, Kenya. I spent time talking with women and used the questionnaire I had developed to pursue some research. I examined families over the generations, as they moved from more rural to the more urban settings. I was interested in discovering the forces related to the ability of women, who were parents and who were professional, to cope effectively with their families and children. They had grown up in the context of traditional lifestyles in which men were dominant and women, in many cases, were subservient. Despite these circumstances, many of these women had done very well in their lives.

At that same time, I was developing a study in which I combined the child and the parent emphasis with a sample from a suburban Maryland area. The focus of this study was on parent-child interaction in two-parent Black and White families of middle-class social status. I examined the interactions and verbal nuances of these families under controlled situations, and the racial attitudes and self-concept data from the children. This was a grant that John and I worked on and it allowed me to take a leave from Howard and just work on the research. I loved that period of my life.

I had another grant (NIMH) in which I was studying middle-class Blacks. This was the early 1970s, and I wanted to reexamine what I had found in Kenya, the intergenerational transfer of mobility, social class status, education, and how that had influenced the stress levels of both mothers and fathers. For this study, I picked a suburban and urban sample and examined the two-parent families and one-parent families. All of the sample was middle-class, with two-thirds of the sample being two-parent families and one-third consisting of one-parent families. Many significant differences existed between the women of the married couples and the single-parent women. I then decided to apply for funding to enable me to study single mothers under NIH.

I looked at single mothers, both working class and middle class. About half of these families had children when they were married, but the family split because of divorce, whereas the other half had children as teenagers and never married. I again looked at mobility, coping strategies, stress levels as well as a lot of different variables. Because, at that time, the government was changing, I felt that if I did not get the data gathered rapidly, I probably would never have an opportunity to do so. This ended up being true because the administration changed. The Republicans came in and money for information about Blacks was cut off. Many of the Blacks who were involved in working on projects or Whites who were working on Black populations found that their monies were cut off when the Republicans got in.

White House Conference on Families

I should mention that I was a participant in the White House Conference on Families, the National Advisory Council planning group, as a

Presidential Appointee of President Jimmy Carter. This was an excellent experience involving two years of going to hear people from all over the country, hearing them testify, hearing pain from a lot of families. This was a significant turning point in my life. I chaired two of the sessions in different cities, with a registered parliamentarian on each side of me. This was when the right-to-life people were building up steam. I became even more interested in families, and became very involved in a lot of organizations. I believe that if things had been different then politically, we might have had some very significant projects, efforts, programs, and policies related to families.

At that point I wrote many grants, seeking to examine the impact of what was happening to families as programs dried up and people became entrenched, but, of course, these efforts were not funded. To do so would allow someone to come in and document some of the things that were going on at the national and local level. So, I returned to seeking faculty grants and received a grant relating to adolescent mothers. It seems the only money that was available was related to Blacks, females, and adolescent pregnancy. A lot of this was stereotypical, of course, in the sense that the only concern of the administration about the Black family was to examine adolescent pregnancy.

We were working on a project with women who were young girls and their grandmothers who were available at Howard University Hospital. This was very good, but very difficult, with the main accomplishment being that we supported several students and they were able to get their degrees. We weren't able to get a lot of data, primarily because our chosen design required mothers who had babies that didn't get pregnant a subsequent time. We lost most of our population because after their first baby, they then had their second and third babies. At that point, I was getting to be much more involved nationally with NCFR, Groves, and with the Society for Research on Child Development. I was selected to the SRCD Governing Council and became involved in national, high level group work for six years that was a great learning experience.

National Council of Family Relations

A bit later, I was elected to the Board of Directors for the National Council of Family Relations primarily because of my previous work for the Ethnic Minority Section. The Ethnic Minority Section was started by Bob Staples and was taken up by Marie Peters, who really put a lot of heart and guts into the program. She deliberately let Staples take over the leadership in Philadelphia, who provided leadership that changed it from a caucus to a section. I was elected Caucus and then Section President, which subsequently led to the NCFR Board. This was very interesting because it was a different structure from SRCD, with people representing sections rather than representing the whole membership. I served on the Board of Directors for a while and then was the Program Vice President. Subsequently, we had a program on ethnicity in Dearborn and I was rewarded the first Marie Peters award. This was really nice because it showed that many people were aware of my hard work for the Section and the Board level.

Groves Conference on Marriage and Family

At the same time, we were active in Groves and there were times when I wondered which one of the professional groups we were working on, because Groves and NCFR tended to flow back and forth in many ways. Groves is an area that I felt particularly close to. We have been able to go back for over 25 years now. We've gotten to be very close, and we've seen people develop, grow up, and we've seen them die. It has been a real family experience. I was invited by Marie Peters, because she wanted to get more Blacks involved. We'd put on a workshop on whatever the topic was that year, related to African American families. This went on for about five or six years, and we would have a different theme and different people, many of which would come in and out and we were able to introduce many other people to Groves. I got to know Marie Peters even better. She was so great in helping the careers of people who were a little bit younger than she was, and my career was definitely helped by Marie. I cannot say enough about her. She was a very self-effacing person. If she had been a different person, she would have been the type who would have gone and gotten all the awards, but instead, she facilitated many other people to advance up the professional career ladder.

I was on the Groves Board of Directors and then I was the Program Vice Chair. We went to the Bahamas, where we did "Groves in the Bahamas." At that point, the program chair and the conference chair was one person, not divided as it is today. Because it was an international group, I had to take care of travel and hotel arrangements and I learned to appreciate all the good Groves people. The decisions became intimately involved. We had to make arrangements for hotel rooms, who was staying with whom, and who was fighting and wanted to change. It was totally interesting and I was energetic. I took on a lot of work and had an excellent secretary, and everything went off nicely. Our travel agent really devoted a lot of time and effort to this and, not only did we have a good time, but we made over $1,000 for Groves. We ended up using the theme "Family Ethnicity: Strengths and Diversity." I was elected to the Groves Board, so overall, at the national level, Groves has really been my professional home.

Writing

I took a leave in 1991 at the end of the summer because my mother unexpectedly died. She had come to my daughter's wedding in June and the minute she stepped off the plane we knew she was seriously ill, though she had not let anybody know. She decided that she was going to go to her granddaughter's wedding, and would not let us take her to a doctor or the hospital until after the wedding. After the wedding, we had to convince her to go to the hospital. She died about six weeks later, but she was there for the wedding. We came home to Michigan after three weeks to go through her things and found just too many things to go through quickly. There were so many things of my father's to go through that we decided that we couldn't do it in the week and a half that we had planned. Consequently, we took a leave of absence and took a standing offer of positions that Michigan State had made a few years earlier.

We decided two weeks before the beginning of the semester that we would take the year to go through my parents' things as we lived in my parents' home. It allowed us to go through my parents' things and we had an emotionally satisfying time. I had come to Michigan two years earlier as a Visiting Professor during the summer, so it was very natural to come back here. We were able to move into my parents' house. One of the things I would say to almost anybody who has a chance to do this at the death of their parents is to go home if you can and go through their things. I had a whole year to go through their things and because they were both professors, they had all sorts of scribblings, and my father had written four books, including *Say Amen, Brother*, and *The Death of an Uncle Tom*. My mother had not written, but she was going to write about English literature. But, of course, one of those things–once she retired, she never got it written. Both my father and my mother had kept files on the books that they were going to write, some related to civil rights. I found so many valuable pieces of information. Articles, they always clipped out articles, and now I know why I still do that. They clipped out articles, wrote all over them, and had written all sorts of notes in many of their books. One of the things I'm finding is that by understanding your parents better, you can then understand yourself a little bit more. So it was a very, very good year.

As far as my writing has been concerned, I have published five books: *Women and Children: Alone and in Poverty* (Pearce & McAdoo, 1981); *Services to Young Families: Program Review and Policy Recommendations* (Parham & McAdoo, 1985); *Black Children: Social, Educational and Parental Environments* (McAdoo & McAdoo, 1985); *Black Families (3rd ed.)* (McAdoo, 1997); and *Family Ethnicity: Strength in Diversity (2nd ed.)* (McAdoo, 1999). Numerous articles and book chapters were also published.

Black Families (McAdoo, 1997) was an edited edition that has become almost a classic used in family courses across the country. It sells itself now. Everybody at every course at the graduate level appears to want to have it. It is quoted in almost every article about Black families that has come out in the last ten years. Two of the people have died and therefore, I don't want to change their articles. When I examine other articles in this book, there is nothing that needs to be changed because the material remains so much on target that it really doesn't need to be updated.

My husband and I edited *Black Children*, which was also a Sage edition. *Black Children* and *Black Families* were Sage focus editions (McAdoo, 2000). The emphasis was on children, examining them carefully, looking at their racial attitudes and the environments in which children are born. We covered educational environments, social environments, and parental environments by soliciting articles. It is a very good experience to edit a book, but a very time-consuming one. We could have written the book much more easily, but it was something that I felt really needed to be done.

Family Ethnicity: Strength in Diversity began as a Groves book, but over the years, as we added or subtracted, we ended up with an edition that is really different from the original that looked at ethnic families of color. I looked at African American, Native American, and Asian American families, plus families of different religious groups. I asked persons from these particular ethnic/religious groups to relate how families are impacted by what we know about the families. What do their families cherish? What do they value? What, in particular, are the heartaches and joys of their particular group?

John's Death

The death of John was doubly hard on me. He was my husband and the father of my children, but he was also my co-author, co-writer, and research partner. It was a good combination. But I wonder if it would have been easier if we had been in different fields. There are so many changes that you must go through just at the death of a spouse that are even more complicated with the death of a co-worker. I would caution students about the consequences of working together very closely. In addition to the difficulty of finding two positions in similar areas within a university, there are the hardships of having your work become too intertwined. But I would not have had it any different than it was. Our being so close meant that we always had things to talk about.

John had leukemia, a slow-acting cancer of the blood that should have taken him many years beyond retirement. But in only 10% of cases it transposes into lymphoma, a fast-acting cancer, for which there is no treatment beyond the regular chemotherapy. So John was teaching his classes spring semester as usual, but he went rapidly downhill during the summer of 1994. That summer was a sad, but good time for my entire family. Everybody, friends and family, came to visit for a while. All of the children came. John insisted that they let him come home to see the beautiful animals and to be able to hold his new grandson, John Lewis IV. He also felt a lot of pain that he did not let us know about until it became severe. Eventually three of us had to sleep in the room with John and we became even closer then. I would be sound asleep and not even hear the activity that was going on around me on the bed until 6:00 the next morning, when I would take over again.

After he died I kept on teaching as usual, for I would not have known what to do with myself. His memorial was Monday evening and I taught a three-hour class on Wednesday morning, fortunately with a guest lecturer. My going to work was my therapy. I went through many changes and am still going through changes. I became interested in grief therapy and writing for a while, but I decided that it was too close to me to really get too involved. It was really interesting to note the changes in the behaviors of friends toward me, though. Many became distant and withdrew. Couples that we had been close to evaporated into thin air. I had to slowly make a new set of friends for myself.

We had just started a five-year research project from NICHD when John became ill, but I was forced to go on with it. Many students were involved and I could not let them down. It has ended up being a really positive element in my life over the years. I finished an article entitled "The Dynamics of African American Father's Family Roles" (McAdoo & McAdoo, 1997-98) that we had been writing about a year after his death. So the work has gone on, though slower than before.

My Research

As far as my research is concerned, it has followed my changes in interest over the years: racial attitudes, self-concept, and then gradually greater focus on families and parent-child interactions, with increasing attention to middle-class families. There are some things about middle-class families that are not getting into the literature because of the overemphasis of the stereotypical view of African Americans as being mothers on welfare, single adolescent mothers, or young boys on dope. A goal of mine has been to examine families, just normal families, middle-class families, working-class families, and place emphasis, not only on their strengths, but on their strategies–for instance, the extended family. At the same time, I provide statistics; I keep my data current to help people realize that there is more than just the negative view presented about African American families. I think this would be one of my major contributions.

As I write about different stages, I find that Black families are just like White families in many ways. There are concerns and conditions that impact families of color much more seriously than for families who are not of color. What I want to try to get a picture of is that within each family setting, there are everyday people doing everyday things. I don't want to examine families as people who don't have things or who have deficits, but look at basically the majority of families who are working-class or middle-class, going to work and raising their children everyday. They are doing what families do all over the world, loving them, hating them, and cuddling up with them. I want to show how Black families are similar to other families, but with a few extra problems because of discrimination and discriminatory practices that are being directed at the families' children.

AUTHOR NOTE

Address correspondence to: Harriette P. McAdoo, 106 Morrill Hall, Michigan State University, East Lansing, MI 48824.

REFERENCES

Billingsley, A. (1968). *Black families in White America*. Englewood Cliffs, NJ: Prentice Hall.

DuBois, W. E. B. (1903). *The soul of Black folk: Essays and sketches*. Chicago: McClurg.

McAdoo, H. P. (Ed.). (2000). *Black children: Social, educational, and parental environments (2nd ed.).* Thousand Oaks, CA: Sage.

McAdoo, H. P. (Ed.). (1999). *Family ethnicity: Strength in diversity (2nd ed.).* Thousand Oaks, CA: Sage.

McAdoo, H. P. (Ed.). (1997). *Black families, (3rd ed.).* Thousand Oaks, CA: Sage.

McAdoo, H. P., & McAdoo, J. L. (Eds.). (1985). *Black children: Social, educational and parental environments.* Beverly Hills, CA: Sage.

McAdoo, H. P. & McAdoo, J. L. (1997-98). The dynamics of African American father's family roles. *Michigan Council of Family Relations, 3*, 1, pp. 7-15.

Parham, T. M. J., & McAdoo, H. P. (Eds.). (1985). *Services to young families: Program review and policy recommendations.* Washington, DC: American Public Welfare Association.

Pearce, D. & McAdoo, H. (1981). *Women and Children: Alone and in Poverty.* Washington, DC: U.S. Government Printing Office. [This monograph was entered in its entirety into the *Congressional Record* in April 1982; reprinted by the Women's Research and Education Institute, Washington, DC; and reissued by the Center for National Policy Review, Catholic University Law School.]

Observing Families: Their Contexts and Consequences

Rand D. Conger

KEYWORDS. Autobiography, family economic stress, family processes, children and adolescence

INTRODUCTION

Over the years, I have emphasized a research strategy that involves observing interactions among family members and studying how the quality of those interactions is affected by social events and conditions outside the home. A subsequent link in this strategy is to examine the consequences of different types of family processes for the developmental course of adults and children. The present task involves turning the camera on myself and attempting to observe how the events and circumstances of my life have influenced my development as a student of the family. Such retrospection, of course, is fraught with the potential for error, primarily because the people we are today affects the kind of lens through which we view the past. But there is one truth about my history about which I am certain. At each point in my life I have had the good fortune to benefit from interactions with a series of exceptional people. Without their influence, I would not enjoy the opportunities I have experienced in my profession. Drawing on this perspective, the following pages consider the pathways I have followed in terms of the people most central to the decisions that have affected my scientific career.

BEING RAISED IN A CHILD-CENTERED HOME

My parents grew up and began their family in Tacoma, Washington, where I was born. My parents put their children first; all six of them, one of whom died as a toddler in a tragic accident. They had more children than they could comfortably afford, but there was never any doubt that their priority was their children's best interests. As I think back to their influence on my life, I try to consider both the social and biological processes that might have been involved. Certainly both genes and social interaction play a role in how parents affect their children, and in each regard my parents likely influenced me in different developmental domains. The traits they clearly shared included their penchant for hard work, the importance they placed on meeting one's responsibilities in life, and their dedication to family and children. Interestingly, they also had enormous respect for people with an advanced education, such as doctors, lawyers and university professors, even though my mother received only a high school diploma and my father never completed high school. Beyond these similar traits and values, however, they provided very different models and motivations in my life.

My mother's central priorities involved the people with whom she was close. My last memory of her is sitting in her small apartment with her family gathered around her shortly before her death. The doctor had let us know that she would not survive more than a few days or weeks, and that we should say our good-byes soon. She sat in her rocking chair, almost deaf and almost blind but with her mind still clear, listening to the cacophony of voices and other noises in a room stuffed with her children and grandchildren. She had a huge smile on her face that reflected the bliss she experienced when her family was around her. Her entire life reflected this dedication to her children and their well-being. She delayed working outside the home until her middle years when her children were well on their way in school. She was active in PTA, regularly communicated with teachers, and was always available to discuss the events and concerns in her children's lives.

Her efforts for her family grew from her conviction that children do best when they know they are loved and monitored, and that what they do has consequences in their lives. Simply put, she demonstrated the characteristics that we try to instill in parents in the educational programs available today. Moreover, these activities came at significant cost to her creature comforts. We were a relatively poor family and she was a bright woman, capable of doing well in the labor force. But her priority was her family, and she chose to spend her time focusing on the lives of her children. For her it was the appropriate choice, as she experienced no greater joy than being with them and, later in life, with her grandchildren. I directly benefited from the attention I received from my mother. When things went poorly for me in school, she was available to provide a helping hand. When I did not know how to solve a social dilemma, she helped to consider alternative solutions to the problem. She was always there when I needed advice or guidance, even long after childhood. And she provided a model of dedication and hard work with an emphasis on close family relationships. Looking back to my mother's influence, there seems little mystery as to why I would be interested in studying families and in how I acquired the work ethic required to pursue that goal.

As I read the above paragraphs, they suggest that I have conveyed a kind of sainthood on my mother. These characteristics shine through, however, even though she experienced all of the frustrations and conflicts that parents do with their children. Moreover, compared to my father, she qualified for sainthood given the equanimity she displayed in response to the machinations of her offspring. Compared with my mother, my father demonstrated a greater range of competing characteristics that appeared to operate in conflict with one another. His attitudes and behaviors reflected significant contrasts of both impulse and conservatism, which resolved in the direction of conservatism as he aged. His impulsiveness is best represented by the time he ran away from home as a teenager to serve as a merchant mariner on a tramp steamer. As with many of his more daring exploits, this one was cut short when he became extremely ill and his parents had to travel from Tacoma, Washington, to San Francisco to bring him home. His conservatism was reflected in a life of hard work that he pursued to maintain the health and well-being of his family. He also was a gifted athlete who considered becoming a professional boxer or a professional golfer. Here genes failed me, as I inherited none of those gifts. He was extremely bright and tested well on standardized examinations, but was too impatient to stay in school and further his education. Throughout his life, however, he read widely and it seems clear that these interests were passed on to me.

In fairness, my father entered adulthood during the economic chaos of the 1930s, married and had children early, and experienced significant economic insecurity until he got a position with the U.S. Postal Service. At the time he went to work for the government, civil service tests alone determined selection for employment. Given the dire economic times, he had to compete with doctors, lawyers, and other extremely well-educated individuals for a position. His views reflected these early experiences and he admonished his children to find economically stable jobs, even at the expense of personal satisfaction. If he had grown up in the modern era, with educational loans widely available and greater economic opportunities, I am sure that he would have gone on for some type of university training. As it was, he frequently worked one or more jobs in addition to his position with the Post Office to assure the economic well-being of his family. After several moves within the postal system, he relocated our family to San Jose, California, where I spent most of my childhood and adolescence. In addition to his devotion to his family, I was always struck by my father's incredible workload as he attempted to make ends meet with a large family and too little income from his primary occupation. I am certain that my professional interest in family economic stress is driven to a significant degree by my father's struggles to maintain a family in the face of economic hardships.

Adolescence and the Early Adult Years

As noted, my parents encouraged all of their children to work hard and to pursue advanced education. These values affected my childhood and adolescent years, as I did reasonably well in school and planned to go on to the university. Although none of my three brothers completed a college degree, my older sister became an elementary school teacher and I gained some understanding from her about the college experience. During high school, then, my sights were set to go on for a college education. Two of my high school instructors, in particular, had a telling impact on these plans and on my future career. One of these teachers offered a course in philosophy in which he encouraged his students to look beyond the relatively insulated environs of suburban San Jose to consider the views of other people in other places and other times. He produced in me an understanding that one must pursue an issue in depth and from multiple perspectives to truly gain a perspective on it. That lesson has aided me in my studies ever since. The second major influence came from an English teacher who admonished her students to consider different pathways for their lives. She extolled the virtues of pursuing lives that are creative and that may make a difference in the broader society. I was especially struck by the notion of doing something creative and initially attempted to express that creativity through a career in music.

As did many of my compatriots, I sought to develop my limited musical talents in the music scene in the Bay Area of the 1960s. I attended San Jose State University part time and played a range of guitar music in the small clubs and coffeehouses that flourished at that time. Eventually I moved from folk and blues guitar to classical guitar and taught and performed in both the San Francisco area and in Denver, where I eventually relocated. During this time I also married and had two children.

Although my marriage eventually ended in divorce, my children remain a mainstay of my life. After several years of part-time schooling and less-than-phenomenal success as an itinerant musician, in 1970 I decided that I needed to find my creativity in some other line of work. That motivation led me to pursue a bachelor's degree in the sociology program at Arizona State University, which proved to be one of the best decisions of my life. Initially I thought that I would pursue a career in social work, and the department offered a minor in social welfare, which could be used to pursue that ambition. That early goal for helping troubled individuals and families has continued to be reflected in research that identifies developmental and social mechanisms that have applied significance. Two extraordinary individuals who fostered my interest in science permanently altered my career direction at ASU, however.

Professor Richard Nagasawa, who was then an assistant professor of sociology, introduced me to the logic of science. In a series of remarkable courses he charted the philosophical underpinnings for contemporary scientific inquiry and revealed the simple but compelling arguments for correlational and experimental research designs. He also introduced his students to the substantial similarities and differences between research aimed at understanding fundamental scientific principles and research designed to evaluate the practical significance of a social program or policy. Before I attended Dick's courses, I viewed science as a dry and laborious activity sure to dull the senses and diminish one's existence; views that were no doubt holdovers from the flower child environment of Northern California. After attending his lectures, I was struck by the power and elegance of this approach to understanding the social world. Professor Nagasawa also aided my development as a social scientist by becoming involved in a senior research project I completed at ASU and by helping me get accepted into his graduate program in sociology at the University of Washington. Thinking in terms of current interest in "turning points" in life, Dr. Nagasawa's instruction, advice and guidance certainly helped turn my trajectory from a career in social work to one in the social sciences.

Equally significant during my undergraduate years at ASU, Professor Peter Killeen, an assistant professor in psychology, provided me with a whole different perspective on human and animal behavior. At that time Peter was primarily involved in research that extended the work of Skinner and Herrnstein, two of his mentors at Harvard University. I was quite taken by the simplicity and power of the behavioral paradigm, which was remarkably effective in predicting and mathematically describing the behavior of experimental subjects in response to environmental contingencies of reward and punishment. In a sense, the behavioral approach in psychology was quite consistent with sociological theory and research that attempted to identify social contingencies that influence the behavior of groups and individuals. Peter generously provided the tutoring and laboratory equipment necessary for me to test a set of behavioral principles involving the "matching law" in an experiment with undergraduates in a small group setting. In the experiment we were able to demonstrate that discussion in a small group conformed to predictions from this behavioral principle. That is, the proportion of verbalizations directed by a targeted individual toward other members of the group was equal to the proportion of reinforcement other group members provided for the content of those verbalizations.

The success of this simple experiment, in which we controlled the rate of reinforcement provided by group members, convinced me that I might be capable of entering the world of social and behavioral science. It taught me something about observing and recording behavioral interactions, a methodology that has played an important role in my work throughout my career. It also convinced me of the importance of contingencies of reinforcement and punishment in social life, although my theoretical views have expanded far beyond this simple paradigm across the years. This undergraduate research project also identified the graduate program I wanted to enter at the University of Washington, where a group of social psychologists had become involved in something called "Behavioral Sociology." The project also led to my first publication during my graduate student days (Conger & Killeen, 1974). In all that he taught me and in all the extraordinary support he provided to allow me to experience the exhilaration of scientific inquiry, I owe a fundamental debt of gratitude to Peter Killeen. Surely, without the influence of Drs. Killeen and Nagasawa, I would not have had the opportunities in the world of social science that I have enjoyed. With these important undergraduate experiences behind me, in 1972 I set off for a graduate career at the University of Washington.

GRADUATE SCHOOL

University of Washington

Despite my aversion to writing course papers and taking examinations, graduate school was quite wonderful. To begin with, after two years in the hot and arid Southwest, the cool climate and lush vegetation of the Pacific Northwest provided a delightful change of scenery. In addition, the Department of Sociology had an outstanding faculty. My primary interests included social psychology, social deviance, and research methodology, areas in which the department excelled. Of special significance was the link that several of the social psychologists in the department had made between contingencies of social reinforcement and the behaviors of individuals and groups. Burgess, Emerson, and Schmidt were all doing important theoretical or empirical work in this area. Burgess's recent edited volume on behavioral sociology was an important factor that attracted me to the University of Washington, along with the fact that they were the first graduate program to offer me an assistantship! My behavior too was related to the significant daily contingencies of life.

It is difficult to untangle all of the important influences during graduate school that shaped my later career. Certainly the wonderful methodological training from sociologists like Blalock, Costner, and Hargins gave me a firm base on which to develop later research projects. The education in social deviance was first rate, with instructors such as Burgess, Costner, Schrag and Weiss. Also important was fellowship support I received for the study of social deviance from the National Institute of Mental Health. Although my major areas of study did not include demography, Professor Sam Preston had an important influence on my approach to sociological inquiry and stands out as the best teacher I ever had in a graduate or undergraduate course. He had a remarkable ability to convey clearly the most complex information and to bring to life the everyday importance of demographic issues. He also helped support my graduate career through a fellowship in demography. I also profited from several courses in the Department of Psychology where I learned a great deal about a psychological approach to both human development and research methodology from some of the best researchers in the country, including Professors Edwards, Robinson, Sackett, and Slaby.

Many of the most important lessons I learned at the University of Washington came from informal discussions as well as from formal coursework. For example, I can still remember a conversation with Phil Blumstein, then an assistant professor of sociology, in which we were discussing the relative merits of different approaches to social psychology. Given my theoretical bent at the time, I was telling him about all of the reasons that a behavioral approach seemed the most rational paradigm for our discipline. My perspective could not have been further from Dr. Blumstein's view on the subject, but he was very kind in his debate with a beginning graduate student. He simply concluded our discussion with the suggestion that it would seem ill-advised to throw out so much that is unique and important in human experience by adopting a singularly behavioral perspective. Of course he was right, and that simple observation motivated me to explore more vigorously other approaches to understanding individual and social behavior. Another important informal influence was the work of Jerry Patterson and John Reid in Eugene, Oregon. They had begun to show how behavior observed in families played an important role in the development of antisocial and delinquent behavior. They became two of my most important mentors at a distance. Their work pushed me toward the study of antisocial behavior in relation to family interactions using an observational approach similar to, but much more elaborate than, the one that Peter Killeen and I had used in our small group experiment at Arizona State.

The most influential faculty member during my graduate career, and the person with whom I worked most closely, was Professor Robert Burgess. Given his interests in the implications of the behavioral paradigm for understanding social behavior, it was natural that I would seek him out as my graduate advisor at the University of Washington. I took a series of courses from him that detailed his views on contingencies of social interaction and eventually developed a dissertation prospectus that drew on but extended this perspective. Early in our association Bob provided important feedback in the development of an article that compared and empirically tested ideas from both social learning and social control theories in the explanation of delinquent behavior. This report presaged current interest in the integration of social control and social learning principles in the explanation of delinquency. That paper eventually was published and continues to be cited from time to time in the criminological literature (Conger, 1976).

By 1974 I had accepted a part-time position as a program evaluator for an agency in Tacoma, Washington, that served families in which a child had been abused or neglected. The federal agency that funded the program became interested in more fundamental studies of social and behavioral processes that increase risk for child maltreatment. Bob and I decided to develop a proposal for the agency that could meet many research goals, including the production of data for my doctoral dissertation. We reasoned that, if funded, the project would give us the opportunity to apply many of the ideas in Patterson's and Reid's work to the problems of abuse and neglect. The study also would allow us to evaluate whether behavioral or social learning principles could help explain the occurrence of these important social problems.

Penn State University

After submitting the grant proposal, Bob accepted a position at Penn State University. Fortunately, the proposal was funded and we shifted the research site from Tacoma to rural Pennsylvania. During 1975, I moved to Penn State to oversee the research project and to begin work on my dissertation.

This project tested my ability to interview, observe, and encode information about family interaction processes and experiences. We observed families in their homes using small digital devices that recorded numbers identified to represent specific forms of behavior between family members, e.g., hostile or supportive actions. Observers scored behaviors in real time as the families engaged in structured games or discussions. This research involved many young children of pre-school age as well as those in the elementary grades. Families were identified by child protective services as either abusive or neglectful of their children. We selected control families from the same communities where the problem families lived. The technology for this early work seems medieval compared to current research practices. Scored behavioral observations were actually entered onto computer cards via teletype and then submitted to analysis. Thus, it took more time to prepare the data for computer entry than to score it in the first place. But the results of the research were extremely important as they demonstrated that it was contingencies in the daily behaviors of parents and children that increased risk for child abuse and neglect. Particularly important was the finding that abusive families generated an environment of interpersonal negativity that primed family members for more serious forms of violence. The central findings of the research were reported in Burgess and Conger (1978).

For my development as a family researcher, my personal interactions with the families in this study were as important as the quantitative findings. In many respects the parents in the study were victims of their own history. Most were poor, had several children, had children at an early age and had themselves experienced harsh punishment or neglect as children. In many instances the abusive or neglectful parents were raising their children as best they knew how and with the best of intentions. In other situations parents suffered from serious emotional, cognitive, or substance abuse problems. As any social worker knows, families identified with a single problem typically have many others, which compound in an interactive fashion. Drawing on these informal observations, we empirically demonstrated the importance of family stress in child abuse in a subsequent article (Conger, Burgess, & Barrett, 1979). These experiences were important as I extended this research during the development of a continuing program of research. Indeed, to a significant degree my later work represents a continuation of this early research on family stress, family process and child development. As planned, I produced a dissertation from the project and, in 1976, moved on to my first academic appointment as an assistant professor of sociology at the University of Georgia.

ACADEMIC APPOINTMENTS

The University of Georgia

I spent five years at the University of Georgia. During this time I attempted to establish myself as an independent scientist concentrating on the study of families and social deviance, especially family influences on antisocial or delinquent behavior. In a sense my work examined deviant families at risk for having deviant children. With a colleague from psychology, Ben Lahey, I was able to secure funding from the National Institute of Mental Health to continue research with abusive families. An important extension of the earlier research was the opportunity to study families of diverse ethnicities, which was not possible in rural Pennsylvania. Another colleague from the Department of Child and Family Studies, Ray Yang, and I also received a grant to study at-risk families in rural areas. We continued to employ the methodology developed in Pennsylvania, using extensive interviews and behavioral observations of families in their homes. The generation of data from these two studies led to some significant findings, but the publications containing these results were actually developed after I left Georgia.

As I look back at this period in my career, there were several positive experiences and achievements, but the record of accomplishment seems quite sketchy or uneven. Although I was involved in the publication of 16 articles or book chapters during this time, and also in the generation of two funded grant proposals, I was still very uncertain as to the exact direction that my work should take. I published some papers on delinquency, on dysfunctional family processes, on observational research methods, and on social theory. However, the work did not have a programmatic quality and I could not identify the organizing base for the empirical or theoretical directions I was pursuing. To compound these difficulties, my marriage came apart during this time. Thus, all the difficulties of a failed marital relationship and childcare in the context of divorce merged with the trials of an assistant professor attempting to secure promotion and tenure. Added to my personal troubles and professional anomie was a fractious sociology department with deeply divided loyalties and ambitions; there were literally opposing groups of faculty in the sociology department who had little respect or trust for one another.

In spite of these difficulties, there were several positive developments as well. First, I began to solidify my research skills such that I became increasingly competent and confident in organizing field projects studying families and children in the community. Second, my understanding of and successful use of observational methods improved and I developed a new observational coding system, which still serves my work today. Third, my theoretical reasoning advanced beyond a simple reliance on a behavioral or social learning perspective and I began to incorporate a broader range of social and behavioral theory into my research. Fourth, I learned a great deal from several important colleagues and friends at the University of Georgia, including, among others, Gene Brody, Rex Forehand, Pat Horan, Ben Lahey, Terry Thornberry, Jim Walters, and Ray Yang. Several of these individuals continue as colleagues and collaborators today. Finally, as a result of my 1976 paper on social control and social learning theories, in 1978 I was asked to consult with Jerry Patterson and John Reid on the interface between sociological and psychological approaches to studying delinquent behavior. They were preparing for a site visit on a grant proposal and the visiting team included both sociologists and psychologists. My trip to Eugene had an enormous and continuing influence on my scientific efforts and Jerry and John have continued to be generous mentors in my research activities since that time.

With these positive advances and under more favorable circumstances, my career might have flourished at the University of Georgia. As I look back now, however, it seems to me that my personal and professional turmoil prevented such a welcome outcome and I look on this time as a period of learning but not exceptional accomplishment. Because I seemed to be stuck in a morass in Georgia, I took advantage of an unexpected opportunity to join the faculty at the University of Illinois at Urbana-Champaign. For reasons I don't clearly understand, several of my colleagues from across the country nominated me for a position as department head for a program in family and human development at the university. At a time when I had no clear professional direction, I was offered a position at double the salary that I had at the University of Georgia, including promotion with tenure. This move turned out to be the most fortunate and most important of my career. Illinois offered a respite from the personal and professional difficulties in Georgia and helped me set a clear direction for my future scientific activities.

The University of Illinois

As head of the Department of Human Development and Family Ecology at the University of Illinois, I had the opportunity to learn about both administration and scholarship at one of the nation's finest universities. Although my tenure at Illinois was only three years, the experience represents another fundamental turning point in my career. In terms of both academic administration and the conduct of scientific inquiry, I was able to interact with and learn from some of the finest scholars in the world from across the university.

From HDFE my approach to science and administration significantly benefited from interactions with Leann Birch, Judy De Loache, and Sonya Salamon. Although I was providing leadership for the department, which grew and improved during that time, I was gaining more than I was giving in the process. Individuals from the sociology department who had a significant influence on my work, knowingly or unknowingly, included Mike Gottfredson, Joan Huber, and John Mirowsky. Most important of all, however, were the lessons I learned in the development of programmatic inquiry from several psychologists, including Steve Asher, John Gottman, and Ross Parke. The opportunity to discuss ideas and approaches to the study of families and children with these individuals has had a telling and continuing impact on my research. Another psychologist and university administrator, Mort Weir, also was generous in his advice regarding the role of a department head. In many ways I enjoyed a postdoctoral training program at Illinois, both in research and university administration.

The move to Illinois also provided several major improvements in my personal life. When I arrived in Urbana, I was a single father. My son, Zachary, then a pre-adolescent, stayed with me, and my daughter, Kim, moved with my ex-wife to Maryland. The years I spent as a single father taught me a lot about the stresses and strains inherent in this family structure; but they also taught me how much more fulfilling life is with one's children than without. Zach was a continuing source of companionship and delight, with all the usual frustrations of the move from childhood to adolescence. My daughter eventually joined us in Urbana, which made life even better. And especially important, I met my current wife, Kathi, while in Illinois. She worked for the Department of Children and Family Services at the time and, for some strange reason, decided to hire on as a stepparent. The quality of my life and our children's lives improved immediately. Kathi has played a remarkable role in creating a home and a family for a recalcitrant crew of Congers. Since our marriage she has gone on to complete her doctoral studies in sociology and we now enjoy both family and profession in our lives together.

Reviewing the record, it seems to me that I enjoyed several significant accomplishments at Illinois. In terms of research, my ideas about families, stress, behavioral interactions, and individual development began to coalesce and move beyond my predominantly behavioral perspective. For example, using data from the studies in Georgia my colleagues and I demonstrated how social cognition, environmental stresses, and emotional functioning come together to influence observable behaviors by mothers toward their young children (Conger, McCarty, Yang, Lahey, & Kropp, 1984a). This initial model played an important role in the development of later research with Iowa families experiencing significant economic hardship. A second paper based on both the Pennsylvania and Georgia samples indicated the importance of an off-time developmental event, the birth of a child at an early age, in predicting risk for aversive maternal behaviors that may exacerbate maladjustment in young children (Conger, McCarty, Yang, Lahey, & Burgess, 1984b). This study also included a replication of effects across three small samples of families, foreshadowing a continuing research interest in the generalizability of findings across diverse populations. Finally, work completed at Illinois increased my facility with observational data and improved my ability to use this technology with later, more ambitious research projects (Conger, Brainerd, Birch, Friedberg, & Navarro, 1986).

In terms of administrative accomplishments, the department I led experienced increases in graduate and undergraduate enrollment and in research productivity. I felt that I had learned something about working with a group of faculty to develop and act upon a strategic plan that improved the usual markers of departmental success. Unfortunately, I had several disagreements with my boss at the time and, in the spirit of my father's impulsiveness and wanderlust, elected to explore other administrative positions. With significant regret about leaving friends and colleagues at the University of Illinois, I accepted an appointment as Associate Dean for Research and Graduate Education in the College of Family and

Consumer Sciences at Iowa State University. My experience at Iowa State demonstrated that I was a better scientist than administrator, and my conviction that I someday wanted to be a dean took second place to the emergence of an exciting program of research that has continued for more than a decade.

Iowa State University

In 1984, I moved with an unhappy wife and son to Ames, Iowa. My daughter stayed in Urbana to pursue her bachelor's degree at the University of Illinois. We left a rich network of friends and colleagues in Illinois and none of us was sure that the move was a good one. I soon learned about disparities in academic cultures inasmuch as the research and graduate training aspirations in my new college were much lower than in my previous department. But I worked for a wonderful dean, Ruth Deacon, who pressed for change and accomplishment within the college. In time, however, it became clear that my skills as a researcher surpassed my patience as an administrator, and I found myself working with a group of faculty to develop projects related to families experiencing the severe economic downturn in agriculture at that time. With the change to a new dean and the receipt of our first grant funding to pursue these research activities, in 1989 I left my role as an associate dean and became a faculty member in the department of sociology. I also became director of a new campus center developed to study social and behavioral influences on the health of rural people.

My shift to a faculty position and to the role of director of a research center gave me the opportunity to pursue research on families of a magnitude that I had never imagined possible. In my previous labor-intensive studies, sample sizes were far less than 100 families and it was difficult to look at subdivisions within these groups, such as differences between boys and girls in developmental processes. In this new program of research we were able to study several hundred rural families using all of the intensive, observational research methodologies and interviewing procedures that characterized my earlier work. Both the National Institute of Mental Health and the National Institute on Drug Abuse provided primary funding to study the experience of rural families who were living through the most difficult economic crisis in Iowa since the Depression years of the 1930s. These agencies supported our initial research with first 75 families and then 450 families in the Iowa Youth and Families Project. NIMH also provided funding for a Center for Family Research in Rural Mental Health, which I have directed since 1990.

Once again, the success of these research activities has depended on the contributions of many exceptional collaborators including faculty members, professional research staff, postdoctoral trainees, and graduate students. With support from several interested consultants (Del Elliott, John Gottman, Jerry Patterson, and Jon Rolf), we launched the IYFP in 1988. The initial group of collaborators provided a complementary set of expertise in the development and execution of the project. As the principal investigator, I had a background in the study of family stress processes and their influence on child and adolescent development. Glen Elder brought his experience in studying economic stress with families of the 1930s, and Fred Lorenz provided remarkable guidance in research and statistical methodology. Paul Lasley taught us all about the special features of rural life, and Ron Simons and Les Whitbeck brought special expertise on competent and problematic adolescent development. In 1991 we added a cohort of single-parent families to the original sample of two-parent families, and the IYFP and single-parent projects were combined in 1994 into the Family Transitions Project. The original cohort of over 500 early adolescents has now reached early adulthood. We have just received funding to continue to follow these young adults as they develop families of their own.

Well over 100 publications have resulted from the study of these families. Findings from the research have contributed to our understanding of family economic stress, sibling relationships, adult health and development, child and adolescent competence and maladjustment, correlates of success and failure in marital and other romantic relationships, family problem solving processes, the influence of family structure, social stress, and physical health and well-being. My primary contributions have related to family economic stress and the influence of family processes on individual and relationship development. Important publications related to economic stress processes have included a book in 1994 (Conger & Elder, 1994) and a series of articles documenting the impact of economic stress on parents and children (e.g., Conger, Conger, Elder, Lorenz, Simons, & Whitbeck, 1992; Conger, Conger, Elder, Lorenz, Simons, & Whitbeck, 1993; Conger, Ge, Elder, Lorenz, & Simons, 1994; Conger, Conger, Mathews, Elder, 1999a; & Conger, Rueter, Elder, 1999b).

As part of this work, we have developed a Family Stress Model of economic hardship, elements of which have been supported by results from our study, and many of these findings have been replicated with urban and minority populations by other researchers. Consistent with our findings, the model suggests that family hardships demoralize parents through daily experiences involving the inability to make ends meet. This demoralization creates conflicts in romantic relationships, disrupts effective parenting practices, and thus jeopardizes the competent development of children and adolescents. Especially important, my colleagues and I have recently demonstrated that the basic model also applies to the experiences of a group of over 800 African American families that we are studying as part of a new project called the Family and Community Health Study. I find this new work extremely satisfying as it again demonstrates that the results from our research with rural white families generalize to a different ethnic group. This research has been extremely fulfilling for me as it links my experiences as a child in an economically stressed family to my role as a social scientist attempting to understand how families cope with significant hardships in their lives. It is especially pleasing that the findings from these studies appear to apply to families in general, and not to just one specific group.

In the space allowed for this autobiography it is impossible to thank all of the people at Iowa State who have done so much to make my work possible. In addition to those already mentioned, however, there is a small group of scientists who began as graduate assistants with the original IYFP that deserves special recognition. Over the years Kathi Conger has proven to be an invaluable colleague in the development of the research on economic stress. Xiaojia Ge has become a project leader in studies of adolescent maladjustment, biological influences on development, and the assessment of change. Jan Melby has considerably improved on my earlier research with observational measures. Martha Rueter created a program of work on family problem solving and has recently made significant contributions to the assessment of mental disorders among the young adults in the project. Equally important, K. A. S. Wickrama has launched a program of research on social influences on physical health, including the intergenerational transmission of health-risk behaviors. I originally advised these scholars in their work, now they instruct me and help me develop further as a family scientist. This circle of influence is especially satisfying as we continue to work together to advance our understanding of individual development in the context of family relationships.

REFERENCES

Burgess, R. L., & Conger. R. D. (1978). Family interaction in abusive, neglectful, and normal families. *Child Development*, *49*, 4, 1163-1173.

Conger, R. D. (1976). Social control and social learning models of delinquent behavior: a synthesis. *Criminology*, *14*, 1, 17-40.

Conger, R. D., Brainerd, D. W., Birch, L. L., Friedberg, P. J., & Navarro, L. A. (1986). Assessing the quality of family observations: A comparative analysis. *Journal of Marriage and the Family*, *48*, 2, 111-122.

Conger, R. D., Burgess, R. L., & Barrett, C. (1979). Child abuse related to life change and perceptions of illness: Some preliminary findings. *The Family Coordinator*, *28*, 1, 73-78.

Conger, R. D., Conger, K. J., Elder, G. H., Jr., Lorenz, F. O., Simons, R. L., & Whitbeck, L. B. (1992). A family process model of economic hardship and adjustment of early adolescent boys. *Child Development*, *63*, 3, 526-541.

Conger, R. D., Conger, K. J., Elder, G. H., Jr., Lorenz, F. O., Simons, R. L., & Whitbeck, L. B. (1993). Family economic stress and adjustment of early adolescent girls. *Developmental Psychology*, *29*, 2, 206-219.

Conger, R. D., Conger, K. J., Matthews, L. S., & Elder, G. H., Jr. (1999a). Pathways of economic influence on adolescent adjustment. *American Journal of Community Psychology*, *27*, 4, 519-541.

Conger, R. D., & Elder, G. H., Jr. (in collaboration with Lorenz, F. O., Simons, R. L., & Whitbeck, L. B.) (1994). *Families in troubled times: Adapting to change in rural America*. Hillsdale, NJ: Aldine.

Conger, R. D., Ge, X., Elder, G. H., Jr., Lorenz, F. O., & Simons, R. L. (1994). Economic stress, coercive family process and developmental problems of adolescents [Special issue on children and poverty]. *Child Development*, *65*, 2, 541-561.

Conger, R. D., & Killeen, P. (1974). Use of concurrent operants in small group research: A demonstration. *Pacific Sociological Review*, *17*, 3, 339-415.

Conger, R. D., McCarty, J. A., Yang, R. K., Lahey, B. B., & Burgess, R. L. (1984a). Mother's age as a predictor of observed maternal behavior in three independent samples of families. *Journal of Marriage and the Family*, *46*, 4, 411-424.

Conger, R. D., McCarty, J. A., Yang, R. K., Lahey, B. B., & Kropp, J. P. (1984b). Perception of child, child-rearing values, and emotional distress as mediating links between environmental stressors and observed maternal behavior. *Child Development*, *55*, 6, 2234-2247.

Conger, R. D., Rueter, M. A., & Elder, G. H., Jr. (1999b). Couple resilience to economic pressure. *Journal of Personality and Social Psychology*, 76, 1, 54-71.

An Interest in Lost Persons

Pauline Boss

KEYWORDS. Autobiography, theory, family stress, boundary ambiguity, ambiguous loss

PREFACE

The personal and professional are woven together in this essay, because that's how my life was–and still is today. Sometimes for reasons beyond my control and more times by volition, my career path was circular, often chaotic, and certainly not linear. This is not an unusual scenario for women. I purposely reveal the twists and turns, so that those who do not fit the mold of "traditional scholar" may be encouraged to press on in spite of social norms or life events. For me, it was difficult to determine whether family was interrupting career or vice versa, because I wanted both. The dialectic of family and work became reality; the constant tension became normal, the delicate balance of family and career. I wouldn't have had it any other way.

FAMILY HISTORY AND EDUCATION

As a child, my favorite radio program was *Mr. Keen, Tracer of Lost Persons*. I never missed a program. I wanted to be a detective like him someday, and in a sense, that is what I have become. The fact that I investigate and study families of missing persons strikes me, in retrospect, as like the Mr. Keen I so admired.

I grew up on a Wisconsin farm in a Swiss immigrant family at the end of the Great Depression. My father had intended to go back to Switzerland, but with no money for a return ticket, he married the girl next door and became a farmer. It would be 30 years before he would see his homeland again (Boss, 1993). His neighbors called him "greenhorn," so

I knew we were different. Inside our family, though, life was happy. Evenings were spent by kerosene lamplight watching my father paint pictures for us, while my mother darned socks. We were poor, but I didn't know it.

The country school my older sister attended was just down the road. I followed her and surprisingly, the teacher let me stay. I was four years old, loved reading, and was eager to listen to all eight classes in the one-room country school. When I was in fifth grade, my family moved to a dairy farm nearer to town, and for the first time, I was able to attend a town school where each class had a separate room. Being a "farm girl," though, meant that I was marginalized by the town kids, so I spent my time studying, a pattern that has stayed with me since.

Near the end of my high school education, the principal called my father in and told him I needed to go to college. Most girls at that time were married right after high school graduation, and I was already wearing an engagement ring. Secretly, I wanted to go to the university, and when my Swiss father said he was willing to borrow money to make that possible, I was euphoric. My fiancé had been drafted and was in Germany at the time, so marriage could be delayed. I took a nanny job in Madison the summer before I was to enroll at the University of Wisconsin, and in my spare time I familiarized myself with the gigantic campus. When fall came, I was in heaven, grateful everyday to be studying at a world-class university. However, the traditionally expected life script kept pulling at me. While I yearned for courses in literature, I majored in Home Economics. While I enjoyed the camaraderie of dormitory life, during the semester break of my sophomore year, I married my high school sweetheart, and moved back to the village, becoming a commuter to stay in school. Some of the Home Economics faculty gave up on me, and there was discussion about withdrawing a much-needed scholarship since married women were considered bad investments.

My hunger for education, though, outweighed all else. For two and a half years, I commuted sixty miles a day, regardless of weather, to attend classes at the university. I would then return home each afternoon to honor the tradition of having supper on the table by six. In June of 1956, I graduated with honors with a Bachelor's degree in Home Economics and Education and a minor in English.

Like elastic returning to its origin, upon graduation I returned full time to my hometown, teaching Home Economics and English in the high school I had attended. After two years of teaching, I became a mother. The next seven years I spent at home being a full-time mother, raising a son and then a daughter. I was doing what is now referred to as

"Martha Stewart living," making difficult and often unnecessary things "from scratch." I loved that period in my life, going to the swimming pool every day with my children in the summer, sledding with them in winter, and having coffees and playgroups with wonderful homemade treats. I have never regretted this period of full-time mothering.

A teacher shortage of the late 1960s produced an unsolicited but irresistible offer to teach Home Economics in a Madison high school. My children were now in elementary school and my parents were eager to have them at the farm after school. So I went back to teaching and back to commuting to Madison. Most of my teaching colleagues at the Madison Memorial High School had their Master's or Doctorate. To keep up, and because I needed to know more about how to teach "Family Life," my largest course, I began graduate school (nights and summers) as a "terminal master's" student in Education. My thesis required research so I interviewed three generations of Amish and Swiss American women (Boss, 1971). I was interested in whether women's roles were changing across the generations, even in these rural groups. My project required field research, or what I called "kitchen table research," and as a budding feminist, I was deeply curious about change in women's roles.

The unexpected happened: I got hooked on research. While I could not verbalize to others that I was continuing for a doctorate, I quit teaching at the High School in Madison and entered the doctoral program in Child Development and Family Studies at the University of Wisconsin. Jane Allen Piliavin, a social psychologist, became my major professor. Since the department's major emphasis area was Child Development, I searched outside the department for courses in family systems. I studied with Carl Whitaker in Psychiatry, Jerald Hage and Bert Adams in Sociology, and E. E. LeMasters in Social Work–professors who emphasized family as a system or organization. These individuals stimulated me to write my first paper on father absence in intact families, an NCFR presentation that I gave in Toronto (Boss, 1972). The Wisconsin professors sustained my interest and energy in what I now see was an ambitious goal given commuting and family demands. While at the university, I lunched with interesting friends, enjoyed my classes, and found the campus to be a haven. Then at four o'clock every afternoon, I drove back to that small rural village and resumed the role of traditional wife and mother.

Fifteen years at the University of Wisconsin-Madison, as an undergraduate, graduate, then assistant and associate professor with tenure changed that life. I saw other possibilities for women. I loved theory, research, therapy, and teaching. Although I continued to love keeping a beautiful home, giving family dinners and attending the children's ball games and concerts, it was time to leave "Martha Stewart" behind. If I couldn't cook it in an hour, I didn't make it. I found a wonderful neighbor woman to help me with the cleaning. The sewing machine gave way to the typewriter. Today, my children, now parents and professionals themselves, tell me they were comforted as they lay in their beds at night, hearing the sound of my typewriter. Even though I was starting a new path, they knew their mother was nearby.

TEACHING

From the start, my teaching was influenced by my enthusiasm for combining research, theory, and application. When teaching abstract theories, I also want students to be able to apply those ideas to real-life situations. Course assignments consistently include application exercises, so that before students leave my courses, they have had opportunities to practice applying the theories introduced in lectures and readings. Each student can apply the theory based on their own unique and diverse life experiences, but they must also be able to apply the theory from a perspective unlike their own. From my experience, students learn and remember best if they apply conceptual frameworks to problems that are uniquely meaningful to them (see Boss, Doherty, LaRossa, Schumm & Steinmetz, 1993). When given theories (rather than just facts), students become armed for a lifetime of professional work with a "map" to guide their work regardless of human diversity.

Having grown up in the 1930s and '40s in a rural, extended, immigrant family, often with a dozen or more kin and non-kin around the supper table, I never felt right reading about the isolated nuclear family as "the normal American family." With the current wave of immigration and migration, continuing to teach a monolithic view of the family is passé, even unethical. Early on, I wrote about the need for less linear views of family development (Boss, 1980). From my personal experience of living with parents with accents, a grandmother who refused to even learn English, and being the first in a family to go to the university, I have a deep empathy for today's immigrant families and their children when I meet them in my classes. I make a special effort that exams are written without tricky wording, because I don't want those for whom English is a second language to be disadvantaged. Texts and readings are checked for readability as well for content that respects differences in family forms, values, and beliefs. While I remain in charge of the class and responsible for what happens there, I consider all of the students a unique source of knowledge, and encourage them to talk about their experiences in large and small groups. At the same time, I ask students to listen respectfully to their peers. A Buddhist talks with a Lutheran; a gay student talks with a heterosexual student; a mother back in school after raising four children talks with a twenty-year-old; a refugee from Southeast Asia talks with a young man who grew up in the safety and comfort of a wealthy suburb; a young man who served in the Navy talks with a pacifist.

My respect for students' unique experiences is high, and in turn, they seem to respect my uniqueness. Instead of suppressing my values, beliefs, and biases, I label them and encourage students to do the same. As teachers, it is not our values that skew classroom teaching, but our refusal to label them explicitly. No human being can sustain a value-free position in the classroom for long, so students have a right to know upfront who we are and for what we stand for. With that made clear, they are more able to think critically about what we teach and how they might apply that knowledge.

When I took in Joe Elder's sociology class in the 1960s at the University of Wisconsin, Alvin Gouldner (1970) was required reading. I have never forgotten Gouldner's idea about domain assumptions–that scholars are influenced by their domain or background assumptions regarding people and society. Whether Marxist or Parsonian, sociologists were according to Gouldner never absolutely value free. Theorists (and I assumed this included family theorists) were necessarily political and ideological. Gouldner therefore thought it essential for theorists, himself included, to explicitly articulate their domain assumptions; this was necessary information to understand intellectual and conceptual schemes so they could be "submitted to the test of evidence" (Gouldner, 1970, p. 35). Fair enough, I thought.

Whatever I learned in my courses in Sociology at Wisconsin, I translated this knowledge into my analysis of families. Indeed, the 1970s Civil Rights and Women's Movements brought new developments in the larger society's discussion of families. Moreover, new waves of immigration, burgeoning technology, the obsolescence of unskilled factory workers, high levels of maternal employment, and even more drastic developments are evident in the hot discourse from left to right about family structure, function, and values. For me, Gouldner's ideas marked my early introduction to postmodernism, but simultaneously, I was learning about the politics of the family and the values debate from other Wisconsin professors in other departments. Ideas about what makes families work (or not work) were coming together for me, personally and professionally, from various disciplines.

Influenced by the University of Wisconsin tradition where the professors I studied with did not hesitate to say upfront what they stood for, I have tried to do the same. With mutual respect for diverse ideas and experiences, classroom discourse is lively. I believe that an active classroom is better than one in which students just sit, take notes, and accept what the professor says as the only truth. From 1974 to the present, I have been privileged to teach and mentor thousands of students, graduate and undergraduate, at the University of Minnesota, recently at Harvard Medical School, and earlier at the University of Wisconsin. Teaching has been for me a two-way street.

RESEARCH AND INQUIRY

Teachers and mentors who influenced my research varied in discipline and style. My doctoral research advisor at the University of Wisconsin-Madison was Jane Allyn Piliavin whose research preference at that time was for laboratory studies in social psychology. Dr. Piliavin insisted I operationalize boundary ambiguity with the indicator of roles. As a result, my *early* research, unlike later work, is limited to roles and role theory and is correctly labeled by Kingsbury and Scanzoni as neo-structure functionalism (Kingsbury & Scanzoni, 1993, pp. 195-217).

For formal coursework in theory building, my professor at the U.W. was Jerald Hage, sociologist and author of *Techniques and Problems of Theory Construction in Sociology* (1972). He was the one who encouraged me to raise the constructs father absence and boundary ambiguity to a higher level of abstraction. It was while studying with him that I came up with the term "ambiguous loss," which still today represents the more general construct resulting from my early work on missing fathers and boundary ambiguity. I recall Professor Hage complimenting me on my ability to think theoretically, my ability to "think like a man," which I didn't yet think to challenge.

Change was afoot, however, because more than any other professor, Carl Whitaker freed up my thinking about change and families as living systems. It was all right to rebel because, among Carl's buddies at that time were Thomas Szasz and R. D. Laing, whose writings Carl gave me to read. As I wrote in the *Family Therapy Networker* (Boss, 1995), Carl Whitaker was deconstruction personified or postmodernism before it was in vogue. I studied with him (and the psychiatric residents) when the University of Wisconsin was a hotbed of anti-establishment fervor, mixing hippies, feminists, and Viet Nam vets together on a campus alive with social and political change. Having just read Betty Friedan (1963), I was returning to college full time, less certain about what I was going toward than what I was leaving behind. What I now saw as my past was an isolated life in a small rural village where I had spent my whole life and where women's roles were limited to "Kinder, Kirche, und Kuche" ("children, church, and kitchen").

Accustomed to working with strong women in his family, Carl provided support for my budding feminism. He valued things then considered only the domain of women–intuition, emotion, intimacy, connections to children, and family. From Carl, I learned to value the symbolic in family boundaries and processes and recognize the flaws in traditionally gendered role prescriptions. His prelim question for me was one I shall never forget: "Are fathers necessary beyond the moment of conception?" I still worry about the answer. In my work on ambiguous loss, it was Carl who encouraged me to expand the operationalization (he would never have used those words) beyond roles. I agreed, but to a doctoral student and then a pre-tenured assistant professor, expansion beyond the indicators of roles was risky. At that time and place, research meant quantification, and roles were easier to quantify than something symbolic.

I graduated with a doctorate in Child Development and Family Studies in 1975 at the University of Wisconsin-Madison. I became an assistant professor in that same department. It was not until I was tenured in 1980 that I came out of the closet as a symbolic interactionist. I was influenced by, among others, the writings of Berger and Luckmann (1966), Goffman (1974), Hess and Handel (1959), and Reiss (1981), and used their perspectives to guide my work, including research with caregivers of Alzheimer's patients.

I finally was in the right circumstances in 1999 to write about ambiguous loss in the way I had always intended, combining both the psychodynamic and symbolic aspects of family boundaries as well as quantitative with qualitative inquiry. Families are psychological entities as well as physical structures and both must be assessed if we are to understand family processes, in this case when there is ambiguous loss (Boss, 1999). Carl Whitaker had consented to writing the preface for this book, but he died before I could write it. I asked no one else to write the preface and he is symbolically present in those pages.

And then there was Reuben Hill. As a consultant with the Center of Prisoner of War Studies, Dr. Hill was asked to come to Madison to consult on my dissertation. We had many lively discussions, and he supported my ideas even when he disagreed with them. Because Reuben Hill had become like Whitaker, a mentor, I asked his advice when Sue Steinmetz and Marvin Sussman invited me to write the family stress chapter for their forthcoming *Handbook of Marriage and the Family* (Sussman & Steinmetz, 1987a). They said I could select my own co-author, so I asked Reuben, "Who should I ask to be co-author?" His answer caught me off guard. "Write it alone!" he said. So I did. However, because women are socialized traditionally, as I had been, they did not easily venture out on their own. Thanks to Reuben Hill, therefore, I established myself as an independent writer in the area of family stress (Boss, 1987a; 1988; 2001).

During my year (1995-96) as Visiting Professor of Psychology at Harvard Medical School, my experience at the Judge Baker Children's Center convinced me that my original inclination to expand the operationalization of my theoretical model to include psychodynamic and symbolic conceptions was correct. These are the more profound indicators of boundary ambiguity when there is ambiguous loss, and more important, this provided the window for change, for interventions or prevention. Being at Harvard provided just the right environment for developing the psychodynamic aspects of the theory. I came to the conclusion that writing the theory of ambiguous loss could be done through narrative discourse–telling stories from my research, therapy, or personal experience that illustrate the theory. Interacting with renowned scholars gave me the courage to proceed with this less didactic way of writing a theoretical book. My perspective since the 1980s and increasingly in the 1990s was, and is, social constructionism. The label neo-structure functionalism no longer fit. Thus, my later writings vary from my early writings. There is a difference. We grow, we learn, we go deeper.

FROM THE UNIVERSITY OF WISCONSIN TO THE UNIVERSITY OF MINNESOTA– AND FINALLY LEAVING MY HOMETOWN

In 1980, I was still commuting to Madison every day, now an associate professor with tenure, and was also practicing family therapy in my hometown. I was recruited that year by Richard Hey at the University of Minnesota to apply for a position in the Department of Family Social Science. Living on the shore of Lake Mendota and being a professor at the University of Wisconsin had been my life's dream. Having just purchased that house on the lake, I, of course, said "No." Dr. Hey was persistent, however, and three months later, when I heard from him again, my life circumstances had changed, and I was ready to move. The Twin Cities, full of theaters, concert halls, and art galleries convinced me that going to the University of Minnesota would be a good move. I joined the faculty of Family Social Science in the fall of 1981. My task was to develop the Marriage and Family Therapy Program, and bring it to accreditation, which I did within five years. I enjoyed working in a department so committed to family studies and a union of theory, research, and application.

WHAT IS MY LEGACY?

If I have a legacy, my hope is that it is "a useful theory." This theory, I hope, is useful for researchers, professionals, and families themselves to better understand families and the individual members that compose families, particularly those experiencing ambiguous losses. I hope my work proves "useful" across a multiplicity of disciplines, and to a more general audience. I hope that this body of work on ambiguous loss and boundary ambiguity is a credit to those who supported the research: the Center for Prisoner of War Studies in the Naval Health Research Institute, the National Institute on Aging, the National Alzheimer's Association, the All- University Council on Aging, the University of Wisconsin Graduate School and Experiment Station; the University of Minnesota Graduate School and Experiment Station.

The book *Ambiguous Loss* (Boss, 1999) summarizes this body of work. Its reception, nationally and internationally, indicates that the theory of ambiguous loss is useful worldwide. That the book is being translated into German, Chinese, and six more languages is a testimony to its universal appeal. Across cultures and races, people struggle with ambiguous losses. I think of Jerald Hage's urging me to raise my ideas about father absence in intact families to a more general level. Having introduced the term "ambiguous loss," I now discovered the phenomenon is more ubiquitous and global than I ever imagined.

Overall, my work has been theoretical, not psychometric. Limiting research on ambiguous loss and boundary ambiguity to quantitative measurement would have lost the symbolic and psychodynamic dimensions I believed were so essential for validity. There are multiple methods for assessing situations of ambiguous loss and resulting boundary ambiguity; the critical task for researchers (and clinicians) is to follow the theoretical map I have provided (Boss, 1999). For those who nevertheless prefer a measurement manual, there is one available (Boss, Greenberg, & Pearce- McCall, 1990). This manual has been requested by researchers from around the world who test the theory with new populations and new types of ambiguous losses.

In addition to my theoretical work on ambiguous loss, I hope my legacy may lie with the many young people I have mentored and advised. They can be found throughout the world, testing ideas in new ways with new people. I hope that their time with me instilled in them a respect for diversity, a hunger for knowledge and creativity, and a zeal for solving problems about families of all kinds. I hope I nurtured in them a passion for writing and then publishing, for we must make our ideas available for review and public discourse. I am particularly happy to have worked with many students who traditionally had not been encouraged to polish, write, and publish their ideas. Part of my legacy, hopefully, will be a fresh battalion of young professors in academe, women and men, who will continue teaching and mentoring those who do not always fit the mold.

Finally, I hope part of my contribution is that I have modeled a way for scholars to publish their findings in a new way. While I continue to support the need for publishing in peer reviewed scientific journals, I also promote the idea that researchers must translate their works for a more general audience and for scholars in other disiplines. The topic of "family" does not belong to one discipline, so it is imperative that our research and theoretical work be readily accessible to others. Getting rid of jargon will help to make cross-disciplinary work easier and at the same time, provide more accessible information for the general public about research that directly affects their human relationships. Indeed, professorial writing for the general public is a risky idea since many academics assume that if you write a trade book you are no longer a serious scholar. I disagree. Writing with a jargon-free vocabulary may challenge academic elitism, but it doesn't have to erode good scholarship. Taxpayers have a right to read our findings, since they so often fund our research. We owe them accessibility.

THE ARTS AND RESEARCH

The arts and sciences for me are not separate worlds. My experience in a theater or concert hall often ignites my ability to see, to hear, and to be. The arts broaden my view of the possibilities of human relationships, and above all, increase the strength of my intuition–a useful tool for researchers as well as therapists. More than a decade age I encouraged the blend of arts and science:

> Hypotheses as well as poems are the product of imaginative thinking. Scientific discoveries happen to people not by magic or luck, but by people being open to discovery, listening to emotions and responding. Like a poet, the researcher as well as the therapist needs the ability to imagine what the truth may be. Each tests it, but in different ways. The poet words a couplet, the therapist tries a strategy, and the researcher tests hypotheses. (Boss, 1987b, p. 147)

Scientific discoveries are rarely premeditated, so we must keep ourselves open to discovery. Music, art, and theater enrich the possibilities of new discovery, new information, and new questions. They help us to know who we are and for what we stand. I emphasize again in this essay the assumption of arts as enrichment for "the person of the researcher," because that idea is so rarely addressed in formal scientific training.

Mentoring

Working with the next generation of family researchers at the University of Minnesota and recently at Harvard Medical School (with Stuart Hauser at the Judge Baker Children's Center), I see that the future of family research is in highly skilled hands. This new generation of scholars will continue to advance the knowledge base. Many are already skilled in the technicalities of research, so my method of mentoring is to focus on "the person of the researcher." I tailor my mentoring to people's specific strengths and needs; I let them know up front what I can offer and what might be better sought from another mentor or technician. I ask questions; I answer their questions–even the one asked routinely by young female researchers, and increasingly by young male researchers: how did you balance being a professor and having a family? I inevitably tell them it is possible if you give up linearity as normality. I often tell them that if they want children and family, they must put them first, for if those we love are diminished by our professional zeal, we will have lost what matters most.

BALANCING WORK AND FAMILY LIFE

I learned the most about how to balance family and professional lives from Carl Whitaker. He let all of us who studied with him know (by his actions, not his words) that his marriage and family came first. We knew we were second, and that provided freedom for us to do the same with our own families. I learned from him that it was not unusual to cut off a meeting when he'd say, "Time to go home. Gotta help Muriel feed the kids." As family therapists and researchers, we must have meaningful relationships outside of our work, for if the families we study or treat become our only passion we will be too needy to do good work.

A Final Thought

My work on ambiguous loss and boundary ambiguity will hopefully make life easier for those who today don't quite fit the mainstream mold–the immigrant families of this century. They know (as my parents did) that education is the way up for their children as they reach for success in a new land. And like the detective, "Mr. Keen," tracer of lost persons, I hope my research and theoretical work may help the uprooted newcomers to live more comfortably with the ambiguity of loved ones left behind or lost.

It has now been twenty years since I left that Swiss-American village in Southern Wisconsin where I was born, raised, and then raised my own children. I still go back to visit since my mother still lives there, but my world is now primarily in the city, and often traveling the globe. It is a wonderful life. The cost is not knowing exactly where I belong. When I was in China in 1988, struggling because *everything* was so unfamiliar to me, I found I felt at home when I arrived on the campus of Beijing University. No matter where I have been in the world–Western Europe, Asia, Southeast Asia, Eastern Europe, England, Ireland, Canada, South and Central America, or the United States, I have found university campuses a haven. The life of a professor is privileged–no matter where one is, no matter where one came from.

AUTHOR NOTE

Pauline Boss is Professor, Department of Family Social Science, University of Minnesota.

REFERENCES

Berger, P.L. & Luckman, T. (1966). *The social construction of reality: A treatise in the Sociology of knowledge.* New York: Doubleday.

Boss, P. (1971). Cross-cultural and cross-generational sex role perceptions of Swiss-American and Amish females. Unpublished master's thesis. University of Wisconsin-Madison.

Boss, P. (1972). Father absence in intact families. Presentation at the annual meeting of the National Council on Family Relations, Toronto, Canada.

Boss, P. (1980). Normative family stress: Family boundary changes across the life-span. *Family Relations, 29*, 4, 445-450.

Boss, P. (1987a). Family stress: Perception and context. In M. Sussman & S. Steinmetz (Eds.), *Handbook on marriage and family* (pp. 695-723). New York: Plenum.

Boss, P. (1987b). The role of intuition in family research: Three issues of ethics. In R. Garfield, A. Greenberg, & S. Sugarman (Eds.), *Symbolic-experiential journeys: A Tribute to Carl Whitaker* (special issue), *Contemporary Family Therapy, 9*, 2, 146-159.

Boss. P. (1988; 2001). *Family stress management: A contextual approach.* Newbury Park, CA: Sage Publications (revision forthcoming).

Boss, P. (1993). The experience of immigration for the mother left behind. *Marriage & Family Review, 19*, 3/4, 365-378.

Boss, P. (1995). "That man Whitaker!" *Family Therapy Networker, 20*, 4, 58-59.

Boss, P. (1996). They did it quietly: the meaning of immigration for women. In H. Ryhner (Ed.), *Jubilaumsbuch 150 jahr new glarus: American's little Switzerland errinnertsich* (pp. 35-102). Glarus, Switzerland: Tschudi AG.

Boss, P. G. (1999). *Ambiguous loss.* Cambridge, MA: Harvard University Press. (German translation, Beck, AG, Munich, in press; Chinese translation, in press).

Boss, P.G., Doherty, W.J., LaRossa, R., Schumm, W.R., & Steinmetz, S.K. (Eds.), (1993). *Sourcebook of family theories and methods: A contextual approach.* New York: Plenum Press.

Boss, P., Greenberg, J., & Pearce-McCall, D. (1990). *Measurement of boundary ambiguity in families.* Minnesota Agricultural Experiment Station Bulletin #593-1990. St. Paul, MN: University of Minnesota, 55108.

Friedan, B. (1963). *The feminine mystique.* New York: New York: W. W. Norton & Co.

Goffman, E. (1974). *Frame analysis.* New York: Harper Colophon Books.

Gouldner, Alvin W. (1970). *The coming crisis of western sociology.* New York: Avon Books (Equinox).

Hage, Jerald. (1972). *Techniques and problems of theory construction in sociology.* New York: Wiley-Interscience.

Hess, R.D. & Handel, G. (1959). *Family worlds: A psychological approach to family life.* Chicago: University of Chicago Press.

Kinsbury, N. & Scanzoni, J. (1993). Structure Functionalism. In P. G. Boss, W. J. Doherty, R. LaRossa, W. R., Schumm, & S. K. Steinmetz, S.K. (Eds.). *Sourcebook of family theories and methods: A contextual approach.* New York: Plenum Press.

Reiss, D. (1981). *The family's construction of reality.* Cambridge, MA: Harvard University Press.

Sussman, M.B. & Steinmetz, S.K. (1987). *Handbook of marriage and the family.* New York: Plenum.

Threads in My Professional Career

Wesley R. Burr

KEYWORDS. Autobiography, research, theory construction, family science

INTRODUCTION

Even though I retired in 1999, I'm still so close to my professional experiences that it's difficult to gain much perspective. It is like trying to look at a forest when it is difficult to see more than a few trees. Also, each time I try to write a part of my history it is like looking at a kaleidoscope I've looked at many times before. Each time I look, the same crystals and marbles are there, with a few pebbles mixed in, but the patterns and overall picture are different. So, this is an attempt to describe some of the things I see this time in an ever-changing picture.

One of the crystals in the glass has been a guiding ideal since my teenage years. I always wanted a career where I would be helping people. I wasn't very interested in an indirect contribution–like through geological exploration to find oil to help the economy. I wanted a more direct connection and impact. I thought about medicine and law, but decided against them even though they had many advantages. My personality didn't match up well with either of them. I didn't like the sight of blood; and I didn't like the ambiguity, complexity, and controversy I saw in law. The other main option I considered was a career in teaching. Since I also didn't care much about wealth, and I wanted to be in a career where there was a sense of purpose and mostly consensus and agreement, being a teacher seemed like a good choice.

In my first several years at college, I planned to teach in the biological sciences, and I came to the family field quite by accident. A friend was going to Brigham Young University as the new dean of the College of Family Living, and he offered me a scholarship if I'd give a new program there in Human Development and Family Relationships (HDFR) a try. I'd always believed that the family is very important, and I didn't have a scholarship to continue studying zoology. The HDFR program seemed to have an interventionist perspective, so I transferred. I enjoyed the first few semesters of study, learned to identify with the field, pursued it, and enjoyed it, and completed my BS and MS degrees at BYU.

When I was deciding in 1962 where to go for a PhD, the choice was between the University of Minnesota and Florida State University. Basically, it was a choice to study with Ivan Nye or Reuben Hill. All the evidence I had suggested that at the time these two schools were the main family oriented programs in the country. I chose to go to the University of Minnesota, and received my doctorate with a major in sociology. This added a sociological perspective onto the interventionist perspective I'd acquired in my BS and MS program. There are some similarities between the two, and a certain amount of compatibility, but there also are number of important differences between those two perspectives. These perspectives added two new crystals to my kaleidoscope, and they have colored everything I've encountered since.

In the middle 1960s the academic culture was quite different than it is today. Now, graduate students need to get involved in the process of submitting manuscripts for publication while they are still in graduate school because it's much more competitive and the expectations are quite different. At the time I went through my doctoral program, the role of doctoral student was defined as being a sponge, where we were to absorb and learn what existed in the field and not to be adding to it. Our goal was to master what was there. Then, after graduation, those who wanted to work in universities should try to add to the field.

During the early part of my career, teaching was my main emphasis. I had taught enough as a graduate assistant and instructor that I felt confident as a teacher. I wasn't at all sure I could do research that would add to the knowledge in the field. Since I didn't know if I was cut out to be a researcher, I chose a professional position in a relatively small school, Portland State University. I reasoned that if I couldn't make a contribution to the research literature at least my teaching would be valued enough that I could still make tenure.

During my first year after graduate school, I found myself thinking about what I might do to try add to knowledge. I talked with my mentors, Murray Strauss and Reuben Hill, rather extensively about it, and eventually decided to try one or two modest papers to try to get some publications in a journal. I used the data from my dissertation to write a couple of papers. I submitted them for the NCFR meetings and to the *Journal of Marriage and the Family*, and they were accepted (Burr, 1970, 1971). This provided some evidence that I could do research that would be a contribution to the field.

After these successes, I sat back in an introspective way for a period of time and said to myself, "OK, if I have the ability to make a contribution, what kind of a contribution should I try to make? Where should I invest my energies? What can I do that would make a difference?" I thought about this for a number of months and observed in this process that I had a number of courses in my doctoral program on theory building, under Reuben Hill primarily, and that was something that was growing and accelerating, and catching a lot of people's attention at the time. I also observed that my best mental skills were in organizing and synthesizing.

A third observation I made at that time was that the literature in the family field had gained an increasingly empirical orientation, so we were getting more and more empirical studies, and people were trying to create empirical generalizations, but there was little integration or cumulativity in it. Thus, there were a large number of relatively unconnected ideas in the literature. Also, a number of people also had written speculative ideas that had not been documented with empirical research, and there were a number of general theoretical perspectives that in many ways weren't very integrated with the empirical literature. My perception at that time was that there was a need to create conceptual clarity where there was considerable conceptual confusion, integrate the empirical findings and theories, clarify explanations, identify similarities and differences, and clarify intervention strategies that were tied to the theories. Another part of this process in my mind was that it was desirable to integrate ideas in the sociological point of view with ideas in the more interventionist approach that I later began calling a familogical or family science approach.

It seemed to me that the theory building movement was attempting to accomplish these tasks by bridging the very abstract theoretical ideas with "middle range" theories, as Robert Merton called them, and also bridge the middle range theories with the expanding empirical findings. It seemed to me that this condition was kind of like a theoretical harvesting, or a vein of ore that had been discovered but needed to be refined. To me it seemed like a golden opportunity, and my penchant for organizing and synthesizing seemed to fit the task fairly well.

This selecting process was a very deliberate activity on my part, and it set the stage for many years of scholarly activity. At the time, Reuben

Hill and Murray Straus were the two mentors that I turned to for advice, and I recall discussing the idea of writing a book with them at the NCFR meetings in 1968. They were both very supportive and encouraging. They also gave me some advice on how to do it. For example, one of their bits of advice was that I had ought to focus first on writing several chapters in the book that could be published as journal articles independently of the book. This would provide some feedback in the process. This kind of a book seemed relatively conducive to that type of approach. So, it seemed like a good idea, and I organized the book in that way. Eventually one of the chapters was published separately in the *Journal of Marriage and the Family* (Burr, 1973).

As I came home from the NCFR meetings in the fall of 1968, I made a decision to try to write a theory book and to put all of my energies in that project. I secured a research grant from Portland State, and began in the spring of 1969 to work on several papers that could also be chapters in a book.

The first feedback I received was from Ken Cannon, a BYU colleague. He was very positive in his feedback, and this helped provide the incentive to go on. The first three chapters of the book were presented at the NCFR meetings in the fall of 1969, and the feedback there was also very positive. I continued to work on the project through 1970, and completed it in early 1971. It was eventually published as *Theory Construction in the Sociology of the Family* (Burr, 1973).

During this period, some of us felt that the professional meetings weren't very conducive to theory building. The pattern at the time was to present completed papers, but we felt it would be helpful to also have some type of forum for discussing theoretical ideas while we were still working on them. We believed this would provide feedback at a time when it could make a difference in the eventual papers and books. Also, we felt that such a forum would stimulate and assist the work of participants other than the presenters. Also, we believed that at that time there was a bias among many of the gatekeepers of the field in favor of empirical papers and against conceptual and theoretical papers. These beliefs led to the formation of the Theory Construction Workshops at the NCFR meetings in 1972.

After I finished the book that was published in 1973, I began to work on another book that was a different but interrelated crystal in my kaleidoscope. My goal in this second book was to write a book that would help us apply the theories that had been "improved" in the 1973 book. I began this second book in late 1972, and worked full time on it during leave in the first half of 1973. This second book was titled *Successful Marriage* (Burr, 1976).

During 1973 a group of us gradually developed the idea of assembling a fairly large team to work in a coordinated way on improving the theories in the field. Reuben Hill, Ivan Nye, Ira Reiss, and I gradually became the coordinators of the project. We discussed it in the Theory Construction Workshop in 1973, and held a conference in the summer of 1974 at BYU to work out a more detailed plan. The plan was then discussed in the NCFR meetings in 1974 and we began the writing phase.

I felt that this project was a great idea and enjoyed working in it from 1973 to 1976. In fact, it was an exhilarating intellectual experience, and I recognized at the time that it would probably be the most significant thing I would ever help with in my career. This project resulted in the two-volume publication *Contemporary Theories About the Family* (Burr, Hill, Nye and Reiss, 1979).

The "Contemporary Theories" volumes made a number of contributions to the field as it became the definitive work on family theories in the 1980s. It also helped the field better understand where we were going with the scientific approach to understanding family life. It appeared at a time when many were questioning the value of the scientific approach, and it probably hastened the development of several other approaches. I believed at the time that the scientific approach was merely a tool, and I still believe it is a useful tool, and I think that most of the alternative approaches that were spawned in the last half of the twentieth century will turn out to be much less useful than it is.

The biggest impact the two volumes had for me was that they helped me see that the directions we were going in the theory building movement were not attaining the goals that I had been seeking. This insight first began to dawn on me when the manuscripts for the two volumes started to come in. In retrospect, I think there were three processes at work that led to the theory building being quite different from what I had wished for. One was that the manuscripts were focused, almost exclusively, on the purpose of understanding and explanation as ends in themselves. It was as though abstract explanations were the intellectual end rather than being a means to the end of intervention. I had tried to have the theoretical ideas deal with generalizations that would be of value to practitioners, but as the years passed the whole business of theory building became relatively independent of the practitioners.

The second source of discontent for me was that the emphasis was primarily on accounting for variance in important dependent variables rather than focusing on how changes brought about through intervention in independent variables could create desirable outcomes. In my 1973 book I had tried to focus on ideas where the main purpose was to think about how specific interventions might lead to desirable outcomes. Whether it was how to cope with stress, how to deal with transitions, or marital satisfaction, the goal was not to explain the natural correlates or causes of those phenomena, but rather to identify phenomena which could be manipulated and changed in order to help families better cope. Hence, my primary emphasis was on trying to think about generalizations that would help us know how to intervene with regard to the independent variables.

The third process that I think contributed to my distress with the theory building movement deals with the difficulties in trying to integrate ideas from different intellectual traditions. At that time, I had a relatively naive and simplistic view of the scholarly process. I assumed there was much more consensus than I now think there was. Oh, I recognized there was considerable controversy, but I thought it was about relatively more minor aspects around the fringes of the field. I assumed a large number of scholars were trying to construct conceptual frameworks and theoretical ideas that were being refined and improved, and I assumed that many scholars had been grappling with that process since the social sciences began emerging in the 19th centuries. I assumed that before the middle of the twentieth century this was mostly a rational rather than an empirical process, and that as it became more of an empirical process it was moving to new heights and being refined and improved by getting multiple levels of abstraction and having very general abstract theories and specific models that were being corroborated with empirical data, and that the empirical data would provide the basis for additional refinements and extension of the theories and that these theories would be the main useful ideas that practitioners would use. I assumed that the development of the theory construction movement was a watershed era that was capitalizing on the large amount of groundwork previously developed, and that we were in the process of creating better order in our ideas and further refinement because we could stand on the shoulders of earlier generations of scholars who had made important contributions. I assumed that the refined theories that we were creating would be welcomed by practitioners as useful, intellectual fruit, and that thereby we would help families be more effective.

I was not very sensitive to the fact that our theories are dependent upon the paradigmatic assumptions in different academic fields. I didn't realize they are largely the manifestations of the unique perspectives of the people who had been developing the theories, and that these change relatively little.

My current view is that there are many different ways of getting ideas in the academic community. We have many ideas from literature, the humanities, arts, theology, and some from the social sciences. The ideas developed in the sociology of the family tradition are so different from those developed in the interventionist approach that has grown out of home economics, family life education and family therapy that all of the attempts to bridge them so far have created little integration. The theory building movement of the 1970s was dominated by scholars who had a "verstehen" rather than "interventionist" approach, and the result was models that had little value to those of us who are primarily interested in improving the quality of family life.

I now suspect that if I had taken a different strategy in my 1973 book, it might have made a difference in what happened later. I organized the chapters in that book around key dependent variables. The result was to then identify factors where we had reason to believe changes would tend to influence the dependent variables. I now wish I had organized it around key intervention areas and tried to identify aspects of family life where we had reason to believe changes would influence various valued aspects of family life. We'll never know whether this other approach would have made much difference because it is now a matter of history, but I suspect it would have. We probably would have discovered earlier that the goals of the interventionists and the verstehenists are so incompatible that we need to do different types of scholarship. I wish I could go back and work on models that would clarify how interventions make a difference, but I'm at the wrong end of my career to do it. I also suspect that some future scholars will do the field a substantial service by this type of systematic theory building.

As I wrestled with the discrepancy between what I had hoped would appear in the theory building movement and what did appear, it gradually became more clear that some of the differences were disciplinary differences. This led to the idea that there is a family oriented perspective or discipline that was emerging from the home economics, family life education and family therapy approaches. It is fundamentally an interventionist orientation, and it is an attempt to use familial processes as the primary processes to pay attention to for explanation and intervention. The discipline is somewhat different from a psychological approach, which relies primarily on psyche issues for explanation and intervention, economics, which uses an economic model to explain, and family sociology, which relies on social phenomena to explain and has little emphasis on intervention.

I believed during the early 1980s, when these ideas were being crystallized, that this was a useful insight that would be appreciated by colleagues because it would clarify some differences that were important that hadn't been identified before. I also discovered that several colleagues shared my views about what was going on. Ivan Nye suggested that what was going on was that a very different family discipline was emerging, and Geoffrey Leigh and I discovered that both of us had begun to write our thoughts in papers. We decided to collaborate and the result was the paper that was presented as my presidential address at the 1981 NCFR meetings and later published as Burr and Leigh (1983). We suggested there was an emerging family discipline. We were totally unprepared for the explosion and controversy these ideas created.

We also underestimated the number of scholars in the emerging family field who are trying to develop new knowledge. There are a large number of people in the family field, but most of them are practitioners rather than researchers, and they remain fragmented in sub-discipline approaches such as family therapy, family life education, marriage enrichment, etc. There are so few scholars who are interested in developing ideas from a familial perspective that the field is not developing as rapidly as we thought it would.

I believe that the postmodern critique that became widespread at about the same time that the 1979 theory volumes appeared was partially prompted by the limited value of the ideas created in the social sciences generally. Our family theories were just like the rest. They had such limited value and utility that we suffered from the same deficiencies as the social sciences generally. If the theories in the family field had been of more value to practitioners and policy makers, the critiques of the last several decades might have been quite different. The post-modern critique also didn't provide new approaches that scholars could agree on, so the result has been a fragmentation and disintegration. This has led to a condition where there are small groups of scholars who have consensus inside their group and so much disagreement between groups that there is little intellectual interchange. Those still involved in the theory movement are just one of a large number of these groups.

During the middle 1980s I found myself in the middle of the discussions and debates about the nature of the disciplines. Many ideas appeared, and eventually there was consensus among one group that the term family science was helpful, but the process couldn't overcome the fragmentation in the field. For example, family therapists prefer to identify with family therapy as their discipline and profession. Family life educators prefer to be known as family life educators, and home economists preferred their unique identity.

During the 1980s I also devoted quite a bit of my time to marriage and family enrichment. I worked at developing enrichment materials and workshops, and trying to develop television programs, package-structured enrichment programs, and we were partially successful. However, I gradually concluded it was difficult to teach an old dog new tricks and I had limited abilities in being an enrichment leader. My strengths were in precise, analytic thinking about abstract ideas and I had limited abilities in their application. I had excellent content, and relatively mediocre form, so in the late '80s I abandoned that foray, and it was one of the less successful aspects of my career.

At about this same time I recognized that the time was right to create a revision to the contemporary theories about the family project. I had taken the main initiative in the original project, and so I decided to do the same with the next version, and submitted a proposal for a follow-up volume to the Theory and Methods Workshop. There was considerable momentum to continue, consensus that it should be done, and scholars who had the ability and interest to assume the leadership roles. I served as the quarterback for the project until an editorial committee was formed, and then turned it over to the next generation.

Since one of the purposes of this article is to share some of the inner experiences of a person stumbling through a career in the social sciences in the last half of the 20th century, I probably ought to share some of the thoughts that led to the decision to withdraw from another exciting theoretical project. That decision was one that I continue to have ambivalence about. On the one hand, it was a very demanding project and I invested thousands of hours. As the book was published I felt that there was something symbolic about the color chosen for the cover. It was a deep red, close to the color of blood, and one thing we talked about during parties and socials about that project was how we put so much blood, sweat, and tears into it that it was an appropriate color.

On the other hand, it was the most exhilarating, interpersonally gratifying, intellectually stimulating activity of my career. I felt very lucky to be a part of it, and I recognized that my involvement in it was partly that I was in the right place at the right time. I felt at the time that it would be the most outstanding thing that I would do in my career, and I still feel that way. When it came time to do another similar type of project, a certain part of my heart, my brain, and desires wanted to be involved as a central figure in it, and another part of me wanted to turn it over to a new generation, to a different group of scholars, and let them do their thing because we needed to do a different thing in the late '80s and in the '90s than we'd done in the middle '70s. So on some days I'm glad I backed out; on other days, I kick myself.

As I was making the decision to not get involved in a substantial role in the next theory building project, I explored a number of alternatives about what I wanted to do, and eventually decided that it would be helpful to the field, and interesting to me, to help create a textbook that would be an introduction to family science. The goal was to help the Introduction to Family Science course get on the same footing in universities as introductory courses in Chemistry, Geology, Humanities, Psychology, Sociology, and Economics. I believe the study of the family is a legitimate field in the academic community and that we have begun developing in the last several decades a sizeable body of ideas that are unique and valuable and can help families better attain their goals. The growth of the field is slower than I ever thought it was in 1981, and it's a smaller field than I thought it was, and I believe that it will prosper in the 21st century, and eventually become a peer with other fields and make important contributions to our society.

I concluded in 1987 that the way I could help the field the best would be to help create a text that would be an introduction to that field, so I decided to spend my time on that project. Several other groups of individuals in my university had tried this before, but they hadn't been successful. My initial decision was to become a member of one of these groups, but eventually things evolved so that I wound up chairing a team of three of us. This resulted in *Family Science* (Burr, Day, and Bahr, 1993). In the initial stages two of us from home management, Kathleen Bahr and Beth Bastion, and two of us from CDFR, Joel Moss and myself, team taught an introductory course so we could better integrate the home management and family relations orientations.

My experience with the *Family Science* textbook proved to be an adventure that was unique among the various projects I've undertaken. I took a sabbatical leave the first six months of 1988, and worked full time on that project at the University of Exeter in England. I wrote several of the chapters, and I discovered while writing on this book that it was relatively difficult to identify a familogical perspective in a way sophomores could understand it, and the articulation, integration, and clarification of the ideas turned out to be considerably more difficult than I anticipated. Thus, this project actually became the most challenging and difficult of my career.

During the last part of my career, I've worked at several different projects. Shirley Klein and I led a team of graduate and undergraduate students in a research practicum, and the volume on *Rethinking Family Stress* (Burr & Klein, 1994) was the result. In some ways it was a delightful project as the team was pleasant to work with and an excellent group of scholars. Part of it also was a lesson in what was going on in the field because the first two chapters were another foray into the theory building arena. We tried to chart some directions that we thought would be helpful for the field, but the result was very different from my 1973 foray. In the 1970s, quite a number of colleagues seemed to care, but by the 1990s it was like talking to a wall. No one seemed to care about the directions that we thought were important.

I also worked with Randy Day, Kathleen Gilbert, and Barbara Settles in co-editing a graduate level text: *Research and Theory in Family Science* (1995).

The last project I worked on was a team of us trying to learn more about the role of kindness in families. We observed that almost all of the widely known theories in the social sciences rest on hedonistic assumptions about human processes, but we believed that the altruistic is very important in understanding family life and in developing programs that can help families be effective. We came to this idea from our observations in our own families and also from our religiously based beliefs, and we were initially surprised at how little attention this aspect of life gets in our theories, research, and intervention programs. Our goal was to develop ways to measure this dimension and then see if empirical data would confirm our theories. We gradually learned that words like love, charity, support, caring, and loving have so many other connotations that they are not good conceptual labels for what we wanted to study. We eventually settled with the term kindness, and happily our data were consistent with our theory. The kindness project is a continuation of the fabric made up of the threads described in the earlier parts of this analysis: trying to improve our theories, testing our theories with data as much as possible, and teaching the ideas in university and lay settings to try to help families be effective.

In sum, it has been quite a journey. I found being family scientist to be a rewarding and frustrating, pleasant and disappointing, stimulating and discouraging activity. I found the association with colleagues and the intellectual stimulation to be exhilarating and exalting and growth producing. I found a career in this field to be one where I was always learning and growing, and dramatic new developments are always occurring. It's been exciting to be a part of it in the last half of the 20th century, and my dream of making some helpful contributions to the field has helped provide meaning and beauty. It is a less vital part of my life than my religious beliefs and experiences and my family experiences because those two parts are closer to the core of Wes Burr, but being a family scientist has been an interesting and mostly enjoyable third part.

AUTHOR NOTE

Wesley Burr is Professor Emeritus, Brigham Young University, Provo, UT.

REFERENCES

Day, R. R., Gilbert, K. R., Settles, B. H., & Burr, W. R. (1995). *Research and theory in family science.* Pacific Grove, CA: Brooks/Cole Publishing Co.

Burr, W. R. (1970). Satisfaction with Various Aspects of Marriage Over the Life Cycle: A Random Middle-Class Sample. *Journal of Marriage and the Family, 32*, x, 27-29.

Burr, W. R. (1971). An Expansion and Test of a Role Theory of Marital Satisfaction. *Journal of Marriage and the Family, 33*, x, 368-372.

Burr, W. R. (1972). Role Transitions: A Reformulation of Theory. *Journal of Marriage and the Family, 34*, 407-416.

Burr, W. R. (1973). *Theory Construction and the Sociology of the Family*, New York: Wiley-Interscience.

Burr, W. R. (1976). *Successful Marriage: A Principles Approach*, Homewood, Illinois: The Dorsey Press.

Burr, W. R., Hill, R., Nye, I. F., & Reiss, I. L. (1979). *Contemporary Theories About the Family*, Volume I and II, New York: The Free Press.

Burr, W. R. & Leigh, G. K. (1983). Famology: A new discipline. *Journal of Marriage and the Family, 45*, x, 467-480.

Burr, W. R., Day, R. D. & Bahr, K. S. (1993). *Family Science*. Pacific Grove, CA: Brooks/Cole Publishing Company.

Burr, W.R. & Klein, S. (1994). *Rethinking Family Stress*. Newbury Park: Sage Publications.

Life Course Reflections

Frank F. Furstenberg

KEYWORDS. Autobiography, adolescence, adolescent pregnancy, fatherhood, longitudinal research

EARLY INFLUENCES

My family encouraged further academic study and supported my decision to pursue a PhD in sociology. I came from a socially committed activist family. My maternal grandfather was a philanthropist and civil rights leader in Baltimore. On the paternal side, my grandfather had emigrated from Sweden, and had moved from work in a watch factory to becoming a jeweler and watchmaker. Despite his rise to the middle class, he never abandoned his socialist leanings.

After completing medical school, my father settled in Baltimore, where he became a politically active physician–an early proponent of national health insurance and a passionate opponent of racial and economic stratification. My mother had received a social work degree from Columbia University in the early 1930s, and shared my father's strong commitment to helping the less fortunate and the disadvantaged. Sociology seemed an appropriate way of combining these activist, political sentiments instilled in my upbringing with a personal predisposition toward academic endeavors, perhaps in my genes.

THE FIELD OF FAMILY STUDIES

The field of family studies has become so much richer in my professional lifetime. It has benefited from the development of social history, gender studies, demography, and public policy. I fell in love with sociology my sophomore year in college. It happened in a course taught by

Ira DeA. Reid, Chair and sole member of the Sociology Department at Haverford College, a small Quaker institution outside of Philadelphia. The only African American on the Haverford faculty, Professor Reid was an imposing man of statuesque build and stentorian tone. Reid had studied with Franklin Frazier, who conducted pioneering research on Black families in the post-Civil War. Though I was mesmerized by Professor Reid's teaching style, I recall having considerable difficulty understanding much of what was discussed in class and a lot of what we read that semester. The course was full of *big ideas*: the link between America's current crises in poverty, work, the family, and international relations. I don't remember everything we read but the list included most of the current critiques of American society that were part of the public discourse at that time: David Riesman's *The Lonely Crowd* (1961); Paul Goodman's *Growing Up Absurd* (1960); Robert and Helen Lynd's *Middletown* (1956); William W. Whyte's *The Organization Man* (1965); and C. Wright Mills' *The Causes of World War III* (1976).

The late 1950s were a heady time in American sociology. Sociologists still wrote for the public and the discipline was far less specialized and academic than it was to become later in the twentieth century. Many practitioners spoke out on what C. Wright Mills referred to as "the link between private troubles and public issues." And sociological training meant reading broadly in the social sciences, including history, economics, anthropology and psychology.

Once I took Professor Reid's course, I never wavered from my intention to become an academic, though I had little idea what that involved. My junior year was spent in Sweden, where I had the good fortune of seeing what late 1950s America looked like from the vantage point of a European social democracy. How peculiar it made our culture and social arrangements appear by contrast to the progressive Scandinavians, who were constantly asking me to explain American patterns of sexuality, race relations, or poverty. When I returned in 1960, I discovered that America was finally awakening to the problems of racial and economic inequality. As did so many other students of my generation, I became more politically active. Sociology seemed to provide a set of tools for examining and addressing the country's ills.

In the early 1960s, graduate training was far less institutionalized than it is today. No official rankings, no well-developed social networks supplying information, no visits to graduate schools, no information on the Web: I made my decision to go to Columbia partly because one of my teachers said that I should spend time living in New York City. I was told that the place to go was Columbia University, which was still enjoying its reputation as the premier institution for studying sociology due to the presence of two giant figures in the field: Robert K. Merton and Paul Lazarsfeld. Merton, a student of Talcott Parsons, had fashioned a series of what he termed "middle-range theories" of social behavior that translated Parsons' grand and abstruse efforts to synthesize the European traditions of Weber, Durkheim, Freud, and Simmel into more modest and lucid essays about the workings of society. Lazarsfeld, in turn, invented ingenious methods to test selected efforts. The students of the Columbia School of Sociology, Lewis and Rose Coser, Seymour Lipset, Peter and Alice Rossi, and James Coleman among others, launched a series of empirical studies at the Bureau of Applied Social Research.

My early interests pointed me in the direction of deviant behavior. Merton sent me to work with one of his students, Richard A. Cloward, who was teaching at the School of Social Work. Cloward had developed the idea that neighborhoods provided "opportunity structures" for deviant as well as conventional behavior. By increasing legitimate opportunities for work and family formation, he believed that youth would be less inclined to engage in antisocial activities. His work brought together ideas from the Chicago School of Sociology and Merton's ideas on anomie. Like many of the current efforts to attack poverty by changing social opportunities, Cloward and his colleagues had designed one of the nation's first anti-poverty programs funded by the Office of Economic Opportunity in the Kennedy/Johnson Administration. Mobilization for Youth was a social experiment and before I knew it, I found myself designing surveys to evaluate changes in family and youth behavior, which ultimately became the topic of my dissertation.

Despite the intellectual ferment, Columbia was not an easy place to be, and the early 1960s was not an easy time to be a graduate student (if there ever is one). The Vietnam War was escalating, and a civil war of sorts was taking place across university campuses as students and faculty were renegotiating relations in and outside the classroom. "Which side are you on?" was a refrain that addressed both foreign and domestic relationships. I left Columbia the year before the campus was barricaded by protesting students and virtually shut down for a whole year by student strikes. I missed that event because in 1966, my wife and I decided that it was time to have a child, which meant finishing my dissertation in a hurry.

Married at 22 and a parent at 26 was not unusual in the early 1960s. But timely parenthood was hardly the reason for this decision. The imminent possibility of being drafted (which would have forced me to leave the country) changed my plans. I remember saying to my thesis advisor, William J. Goode, that I would be ready to defend in the spring of 1967. A man of immense critical sensibilities and uncommonly good sense, Si Goode replied that he wasn't sure that I was ready. "Well, if you won't be there," I countered, "I'll find someone else who will." Si relented and I completed my thesis in 1967 in nearly record time for Columbia. On the other hand, my dissertation deservedly never became a classic.

While I was writing my dissertation, I became involved in an evaluation of one of the nation's first comprehensive care programs for teenage mothers. Here is how it happened. One day, my mother, who was a social worker at Sinai Hospital in Baltimore, called me. She said she needed some questions for an evaluation study that they were planning to undertake on the program. Fully informed by my single course on research evaluation, I explained that it was impossible to write questions without fully understanding the program's goals and services. She replied, "But I need the questions on Monday." Being a good son, I wrote a set of questions with a long disclaimer about why it was unprofessional to do what I had done. Next thing I knew, I was invited down to Baltimore to give my first lecture on evaluation. So I began what has come to be known as The Baltimore Study–a 30-year longitudinal investigation of the lives of the teenage mothers, their children, and now, their children's offspring (Brooks-Gunn, Guo, Furstenberg, 1993; Elo, King, & Furstenberg, 1999; Furstenberg, 1971a, 1971b, 1976a, 1976b, 1976c, 1980, 1988, 1999a; Furstenberg, Jr., Brooks-Gunn, & Morgan, 1987; Furstenberg & Crawford, 1978; Furstenberg, Levine, & Brooks-Gunn, 1990; Furstenberg, Lincoln, & Menken, 1981).

In the meantime, I had taken a job at the University of Pennsylvania, where I had been hired on the basis of a strong recommendation from Goode (who has since told me that he thought that I probably would not amount to anything because I enjoyed life too much) and a single published article entitled "Industrialization and the American Family: A Look Backward" (Furstenberg, 1966). The article, a slightly revised course paper, would not have happened were it not for the fact that Robert Merton happened to mention in a lecture that he published his first article at the age of 24. Twenty-four at the time, I thought I'd better do something about it. So I sent the paper to the *American Sociological Review*. Drawing on historical data from travelers' diaries in the 19th century, it demonstrated that the nuclear family existed well before industrialization, a fact that was still contested in the 1960s.

In the late 1960s, it was still unusual for a graduate student to publish an article. After all, it was a time when faculty were commonly hired before completing a dissertation and without giving a formal job talk. No job announcements and no equal opportunity employment, it was still the era of the old boys' network. Penn was not an especially promising department, though it had a strong reputation in criminology and demography. Neither a criminologist nor a demographer, I seemed to be equally satisfactory (or unsatisfactory) to both camps.

My pre-tenure years were difficult, to say the least. In those years, junior faculty at Penn did most of the teaching and were not even invited to faculty meetings. At the end of my second year, I resigned to take a job in the federal government. Persuaded by the Chair to go on leave instead (it was already April when I told him of my decision), I went off to Washington in 1969 to the National Institute for Law Enforcement and Criminal Justice. To my utter astonishment, I found government much worse than academia (Furstenberg, 1971c).

After a month, I wanted to return to academia and started looking for another position. The academic market place was suffering its first real retrenchment as the Vietnam War was escalating and as the economy was discovering that it could not afford "both guns and butter." No job offer materialized. In 1970, the year I turned 30, I returned to Penn with my tail between my legs and buckled down to work.

Work was painfully slow. I was still collecting data on the Baltimore Study and had not really developed a sustained line of inquiry. Initially, I was turned down for tenure but managed to squeak by in 1972, at the end of my fifth year at Penn, the point at which tenure decisions were made in those days. I was relieved but also felt unsure that I merited the promotion. My colleagues were hardly overwhelming in their enthusiasm of my future promise. I set about to prove them wrong though it was some years still before I reached professional maturity–when I had a clear idea of my research agenda and a real sense of mission.

In the 1970s, I began to explore new areas and to experiment with different techniques of research. As a result of my friendship with John Modell, I did several papers in social history (Furstenberg, 1971d; Furstenberg, Strong, & Crawford, 1979; Furstenberg & Thrall, 1971; Modell, Furstenberg, & Hershberg, 1976). Glen Elder became a mentor and friend; I acquired an interest in life course research and began to take up demographic studies (Cherlin & Furstenberg, 1983; Furstenberg, 1971e, 1988; Furstenberg, Nord, Peterson, &, Zill, 1983; Cherlin, Furstenberg, Chase-Lansdale, Lindsay, Robins, Morison, & Teitler, 1991; Iversen, Furstenberg, Belzer, 1999; Jacobs & Furstenberg, 1986).

The publication of *Unplanned Parenthood* in (Furstenberg,1976a) freed me to move away (or so I thought at the time) from the area of adolescent parenthood.

I began to collaborate with Graham Spanier on a study of the transition from divorce to remarriage (Furstenberg & Nord, 1985; Furstenberg, Nord, Peterson, Zill, 1983; Furstenberg & Seltzer, 1986; Furstenberg, & Spanier, 1984a, 1984b, 1987; Spanier & Furstenberg, 1982). I started doing qualitative research and read widely in the Chicago School Studies of Sociology.

At the time, I felt unsettled and at sea. Now I recognize that the post-tenure period is a time of great potential growth and professional development. A young scholar has an opportunity to recast his or her academic identity and begin to shed the unwanted burdens of early professional socialization. As you approach the second third of your career–the middle years–it is absolutely essential to be certain that you are doing the work that you want to do and are setting your own agenda.

One of the great satisfactions in the middle career is beginning to train students who are experiencing the same sorts of dilemmas that you had in earlier years. Many of these students in time become collaborators and friends as their careers begin to unfold. There comes a point in an academic career when it becomes more pleasurable to see your younger colleagues and students publish than it is to write another article yourself, though I confess that I still get than charge from looking a fresh data analysis. I'm inclined to stop whatever I am doing and look at the results. It also becomes less of a burden to write and more fun. The fear of rejection and the perception of critical response for not doing enough are deeply etched in the scholarly superego, but the terrors that they invoke diminish in time. With experience and time, you learn to suspend these feelings so that you let go more when you write. As a mature scholar, you begin to find a voice and develop a longer-range view that provides perspective on your work. You neither dismiss it as being trivial nor overstate its importance but come to consider as merely a link in the chain of discovery.

The stakes of our work have increased as the public perceives that the family is threatened by broader social and economic forces and that children's development is being compromised by the growing demands on the family to provide resources that it often does not possess. My own work has accordingly become more interdisciplinary and more aimed at the linking the macro-level changes in society with the everyday experiences of parents, children, and the surrounding cast of characters who used to lend a hand, but are often no longer available for support–kin, neighbors, and the surrounding community.

Recently, I have begun to think more about the peculiar properties of American culture and social institutions that give our family life its distinctive qualities. We are a society that gives immense latitude to parents, and many Americans find the idea that "it takes a whole village to raise a child" either anomalous or repugnant. More and more social scientists have been drawn into the "culture wars" over the family. I would argue that the dialogue and controversy have both positive elements and potential dangers for how we function in society. It is necessary to walk a fine line between partisanship and detachment. In our role as social scientists (as opposed to interested citizens), we must be prepared to have our cherished beliefs challenged by the evidence. Yet, we cannot be so detached and removed from social debates that we become deluded that the evidence will simply speak for itself. Thus, we are ultimately thrust into the ambiguous role of participant observers in our own society.

As I entered the final third of my career, I began to think more about how to operate in this delicate terrain between scholarship and social action. I have no wish to give up my role as a researcher who must be willing not to develop a strong stake in a particular outcome, who is prepared to follow the evidence wherever it leads, and to speak out against those who wish to distort the findings of research to suit their political purposes. At the same time, I cannot afford to turn a deaf ear on the very real suffering that takes place in America and the larger world because of injustice and inequity. Sociologists have always had a role simply giving a voice to the unheard and explaining their perspective on the world. Understanding the circumstances of the inner-city poor, rural families under siege, street children, abused spouses, and those in unfortunate or unfamiliar settings provokes policy makers to make room on their agendas and gets the public stirred up to support action (Cherlin & Furstenberg 1986, 1992, 1994; Foster & Furstenberg, 1998, 1999a; Furstenberg & Cherlin, 1991; Furstenberg et al., 1999; Furstenberg & Weiss, 2000).

We have made smaller strides in learning how to devise effective policies, develop successful programs and services, and couple political actions with promising solutions. Our most prestigious journals and training programs are more inclined to talk about research in the abstract than on the ground. Could it be otherwise? Will we become better able to integrate so-called basic and applied research in the next century? I don't think we can afford the luxury of being so detached in the future. Our science may improve when we are actually put to the test of trying to alter the institutions and practices that we study.

AUTHOR NOTE

Frank F. Furstenberg is Professor of Sociology, Department of Sociology, University of Pennsylvania, 3718 Locust Walk, Philadelphia, PA 19104-6299.

References were assembled by the editors and added to the text.

REFERENCES

Brooks-Gunn, J., Guo, G., & Furstenberg, F. F., Jr. (1993). Who drops out of and who continues beyond high school? A 20-year follow-up of black urban youth. *Journal of Research on Adolescence*, *3*, 3, 271-194.

Cherlin, A. & Furstenberg, F. F., Jr. (1983). The American family in the year 2000. *Futurist*, *17*, 3, 7-14.

Cherlin, A. & Furstenberg, F. F., Jr. (1986; 1992). *The new American grandparent: a place in the family, a life apart*. Cambridge, MA : Harvard University Press.

Cherlin, A. & Furstenberg, F. F., Jr. (1994). Stepfamilies in the United States: A reconsideration. *Annual Review of Sociology*, *20*, 359-381.

Cherlin, A. J., Furstenberg, F. F., Jr., Chase-Lansdale, P., Lindsay, K. K. E., Robins, P. K., Morison, D. R., & Teitler, J. O. (June 7,1991). Longitudinal studies of effects of divorce on children in Great Britain and the United States. *Science*, *252*, 5011.

Elo, I. T., King, R. B., & Furstenberg, F. F., Jr. (1999). Adolescent females: Their sexual partners and the fathers of their children. *Journal of Marriage and the Family*, *61*, 1, 74-84.

Foster, E. M. & Furstenberg, F. F., Jr. (1999). The most disadvantaged children: Trends over time. *Social Service Review*, 73, 4, 560-578.

Foster, E. M. & Furstenberg, F. F., Jr. (1998). Most disadvantaged children: Who are they and where do they live? *Journal of Poverty*, 2, 2, 23-47.

Furstenberg, F. F., Jr. (1966). Industrialization and the American family: A look backward. *American Sociological Review*, *31*, 3, 326-337.

Furstenberg, F. F., Jr. (1971a). Preventing unwanted pregnancies among adolescents. *Journal of Health and Social Behavior*, *12*, 4, 340-347.

Furstenberg, F. F., Jr. (1971b). Birth control experience among pregnant adolescents; The process of unplanned parenthood. *Social Problems*, *19*, 2, 192-203.

Furstenberg, F. F., Jr. (June, 1971c). Political intrusion and governmental confusion: The case of the National Institute of Law Enforcement and Criminal Justice. *American Sociologist*, *6*, Supp, 59-61.

Furstenberg, F. F., Jr. (1971d). Public reaction to crime in the streets. *American Scholar*, *40*, 4, 601-610.

Furstenberg, F. F., Jr. (1971e). Mobility of orientation in the family. *Social Forces*, *49*, 4, 595-602.

Furstenberg, F. F., Jr. (1976a). *Unplanned parenthood: the social consequences of teenage childbearing*. New York: Free Press.

Furstenberg, F. F., Jr. (1976b). The social consequences of teenage parenthood. *Family Planning Perspective*, *8*, 4, 148-164.

Furstenberg, F. F., Jr. (1976c). Premarital pregnancy and marital instability. *Journal of Social Issues, 32*, 1, 67-86.

Furstenberg, F. F., Jr. (1980). Burdens and Benefits: The Impact of Early Childbearing on the Family *Journal of Social Issues, 36*, 1, 64-87.

Furstenberg, F. F., Jr. (1988). When will teenage childbearing become a problem?: The implications of western experience for developing countries. *Studies in Family Planning, 29*, 2, 246-253.

Furstenberg, F. F., Jr. (1999a). *Managing to make it: urban families and adolescent success*. Chicago: University of Chicago Press.

Furstenberg, F. F., Jr. (1999b). Is the modern family a threat to children's health? *Society, 36*, 5, 31-37.

Furstenberg, F. F., Jr. (1999c). When will teenage childbearing become a problem: The implications of Western developing countries. *Studies in Family Planning, 29*, 2, 246-253.

Furstenberg, F. F. Jr. et al. (1999). *Managing to make it: Urban families and adolescent success*. Chicago: University of Chicago Press, 1999.

Furstenberg, F. F. Jr., Brooks-Gunn, J. & Morgan, P. (1987). Adolescent mothers in later life Cambridge: Cambridge University Press.

Furstenberg, F. F., Jr. & Cherlin, A. J. (1991). Divided families: What happens to children when parents part. Cambridge, MA: Harvard University Press.

Furstenberg, F. F. Jr. & Crawford, A. G. (1978). Family support: Helping teenage mothers to cope. *Family Planning Perspective, 10*, 6, 322-333.

Furstenberg, F. F., Jr., Levine, J. A., Brooks-Gunn, J. (1990). The children of teenage mothers: Patterns of early childbearing in two generations. *Family Planning Perspectives, 22*, 2, 54-61.

Furstenberg, F. F., Jr., Lincoln, R., & Menken, J. (Eds.) (1981). *Teenage sexuality, pregnancy, and childbearing*. Philadelphia: University of Pennsylvania Press.

Furstenberg, F.F., Jr. & Nord, C.W. (1985). Parenting apart: Patterns of childrearing after marital disruption. *Journal of Marriage and the Family, 47*, 4, 893-904.

Furstenberg, F.F., Jr., Nord, C.W., Peterson, J.L., & Zill, N. (1983). The life course of children of divorce: Marital disruption and parental contact. *American Sociological Review, 48*, 5, 656-668.

Furstenberg, F. F., Jr. & Seltzer, J. A. (1986). Divorce and child development. *Sociological Studies of Child Development, 1*, 137-160.

Furstenberg, F. F., Jr. & Spanier, G. B. (1984a; 1987). *Recycling the family: Remarriage after divorce*. Beverly Hills/Newbury Park, CA: Sage Publications.

Furstenberg, F. F., Jr. & Spanier, G. B. (1984b). The risk of dissolution in remarriage: An examination of Cherlin's hypothesis of incomplete institutionalization. *Family Relations, 33*, 3, 433-441.

Furstenberg, F. F., Jr., Strong, D., & Crawford, A.G. (1979). What happened when the census was redone: An analysis of the recount of 1870 in Philadelphia. *Sociology and Social Research, 63*, 3, 475-505.

Furstenberg, F. F., Jr & Thrall, C. A. (1971). Counting the jobless: The impact of job rationing on the measurement of unemployment. *Annals of the American Academy of Political and Social Science, 418*, (March) 45-59.

Furstenberg, F. F., Jr. & Weiss, C. C. (2000). Intergenerational transmission of fathering roles in at risk families. *Marriage & Family Review, 29*, 2-3, 181-201.

Goodman, Paul. 1960. *Growing up absurd: Problems of youth in the organized system.* New York: Random House.

Iversen, R. R., Furstenberg, F. F., Jr. & Belzer, A. A. (1999). How much do we count?: interpretation and error-making in the decennial census. *Demography, 36*, 1, 121-134.

Jacobs, J. A. & Furstenberg, F. F., Jr. (1986). Changing places: Conjugal careers and women's marital mobility. *Social Forces, 64*, 3, 714-732.

Lynd, R. S. & Lynd, H. M. (1956). *Middletown: A study in American culture.* New York: Harcourt, Brace & World.

Mills, C. W. (1976). *The causes of world war three.* Westport, Conn: Greenwood Press.

Modell, J., Furstenberg, F. F., Jr., & Hershberg, T. (1976). Social change and transitions to adulthood in historical perspective. *Journal of Family History, 1*, 1, 7-32.

Riesman, D. (1961). *The lonely crowd.* New Haven: Yale University Press.

Spanier, G. B. & Furstenberg, F. F., Jr. (1982). Remarriage after divorce: A longitudinal analysis of well-being. *Journal of Marriage and the Family, 44*, 3, 709-720.

Whyte, W. H. (1956). *The organization man.* New York: Simon & Schuster.

Everyday Life in Family Scholarship and Family Life: Sketches and Interpretations

Barbara H. Settles

KEYWORDS. Autobiography, family life education, international, future of families

INTRODUCTION

Twice I have been asked to compose an autobiographical remembrance. When I was in high school there was a craze for creative writing and performance. The trick was to be forthcoming and interesting enough to get a good grade, but not so transparent as to provide the teachers' lounge with juicy gossip. The second is this essay and the challenge is to pull from my stories those events that may be interesting to a family scholar and to understanding how my career has been shaped. I love to do watercolor sketches, which pick up on the color and impression of the moment, and hope these short anecdotes will give a feel for what was important to me in my decisions. I will give a few key dates and events that tie together the order and sequence of how things evolved, then review several themes of importance to me in my work and note how the personal and professional have been linked.

SOCIAL CHANGE, MOBILITY AND EDUCATION

I was born at the end of the depression in 1937 and was for seven years my father's oldest "son," with my sister born in 1941 and my brother in 1944. My father gave me the impression that I could do anything any boy could do. My daddy had missed the First World War by being too young and the second by being too old. My mother was a decade younger than he. My family was rather the classic tale of American ambitions, whereas my mother's family was a long-time Appalachian family. My great-grandmother was a McCoy and my grandmother an Adkins, and it was said that they never went down to visit their relatives in Kentucky because of historic animosities. My granddaddy died from pneumonia at the end of WWII, so my memory of him is mostly pictures in my mind. He looked the part of the mountaineer sitting by the fire, or plowing with a mule and feeding the hog. My grandmother was proud to say at a Thanksgiving dinner that all her children had taught school. She had seven children all born in January or February to avoid milk fever and lost one to whooping cough. She was a midwife to women further up in the hollows. They built a house in town and my granddaddy worked for the schools as groundskeeper and janitor during the depression. My mother had hoped to go to Berea College but was too well-off to qualify and worked her way through college at Marshall doing housework and childcare. My father's family, the Hallidays, came to the United States from the Cotswold area of England early in the century. His dad was a butcher who suffered from diabetes and died before there was any treatment. His mother, a Rowels, while not highly educated, was an avid reader. She read to her four boys and a girl romance novels just to keep them home as teenagers.

My daddy started elementary school when he was four and had graduated from high school when he was fourteen. His family needed his paycheck and Ohio State University did not think he was old enough to matriculate and told him to come back when he was 18. By the time he was 18, he had been discovered sweeping up in the shop by a manager who got him a job in purchasing. He gravitated to the crowd that was involved in university and political life and shared a house with a group of young professors who were later administrators of the university. He felt the lack of formal education. He often kidded me, as I pursued an academic career, that professors, as he had known them, had a hard time balancing their checkbooks and counting points when playing bridge.

My daddy and mother chose to buy a stone cottage out in the country. The lifestyle of gardening, raising chickens, grass cutting, and entertaining for Sunday dinner were their pleasures. I went to the university preschool when my mother taught a college class and later went to a private kindergarten. My public grade school was double grades through eighth grade, so my father ran for school board to assure there were a junior high school and a new high school complex. My fifth and sixth grade teacher was inspirational and she came to my doctoral graduation. She was an

American history buff and she kept me busy by having me tutor others. Ohio State University (OSU) was the dominant player throughout my elementary and secondary education and my teachers. College was pragmatic, based on Dewey and Bode, with a touch of Carl Rogers and learning theory and in family classes Duvall and Hill reigned supreme. I loved OSU. It was huge, and classes were great.

One of my father's friends knew how the sorority rush process worked. If it had been me alone I would not have accepted the right invitations and been an independent. One serendipitous happening my sophomore year occurred when two sorority sisters asked if I would be willing to date someone a little younger than me. I was cross with my current beau, so I accepted their offer and met my lifelong love, Andy. Because he was in a five-year engineering program and a year behind me I had a little less pressure to get married early. After seven years we married at the ages of 24 and 23.

My husband's family was quite mobile too. His mother was born in Poland and immigrated when her mother came in search of her husband. They had refused to go to Russian schools, and assimilation here was important. Andy's mother did housework in high school and her employer helped her go to Miami University for the two-year teacher certification program. His grandfather worked for the paper plant and his dad used the University of Cincinnati work-study program in engineering. The background that was never discussed was that both grandparents were raised in Shakertown as orphans who got back together after leaving at their 18th birthday.

Andy went to OSU in engineering. He became focused on physics and took advanced courses for graduate credit his fourth year and fifth year and had many courses to apply to a PhD program. We had no idea how academic and research careers were developed. I remember my fiancé and my mother cornering me on the front porch on a summer's evening to tell me that neither one of them wanted to be blamed if I did not do what I wanted to do for a career. They indicated that I should go to graduate school and that this goal would not happen unless I made an appointment with the dean and filled out the application. Andy made fallback plans in case we failed.

I read the university bulletin to understand the rules. I was scheduled to graduate with my master's degree at the end of winter session and had a stipend only for spring, with no other job in view. Fortunately, my advisor assumed I was going on for my PhD, so my stipend was renewed and we started taking French for the language exam. Because of Sputnik, there were more stipends and good summer employment that allowed us both to attend full-time. The summer we married he had a job out in New Mexico at the Sandia Research Laboratory, which allowed us to rent an apartment and pay our fees that were due before our first paycheck came for our assistantships. We were not as poor as our parents had been, but everyday we were living on graduate assistantships that had not been adjusted since the depression. Andy's Aunt Sophie gave him $500.00 for a wedding present and we were "rich" for several years. We always repaid to a fund her money when we used it for deposits.

My theory of women's options was built from an observation that most of the people who finished degrees did not have children before they completed their studies. In my graduate program I wrote a paper on women's roles that was based on Kilpatrick's typology of risk and combinations of women's commitments. High commitment to work, fertility, and spousal companionship was risky, but had a high payoff. With someone to marry, my theory was to postpone children and be satisfied with two children. My husband had assumed that we would be a dual-career couple.

Most of my major life decisions were made before the advent of the second women's movement so I was often surprised at the issues raised, which I thought had already been addressed. My feminism was based on nineteenth-century women's rights and abolition movements. Growing up in Ohio for me involved having real pride in the Civil War, the Underground Railroad, and abolition. Although Ohio State suffered from provincialism, they had been educating women, blacks, and international students for many years. I remember the fifties and sixties as having room for aspirations and social consciousness.

HOME ECONOMICS IN MY PROFESSION AND PERSONAL LIFE

Home economics arose as an interdisciplinary study early in the 20th century as science and engineering with the goal of producing applications that could change homemaking radically. A primary theme was that rational thought and problem solving could provide individuals and families with the knowledge to choose from available options those technologies and products that would best advance their goals. Within this paradigm, the ordinary person could share in the culture and advance their position within the class structure (Settles, 1995). The name "Home Economics" has faded from academe and home economists have been redesignated in higher education. The new family studies and family science departments have prospered and expanded. The profession was a major route to mobility for my family with my mother, her sister, my sister, and three of my cousins following suit. My first position, in 1959, as a home economics extension agent had great respect in the community and was well paid. Youth and inexperience were overlooked, as my recent education was modern and useful.

My studies at the university had a strong basis in science, social sciences and the arts with wonderful teachers throughout the university. I was fortunate to have Dr. Bea Paolucci for my education methods course. She went on to Michigan State to specialize in home management and we later became reacquainted in the NCFR theory and methodology workshop. Through a course in household equipment, Ruth Beard presented dynamic demonstrations of the principles of physics and engineering applied in the least intimidating way. One of my art courses was based on what became the content of that book *Color Me Beautiful*. My house plans were put in the sample book for engineering drawing. Chemistry, bacteriology, psychology, sociology, and art history were all taught by the top professors. I worked for Dr. Everett Rogers who was doing research in rural development. His theory about the adoption of new technologies was one that I have used many times in my own work.

As an undergraduate I spent an exchange term at the Merrill-Palmer School in Detroit, which was on the cutting edge of family and developmental studies. Such leaders as Richard Kerckoff, Hy Rodman, Keith Osburn, Betsy Meadows, and Dorthey Lee were my teachers. The style and approach of the program was much like being in graduate school, including the Dewey "learn by doing" techniques. Even at that time, their child development labs included toddlers and parents. For our class on work and human development we were put in touch with such leaders as George Romney, auto executive, before his political career began, and Ruth Roman, the actress, who was on tour. High tea and great speakers, field trips and living together were among the features, which built close ties and lots of intellectual talk.

My economics professor, Dr. Meno Lovenstein, was a charismatic teacher. The story of his major career shift influenced my own view of university life. After I graduated he married a colleague and built a lovely home in Columbus. At this time, universities were beginning the quest for quick institutional fame and the legislature had provided the state universities with money for a few super-grade professors. Dr. Lovenstein had done a great deal of public lecturing and university development work and was a long-term member of the OSU faculty. When he asked about these new professorships he was told that he would not be likely to move because of his family and home and so they did not need to hold him. A few months later he had one of the super-grade professorships at Ohio University and rolled out his house plans before his chair and said that he was constructing it on a bigger property where his kids could have ponies. It is the perception of vulnerability, not simply discrimination, which gives rise to a lack of appreciation and support.

Home economics offered an open and unstructured graduate program so I was able to pursue a family studies emphasis with lots of sociology, educational psychology, and developmental work. My advisor was new to the university and although I came back to my undergraduate university I do not believe I had more than one teacher with whom I had studied before. Dr. Christine Hillman was very special to me. She had a bold and clear mind and encouraged me to learn on my own and be a serious scholar. Her own career was somewhat curious. She had finished her doctorate at Case Western in Cleveland after she was married and was encouraged by her husband, who was a self-taught man who had risen in the insurance business. He could live anywhere in his territory in the Midwest, so she was able to take a position at the Extension Graduate Center at University of Wisconsin and then come to OSU as a full professor to lead the graduate program. She ran for president of NCFR one year and belonged to the Groves Conference. She sponsored me for the Groves Conference. At least a dozen dissertations were written under her direction. Her own career was cut short when she departed from OSU due to her husband's promotion. She moved to Boston without securing a position, because his company added the amount of her OSU salary to her husband's wages. Her early death left me without her sponsorship and advice.

I have been active in the national organization (now the American Association of Family and Consumer Sciences), paid my dues, was recognized at their 75th anniversary celebration for leadership and was invited to present a futures paper for the Massachusetts Avenue prize. Even at my advanced age I am somewhat a radical in this group. I served as president of the local group, Delaware Association of Family and Consumer Sciences, a constructive link with other educational groups that serve our area. Recently the role of international home economics has been of interest to me in Central America, including participation in the recent regional International Home Economics Association meeting in Puerto Rico (Settles & Barboni, 1998) and a conference on Family and Sustainable Development in Panama in 2001.

SOCIOLOGY AS A FIELD AND MY PROFESSIONAL COMMITMENT

During my doctoral work I came to appreciate the value of sociological methods and theories in family and community studies. Dr. Russell Dynes was on my committee and was a mentor. (He and I have crossed paths many times with his coming to University of Delaware subsequent to his work with ASA as executive director.) John Cuber, Al Clarke, and Merton Oyler were working in areas of child and family studies. Cuber and Harroff had just completed their study of *The Significant Americans* in which they used a qualitative approach. At that time most sociologists were convinced that objectivism was the route to science with structural functionalism being preferred. I read Busman's arguments against Parsons because my advisor had known him in Cleveland. Because my assistantship was funded by the agricultural experiment station I had help in the latest programs, the California biomedical series. Dr. Dynes suggested examining the tools I borrowed from other studies to see if they were reliable. At my defense I remember being asked to discuss the good stuff, that is, the comments and ideas the families had given me that were not in the objective measures. It was not the fashion then to write about those data.

I joined the sociology honorary, the Rural Sociological Society, as well as the American Sociological Association in graduate school. In the family section of ASA I have served on the Council and have been in the aging and life course section and the sex/gender section. More recently I have been active in the International Sociological Association as president of the Committee on Family Research. I have found many colleagues and professional support within the sociological networks.

FAMILY STUDIES AS THE INTERDISCIPLINARY CONNECTION

The National Council on Family Relations has been a meeting place for all the many professions in service to families, with high quality research and evaluation. From its beginning, it was an inclusive rather than an exclusive group. When I began to attend in the sixties many of the founders were still active. The "names" I wanted to meet were often sitting by themselves ready to talk, and I also met many of the up-and-coming new lights the same way. Being shy is an advantage in academe. NCFR still is an open crossroads for communication in family science, where I can meet new professionals for the first time as well as keeping up with old friends.

Throughout my life as a student of the family I have found the associations of professionals to be absolutely crucial to my functioning and growth. I am happy to serve in most of them as an officer or committee chair. I have gifts for bringing people together for scholarly interchange, finding support for activities, thinking ahead for the direction of the field in-service education needs. My first major responsibility was as program chair for NCFR in 1979, for which I chose the theme of *Everyday Life in Families*. I enjoyed serving as Vice President for Public Policy for NCFR and remain interested in seeing the organization be a more effective voice for the scholarly knowledge in family science and its implications for policy. Working with such leaders as M. Feldman, C. Chilman, B. Chandler, R. Rubin, E. Anderson, N. Kingsbury, P. Knaub, K. Bogenscheider, L. Koepke, K. Troost, M. A. Hollinger, P. Langley, P. Monroe, and many others on these issues has been exciting and productive.

The Family Science Association is an outcome of the discourse on the field. It was founded to promote several activities, an annual Teaching of Family Science conference and the specialized journal *Family Science Review* (now *Journal of Teaching Marriage and Family*) that were too small to be supported within the NCFR structure. My role, first as treasurer and corporate member, has been to set up systems and support, which have helped the group develop ongoing mechanisms for these activities based on a small membership and participant base.

In my practical work both in Delaware and nationally and internationally I see that family studies has a vulnerable place in academic life. To be a family scholar carries with it the responsibility to care about and attempt to influence some institutionalization of the studies and education in the field (Settles, 1999a). We cannot assume that the field we love and that has been so good for us will continue to thrive unless we attend to both institutional and disciplinary politics. Even sociology is being folded into larger units or even dropped in general education reform (Settles, 1998). Interdisciplinary work requires cross-disciplinary appreciation (Liprie & Settles, 1996) and efforts to gain recognition for the accomplishments and findings (Settles, 1993a). Interdisciplinary efforts often suffer from the tensions the disciplines bring to them as teams of specialists. I will not attempt to explain how much effort has been spent in my own department dealing with the persistence of these differences in perspective.

GETTING STARTED AND MAKING A CAREER

While my husband was still in school, I obtained a job at Otterbein College that was half-time home economics and half-time sociology.

Otterbein had been in the forefront of the abolition movement in the nineteenth century and remained socially conscious. The custom of religious convocation had evolved into a program for important speakers such as Father Drinan and Gore Vidal followed by meetings with these speakers. Buses left each week for the marches and demonstrations of the era.

My mother heard from her former colleague in graduate school that a part-time position was available at Otterbein College in home economics in foods and nutrition. While it was out of my current field I jumped at the chance. Mrs. Mable Joyce, chair, and Mrs. Margaret Gill were the department. I needed more than part-time wages, and she was able to connect me with Dr. Albert Lovejoy, who was the Sociology Department. I was hired across the departments to teach nutrition, food preparation, and demonstration methods in home economics and in sociology to teach introductory sociology, family and research methods. Lovejoy was interested in family studies and studied at Merrill-Palmer School. He referred me to a research and evaluation project in inner-city Columbus that focused on at-risk youth with a program of youth involvement and leadership. Not only did I have a nice stipend to do the work but also it provided my students with a practical research project. I received my tenure early, but not the promotion to Associate Professor, because it was explained to me that my short skirts and long hair were a bit too much for the board.

We had few models for long-term success with dual careers. One academic couple I admired because they had persevered in graduate school and had real positions fell apart over his indiscretions with grants and employees. There was much talk about needing faculty while universities expanded, but for us the pickings seemed mighty slim. When my husband graduated in 1968, the field of physics was collapsing in universities and the Vietnam War was heating up. It was the era before affirmative action, and academic jobs were secretly filled by networks of academics.

Andy's mentor was no more sophisticated than mine in career placement. He had come back from World War II to graduate school and had risen to professor of physics. Our one national job search was not an easy effort. Our collection of refusal letters and insults still amuses and angers us. We were simply not taken as serious people in our search for two real careers. I was frightened we might end up some place like Los Alamos, which was well known for radiation badges, neurotic wives, and contract bridge as distraction. By April 1968 we were deciding to come to Dupont for Andy and either University of Delaware or Glassboro State (now Rowan University) for me. I chose slightly lower pay at Delaware for the title of Associate Professor as there was a master's program. My daddy was pleased that my husband finally had a real job and we had a wonderful party for Andy's graduation. It was the last time I saw my dad; he died of a heart attack the first day of autumn.

I had not been paying much attention to myself, so when I went to select a new doctor for Delaware, I was a little surprised to find myself so far along in pregnancy that it could be detected by exam, not a lab test. I was happy, but frightened. There was no sick leave and maternity leave was unknown. The university was undergoing a major transition. Over 100 professors were hired that year, and the emphasis was now on research and graduate education after many years of liberal arts and engineering focus. Policies and procedures at the university were typical of small colleges with strong presidents and weak departments. Little was written down and what was written was not followed. My classes that fall were responsive and students told everyone I was a fine teacher. When I finally got an appointment to see my Dean it was a most bizarre conversation. First there was some discussion that it would be proper for me to resign, as the public school teachers were required to do. Next there was a statement that I would have to pay for any substitute I might require. This was followed by a long lecture on the fact that I could not be promoted if I left my hair long and loose and wore provocative clothing (i.e., short skirts). I said that I had not moved halfway across the country to quit working. I reminded her that two of my classes were at night when my husband was home. She said that I should be at work at my office everyday for advising and other duties. I did make a standing appointment with a hairdresser so my hair was done each Monday up high on my head into what is now called "Jersey Hair." Wrapped in toilet tissue at night it would last until Friday.

My administrator was not the only one who found my situation inappropriate; many colleagues were at a loss for words or were clearly disapproving. I followed my advisor's earlier advice to wear regular clothes as long as I could and not bring up the subject. My advisor received a call from my Dean to tell her how awful I was to have done this terrible thing and that she should not write such glowing descriptions of me in future. I was 30 and thought my husband and myself ready to be parents. My baby was a dear and waited to be born until the day before spring break. My mother arrived early in March to clean my apartment and worry about me and she was more than pleased to meet one of my classes. She checked out the young women in my apartment building from our college who were to help me out with baby-sitting and was ready to go home soon after we came home from the hospital. My husband had two approved days off from work, one for the day the baby was born and one to take me home. I got by without any approved days. My graduate assistant was allowed to give a diagnostic test for my classes on Monday and I returned to classroom on Wednesday following spring break. Luckily both my pregnancy and recovery were uneventful and Alex, my first son, was healthy and cheery.

HAPPILY EVER AFTER

I spent so much of this essay on how we began our careers because these decisions were so critical and made under such high stress. In retrospect we were fortunate not to know how much we had riding on those choices. Andy spent his career working at Dupont and this is my 32nd anniversary at University of Delaware. We had a second son, Mark, two years after Alex was born. He came more properly for the academic mother, in July, and was also a healthy and delightful child.

While we have had interesting and generally pleasant experiences, it would be silly to think that our lives were only happily ever after. In fact, maintaining a dual-career pattern as well as maintaining one's nuclear and extended family are amazing challenges even today.

TIME AND TIMING

Academic time, company time, and school time are often not compatible. We took our big vacations at Christmas because it was the only time we all could get away from our respective obligations. Academic life has regular peaks and valleys of activity during the terms, with graduate instruction being essentially an evening activity. The academic professional has flexibility but is never actually free. To fill the schedule with meetings and commitments, office hours, and projects is far too easy. We have projects at different stages of completion so we can switch from one to another when we are stuck or waiting for another person to complete their contribution and finishing is a scary surrender. The seven-year cycles of tenure and sabbatical are sufficiently malleable that one may be surprised at how quickly they come around.

Summer has shifted its meaning over the years in our institution. I was shocked my first summer at Delaware when my college wanted my keys back for my office, even though I was teaching summer school. Nine-month contracts were nine months, with professors pursuing different jobs or avocations in the summer. Now you keep up with your research and graduate students and keep the office informed about how to find you. The press to be at the office has slacked, as faculty can answer their e-mail and word-process their work anywhere.

In contrast, chemical companies run continuous shifts 24 hours, 7 days a week in the plants and treasure the early morning hours. My husband's expertise in lasers was respected because nonintrusive measurement did not shut down the process. He often worked 3 straight shifts in the plant and flew home to get to work on time here the next day. Decisions made by 8:00 a.m. were morally superior to late afternoon meetings and plans. However, one is not supposed to carry home the company secrets, so there is a break between the family and the workplace. Even though one may build up vacation days, taking long vacations is a risk in industry. Maybe they can get along without you or transfer or downsize you.

Finding appropriate support services requires effort. We were pleasantly surprised to find an adequate day care center, the Newark Day Nursery that was receiving consultation from our child development program. My husband became the treasurer of the board and made sure the teachers had good compensation and materials budgets. I paid for overtime when faculty meetings scheduled late in the day ran over. Later the YWCA provided great afterschool care, right across the street from my office.

While our new president and his provost were committed to change within the university, it did not arrive all at once. The president, who came to the university the year I arrived, decided to do a long-term planning project in which university committees were formed to look at different issues. In this exercise, the faculty got to know each other and discovered that the rules of the university and the pay scales were different and not equitable in the various colleges. This knowledge provided the momentum for organizing an AAUP union in which I served on the first bargaining team and later served as president and national council member. While productivity in research and publication became more important, my college did not improve labs or typists or support services for housing and operating the research grants.

Dupont had its own culture and recreational facilities that were more fifties than seventies, ballroom dancing, golf, and tennis. My husband had everything for his lab and reports, but the work setting required that anything scholarly should be kept secret. In contrast, in academe the goal was for me to be disseminating my work. Writing and publishing were abstractly what it was about, but actually if I could get a paper accepted on the basis of an abstract and write it on a yellow pad my department might get it typed before the following year's meeting. In high school I had made a critical mistake in not learning to type. This turned out to be a handicap for a professor in a rapidly changing milieu.

ORGANIZATIONAL CULTURE AND CHANGE

Our attitudes toward each of the organizations' likelihood for change were different, too. I was promptly reviewed for tenure and received it. I exercised my academic freedom and became involved in building the union, working on sex education, women's studies, family studies as a major, developing the department and its graduate program, and generally being an activist on campus. I took my turn on the university committees and college committees that are so important to faculty governance and opportunity for women and minorities. I wanted to build an institution I could be pleased to be associated with throughout my career. It was unlikely that we would ever move if Andy were content in his job. The lifetime employment opportunity was still an expected part of company life.

Even before I had tenure I had to stand and be counted. The summer after Alex was born I was to teach a graduate level course on sex education for public school teachers. Suddenly the John Birch Society and other organizations opposed to sex education in schools started a campaign against sex education in the schools with the state legislature, and I received a request for my syllabus, films, and references for the committee considering legislation. This time, however, the university dean, provost, and president and I were on the same side. The university, although a Land Grant university, has jealously preserved its independence and endowment. So the provost wrote a letter refusing the request but inviting the critics to drop in on my class anytime that summer. Not exactly the protection I hoped for, but I went ahead and taught what I saw as important. I have done so ever since and served again last year on a committee to review if what we were teaching in sex education was appropriate. There are always questions about the topics related to family and one must defend academic freedom for students and faculty (Settles, 1999a). The paternalism and security offered by major companies in the sixties gave way to continuous reorganization and training in whatever current management styles were in vogue. As a research and technical consultant, my husband was usually busy and had several different major projects that were significant contributions.

Our theory about it being better to have one's children after grad school worked well for us. We enjoyed them and found family life an excellent relief from stress and pressures at work. Every stage was interesting to us and our children were interested in everything. They were good travelers and entertained other adults like their grandparents with enthusiasm. My husband and I liked doing what kids need. I was a Cub Scout den mother and a driver to music lessons and afterschool programs. My husband liked camping on the ground in the winter with the Boy Scouts. We discovered the Chesapeake Bay and bought a sailboat for weekend retreats. The Pretendre was designed to be a race boat and was fully equipped, but it did not like the light and variable winds of the Chesapeake. We learned as a family how to be patient and to support each other. By the time our children reached their teenage years, we were able to win many of our club races. We still take occasional vacations together sailing in some far-away islands.

Even though I study family and parenting, I was a little taken aback about how quickly the boys were their own persons. Alex and Mark, now grown men, are two of my favorite confidants and friends. They have wonderful judgment and are especially empathetic. However, I would have to say that many of those characteristics were seen even as youngsters. Even in preschool their personalities they were clearly independent. While they were their own selves, they cared for each other and us. As parents our greatest task was to estimate their needs for challenge. Intelligence and insight can be severe gifts. Often students who are bright are ignored when some instruction could be helpful. While their dad and I can cover a lot of areas of study we were not perfectly matched for their needs for instruction. We had to advocate for them in elementary and middle school to get the right challenges and the coaching they needed from others.

DECADES AND DECISIONS

The decades do not usually work out for organizing how things went historically, but we often try to see them that way. It seems to me that the sixties ran up to about 1974 and so forth. When I came to Delaware I was the first full-time faculty member to specialize in family studies. There was uncertainty that there would be enough for me to do, although the teaching load was higher than it is now (with 3 courses and unlimited class size quite normal). A small master's program had been built in home economics education and recently expanded to child development, so I taught a graduate-level family course and a research methods course for the college. I did the capstone core course in family relationships so my undergraduate classes were large. The development of Headstart and a reform in children's services in the state helped the graduate program to grow with more stipends provided by the state. In the seventies I was on many committees as well as serving as an advisor to fourteen students who sought more general gender and family studies work or were interested in day care (B. Wiebe, J. Schmidt, I. H. Talley, R. R. Blum, N. Clouser Edwards, D. Trumbower, P. Koch, M. B. Good, I. W. Zych, E. E. Zannino, A. Newswenger, L. Wiley, J. H. Cripps and B. McCauley).

Both sex education and women's studies were beginning to become interdisciplinary movements on our campus. The university has had a consistent need to improve its service to African American students and other ethnic groups, as one of the universities under judicial review. Throughout my career I have been involved in supporting diversity and promoting opportunities.

Family life education projects are in every stage of my work and have included my close association and friendship with Mary Lou Liprie, whose background in home economics education and adolescent development provides complementary interests and commitments. We have been colleagues in providing in-service teacher education and products for family life education. We have presented many courses, programs, and papers together and been a sounding board for ideas and projects for each other. We keep each other from going crazy when the everyday stresses of an educational institution, family, and friends are extreme. One of our best cooperative ventures was creating a series of videos for teaching about the roots of family studies for our new doctoral program in the '80s (Settles & Liprie, 1982, 1983, 1984, 1986, 1987). We found bits and pieces of funding to bring scholars to campus to speak and then to produce videotape. We ended up with archival and edited tapes for Jessie Bernard, Paul Glick, Mary Calderone, Marvin Sussman, Irma Ayers (Dean Emeriti of our college), and Lois Hoffman (Ivan Nye was not up to the trip so he is discussed but not included). It would be fun to do more interviews, but it requires much more money and dedicated time for current production values. Our current emphasis has moved to linking curriculum and research in adolescent decision making to improve family life education in secondary schools (Settles, Grasse-Bachman, & Liprie, 2000; Settles, Davis, Hanks, III, D. E., & Grasseman-Bachman, 1999).

I met Sue Steinmetz at the 1971 NCFR and ASA meetings, where we were involved in the founding of the theory workshop. We rode back on the plane to Philadelphia with her. She lived less than twenty minutes from my house and was at that time teaching part time everywhere in the region and doing graduate work at Temple. We had begun to build the department by hiring several young professors and one senior professor in child development and early childhood education, but family life had not yet been expanded. I wanted to do more research, but could not buy out without a person on staff. The students were pleased with her teaching; she was able to complete her studies by returning to Case Western Reserve University to work with Marvin Sussman and Jetsy Sprey; she received tenure at Delaware and was promoted to Professor. Our lives have been intertwined both personally and professionally ever since. Sue's love of editing and publishing has been a key element in both of our careers.

A major turning point at work for me was securing a series of research grants from 1975 to 1979 with Judy Van Name, Penny Diener, and Joseph Lucca. The theme was the costs and demands on parents in foster care, with special-needs children and with children with chronic illness. Having outside funding let me develop a different approach to dealing with the chronic resource problems in the department. I was able to develop independent support services and to gather an excellent group of students together to learn and produce some fine scholarly work, advising ten theses at both the undergraduate and graduate level (L. MacRostie, G. Green, M. J. Graf, K. Schmidt, B. Carlough, B. Frumpkin, T. Cristofish, B. Zimney, J. Grymes and C. Paris). As with any group project there were plenty of problems. Doing fieldwork in foster care was difficult due to the primitive state of the records and support systems (Settles, Culley & Van Name, 1976a, b; Van Name, Culley & Settles 1977; Van Name & Settles, 1977). It was a little easier with hospitals in the chronic illness project, but they also wanted to shape who we would talk to and what we would talk about with their clients.

Concepts from my work with special-needs children were useful in understanding the mental strain that changing medical practices and advice often cause for families. Our respondents were frightened about their dependence on an expert who could not be easily replaced if they were at odds with him or her. They blamed themselves for not doing things that were not known earlier. They tended to maintain every intervention they had been given (Settles & Lucca, 1981). Perhaps it was magical thinking, but doing something was preferable to waiting to see if things changed on their own.

In 1980, we were able to bring Marvin Sussman to the department as our first UNIDEL Professor. He had been a mentor to many new scholars. As a creative thinker, he added momentum to expansion of our graduate program and research support. I enjoyed working with him as membership chair when he was president of Groves and appreciated his willingness to include me in professional meetings and presentations before I was well established. He has left a permanent legacy for our program.

Real life and research may be a single process. I have always tried *not* to study my navel. When I did my dissertation I was delighted to pursue an aspect of my advisor's grant to study families with young children (Settles & Hillman, 1969). Many of my other colleagues chose to study themselves. While I never looked for such projects, we experienced another overlap with real life when my next large group of grants on a different theme were initiated. The early Reagan era created a shift in grants for social science research, discouraging for anyone who was not committed to their policy-driven projects. Even the peer review process was, for a time, shaped to include political action members in the review committees. I chose international work as an alternative and made use of training in language. I worked with the Agency for International Development project and Women in Development programs to retrain and took my second sabbatical in Panama. When I returned from my sabbatical trip I discovered that our doctoral program proposal had been approved. Suddenly we were to have a full doctoral operation the next fall.

In 1985 I saw an RFP from the Administration on Aging that I could relish. It combined both research and program development initiative to encourage adults in midlife to look ahead and plan for their long-term futures. While its purpose was relieving the government of responsibility for old age support and assistance, the concepts were reasonable ideas for families anyway. Using a conceptual framework on choice, I first presented these ideas in the family life education section at NCFR and later developed them in a chapter entitled "A Perspective on Tomorrow's Families" in *The Handbook on Marriage and the Family* (Settles, 1986).

Before the project began, a major turning point in our family set a new context for my research. My husband had a bad case of flu and his physician sent him for a chest X-ray. They found a mass high in the chest. All our information gathering, weighing, and seeking of informed opinion were to be tested. Coping with fear and danger and finding strength to meet the unknown and the interventions, treatments, and side effects were our daily challenge for years. The first two weeks we went from numb to crazed, but did things that led to better outcomes. We told our friends and my graduate students what was happening and found network contacts that linked us with the best programs and led us to oncology at Johns Hopkins. We asked questions and kept records as in a research project. Becoming more assertive in both the medical aspects and our real lives resulted in better outcomes.

Our children were our mainstays in this storm. They were in high school and it was difficult for the teachers to support them. They stopped talking to them, according to the guidance counselor, because they were frightened they might say something wrong. There was an immediate assumption that the boys would not be able to do their work at school and would, of course, have to accept lower grades. They did not see that our sons' success was critical to my husband's recovery. We found out what they needed to do for their studies and provided the missing support. Later when the cancer recurred our sons were even more important in helping us. During Andy's bone marrow transplant I lived in the house for patients' families beside the hospital and commuted to Delaware to teach my classes. My older son kept track of my younger son's graduation activities and needs and they managed their everyday lives. They both became platelet donors and contributed blood regularly, which was a close match to my husband's with few antibodies. We were proactive in the medical treatment and with the changes to everyday life. We managed our parents' aging needs as well. We are grateful to the many friends and acquaintances who were supportive throughout this long process.

The research on "Interactive Planning for Family Futures" overlapped all these events. There were resources to support many of our new doctoral students' work and master's and undergraduate theses. Among the topics were demographic analysis of Delaware (Cannon, 1987), filial responsibility for early retirees (Jackson, 1988), early retirement (Hanks, 1989), family futures presentation evaluation (Foulke, 1989), social support (Berke, 1991), parenting inputs for normal and handicapped children (Lucca, 1991), health planning (Rock, 1992), and future housing arrangements (Flexman, 1993) (see Dissertation Abstracts and University of Delaware Library). My long-term colleague Judith Van Name helped us with our study and used this data for her dissertation at Virginia Tech. Ideas about risk management and information integration with previous decisions and plans were useful. I developed a model for examining the unwinding of decisions and making new commitments (Settles, 1993b). Large-scale risk management theory and ethical issues in family dependency and vulnerability of individuals to care givers were important to the project (Hanks & Settles, 1989, 1990).

The Family Futures project yielded several tested products for intervention programs: Video (Foulke & Settles, 1988), Computer game and simulation (Settles & Berke, 1990), and Peer manual (Settles & Foulke, 1989). While I was, at first, the test person for whether the computer game was friendly enough to the non-technical person, I had a turning point in my own professional life as I started using word processing and actually radically increased my publication and writing program. Many other students and faculty were involved in reviewing and developing various aspects of these studies and educational materials. A community advisory committee helped us identify collaborators, test sites, audiences, and utility of concepts and products. Because of our collaborative relationships with agencies, business, schools, volunteer organizations, and professional groups, we were able to stretch the grant funds to produce extremely sophisticated products and several extra research projects. Dr. Mary Lou Liprie participated in the team throughout and we expanded the focus to look at adolescents' participation in their families' decisions. I obtained funding from the State Department of Public Instruction to adapt the teaching materials (Settles, 2000a). Later it was translated into Spanish with support of the State of Delaware and the Hewlett Foundation through the Partners of the Americas.

Family science is a lively enterprise with many aspects and participants. I became a part of the team (Randy Day, Kathy Gilbert, Barbara Settles, and Wes Burr) that put together an advanced undergraduate text, *Research and Theory in Family Science* (1995) (see also Settles, 1993c, 1995). We received great deal of helpful advice from the NCFR section on the family discipline. Family life education has taken on an increasingly important role in the field and research as evaluation has become more complex and process oriented. The value of multiple coordinated interventions, including education, social and material support, therapy, modeling and community action are being seen as reinforcing (Settles, Hanks III, Grasse-Bachman & Davis 1998; Settles, Hanks, III, Grasse-Bachman & Davis, 1999). Understanding how to reach at-risk and marginal families has had some new approaches. Hanks, III (1995) developed an innovative educational involvement of fathers of children born to teenage mothers and Stigile (1999) evaluated prison family life programs. James Davis and I recently had the opportunity to be the evaluation specialists for a five-year preschool parent outreach program funded by the U.S. Center for Substance Abuse through the State of Delaware. The Families and Centers Empowered Together (FACET) project provided support for data gathering on all aspects of the intervention. This included organizational and process changes in delivering the program as well as family, child, and staff measures. In contrast to traditional educational models that separate evaluation from the project, the process evaluation components included regular feedback and fine tuning for the program (Franyo & Settles, 1996; Settles, Davis, Grasse-Bachman, Janvier & Rosas, 2000).

Running concurrently with these family life education and planning projects I have had a continuing interest in theoretical issues in understanding family policy and exploring definitions of family (Settles, 1986, 1999b; Settles, Peterson, Steinmetz & Sussman, 1999), gender (Settles, 1993c), immigration and mobility (Settles, Hanks, III & Sussman, 1993; Settles, 2001a & b; Nauck & Settles, 2001; Sussman & Settles, 1993), work, benefits and care giving (Flexman, Berke & Settles, 1999), family programs (Settles & Robles, 2000), and political dynamics (Settles, 2000b). I am concerned about how families manage their interface with agencies and the extent to which policy and definition ration access to support.

I found myself able to participate actively in international family conferences and projects. The Committee on Family Research of the International Sociological Association meetings were more accessible. We also organized a conference on gender and families in Annapolis and later when I was elected to be President of the committee, I helped organize many conferences around the world. This group of colleagues is so large as to be difficult to pick out all the influences (such as J. Trost, J. Aldous, B. Adams, J. Peres, R. Katz, B. Nauck, C. Harvey, T. Le Roux, and many more). This spring, 2001, we had another CFR conference here at University of Delaware for CFR on "Families Interacting with Caregiving Institutions." When my husband took early retirement, we were able to take advantage of Delaware's international program and devoted a semester to teaching in Costa Rica. We celebrated the International Year of the Family with the Groves Conference on Marriage and the Family in San Jose, Costa Rica that semester. We brought many scholars and students from Central America as well as a good representation of our own Groves members together in a bilingual conference with the support of the Costa Rican First Lady's office (I dare not try to list the Groves members who have been my mainstay throughout my career as the whole membership list is needed). In addition, through my work in the Delaware/Panama Partners of the Americas I have been able to be active in encouraging family life education and working with teachers both here and there. My colleagues in Panama and Costa Rica have been a great encouragement to me in seeing how small projects can make big changes (especially T. de Barboni, A. Jovane, H. Pitti, R. de Mock & I. Robles).

When I corrected the earlier draft of this sketch, I was planning for my sabbatical with an objective to link the policy and the international aspects of my work together. My husband and I spent the first half of the year 2000 in the south of France working on these topics, traveling to some European campuses and enjoying the quiet countryside. Two outcomes from this period were completing many projects that had been 95% done for sometime and starting some new lines of development in policy and international work. Returning to the turmoil of regular campus life, I found myself finding many new students and colleagues to start new projects and see many opportunities for the future. At our university, a commitment to community development and family policy has been made clear by developing a center within our new College of Human Resources, Education, and Public Policy, and support for graduate study in family policy is broadly available. My expectation is to continue working on the issues affecting families as they shape their futures in the context of the local and global community.

At this point I realize that this recital of some of my favorite stories risks being like the annual *New Yorker* New Year's poem where as many names as one can put into a short space are welded together. Then one begins to think of all those who were forgotten and their significance for you not addressed. My great fortune is to have known several generations of family scholars and to have spent many moments chatting in the hallways and back of conference sessions with the best and brightest minds. I enjoy seeing my former students and younger colleagues moving along in their own careers and like to think I have been of some help. I also treasure those friends, both older and younger, who have given me so much of their wisdom and insight. It seems that there are a few more great adventures to be undertaken and projects that need to be proposed.

AUTHOR NOTE

Barbara H. Settles is Professor, Individual and Family Studies, University of Delaware, Newark, DE 19711.

REFERENCES

Culley, J. D., Van Name, J. B., & Settles, B. H. (1976). Measuring the indirect costs of foster family Care. *American Public Welfare*, *34*, 4, 6-13.

Day, R., Gilbert, K., Settles, B. H., & Burr, W. (Eds.). (1995). *Advanced family science*. Pacific Grove, CA: Brooks/Cole Publishing.

Flexman, R., Berke, D. L., & Settles, B. H. (1999). Negotiating family: The interface between family and support groups. In B. H. Settles, S. K. Steinmetz, G. W. Peterson, & M. B. Sussman (Eds.), *Concepts and definition of family for the 21st Century* (pp.173-190). NY: The Haworth Press, Inc.

Foulke, S., & Settles, B. H. (1988). *Interactive Planning for Family Futures* [Video]. University of Delaware. The Administration on Aging, USDHHS.

Franyo, G. A., & Settles, B. H. (1996). Preschool lending libraries: What works? *Early Child Development and Care*, 115, 1, 65-75.

Hanks, R. S. & Settles, B. H. (1989). Theoretical and ethical issues in a family care-giving relationship. *The Journal of Applied Social Sciences*, 13, 1, 9-39.

Hanks, R. S. & Settles, B. H. (1990). Theoretical and ethical issues in a family caregiving relationship. In D. E. Bugal & A. Blum (Eds.), *Aging and caregiving* (pp. 98-120). Newbury Park, CA: Sage.

Liprie, M. L., & Settles, B. H. (1996). Interdisciplinary programming, 1985-1994. *Review and synthesis of home economics education research*. AHEA Yearbook.

Nauck, B., & Settles, B. H. (Eds.). (in press 2001). Migrant and ethnic minority families (Special issue). *Journal of Comparative Family Studies*.

Settles, B. H. (1986). A perspective on tomorrow's families. In M. B. Sussman & S. K. Steinmetz (Eds.), *Handbook on marriage and family* (pp. 157-180). Plenum Press, NY.

Settles, B. H. (1993a). Finding multiple publication outlets for family science research and development: A case study of project dissemination. In R. S. Hanks, L. Matocha, & M. B. Sussman (Eds.), *Publishing in journals on the family: Essays on publishing* (pp. 183-200). Binghamton, NY: The Haworth Press, Inc.

Settles, B. H. (1993b). Expanding choice in long term planning for family futures. In B. H. Settles, R. S. Hanks, & M. B. Sussman (Eds.), *American families and the future: Analyses of possible destinies* (pp. 1-36). Binghamton, NY: The Haworth Press, Inc.

Settles, B. H. (1993c). Gender issues in global perspective. In K. Altergott (Ed.), *One world, many families* (pp. 38-42). Minneapolis, MN: National Council on Family Relations.

Settles, B. H. (1995). Families in everyday life. In R. Day, K. Gilbert, B. H. Settles, & W. Burr (Eds.), *Research and theory in family science* (pp. 154-170). Pacific Grove, CA: Brooks/Cole Publishing.

Settles, B. H. (1998). Putting families in family policy and programs: Local, regional, national and international options. In K. Matthijs (Ed.), *The family: Contemporary perspectives and challenges* (pp. 263-283). Leuven, Belgium: Leuven University Press.

Settles, B. H. (1999a). Definition of the family: professional and personal issues. In B. H. Settles, S. K. Steinmetz, G. W. Peterson, & M. B. Sussman (Eds.), *Concepts and definition of family for the 21st Century* (pp. 209-224). NY: The Haworth Press, Inc.

Settles, B. H. (1999b). The future of families. In M. B. Sussman, S. K. Steinmetz, & G. W. Peterson (Eds.) *Handbook on marriage and the family* (2nd ed) (pp. 143-176). NY: Plenum.

Settles, B. H. (2000a). Language and multicultural issues in adapting family life education and evaluation: A model for collaborative development. In Settles, B. H., & Robles, I. V. (Eds.), *Building support for the well being and future of the family* (pp. 84-95). *Family Science Review*, 13(3&4).

Settles, B. H. (2000b). Sociology of the family: Global advances and challenges. In S. Quah, & A. Sales (Eds.), *The international handbook of sociology* (pp. 173-196). Thousand Oaks, CA: Sage Publications.

Settles, B. H. (in press, 2001a). Being at Home in a Global Society: A Model for Families' Mobility and Immigration Decisions. Revised Paper from presentation at the International Sociological Association's Committee on Family Research XXXVI the Seminar on Migrant and Ethnic Minority Families. Berlin, Germany, June 14-20, 1999. *Journal of Comparative Family Studies.*

Settles, B. H. (in press, 2001b). Conflicts between Family Strategies and State Policy in a Global Society. Revised Paper from presentation at the International Sociological Association's Committee on Family Research XXXVI the Seminar on Migrant and Ethnic Minority Families. Berlin, Germany, June 14-20, 1999. *Journal of Comparative Family Studies.*

Settles, B. H., & Barboni, T. (1998). Developing On-Going Family Life and Prevention Programs in Panama, Costa Rica and Delaware. In N. B. Leidenfrost (Ed.), *Proceedings of International Federation for Home Economics Americas Region Conference* (pp. 105-111). University of Puerto Rica-Mayaguez, PR Campus.

Settles, B. H., & Berke, D. L. (1990). Relocation: Jane and the Job. An interactive teaching program on decision [Computer software]. University of Delaware and Administration on Aging, USDHHS.

Settles, B. H., Culley, J. D., & Van Name, J. B. (1976a). Estimating costs in foster family care. *Children Today*, 5,6 19-21.

Settles, B. H., Culley, J. D., & Van Name, J. B. (1976b). Understanding and Measuring the Cost of Foster Care. Newark, DE: Bureau of Economic and Business Research, University of Delaware.

Settles, B. H., Davis, J. E., Grasse-Bachman, C., Janvier, K. A., & Rosas, S. R. (2000). Developing community and peer support for young parents: Process and outcome evaluation inputs in prevention programs. In Settles, B. H., & Robles, I. V. (Eds.), *Building support for the well being and future of the family* (pp. 182-196). *Family Science Review*, 13(3&4).

Settles, B. H., Davis, J. E., Hanks, III, D. E., & Grasse-Bachman, C. J. (1999). Family life education and prevention programs: A cross-cultural program development model. In R. Richter & S. Supper (Eds.), *New qualities in the life course: Intercultural aspects* (pp. 219-236). Vienna, Austria.

Settles, B. H., & Foulke, S. (1988). *Interactive planning for family futures* [video]. University of Delaware. The Administration on Aging, USDHHS.

Settles, B. H., & Foulke, S. R. (Eds.). (1989). *Family futures: A manual for peer leadership.* (Available from B. H. Settles, Department Individual and Family Studies, Newark, DE: University of Delaware).

Settles, B. H., Grasse-Bachman, C., & Liprie, M. L. (2000). Expanding choices for underserved adolescents: A resource program for family life education. In Settles, B. H., & Robles, I. V. (Eds.), *Building support for the well being and future of the family* (pp. 68-77). *Family Science Review*, *13*(3&4).

Settles, B. H., Hanks, D. E., III, & Sussman, M. B. (Eds.). (1993). *Families on the move: Migration, immigration, emigration, and mobility.* Binghamton, NY: The Haworth Press, Inc.

Settles, B. H., Hanks, D. E., III, Grasse-Bachman, C. J., & Davis, J. E. (1998). Building bridges of inclusiveness in multiculturally diverse groups: The challenge for family life education and prevention. In S. C. Ziehl (Ed.), *Multicultural diversity and families* (pp. 397-454). Grahamstown, South Africa: Rhodes University.

Settles, B. H., Hanks, D. E., III, Grasse-Bachman, C. J., & Davis, J. E. (1999). Family Life education and prevention programs: A cross-cultural program development model. In R. Richter & S. Supper (Eds.), *New qualities in the life course: Intercultural aspects* (pp. 219-236). Würzburg, Germany: Ergon-Verlag.

Settles, B. H., & Hillman, C. S. (1969). Younger families in the rural fringe. *Journal of Cooperative Extension*, 7, 35-42.

Settles, B. H., & Liprie, M. L. (1982, 1983, 1984, 1986, 1987). *Contemporary Issues in Family Studies, Retrospective and Prospective* [Video Series]. University of Delaware, Newark, DE 19716.

Settles, B. H., & Lucca, J. (1981). Effects of Children's Disabilities on Parental Time Use. *Physical Therapy*, 61(2), 196-201.

Settles, B. H., & Robles, I. V. (Eds.). (2000). Building support for the well being and future of the family. *Family Science Review*, 13, 3&4.

Settles, B. H., Steinmetz, S. K., Peterson, G. W., & Sussman, M. B. (Eds.). (1999). *Concepts and definition of family for the 21st Century*. NY: The Haworth Press, Inc.

Sussman, M. B., & Settles, B. H. (1993). Worldwide contemporary issues in family mobility and immigration. In B. H. Settles, D. E. Hanks III, & M. B. Sussman (Eds.), *Families on the move: Migration, immigration, emigration, and mobility* (pp. 209-232). Binghamton, NY: The Haworth Press, Inc.

Van Name, J. B., & Settles, B. H. (Eds.). (1977). *Measuring the cost of foster family care*. DHEA NO. (OH DS) 77-0126; ERIC EJ164805.

Van Name, J. B., Culley, J. D., & Settles, B. H. (1997). Measuring the cost of caring for a foster child. *Child Welfare*, LVI(7), 431-439.

Index

